HANDBOOK OF
Nutrition
in the Aged
FOURTH EDITION

HANDBOOK OF
Nutrition
in the Aged

FOURTH EDITION

Edited by

Ronald Ross Watson

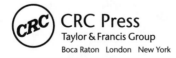

CRC Press
Taylor & Francis Group
Boca Raton   London   New York

CRC Press is an imprint of the
Taylor & Francis Group, an **Informa** business

CRC Press
Taylor & Francis Group
6000 Broken Sound Parkway NW, Suite 300
Boca Raton, FL 33487-2742

© 2009 by Taylor & Francis Group, LLC
CRC Press is an imprint of Taylor & Francis Group, an Informa business

No claim to original U.S. Government works
Printed in the United States of America on acid-free paper
10 9 8 7 6 5 4 3 2 1

International Standard Book Number-13: 978-1-4200-5971-7 (Hardcover)

Library of Congress Cataloging-in-Publication Data

Handbook of nutrition in the aged / editor, Ronald R. Watson. -- 4th ed.
    p. ; cm.
  Includes bibliographical references and index.
  ISBN 978-1-4200-5971-7 (hardcover : alk. paper)
  1. Aging--Nutritional aspects--Handbooks, manuals, etc. 2. Older people--Nutrition--Handbooks, manuals, etc. 3. Nutrition disorders in old age--Handbooks, manuals, etc. I. Watson, Ronald R. (Ronald Ross)
  [DNLM: 1. Nutrition Physiology. 2. Aged. 3. Aging--physiology. 4. Dietary Supplements. 5. Nutritional Requirements. WT 115 H2365 2009]

QP86.C7 2009
613.2084'6--dc22
                                       2008038181

Visit the Taylor & Francis Web site at
http://www.taylorandfrancis.com

and the CRC Press Web site at
http://www.crcpress.com

Contents

SECTION I   Nutritional Requirements for Health in the Aged

SECTION II   Nutrition and Promotion of Health

SECTION III   *Bioactive Foods as Nutrients in Health Promotion*

SECTION IV   Fruits and Vegetables to Prevent Illness

Preface

Nutrient requirements for optimum health and function of aging physiological systems often are quite distinct from those required for young ones. Recognition and understanding of the special nutrition problems of the aged are being intensively researched and tested, especially due to the increases in the elderly in the general population. In developed countries, economic restrictions and physical inactivity during aging can significantly reduce food intakes, contributing to nutritional stresses and needs. Many disease entities and cancers are found with higher frequency in the aged. Cancer, trauma, or infectious disease can alter intakes or requirements for various nutrients. Thus, specific foods and nutritional supplementation may be helpful in treatment of aged adults, including cancer patients.

Many adults and elderly are using foods and nutrients well above the recommended daily allowance, which may not always be needed for optimal health. Thus, dietary alcohol and high calorie intakes associated with causation and exacerbation of alcoholism or diabetes, respectively, will form a section of health promotion in seniors. To some extent, treatment of these conditions with diet or nutritional supplements is a unique problem in the aged.

The major objective of this book is to review in detail health problems occurring with significant frequency in aging adults and nutritional therapies to overcome them. The effects of the aging processes, changes in social status, and financial conditions significantly affect the approaches to treatment and study of nutritional and health problem in the aging adult and the elderly. In summary, to understand their health problems, increasing numbers of older adults and elderly in the population require detailed study and directed research using nutritional therapies.

This book, the 4th edition, was created by enhancing and updating key chapters by the authors who wrote them in the 3rd edition. Some new topics and chapters are included:

- Nutrition and Nutritional Needs
- Undernutrition
- Mechanistic Studies of Nutrition in the Aged
- Nutritional Therapies and Supplementation

Acknowledgments

Special appreciation is extended to the National Health Research Institute (non-profit) http://www.naturalhealthresearch.org. Its support for educating scientists and the lay public about nutrition in foods and dietary supplements stimulated the idea for this book. The institute provided support for Bethany L. Stevens, the editorial assistant. Her excellent work with the authors and publishers greatly supported the editors in their work. Dr. Ronald R. Watson is particularly thankful for decades of research support by H. B. and Jocelyn Wallace through the Wallace Research Foundation, facilitating his studies of dietary supplements including nutrients in health promotion. This research support encouraged a longstanding interest in nutrition in healthy aging that led to the editing of this book. The assistance of Nguyen T. Nga, library specialist at the Arizona Health Sciences Library, is very much appreciated.

Editor

Ronald Ross Watson, Ph.D., has worked at researching the role of bioactive nutrients, dietary supplements, and alternative medicines for 30 years. Dr. Watson has been and currently is funded to do such research by grants from the U.S. National Institute of Heart, Lung and Blood, and companies and private foundations to study effects of nutrients and dietary supplements to modify age and autoimmune diseases. He has recently completed several successful clinical trials in osteoarthritis patients using bioactive nutriceuticals. Dr. Watson has edited 62 scientific books, including several dealing with heart disease and conditions such as aging and AIDS that promote immune dysfunction as well as heart disease.

Dr. Watson is currently professor, Health Promotion Sciences, Mel and Enid Zuckerman College of Public Health and the Sarver Heart Center in the School of Medicine, University of Arizona in Tucson.

List of Contributors

Aránzazu Aparicio, MSc, PhD
Departamento de Nutrición
Facultad de Farmacia
Universidad Complutense
Madrid, Spain

Geertruida E. Bekkering, PhD
Department of General Practice
Katholieke Universiteit Leuven
Comprehensive Cancer Institute
Leuven, Belgium

Laura Mª Bermejo, MSc, PhD
Departamento de Nutrición
Facultad de Farmacia
Universidad Complutense
Madrid, Spain

Meredith C. Bogert, DMD
Department of Restorative Dentistry
Temple University School of Dentistry
Philadelphia, Pennsylvania

Sarah L. Booth, PhD
Vitamin K Laboratory
USDA Human Research Center on Aging
Tufts University
Boston, Massachusetts

Patrice Brocker, MD
Professor of Geriatrics,
Université de Nice Sophia-Antopolis
Nice, France

Zhao Chen, PhD
Mel and Enid Zuckerman College of
  Public Health
University of Arizona
Tucson, Arizona

William G. Christen, ScD
Brigham and Women's Hospital
Harvard Medical School
Boston, Massachusetts

Jessica Coppola, PhD
Department of Family and
  Consumer Sciences
Sacramento City College
Sacramento, California

Laurie Drozdowski, MSc, PhD
Division of Gastroenterology
University of Alberta
Edmonton, Alberta

Alia El-Kadiki
Chemical Pathology Department
Royal Hallamshire Hospital
Sheffield, United Kingdom

Reza Ghiasvand, PhD
Medical Sciences
University of Tehran
Tehran, Iran

Charles K. Herman, MD
Pocono Health Systems
East Stroudsburg, Pennsylvania
and
Albert Einstein College of Medicine
New York

Saeed Hosseini, MD, PhD
EMRC
Tehran University of Medical Sciences
Tehran, Iran

Claudiu Iordache, MD, MSc
Division of Gastroenterology
University of Alberta
Edmonton, Alberta

Vijaya Juturu, PhD, FACN
Nutrition 21 Inc.
Purchase, New York

Eliane Kellen, MD, PhD
Department of General Practice
Katholieke Universiteit Leuven
Comprehensive Cancer Institute
Leuven, Belgium

Kathleen LaPoint, MS
Department of Nutrition
University of North Carolina-Greensboro
Greensboro, North Carolina

Baowan Lin, MD
Department of Neurology
Miller School of Medicine
University of Miami
Miami, Florida

Roger B. McDonald, PhD
Department of Nutrition
University of California
Davis, California

Michael K. McIntosh, PhD, RD
Department of Nutrition
University of North Carolina-Greensboro
Greensboro, North Carolina

Susanne U. Mertens-Talcott
Department of Nutrition and Food Science
Texas A&M University
College Station, Texas

John A. Milner, PhD
Nutritional Science Research Group
National Cancer Institute
National Institutes of Health
Rockville, Maryland

Marthe J. Moseley, PhD, RN, CCRN, CCNS, CNL
Clinical Nurse Specialist, Critical Care
South Texas Veterans Health Care System
San Antonio, Texas
and
Rocky Mountain University of Health
  Professions
Provo, Utah

Giuliana Noratto
Department of Nutrition and Food Science
Texas A&M University
College Station, Texas

Rosa M. Ortega, PhD
Departamento de Nutrición
Facultad de Farmacia
Universidad Complutense
Madrid, Spain

Lisbeth Pacheco
Department of Nutrition and Food Science
Texas A&M University
College Station, Texas

Elena Rodríguez-Rodríguez, PhD
Departamento de Nutrición
Facultad de Farmacia
Universidad Complutense
Madrid, Spain

Stéphane M. Schneider, MD, PhD
Nutritional Support Unit
ARCHET University Hospital
Nice, France

Vidyasagar Sriramoju
Institute for Ultrafast Spectroscopy and Lasers
The City College of New York
New York, New York

Jeffrey Stanaway
Healthy Aging Lab
Mel and Enid Zuckerman College of Public
  Health
University of Arizona
Tucson, Arizona

Craig S. Stump, MD, PhD
Section of Endocrinology, Diabetes and
  Hypertension
University of Arizona
Tucson, Arizona

David R. Thomas, MD, FACP, AGSF, GSAF
Division of Geriatric Medicine
St. Louis University Health Sciences Center
St. Louis, Missouri

Alan B. R. Thomson, MD, PhD
Division of Internal Medicine
University of Alberta
Edmonton, Alberta

Elaine B. Trujillo, MS, RD
Nutritional Science Research Group
National Cancer Institute
National Institutes of Health
Rockville, Maryland

Jennifer Truong, MD
Vitamin K Laboratory
USDA Human Nutrition Research Center on
  Aging
Tufts University
Boston, Massachusetts

Rosemary Walzem
Department of Nutrition and Food Science
Texas A&M University
College Station, Texas

Sheldon Winkler, DDS
Maurice H. Kornberg School of Dentistry
Temple University
Philadelphia, Pennsylvania
and
College of Dental Medicine
Midwestern University
Glendale, Arizona

Trudy Woudstra, MSc, MD
Division of Gastroenterology
University of Alberta
Edmonton, Alberta

Hilary A. Wynne, MA, MD, FRCP
Care of the Elderly Services
Royal Victoria Infirmary
Newcastle upon Tyne, United Kingdom

Hussein Naji Yassine, MD
Division of Endocrinology
Section of Endocrinology, Diabetes and
  Hypertension
Tucson, Arizona

Jianping Ye, MD
Pennington Biomedical Research Center
Louisiana State University System
Baton Rouge, Louisiana

Jun Yin, MD, PhD
Pennington Biomedical Research Center
Louisiana State University System
Baton Rouge, Louisiana

Section I

Nutritional Requirements for Health in the Aged

1 Nutrition and Electrolytes in the Elderly

Marthe J. Moseley

CONTENTS

Nutrition plays a pivotal role in health promotion, disease prevention, and chronic disease management. The normal physiologic changes of aging place the elder at risk for potential complications regarding altered nutritional state and electrolyte imbalance. The most important principle in limiting the possibility of complications at any time throughout the age span is prevention.

1.1   INTRODUCTION

The population of older persons has risen dramatically and will continue to grow rapidly throughout the world. The size and character of the elderly population in the United States is rapidly changing. During the 20th century, the U.S. population under age 65 tripled, but those 65 and older increased by a factor of 11 (American Geriatric Society [AGS] 2006). Those persons who are 65 or older numbered 37.3 million in 2006, representing 12.4% of the U.S. population. By 2030, about one in every five Americans (20%) will be a senior citizen, with about 71.5 million older persons, more than twice their number in 2000. People 65 and older represented 12.4% of the population in the year 2000 but are expected to grow to 20% of the population by 2030. In 2005, the 65–74 age group (18.6 million) was over 8.5 times larger than in 1900, but the 75–84 group (13.1 million) was 17 times larger and the 85+ group (5.1 million) was 42 times larger (AGS, 2006).

Data from the Department of Health and Human Services (2006) reports the following information. In 2003, persons who reached age 65 had an average life expectancy of an additional 18.4 years (19.8 years for females and 16.8 years for males). A child born in 2004 could be expected to live 77.9 years, which is about 30 years longer than a child who was born in 1900. Much of this increase occurred because of reduced death rates for children and young adults. However, during the period of 1983–2003, reduced death rates were also noted for the population aged 65–84, specifically for men. with a reduction of 29.4% for men aged 65–74 and a reduction of 22.3% for men aged 75–84. Life expectancy at age 65 increased by only 2.5 years between 1900 and 1960, but had increased by 4.3 years from 1960 to 2004. Over 2.0 million persons celebrated their 65th birthday in 2005 and, in the same year, about 1.8 million persons 65 or older died. Census estimates showed an annual net increase of almost 500,000 in the numbers of persons 65 and over. There were 70,104 persons aged 100 or more in 2005 (0.19% of the total population), which had increased 88% from the 1990 data of 37,306.

1.2 BACKGROUND

The Department of Health and Human Services (2006) also reported statistics in terms of health and health care. In 2005, 38.3% of noninstitutionalized older persons described their health as excellent or very good. There was little difference between the sexes on this measure, but African Americans (22.8%), older American Indians/Alaska Natives (24.2%) and older Hispanics (28.4%) were less likely to rate their health as excellent or good than were older whites (40.9%) or older Asians (34.9%). Most older persons have at least one chronic condition and many have multiple conditions.

In other areas of lifestyle, reports reflected disease prevention behaviors and at-risk behaviors (DHHS 2006). Almost 60% of elders reported that they received an influenza vaccination in 2005 and 56% reported that they had received a pneumococcal vaccination. About 24% (of persons 60+) report height/weight combinations that place them among the obese, yet over 25% of persons aged 65–74 and 17% of persons 75+ report that they engage in regular leisure-time physical activity. Only 9% of elders reported that they are current smokers and 4% reported excessive alcohol consumption. Elders reported at 2.6%, that they had experienced psychological distress during the past 30 days.

Elderly persons experience more frequent hospitalizations (DHHS 2006). In 2004, over 13.2 million persons, aged 65 and older, were discharged from short-stay hospitalizations, a rate of 3,629 for every 10,000 persons aged 65+. This rate was considered to be more than two and one half times the comparable rate for persons of all ages (1,384 per 10,000). The reportable average length of hospital stay for persons aged 65+ was 5.6 days, which had decreased by 5 days since 1980. In 2003–2004, older persons averaged more doctor office visits, with 6.1 visits for elders aged 65–74, and 7.6 office visits for persons over 75. Over 96% of older persons reported access for medical care, yet 2.4% stated a failure to obtain needed medical care during the previous 12 months, citing financial barriers as the reason—thus supporting the link between poverty and poor health (Braveman 2007; Wilcox 2007).

1.3 IMPORTANCE OF ADEQUATE NUTRITION

Adequate nutrition status has been recognized as an important factor in both the prevention and treatment of chronic disease, in elders undergoing surgery (perioperative condition), and in any elder with alterations in immune function. The elderly are particularly prone to inadequate nutritional status partly due to age-related physiologic (Resnick 2005) and social changes (Metzler 2007), development of chronic diseases, use of medications (Hayes 2005), and decreased mobility. These factors may lead to subclinical malnutrition, which is not easy to recognize or separate from changes resulting from the aging process itself (Amella 2006). If undetected, subclinical malnutrition among older people may result in more rapid deterioration of health and early death.

It is important to distinguish age-related changes from those associated with a chronic disease or acute illness. Age-related changes in the gastrointestinal system, clinical implications and interventions related to these changes are important for discussion (Amella 2006; Beers 2005b; Mick 2007; Resnick 2005). Gastrointestinal age-related changes include a decrease in liver size, less efficient cholesterol stabilization and absorption, fibrosis and atrophy of salivary glands, decreased muscle tone in the bowel, atrophy of and decrease in the number of taste buds, slowing in esophageal emptying, decreased hydrochloric acid secretion, decreased gastric acid secretion, atrophy of the mucosal lining, and decreased absorption of calcium all as part of physiological aging. The clinical implications of these physiological changes include a change in oral intake due to a reduction in appetite, discomfort after eating related to the slowing of the passage of food, decreased absorption of calcium and iron, altered drug effectiveness, and increased risk of constipation, esophageal spasm, and diverticular disease. The problems in digestion influence the active transport mechanisms in the conversion of substrates of digestion. The decrease in hydrochloric acid, digestive enzymes, and bile may contribute to incomplete digestion of nutrients, thereby contributing to electrolyte alterations. Possible interventions to diminish the effects of the clinical implications include the encouragement of the elder to eat small, frequent meals to avoid discomfort and improve intake and the encouragement of fluid intake and fiber to improve bowel function.

Older adults who have diagnosed co-morbidities are at higher risk for under-nutrition or malnutrition (Alamoudi 2001; Beers, 2005b; Resnick 2005). Poor nutrition is not a natural concomitant of aging (Amella 2007), however the age-related changes discussed previously highlight the complexity of the multidimensionality of the issues surrounding nutrition (Beers 2005b). For example, either persons who have a body mass index (BMI) less than 19 (considered underweight) and those who with a BMI greater than 25 (considered overweight) often have a greater potential for loss of muscle mass, a compromised immune system and increased incidence of complications and premature death (Amella 2006). The progression to malnutrition is often insidious and often undetected (Amella 2007). The healthcare provider plays a key role in prevention and early intervention of nutritional problems.

Nutrition plays a pivotal role in health promotion, disease prevention, and chronic disease management. Older adults experience a variety of nutritional problems connected to age-related changes, including a decrease in total body protein, a reduction in total body water, a loss in bone density, and an increase in the proportion of total body fat with a redistribution of fat stores. Cumulatively, these changes place a substantial number of elderly at high risk for poor nutrition status.

Many elderly patients requiring hospitalization show signs of malnutrition on admission to the hospital or develop malnutrition during hospitalization. Malnutrition from any cause impacts on the recovery and rehabilitation after surgery and is not limited to protein-calorie deficiency but also low intakes of iron, vitamins, and minerals.

Beers (2005b) addressed the importance of the role of leptin, a recently discovered protein hormone produced by fat cells that contributes to decreased food intake and increased energy metabolism. Beer noted that in normal younger adults, an increase in body fat triggers an increase in leptin levels and a decrease in body fat triggers a decrease in leptin levels. However, abnormally elevated leptin levels are strongly correlated with decreased body fat. In elderly women, leptin levels decline with the decline in body fat that occurs after age 70. But in elderly men, leptin levels increase despite the decline in body fat related to the decline in testosterone levels that occur at the same age. The importance of leptin in decreasing food intake with age is unknown. Yet, postmenopausal women with high leptin levels tend to eat somewhat less than those with low leptin levels.

Management of perioperative care in geriatric patients is typically more complex than in younger patients, due to changes associated with advancing age. One in four elderly suffer from malnutrition, which is costly in the surgical patient because it leads to impaired immune system, poor wound healing, infections, complications, multisystem organ failure, prolonged hospitalizations, catastrophic costs, and death. Factors critical for obtaining the best outcomes from surgical treatment of elderly patients include avoidance of disturbances in nutritional and electrolyte status (Tonelli 2005).

Immune response, typically a protective pattern, is impaired in old age, resulting in an augmented risk of infection (Mick 2007). Nutrition is a significant determinant of immunocompetence. Functional adaptations include decreased lymphocyte proliferation, reduced production of interleukin-2, impaired mixed lymphocyte reaction, and decreased natural killer cell activity. Beers (2005c) reported that an increased number of cytokines (eg, tumor necrosis factor, interleukin-2, interleukin-6) decreased food intake. Some elderly persons had elevated levels of these cytokines, which may contribute to anorexia. Stressors, often defined as surgery, infection, or burns, usually resulted in cytokine release, which inhibited the production of albumin and caused it to move from the intravascular space to the extravascular space, explaining the decreased albumin level which is more rapid in elderly patients. The most susceptible elderly patients have usually been underweight, but with a recent history of rapid weight loss even those who appear to have ample fat and muscle mass are susceptible.

1.4 DETECTION OF NUTRITIONAL RISK

The Mini Nutritional Assessment (MNA) (Guigoz 1994), a validated nutritional screening device for elderly persons, has been translated into numerous languages available at the Hartford Institute for Geriatric Nursing site. The MNA is an assessment tool to identify patients who are at risk from malnutrition or who are already malnourished. It is completed at regular intervals in the community or in the hospital setting (Guigoz et al. 1994; Nestle 2007). The tool contains two sections: screening and assessment.

The screening section of the MNA (Nestle 2007) consists of questions on food intake, weight loss, mobility, stress, neuropsychological problems, and BMI. Scoring for responses ranges from 0 to 2 or 3, depending on the choices offered. Within each subsection, questions are posed for the patient if he or she is able or the information is obtained from the medical record. In addition, information can be obtained from the care provider. Some indication of mental state of the patient is required, thus, if the patient is severely confused, accuracy is determined by validating professional judgment with someone from the health care team. The scores from this section are summed. If the score is 12 points or greater, the elder is not at risk and no further testing is required. If the score is 11 points or less, the elder might be at risk from malnutrition and the additional assessment section should be completed.

The additional assessment is the section that includes aspects addressing independent living, use of prescription drugs, presence of pressure ulcers, number of full meals eaten daily, selected consumption of products as markers for protein intake, consumption of fruits and vegetables per day, fluid consumption per day, mode of feeding, personal view of nutritional status, comparison of health status with other people of the same age, and measurements of both mid-arm circumference and calf circumference (Nestle 2007). The points from the assessment section of the MNA are summed. Then this total is added to the screening scores to give the total assessment score (maximum score 30 points). The score range of greater than 23.5 points requires no further action. Scoring points less than 23.5 recommends that the elder be referred to a dietitian.

In the situation where no dietitian is available, some advice on how to improve nutritional intake is recommended to include: increasing consumption of energy/protein-dense foods, supplementing food intake with additional snack and glasses of milk, ensuring adequate fluid intake of 6–8 cups per day, and seeking need for oral nutritional supplements if nutritional intake cannot be improved by diet alone (Nestle 2007). Conversion charts available in the MNA user guide include pictures on how to measure the correct circumferences.

The Merck Manual of Geriatrics identifies predictors for persons at risk of malnutrition (Beers 2005b). Weight loss is the single best factor for predicting such persons, and a BMI < 21 kg/m^2 (weight/height^2) suggests a problem in the elderly. Midarm circumference or midarm muscle circumference helps to detect muscle mass changes in persons retaining fluid. Albumin is an excellent measure of protein status. Healthy ambulatory elderly persons have serum albumin levels > 4 g/dL. In hospitalized elderly persons albumin levels < 3.2 g/dL are highly predictive of mortality. Cholesterol levels < 160 mg/dL in nursing home residents predict mortality reflective of malnutrition. However, acute illness associated with cytokine release can also lower cholesterol levels. Anergy is a failure to respond to common antigens, such as mumps, injected into the skin. Anergy can occur in healthy as well as in malnourished elderly persons, but the combination of anergy and signs of malnutrition correlate more strongly with a poor outcome than do either one alone.

In elders who are identified as having a poor nutritional status, screening and assessment identify the need for additional support. Based on the Hartford Institute (Amella 2007) best practices overview, older adults are at risk for alterations in nutritional status; estimates for malnutrition in older adults were as follows: 40–60% of hospitalized older adults were malnourished or at risk for malnutrition; 40–85% of nursing home residents had malnutrition, and 20–60% of home care patients were malnourished. In the same overview, it was noted that older adults who were malnourished were more likely to experience longer lengths of hospital stay and costs, diminished muscle strength, poor wound healing, development of pressure ulcers, increased infections, postoperative complications, functional impairment, and death.

1.5 OPTIMAL INTERVENTION

Risk factors are identified through purposeful screening and assessment. Intervening based on identification of risk factors in older adults who are at risk for undernutrition due to dietary, economic, psychosocial, and physiological factors that include: dietary intake (little or no appetite, problems with eating or swallowing, eating inadequate servings of nutrients, eating fewer than two meals a day. Limited income and isolation may cause restriction in the number of meals eaten per day or reduction in the dietary quality of meals eaten. Older adults who live alone may lose the desire to cook because of the decreased appetite of widows, difficulty cooking due to disabilities, lack of access to transportation to buy food, diagnosis of chronic illness or presence of chronic conditions that can affect intake. Disability can hinder the ability to prepare or ingest food, depression can cause decreased appetite, poor oral health impairs ability to lubricate, masticate, and swallow food, and use of medications (Hayes 2005), specifically antidepressants, antihypertensives, and bronchodilators can contribute to dry mouth, which impairs oral health.

Once assessment is made and a plan is completed, Hartford Institute of Geriatric Nursing (Amella 2007) recommends a holistic assessment to include: clinical history, social history, drug–nutrient interactions, functional limitations, psychological assessment, and a mini-nutritional assessment—all combined to determine risk. If the risk continues, the complete in-depth assessment ensues to include: food intake, mobility, BMI, history of weight loss, psychological stress or acute disease, and dementia or psychological conditions. If a score of 11 points or less is summed, then an in-depth assessment is done to include: assessment of dietary intake, documentation of intake with a calorie count (dietary intake analysis), and anthropometry by obtaining an accurate weight and height through direct measurement. If the patient is unable to stand erect to measure stature, knee-height measurements are taken to estimate height using special knee-height calipers. Height is not estimated in older adults because of the potential of shortening of the spine with advanced age. A self-reported height may be off by as much as 2.4 cm. The current weight and weight history are obtained using usual body weight, history of weight loss—whether intentional or unintentional and over what period of time. A loss of 10 pounds over a 6-month period is a red flag indicating need for further assessment. BMI is calculated to determine if weight for height is within normal range 22–27. BMI below 22 is a sign of undernutrition. Visceral proteins are then monitored. Albumin, transferrin, pre-albumin and retinol-binding protein are protein levels monitored to assess nutritional status and progress with nutritional repletion. Albumin is the most widely available level and usually is the most affordable.

1.5.1 Ongoing Nutritional Evaluation

Monitoring ongoing weight changes is a large part of evaluating nutritional status in older adults. In general, an older person who unintentionally loses 10 pounds or more in a 6-month period remains at risk of malnutrition. A similar guideline, used by Medicare-certified nursing homes, is weight loss of 5% or more in the past month or 10% or more in the past 6 months. This degree of weight loss increases risk of functional limitations, increased healthcare costs, and need for hospitalization.

BMI is also sometimes used to estimate body size and reevaluate nutritional status on an ongoing basis. BMI is defined as body weight in kilograms divided by height in meters squared (kg/m2). A BMI below 18.5 kg/m2 suggests underweight nutritional status, while a BMI above 30 kg/m2 suggests obesity.

Another method of reassessment is to determine ongoing adequate intake. Inadequate nutritional intake has been defined as an average or usual intake of food-group servings, nutrients, or energy below a threshold level of the recommended daily allowance (RDA). The thresholds have generally been set at 25% to 50% below the RDA, because it is difficult to accurately assess dietary intake and because actual need varies somewhat from person to person. Older adults with daily intakes at or below screening thresholds are further evaluated for malnutrition and any underlying disease.

1.6   FLUID NEEDS

Dehydration is the most common fluid problem in older people (Bossingham 2005; Mentes 2006). As one ages, our bodies lose some ability to regulate fluid levels. As the sense of thirst is often reduced, elderly people tend to drink fewer fluids. In addition, certain conditions also reduce the ability to recognize thirst or need for fluid (Mentes 2006). It is common to need more fluid than usual during fever or infection, as well as when taking diuretics or laxative medications. Common signs of dehydration are less urine output, low-grade fevers, constipation, dry gums, and confusion (Bossingham 2005).

In general, older adults need to take in 1 ounce (30 mL) of fluid per kg (about half an ounce per pound) of body weight per day. For example, a 150-pound person needs 75 ounces of fluid every day. Ways to take in fluid include drinking liquids (nonalcoholic) or eating moist foods such as fruits and vegetables. If an elder becomes over- or under-hydrated (by taking in too much or not enough fluid), the results of clinical tests may be affected and result in an inaccurate assessment of health status (Mentes 2006).

1.6.1   PERIOPERATIVE PLAN

A plan of care for the perioperative (before, during and after surgery) elder includes determination and assessment of nutritional status. During the preoperative phase assessment, the mortality rate is significantly higher in patients who have lost > 20% of body weight before surgery (Beers 2005a). Nutritional status is assessed by standard instruments, such as the MNA or Subjective Global Assessment. Serum albumin is measured in patients with chronic disorders, signs of undernutrition, or poor wound healing. A value < 3.5 g/dL indicates higher risk of complications and mortality.

Many experts believe that nutritional support should be provided to all patients preoperatively, preferably using the GI tract, to the limit tolerated by the patient (Beers 2005a). Some data suggest that, in severely malnourished patients, preoperative use of total parenteral nutrition (TPN) decreases complication rates and does not increase infection rates.

In the postoperative phase, fluid and electrolyte imbalances can cause alteration in the elderly (Tonelli et al. 2005); the ability to maintain homeostatic levels of fluids and electrolytes is reduced (Beers 2005c). In addition, the margin between too little and too much fluid is relatively narrow. Overexpansion of the extracellular compartment from excess fluid administration may be dangerous, as cardiopulmonary reserves are limited in the elderly. During the early postoperative period, the body normally retains water and sodium, and the elderly may have difficulty eliminating the excess fluid.

Initially, the amount of IV fluids is adjusted to optimize outcomes. Saturated venous oxygen (SVO2) values, stroke index, pulmonary artery occlusive pressure and central venous pressure are monitored and trended. If central measures of fluid status are not accessible for trending, then blood pressure, pulse, and urine output measurements are closely monitored to help determine fluid requirements. Enough fluids are given to replace insensible fluid losses and measured or estimated through external losses to produce a urine output of 0.5 mL/kg/hour, or about 30 mL/hour (Beers 2005c).

When external losses are minimal, fluid requirements are usually 1500 to 2500 mL for 24 hours (Beers 2005c). However, more fluids may be needed if third-space sequestration of fluids is excessive. The sequestered fluid is usually mobilized on the 3rd to 5th day after surgery.

Electrolyte replacement must include potassium, which is replaced as 20 to 100 mEq/day intravenously or by mouth to replace losses calculated as approximately two thirds lost in urine and one third lost from the gastrointestinal tract. If potassium replacement is inadequate, postoperative ileus (POI), or impairment of bowel motility, may be prolonged, and resistant metabolic alkalosis may develop (Ezri et al. 2006). POI delays return to feeding and can prolong hospitalization. Calcium and magnesium may also be replaced, but usually are determined based on the serum levels.

Hyponatremia, or low blood sodium, is common among elderly patients, particularly among men undergoing transurethral resection of the prostate because hypotonic irrigation solution is absorbed through the open venous sinuses of the prostate (Beers 2005c). Symptoms appear when the sodium level is < 130 mEq/L, and confusion or a seizure may occur a few days after surgery.

The patient's total body sodium content and total body free water content may be increased, normal, or decreased (Beers 2005c). Pulmonary edema, excessive peripheral edema, or evidence of major third-space losses suggests increased total body sodium content. If hyponatremia is due to inadequate sodium intake, 0.9% sodium chloride solution should be given cautiously, avoiding increases in sodium > 10 mEq/L in a 24-hour period.

Beers (2005c) has suggested early, aggressive nutritional support be given to patients with malnutrition—most notably to those with septic complications and those who have lost > 10% of their premorbid weight. Supplemental oral feedings, tube feedings, or total parenteral nutrition may be given, depending on the patient's condition. If anorexia or dysphagia makes oral feeding difficult but gastric and intestinal motility and absorption are normal, enteral feedings may be given by continuous drip. In such cases, the enteral route is preferable to the parenteral route because it causes fewer complications, costs less, and may have a trophic effect on the intestine (Beers 2005c). TPN is used when intestinal motility or absorption is abnormal.

Beers (2005c) has suggested that postoperative metabolic rate briefly increases. Measured by oxygen consumption, it is usually to 20% to 40% more than the normal basal metabolic rate, unless a complication such as sepsis develops. Age, sex, height, and weight affect the basal caloric requirement, but body temperature, protein losses through wounds, and muscular work related to physical activity do not. A total daily caloric requirement of 1.2 to 2 times the basal metabolic rate is generally adequate.

An admixture of substrates including carbohydrates, proteins, and fats is used to meet the patient's metabolic needs and to produce a positive nitrogen balance (Beers 2005c). For most elderly patients, protein infused at 0.5 to 1.0 g/kg/day is sufficient to maintain a positive nitrogen balance, increasing to 1.5 to 2.5 g/kg/day if needed.

Parenteral or enteral administration of fats is given to meet the patient's total caloric requirement. Fats supply essential fatty acids and enough calories to minimize the mobilization of endogenous proteins for energy and gluconeogenesis (Beers 2005c).

1.8 ROUTE SELECTION

Overall, undernutrition is poorly recognized and treated in elderly persons. If nutritional support is indicated, the most appropriate route must be determined. A nutrition support consultation may be indicated for older individuals who, because of anatomical, physiological, or mental health problems, cannot meet their nutritional needs by eating a nutritionally balanced diet. Nutrition support consultation may provide for interventions that include altering usual food intake by modification of nutrient content or optimizing nutrient density or food consistency or form. The goal of nutritional support is to maintain adequate nutritional state, to determine and institute dietary modifications needed for prevention of energy and nutrient deficiencies and for management of the elder with the most efficient method possible.

The enteral route is the preferred route and the optimal route for nutrition administration. The estimation of the nutrient balance accomplished when completing the calorie count might reveal at least 50% ingestion of nutritional needs; supplementation may be sufficient to increase intake to an optimal nutrient level. If, however, less than 50% of nutritional needs is ingested, tube feedings may become a necessity. Tube feedings can be instigated if gastric output is not more than 600 ml per day on gravity drainage. In the hospital or acute care setting the gastric residuals are obtained every 4 hours to determine that the residual does not exceed 50% of the volume infused. At the start of gastric feedings, rates are initially slow to determine tolerance. Increases by 20 to 25 ml/hour are completed every day until the patient's nutrient requirements are met. Other options for feeding access include nasoenteric tubes or jejunostomies in the compromised elder. It is well known and documented that bowel rest causes intestinal mucosa atrophy with increased permeability to bacteria and endotoxins, thus the phenomenon of bacterial translocation. As a result of this, all nutritional needs cannot be met intestinally. Whenever possible, the intestine should be stimulated with some amount of enteral nutrition as a preventive measure. A balanced diet administered continuously over 24 hours in the elderly includes an optimally balanced polymeric formula.

Adverse effects such as abnormal electrolytes, altered glucose levels, or even aspiration pneumonia may result from the feeding of a malnourished elderly person (CREATE 2005). In addition, the presence of food in the gut can cause a significant drop in blood pressure, which is associated with falls and syncope, or loss of consciousness. The decrease in blood pressure results from carbohydrate, which releases the vasodilatory calcitonin gene-related peptide (Beers 2005b).

1.9 WATER AND ELECTROLYTE BALANCE

Total body water accounts for 60% of body weight. Water content reaches approximately 50% with a decline in age. This reduction in body water is associated with a decrease in lean body mass, as water composes approximately 70% of muscle tissue.

Age, body size, fluid intake, diet composition, solute load presented for renal excretion, metabolic and respiratory rates, body temperature, and presence and extent of abnormal fluid losses in part determine fluid and electrolyte balance (Mentes 2006; Tonelli et al. 2005). The body gains water via the gastrointestinal tract (GI) with additional water produced as a result of oxidation. Oral intake encompasses approximately two thirds of the intake and is usually in the form of pure water or some other beverage, and the remainder is via ingested food. Water is mainly lost through the skin, lungs, GI tract, and kidneys. These fluid losses are coupled with varying losses of electrolytes, which must also be replaced.

The kidneys primarily regulate homeostasis, the maintenance of body fluids. There is a progressive decrease in kidney function, in particular the glomerular filtration rate (GFR), as a result of aging, equivalent to the decline in muscle mass explanatory of the normal creatinine associated with aging (Bennett et al. 2004; Mentes 2006).

Cardiac output (CO) in part determines renal blood flow and GFR. Thus, any alteration in CO that results in a decrease CO will result in a reduced renal blood flow and GFR. Acute renal failure (ARF) is one indicator for increased mortality in the elder person, indicated by a rise in the blood urea nitrogen (BUN) and creatinine, with or without oliguria. Immediate evaluation of the cause of increased BUN or creatinine to correct or remove reversible factors is a priority (Bennett 2004).

Elderly individuals are at increased risk for dehydration because of age-related physiologic changes (Amella 2007; Bossingham et al. 2005). These include altered thirst perception, reduced total body water (TBW) as a portion of body weight, body composition changes (i.e., higher proportion of fat to muscle), impaired renal conservation of water, decreased effectiveness of vasopressin, and increased prevalence of multiple chronic diseases.

Research-based (Amella 2007) risk factors for dehydration include:

- Age of 85 years and older
- Female gender
- Functionally semi-dependent elders who are cognitively impaired yet have mobility, and those who are physically unable to meet their needs but who can express them
- Functionally independent
- Elders with a decrease in activities of daily living (ADLs)
- Diagnosis of Alzheimer's disease or other dementias
- Presence of four or more chronic conditions (Bennett et al. 2004)
- Bedridden
- Daily intake of more than four medications
- Presence of fever
- Few fluid ingestion opportunities
- Poor oral intake
- Communication difficulties (Price et al. 2006).

These factors are taken into account in planning intervention measures.

1.10   INTERVENTION MEASURES

A practical approach to fluid and electrolyte balance in the elderly is considered in context of a collaborative team approach. Hartford's (Amella 2007) approach is in care strategies. Refer the elder to a dietitian if at risk for undernutrition or has undernutrition. Consult with a pharmacist to review the patient's medications for possible drug–nutrient interactions (Hayes 2005). Consult with a multidisciplinary team specializing in nutrition. Consult with social worker, occupational therapist, speech therapist as appropriate. Alleviate dry mouth to include: avoidance of caffeine, alcohol and tobacco, and dry, bulk, spicy, salty or highly acidic foods. If the elder does not have dementia or swallowing difficulties, offer sugarless hard candy or chewing gum to stimulate saliva. The lips are kept moist with petroleum jelly, frequent sips of water are offered. The elder needs to maintain adequate nutritional intake. Daily requirements for healthy older adults include: 30 kcal per kg of body weight, with no more than 30% of calories from fat; 0.8 to 1 g/kg of protein per day; caloric, carbohydrate, protein and fat requirements may differ depending on the degree of malnutrition.

The nutrition plan strives to improve oral intake. Mealtime rounds determine how much food is consumed and whether assistance is needed. Limit health care team breaks to before or after patient mealtimes to ensure adequate staff available to help with meals. Encourage family members to visit at mealtimes and ask family to bring favorite foods from home when appropriate; ask about patient food preferences and honor them and suggest small frequent meals with adequate nutrients to help patients regain or maintain weight. In addition, nutrition snacks are offered to the elder.

Consideration is given to the environment (Amella 2007). All bedpans, urinals, and emesis basins are removed from rooms before mealtimes. Analgesics and antiemetics are administered on a schedule that will diminish the likelihood of pain or nausea during mealtimes. Meals are served to elders in a chair if they can get out of bed and remain seated. A more relaxed environment is created by sitting at the patient's eye level and making eye contact when feeding. Late food trays are ordered or food is kept warm if the elder is not in his or her room during mealtimes. Interruptions are made for patient rounds and nonurgent medical procedures are rescheduled to not conflict with mealtimes. In addition, patients are assisted with mouth care and placement of dentures before food is served. Older adults are scheduled for tests or procedures early in the day to decrease the length of time they are not allowed to eat and drink.

Hydration management is the ongoing management of oral intake (Amella 2007; Mentes 2006). Care strategies include calculating a daily fluid goal that is individualized and providing fluids consistently throughout the day. Fluid intake is planned as 75% to 80% delivered at meals and 20% to 25% delivered during nonmeal times along with offering a variety of fluids based on the elder's preferences. Plans are made for at-risk individuals in nursing homes. Plans are standardized for risk of underhydration. Fluid rounds are scheduled midmorning and late afternoon. Plans for afternoon gatherings where patients can meet for additional fluids, nourishment, and socialization are included. Modified fluid containers are used based on the elder's ability to hold a cup or to swallow. Varieties of fluids are offered and encouraged as ongoing intake throughout the day. "Sip 'n' go" interventions are used to encourage reluctant elders to drink a standardized amount of fluid. For this intervention, anyone who enters the elder's room while that elder is awake offers at least 2 ounces (60 mL) of water or other beverage of choice.

Fluid regulation is documented and trended. Cognitively intact elders who are visually capable are taught to regulate fluid intake by comparing the color of their urine to a standardized urine color chart. For those individuals who are cognitively impaired, caregivers are taught how to use the color chart. In most settings, at least one accurate intake and output recording should be documented and include the amount of fluid consumed, intake pattern, difficulties with consumption, and urine specific gravity and color. Accurate calculation of intake requires knowledge of the volumes of containers used to serve fluids, which should be posted in a prominent place on the care unit. Health-care providers over- or underestimate the volumes of common vessels.

Any older adult who develops a fever, vomiting, diarrhea, or a non-febrile infection is closely monitored by implementing intake and output records and provision of additional fluids as tolerated (Bennett et al. 2004; Mentes 2006). Elders who can accept nothing by mouth (NPO) are given special consideration to shorten the NPO time and are provided with adequate amounts of fluids and food when the NPO status is completed.

1.11   CONCLUSION

Physiologic changes associated with the normal process of aging place the elder at risk for complications, particularly during illness. Prevention is the most important principle in limiting the possibility of complications. The goals for the elderly person include maintaining nitrogen balance, sustaining intravascular volume, and preserving electrolyte status. Attention must be placed on screening for risk and assessment to prevent untoward events from occurring. Awareness with the circumstances of the elderly plus routine and regular screening offers the best guarantee for timely identification of nutritional risk and electrolyte imbalance, which leads to prompt appropriate intervention. Nutritional and electrolyte status maintenance in the elderly improves health status and quality of life.

ACKNOWLEDGMENT

A special thank you to the South Texas Veterans Health Care System elderly veterans who choose to receive care within the Veterans Administration system.

REFERENCES

Alamoudi, O.S.B. 2001. Electrolyte disturbances in patients with chronic, stable asthma: Effect of therapy. *Chest*, 120(2), 431–436.
Amella, E.J. 2007. Assessing nutrition in older adults. The Hartford Institute of Geriatric Nursing. Issue Number 9. http://www.hartfordign.org/publications/trythis/issue_9.pdf (accessed November 30, 2007).
Amella, E.J. 2006. Presentation of illness in older adults: If you think you know what you're looking for, think again. *AORN J.*, 83(2), 372–389.
American Geriatrics Society (AGS). 2006. Trends in the elderly population. AGS Foundation for Health in Aging. http://www.healthinaging.org/agingintheknow/chapters_print_ch_trial.asp?ch=2 (accessed November 28, 2007).

Beers, M.H., ed. (2005a). Assessment and minimization of surgical risk. *The Merck Manual of Geriatrics*. 3rd ed. http://www.merck.com/mrkshared/mmg/sec8/ch61/ch61a.jsp (accessed November 30, 2007).

Beers, M.H., ed. (2005b). Protein–energy undernutrition. *The Merck Manual of Geriatrics*. 3rd ed. http://www.merck.com/mrkshared/mmg/sec8/ch61/ch61a.jsp (accessed November 30, 2007).

Beers, M.H., ed. (2005c). Perioperative care *The Merck Manual of Geriatrics*. 3rd ed. http://www.merck.com/mrkshared/mmg/sec8/ch61/ch61a.jsp (accessed November 30, 2007).

Bennett, J.A., Thomas, V., and Riegel, B. 2004. Unrecognized chronic dehydration in older adults: Examining prevalence rate and risk factors. *J. Geront. Nurs.*, 30(11), 22–28, 52–53.

Bossingham, M.J., Carnell, N.S., and Campbell, W.W. 2005. Water balance, hydration status, and fat-free mass hydration in younger and older adults. *Am J. Clin Nutr*, 81, 1342–1350.

Braveman, P. 2007. Do we have real poverty in the United States of America? *Prev. Chronic Dis.*, 4(4). http://www.cdc.gov/pcd/issues/2007/oct/07_0124.htm Accessed November 30, 2007.

CREATE-ECLA Trial Group Investigators. 2005. Effect of glucose-insulin-potassium infusion on mortality in patients with acute ST-segment elevation myocardial infarction: The CREATE-ECLA randomized controlled trial. *JAMA*, 293(4), 437–466.

Department of Health and Human Services (DHHS). 2006. Administration on aging. Statistics on the aging population. http://www.aoa.gov/PROF/Statistics/statistics.asp (accessed November 28, 2007).

Ezri, T., Lerner, E., Muggia-Sullam, M. Medalion, B., Tzivian, A., Cherniak, A., Szmuk, P., and Shimonov, M. 2006. Phosphate salt bowel preparation regimens alter perioperative acid-base and electrolyte balance. *Can. J. Anesth.*, 53(2), 153–158.

Guigoz, Y. Vellas, B.J., and Garry P.J. 1994. Mini nutritional assessment: A practical assessment tool for grading the nutritional state of elderly patients. *Facts Res. Gerontol.*, 4 (suppl. 2): 15–59.

Hayes, K. 2005. Designing written medication instructions: Effective ways to help older adults self–medicate. *J. Gerontol. Nurs.*, 31(5), 5–10.

Mentes, J. 2006. Oral hydration in older adults. *AJN*, 106(6), 40–49.

Metzler M. 2007. Social determinants of health: what, how, why, and now. *Prev. Chronic Dis.*, 4(4). http://www.cdc.gov/pcd/issues/2007/oct/07_0136.htm (accessed November 30, 2007).

Mick, D.J. 2007. Gerontological issues in critical care. In R. Kaplow and Hardin, S.R. *Critical care nursing: Synergy for optimal outcomes.* Sudbury, MA: Jones and Bartlett. p. 82–83.

Nestle Clinical Nutrition. 2007. Mini Nutritional Assessment (MNA) User Guide. http://www.mna-elderly.com/clinical-practice.htm (accessed November 30, 2007).

Price, J.F., McDowell, S., Whiteman, M.C., Deary, I.J., Stewart, M.C., and Fowkes, G.R. 2006. Ankle brachial index as a predictor of cognitive impairment in the general population: Ten-year follow-up of the Edinburgh artery study. *J. Am. Geriat. Soc.*, 54(5): 763–769.

Resnick, B. 2005. The critically ill older patient. In P.G. Morton, D.K. Fontaine, C.M. Hudak, and B.M. Gallo. *Critical care nursing: A holistic approach.* Philadelphia, PA: Lippincott Williams and Wilkins. p. 150–174.

Tonelli, M. Sacks, F., Pfeffer, M., Gao, Z., Gurhan, G., Cholesterol and Recurrent Events (CARE) Trial Investigators. 2005. *Circulation*, 112, 2627–2633.

Wilcox, L. 2007. Health, wealth, and well-being. *Prev. Chronic Dis.*, 4(4). http://www.cdc.gov/pcd/issues/2007/oct/07_0147.htm (accessed November 30, 2007).

2 Vitamins and Health in Older Persons

David R. Thomas

CONTENTS

Evidence of epidemiological associations of vitamins and disease states has been found for nine vitamins (Table 2.1).[1] Inadequate folate status is associated with neural tube defect and some cancers. Folate and vitamins B-6 and B-12 are required for homocysteine metabolism and their deficiency is associated with coronary heart disease risk. Vitamin E and lycopene may decrease the risk of prostate cancer. Vitamin D is associated with decreased occurrence of fractures when taken with calcium.[2] Zinc, beta-carotene, and vitamin E appear to slow the progression of macular degeneration, but do not reduce the incidence.

In observational studies (case-control or cohort design), people with high intake of antioxidant vitamins by regular diet or as food supplements generally have a lower risk of myocardial infarction and stroke than people who are low consumers of antioxidant vitamins. The associations in observation studies have been shown for carotene and ascorbic acid, as well as tocopherol. In randomized controlled trials, however, antioxidant vitamins as food supplements have no beneficial effects in the primary prevention of myocardial infarction and stroke.

TABLE 2.1

Examples of Epidemiological Associations of Diet, Vitamins, or Supplements with Specific Diseases

Study	Population	Condition	Association	Results	95% CI
Kittner et al. 1999	167 women aged 15 to 44 years vs. 328 women without a stroke	First ischemic stroke	Plasma homocysteine level > 7.3 mu mol/L	Odds ratio 1.6.	1.1 to 2.5
Cancer Prevention Study 2000	26,593 male smokers, aged 50 to 69 years	Cerebral infarction	Dietary intake of p-carotene	Relative risk 0.77	0.61 to 0.99
Cancer Prevention Study 2002	26,593 male smokers, aged 50 to 69 years	Cerebral infarction	Lycopene, lutein, zeaxanthin, vitamin C, flavonols, flavones, vitamin E	No association	
Robinson et al. 1998	750 patients vs. 800 controls	Coronary artery disease	Homocysteine concentrations >80th percentile of control subjects	Increased risk	
Robinson et al. 1998	750 patients vs. 800 controls	Coronary artery disease	Red cell folate <10th percentile of controls	Increased risk	
Robinson et al. 1998	750 patients vs. 800 controls	Coronary artery disease	Vitamin B-6 < 20th percentile of controls	Increased risk	
Anderson et al. 2000	1412 patients	Coronary artery disease	Plasma total homocysteine levels	Higher 3-year mortality	15.7% vs. 9.6%
Muntwyler et al. 2002	83,639 male U.S. physicians with no history of CVD or cancer.	Cardio-vascular disease or cardio-vascular mortality	Self-reported use of vitamins E, C, or multivitamins	No association	
Hung et al. 2004	71,910 female participants in the Nurses' Health study and 37,725 male participants in the Health Professionals Follow-up Study, free of chronic disease	Incidence of cardio-vascular disease, cancer, or death	Total fruit and vegetable intake by dietary questionaire	Relative risk for major chronic disease of 0.95 for highest quintile vs. lowest. Relative risk for greater than 5 servings daily 0.88 for cardiovascular disease and 1.00 for cancer	0.89 to 1.01 for major chronic disease; 0.81 to 0.95 for cardio-vascular disease; 95 to 1.05 for cancer
Chen et al. 2002	15,317 men and women >20 years of age	Hypertension	Lower levels of vitamin A and vitamin E	Higher risk of hypertension	43% vs. 18%

TABLE 2.1 (CONTINUED)
Examples of Epidemiological Associations of Diet, Vitamins, or Supplements with Specific Diseases

Study	Population	Condition	Association	Results	95% CI
Chen et al. 2002	15,317 men and women >20 years of age	Hypertension	Higher levels of alpha-carotene and beta-carotene	Lower risk of hypertension	16% vs. 11%
Chen et al. 2002	15,317 men and women >20 years of age	Hypertension	Higher levels of vitamin C	Lower diastolic pressure	
Tabak et al. 1999	Finland (n = 1248), Italy (n = 1386), and the Netherlands (n = 691) middle aged men	Pulmonary	Higher intake of fruits, vegetables	Higher forced vital capacity	53 to 118 ml
Tabak et al. 1999	Finland (n = 1248), Italy (n = 1386), and the Netherlands (n = 691) middle aged men	Pulmonary	Higher intake of vitamin C, beta carotene	No association	
Tabak et al. 1999	Finland (n = 1248), Italy (n = 1386), and the Netherlands (n = 691) middle aged men	Pulmonary	Higher intake of vitamin E	No association	
Nomura et al. 2003	9,345 Japanese-American men	Bladder cancer	Alpha-carotene, beta;-carotene, lutein plus zeaxanthin, beta;-cryptoxanthin and total carotenoids	No association after adjusting for smoking	
Luchsinger et al. 2003	980 elderly subjects free of dementia at baseline, followed for mean 4 years	Alzheimer's disease	Carotenes and vitamin C, or vitamin E in supplemental or dietary (nonsupplemental) form or in both forms	No association	

2.1 EPIDEMIOLOGICAL ASSOCIATIONS

Table 2.1 summarizes examples of the epidemiological associations of vitamins with specific disease states.

The epidemiological data suggests a clear association between elevated homocysteine levels and higher risk of stroke and cardiovascular disease. An association has been shown for carotid disease (five studies), coronary disease (two studies), peripheral vascular disease (one study), and aortic atherosclerotic disease (one study). An increased risk of cardiovascular disease with high levels of homocysteine levels has been shown in 10 of 13 case-control studies and one cohort study. A decreased risk for cardiovascular disease was also shown with high levels of folate (three of five prospective and one of two retrospective studies) and vitamin B_6 (two of two prospective and two of two retrospective studies) but not with high levels of vitamin B_{12} (one prospective and two retrospective studies).[3] The risk of stroke is also higher for persons who consume fewer fruits and vegetables. Folate levels, which are dependent on homocysteine levels, are also predictive of cardiovascular risk. Whether or not decreasing homocysteine levels by dietary or pharmacological interventions is not known. Low levels of vitamin B6 have been associated with cardiovascular risk and hyperlipidemia.

Other studies have not supported a link between supplemental vitamins and disease. The self-reported intake of vitamins E, C, or multivitamins was not associated with decreased incidence of cardiovascular disease or cardiovascular mortality after adjusting for known cardiovascular risk factors in a large observational study of male physicians.[4]

Lung function studies illustrate the sometimes confusing data from epidemiological surveys. Forced expiratory volume was associated with intake of vitamin E in Finland, but only with dietary intake of fruit in Italy, and only with beta-carotene intake in the Netherlands. But in all three countries, men with above-average intakes of both fruit and vegetables had a higher forced expiratory volume than those with a low intake of both foods. However, after adjustment for energy intake, the association of all three antioxidants disappeared.[5] Differences across populations, even over relatively small distances, confound these studies.

Micronutrient intake, including lutein, zeaxanthin, anhydrolutein, alpha-cryptoxanthin, beta-cryptoxanthin, lycopene, dihydrolycopene, alpha-carotene, beta-carotene, total carotenoids, retinol, alpha-tocopherol, beta-tocopherol, gamma-tocopherol, delta-tocopherol and total tocopherols, were examined in men who developed bladder cancer after 20 years of surveillance and compared to age-matched controls. There were statistically significant inverse linear trends in risk for alpha-carotene, beta-carotene, lutein plus zeaxanthin, beta-cryptoxanthin and total carotenoids. However, after adjustment for pack-years of cigarette smoking, none of the inverse trends remained significant.[6]

Baseline intake of carotenes and vitamin C, or vitamin E in supplemental or dietary (nonsupplemental) form or in both forms, was not related to a decreased risk of dementia of the Alzheimer's type after 4 years of follow-up.[7]

2.2 RANDOMIZED CONTROLLED TRIALS

The use of various dietary supplements, including vitamins, to prevent or delay disease or aging rests for the most part on epidemiological associations. It does appear from this data that a diet rich in vitamins is associated with a tendency to improved health. However, the results from controlled trials is dismal. The discrepancy between different types of studies is probably explained by the fact that dietary composition and supplement use is only a component in a cluster of healthy behaviors. An alternative hypothesis is that there are as yet unknown essential organic compounds in certain foods.

Table 2.2 summarizes examples of randomized controlled trials and meta-analytical reviews for vitamins and specific diseases. The data from randomized controlled trials shows (with a few exceptions) that supplementation with vitamin supplements has not had much effect on disease states. The use of mineral and vitamin supplements has been shown to slow the progression, but not

TABLE 2.2

Examples of Controlled Trials of Vitamins or Supplements on Specific Diseases

Study	Population	Condition	Intervention	Results	Effect
MRC/BHF Heart Protection Study 2002	20,536 subjects followed 5 years	Coronary heart disease, vascular occlusive disease, diabetes mellitus, hypertension	Vitamin E 600 mg/d, plus vitamin C 250 mg/d, plus beta-carotene 20 mg/d or placebo	All-cause, vascular, or nonvascular mortality, or secondary measures including major coronary events, stroke, revascularization, and cancer.	No difference
The SU.VI. MAX Study 2004	13,017 persons, age 45–60, followed 7.5 years	Cancer, cardiovascular disease or Cardiovascular mortality	120 mg ascorbic acid, 30 mg of vitamin E, 6 mg of beta carotene, 100 microg of Selenium, 20 mg of zinc vs placebo	Total cancerincidence 4.1% vs. 4.5%; ischemic cardiovascular Disease incidence 2.1% vs. 2.1%, all-cause mortality 1.2% vs. 1.5%	No difference; may have small protective effect in men
HOPE trial 2005	3,994 persons, >55 yrs with CVD or DBM, followed 7 years	Cardiovascular events and cancer	Vitamin E 400 IU/d vs. placebo	Cancer incidence 11.6% vs. 12.3%; cancer deaths 3.3% vs. 3.7%; major cardiovascular events 21.5% vs. 20.6%.	No difference. Higher risk of CHF and hospitalization for CHF
Heart Protection Study 2002	15,000 men aged 40 to 80, followed 5 years	Cardiovascular disease	Daily combination of vitamin E (600 mg), vitamin C (250 mg), and [beta]-carotene (20 mg)	Incidence	No significant reduction
Women's Health Study 2006	39,876 healthy women age >45 years	first nonfatal myocardial infarction, nonfatal stroke, or cardiovascular death and total invasive cancer	600 IU of vitamin E on alternate days	24% reduction in cardiovascular death (RR, 0.76; CI, 0.59–0.98); no effect on total mortality	No difference in myocardial infarction, stroke, or cancer.
Jamison	2056 persons, >21 yrs with CKD, followed 3.2 yrs	CKD all-cause mortality	40 mg folic acid, 100 mg pyridoxine (B6), and 2 mg cyanocobalamin (B12) vs. placebo	Relative risk 1.04, (CI, 0.91–1.18)	No difference mortality, myocardial infarction, stroke, amputation, time to initiation of dialysis
Meta-analysis 2005	135, 967 participants in 19 clinical trials	All-cause mortality	Vitamin E >400 IU/d	39 deaths per 10,000 persons (3 to 74 per 10,000 persons; P = 0.035)	Higher mortality

TABLE 2.2 (CONTINUED)

Examples of Controlled Trials of Vitamins or Supplements on Specific Diseases

Study	Population	Condition	Intervention	Results	Effect
Mullan et al. 2002	30 patients, 45 to 70 years old, with type 2 diabetes, followed 4 weeks	Hypertension	500 mg of ascorbic acid daily	Mean systolic 9.9 mm Hg, mean diastolic 6.0 mm Hg.	Reduced systolic blood pressure
Kim et al. 2002	439 subjects followed 5 years	Hypertension	500 mg of vitamin C daily	Blood pressure	No reduction
Pfeifer et al. 2001	148 women, mean age 74 years followed 8 weeks	Hypertension	1200 mg calcium plus 800 IU vitamin D3 or 1200 mg calcium/day	Decrease in systolic blood pressure of 9.3%	Improved
Ram et al. 2003	Six trials	Asthma	Vitamin C supplementation	Asthma outcome	No difference
Caraballoso et al. 2003	109,394 subjects	Lung cancer	Beta-carotene, alone or combination with alpha-tocopherol or retinol, or alpha-tocopherol alone	Cancer incidence	No reduction
The Beta-Carotene and Retinol Efficacy Trial 1996	18,314 subjects, 45 to 74 years, at high risk, followed 4 years	Lung cancer	[Beta]-carotene and retinyl palmitate compared with placebo	28% (4%–57%) higher cancer incidence and 17% (3%–33%) higher total mortality in the supplemented group	Worse outcome
Virtamo et al. 2003	25,390 persons followed 6 years	Prostate cancer	Alpha-tocopherol	Relative risk 0.88 (0.76–1.03)	No difference
Virtamo et al. 2003	25,390 persons followed 6 years	Prostate cancer	Beta carotene	Relative risk 1.06 (0.91–1.23)	No difference
Cole et al. 2007	1021 persons with recent history of colorectal adenomas	Incidence of colon polyps in next 6 to 8 years	1 mg per day folic acid vs. placebo	Polyps 44.1% for folic acid and 42.4% for placebo at 3 years (risk ratio 1.04; CI, 0.90 to 1.20). Polyps 41.9% for folic acid vs. 37.2% for placebo at 6 years.	Higher risk with folic acid

TABLE 2.2 (CONTINUED)

Examples of Controlled Trials of Vitamins or Supplements on Specific Diseases

Study	Population	Condition	Intervention	Results	Effect
Alzheimer's Disease Cooperative Study 1997	341 subjects followed 2 years	Alzheimer's dementia	Vitamin E 1000 mg twice a day, selegiline 5 mg twice a day, both or placebo	Time to either death, institutionalization, decline in activities of daily living, or progression to severe dementia	Reduced in vitamin E group (670 days) and selegiline group (655 days) compared with placebo group (440 days), higher mortality 1.08 (1.01 to 1.14)
Rodriguez-Martin 2003	50 subjects, followed 1 year	Alzheimer's dementia	Thiamine supplementation	Cognitive status	No benefit
Lerner et al. 2002	15 subjects	Schizophrenia	Vitamin B6 400mg vs. placebo	Mental status	No difference
Taylor et al. 2003	247 subjects	Depression	Folic acid	Reduction in depression scores	2.65 points, CI 0.38 to 4.93
Christen et al. 2003	22,071 male US physicians aged 40 to 84 years, followed 1 year	Cataract	Beta carotene 50 mg on alternate days vs. placebo	Incidence	No benefit
Evans 2003	4119 subjects in 7 trials	Age-related macular degeneration, progression to advanced disease	Antioxidant and zinc supplementation	Risk ratio 0.72 (0.52 to 0.98)	Less risk
Evans 2003	4119 subjects in 7 trials	Age-related macular degeneration	Vitamin E, beta carotene or both.	Prevention	No benefit
Girodon et al. 1999	725 institutionalized elderly subjects >65 years, followed 2 years.	Antibody titers, respiratory infections, urinary tract infections, survival rate.	Trace elements (zinc and selenium sulfide) or vitamins (beta carotene, ascorbic acid, and vitamin E) or a placebo	Antibody titers after influenza vaccine were higher in groups that received trace elements alone or associated with vitamins, but the vitamin group had significantly lower antibody titers.	Higher titers with minerals but low with vitamins

TABLE 2.2 (CONTINUED)

Examples of Controlled Trials of Vitamins or Supplements on Specific Diseases

Study	Population	Condition	Intervention	Results	Effect
Chandra et al. 1992	96 subjects	Infection-related illness, days taking antibiotics, nutritional deficiencies	Vitamin A 400 units, beta-carotene 16 mg; thiamine 2.2 mg; riboflavin 1.5 mg; niacin 16 mg;vitamin B6 3.0 mg; folate 400 microg; vitamin B12 4.0 microg; vitamin C80 mg; vitamin D 4 microg; vitamin E 44 mg; iron 16 mg; zinc 14 mg; copper 1.4 mg; selenium 20 microg; iodine 0.2 mg; calcium 200 mg; and magnesium 100 mg. vs. placebo (calcium, 200 mg, and magnesium, 100 mg).	23 (23 to 28) vs. 48 fewer infection-related illness days; 18 (12 to 16) vs. 32 fewer days taking antibiotics	Improved
El-Kadiki et al. 2005	8 trials in older adults	Days with infection, at least one infection, incident infections	Any combination of vitamin or mineral supplements	14 (10 to 18) fewer days with infection; at least one infection 1.10 (0.81 to 1.50) ; incident infections 0.89 (0.78 to 1.03	Fewer days with infection, no difference in incident infections
Gillespie et al. 2003	Frail elderly subjects	Hip fracture and vertebral fracture incidence	Vitamin D3 supplementation along with calcium	Risk ratio 0.74 (0.60 to 0.91)	Less risk
Gillespie et al. 2003	Frail elderly subjects	Hip fracture and vertebral fracture incidence	Vitamin D3 supplementation alone without calcium	Risk ratio 1.20 (0.83 to 1.75)	No difference
Gillespie et al. 2003	In healthy younger, ambulatory subjects	Hip fracture	Vitamin D3 supplementation along with calcium	Risk ratio 0.36 (0.01 to 8.78)	No difference
Gillespie et al. 2003	In healthy younger, ambulatory subjects	Non-vertebral fracture	Vitamin D3 supplementation along with calcium	Risk ratio 0.46 (0.23 to 0.90)	Less risk

TABLE 2.2 (CONTINUED)
Examples of Controlled Trials of Vitamins or Supplements on Specific Diseases

Study	Population	Condition	Intervention	Results	Effect
Trivedi et al. 2003	Community-dwelling, 65–85 years	First non-vertebral and vertebral fracture	Vitamin D3 v. placebo	Relative risk 0.78 (0.61 to 0.99)	Less risk
Bischoff-Ferrari et al. 2004	5 RCT with 1237 persons	Falls	Vitamin D vs. placebo	Odds ratio for 0.78; (CI, 0.64–0.92)	Decreased risk 22%

prevent, age-related macular degeneration. Folate may have some role in the treatment of depression, although the trials have been small in numbers. Vitamin C may, or may not, have an effect on hypertension, but the longest trials were only 2 months in duration.

Randomized controlled trials of specific supplements also have failed to demonstrate a consistent or significant effect of any single vitamin or combination of vitamins on incidence of or death from cardiovascular disease.[8] After an initial enthusiasm for antioxidants in the secondary prevention of cardiovascular disease, recent reports from several large randomized trials have failed to show any beneficial effects. Thus, the apparent beneficial results of high intake of antioxidant vitamins reported in observational studies have not been confirmed in large randomized trials.[9]

Vitamin E plus vitamin C plus beta-carotene showed no difference in all-cause, vascular, or nonvascular mortality, or secondary measures including major coronary events, stroke, revascularization, and cancer compared with placebo.[10] Four placebo-controlled trials have not shown a benefit of beta-carotene, alone or combination with alpha-tocopherol or retinol, or alpha-tocopherol alone on the development of lung cancer. For people with risk factors for lung cancer, no reduction in lung cancer incidence or mortality was found in those taking vitamins alone compared with placebo. For people with no known risk factors of lung cancer, none of the vitamins or their combinations appeared to have any effect. In fact, in combination with retinol, a statistically significant increase in risk of lung cancer incidence was found compared with placebo.[11]

Antioxidant vitamins and zinc had reduced progression to advanced disease in age-related macular degeneration, but has not been demonstrated to be effective for prevention.

Six controlled trials on supplementation of vitamin C in persons with asthma showed no appreciable benefit on asthma outcome.[12] Trace elements, but not vitamins alone, have been shown to produce higher antibody titers after influenza vaccination in older persons, but had no effect on infection rate or survival.

Vitamin D supplementation, along with calcium, has been demonstrated to reduce hip fracture rate in older persons. A randomized controlled trial of persons aged 65–85 years living in the general community (n = 2686), evaluated 100,000 IU oral vitamin D3 (cholecalciferol) supplementation or matching placebo every 4 months over 5 years. Relative risks for fracture of the hip, wrist or forearm, or vertebrae in the vitamin D group compared with the placebo group were 0.78 (95% confidence interval 0.61 to 0.99 for any first fracture and 0.67 (0.48 to 0.93) for first hip, wrist or forearm, or vertebral fracture. The relative risk for total mortality in the vitamin D group compared with the placebo group was 0.88 (0.74 to 1.06). Supplementation every 4 months with 100,000 IU oral vitamin D may prevent fractures without adverse effects in men and women living in the general community.[13] Two trials found that 400 IU of vitamin D did not significantly reduce fracture risk,[14,15] but trials using 700 to 800 IU/d of vitamin D did show significant reductions in observed fractures, suggesting that the effect may be dose dependent.[16,17,18]

In a meta-analysis of five randomized controlled trials with 1237 elderly individuals, the effect on falls of treatment with different vitamin D analogues for 2 months up to 3 years was evaluated.[19]

Four trials administered either vitamin D 800 IU/d plus 1200 mg/d of calcium[20,21] or an active vitamin D analogue and no calcium supplements.[22,23] The lowest dose of vitamin D was 400 IU/d, but reported calcium intake from dairy products was high at 800 to 1000 mg/d in that trial. Taken together, vitamin D reduced the risk of falling by 22% (corrected odds ratio (OR), 0.78; 95% confidence interval, 0.64–0.92) compared with patients receiving calcium or placebo. From the pooled risk difference, the number needed to treat (NNT) was 15 (95% CI, 8–53). It should be noted that none of these trials involved residents in long-term care settings. In a second meta-analysis of three studies involving 613 participants treated with cholecalciferol, a non-significant corrected OR of falling was observed. (0.83, 95% CI, 0.65–1.06). However, after excluding the trial with a 400 IU dose, the two trials with 259 subjects using 800 IU of cholecalciferol demonstrated a corrected OR of falling of 0.65 (95% CI, 0.40–1.00), which approached statistical significance. For the two studies involving 626 participants who used active vitamin D, the corrected OR for falling was 0.71 (95% CI, 0.55–0.92). Thus, a dose of 400 IU of vitamin D suggests that this dose may not be clinically effective in preventing falls in the elderly.[24] Older ambulatory subjects (n = 139) with a history of falls and 25-hydroxyvitamin D levels less than or equal to 12 microg/l, were randomized to receive a single intramuscular injection of 600,000 IU of ergocalciferol or placebo. Aggregate Function Performance Time (AFPT), choice reaction time, and postural sway measures improved in the intervention group and deteriorated in the control group. There was no significant difference in muscle strength change between groups. A significant correlation between change in AFPT and change in 25O HD levels was observed. However, there was no significant difference in the number of falls or persons falling between two groups. Vitamin D supplementation, in fallers with vitamin D insufficiency, had a significant beneficial effect on functional performance, reaction time and balance, but not muscle strength.[25]

2.3   RISKS

If the results of these randomized controlled trials were not disappointing enough, the data showing potential harm from vitamin and mineral supplements is alarming. β-carotene and retinyl palmitate in combination produced a statistically significant increase in risk of lung cancer incidence compared with placebo.[26] In a meta-analysis of participants in randomized controlled trials using vitamin E, nine of 11 trials showed an increased risk for all-cause mortality at a vitamin E dose greater than or equal to 400 IU/day.[27] No increase in all-cause mortality was seen for doses less than 400 IU per day in these trials, but a dose–response analysis showed that a statistically significant relationship between vitamin E dosage and all-cause mortality began at a dose greater than 150 IU/day. A similar increase in mortality has been described in very high dose vitamin E (2000 IU/day) supplementation in persons with Alzheimer's dementia.[28]

Serious adverse events have been reported. Toxicity may result from excessive doses of vitamin A during early pregnancy and from fat-soluble vitamins taken anytime.

There is some concern that Vitamin E plus vitamin C plus beta-carotene may blunt the protective HDL2 cholesterol response to HDL cholesterol-targeted therapy.[29]

2.4   VITAMINS AND OLDER ADULTS

Aging is associated with increased risk for low vitamin consumption. In the United States, total energy intake decreases substantially with age, by 1000 to 1200 kcal in men and by 600 to 800 kcal in women in the seventh decade. This results in concomitant declines in most nutrient intakes. Lower food intake among the elderly has been associated with lower intakes of calcium, iron, zinc, B vitamins and vitamin E. This low energy intake or low nutrient density of the diet may increase the risk of diet-related illnesses. Fifty percent of older adults have a vitamin and mineral intake less than the recommended daily allowance (RDA), while 10–30% have subnormal levels of vitamins and minerals.[30] Populations at high risk for inadequate vitamin intake include elderly people, vegans, alcohol-dependent individuals, and patients with malabsorption.

Older adults tend to consume fewer energy-dense sweets and fast foods, and consume more energy-dilute grains, vegetables and fruits. Daily volume of foods and beverages also declines as a function of age. Physiological changes associated with age, including slower gastric emptying, altered hormonal responses, decreased basal metabolic rate, and altered taste and smell may also contribute to lowered energy intake. Other factors, such as marital status, income, education, socioeconomic status, diet-related attitudes and beliefs, and convenience likely play a role as well.[31] Many age-related nutritional problems may be remedied to some extent by providing nutrient-dense meals through home delivery or meal congregate programs.[32]

2.4.1   VITAMINS AND HEALTH

2.4.1.1   The Vitamin A and Carotenoid Family

The carotenoids are a diverse group of more than 600 naturally occurring pigments. Natural sources include yellow, orange, and red plant compounds, such as carrots and green leafy vegetables. Humans must depend on dietary intake exclusively for these micronutrients as they cannot be synthesized. Beta-carotene and lycopene are the major dietary carotenoids. Lycopene is a natural pigment synthesized by plants and microorganisms but not by animals. It occurs in the human diet predominantly in tomatoes and processed tomato products. It is a potent antioxidant and the most significant free-radical scavenger in the carotenoid family. There is no known deficiency state for carotenoids themselves and no recommended daily intake. Beta-carotene can be converted to vitamin A, whereas lycopene cannot. All of the carotenoids are antioxidants, and approximately 50 are considered vitamins because they have provitamin A activity. Vitamin A refers to preformed retinol and the carotenoids that are converted to retinol. Preformed vitamin A is found only in animal products, including organ meats, fish, egg yolks, and fortified milk. More than 1,500 synthetic retinoids, analogs of vitamin A, have been developed. The current recommended daily intake (RDI) for vitamin A is 1500 micrograms/L (5000 IU).

2.4.1.2   Vitamin C

Vitamin C (ascorbic acid) is a water-soluble vitamin widely found in citrus fruits and raw leafy vegetables, strawberries, melons, tomatoes, broccoli, and peppers. Humans cannot synthesize vitamin C and a deficiency results in scurvy.

2.4.1.3   Vitamin E

Vitamin E occurs in eight natural forms as tocopherols (alpha, beta, gamma, and delta) and tocotrienols (alpha, beta, gamma, and delta), all of which possess potent antioxidant properties. Gamma-tocopherol is the predominant form of vitamin E in the human diet, yet most studies have focused on alpha-tocopherol, which is the type found in most over-the-counter supplements. One reason for this is that alpha-tocopherol is biologically more active than gamma-tocopherol. Vitamin E deficiency is rare and is seen primarily in special situations resulting in fat malabsorption, including cystic fibrosis, chronic cholestatic liver disease, abetalipoproteinemia, and short bowel syndrome.

2.4.2   OTHER ESSENTIAL VITAMINS

2.4.2.1   Vitamin B12

Vitamin B12 deficiency occurs in from 5% to 20% of older persons,[33] but it is often unrecognized because the clinical manifestations are subtle.[34] Causes of the deficiency include malabsorption of the vitamin (60% of all cases), pernicious anemia (15%–20% of all cases), and insufficient dietary intake. Measurement of vitamin B_{12} and folate concentrations will determine anemia due to these causes in the majority of cases. Confirmation of vitamin B_{12} deficiency in those patients who have values in the lower normal range should be obtained, since about 50% of patients with subclinical disease may have normal B_{12} levels. A more sensitive method of screening for vitamin B_{12} deficiency is measurement of serum methylmalonic acid and homocysteine levels, which are increased early in vitamin B_{12} deficiency. A homocysteine level will be elevated in both vitamin B_{12} and folate deficiencies, but a methylmalonic acid level will be elevated only in vitamin B_{12} deficiency. Renal failure is the only other confounding cause of an elevated methylmalonic acid concentration.

2.4.2.2   Folic acid

Folate, along with vitamins B-6 and B-12, are required for the conversion of homocysteine to methionine. Increases in homocysteine have been associated with increased coronary heart disease risk in observational trials; inadequate folate status associated with neural tube defect in children,[35] and with colon cancer.[36] Folate occurs naturally in a variety of foods, including liver; dark-green leafy vegetables such as collards, turnip greens, and Romaine lettuce; broccoli and asparagus; citrus fruits and juices; whole-grain products; wheat germ; and dried beans and peas, such as pinto, navy and lima beans, and chickpeas and black-eyed peas. Effective in 1998, the Food and Drug agency requires manufacturers to add from 0.43 mg to 1.4 mg of folic acid per pound of product to enriched flour, bread, rolls and buns, farina, corn grits, cornmeal, rice, and noodle products.

2.4.2.3   Vitamin D

Vitamin D occurs naturally in animal foods as the provitamin cholecalciferol. This requires conversion in the kidney to the metabolically active form, calcitriol. Vitamin D is not a true vitamin, since humans are able to synthesize it with adequate sunlight exposure. By photoconversion, 7-dehydrocholesterol becomes previtamin D3, which is metabolized in the liver to 25-hydroxyvitamin D3, the major circulating form of vitamin D. In the kidney, this is converted to 2 metabolites, the more active one being 1,25-dihydroxyvitamin D3. Food sources include fortified milk, saltwater fish, and fish-liver oil.

2.4.2.4   Thiamin

Thiamine pyrophosphate is a coenzyme for pyruvate dehydrogenase, α-ketoglutarate dehydrogenase, and transketolase. The deficiency of thiamine results in beriberi, a syndrome that includes symptoms of weight loss, emotional disturbances, impaired sensory perception, weakness, and heart failure. Thiamine is found in fortified breads, cereals, pasta, whole grains (especially wheat germ), lean meats (especially pork), fish, dried beans, peas, and soybeans. Dairy products, fruits, and vegetables are not very high in thiamine, but when consumed in large amounts, they become a significant source.

2.4.2.5   Pyridoxine

Vitamin B6, or pyridoxine, has been associated with cardiovascular risk and hyperlipidemia. Vitamin B_6 is found in a wide variety of foods including fortified cereals, beans, meat, poultry, fish, and some fruits and vegetables.

2.4.2.5   Riboflavin

Deficiency is rare in the United States due to widely available sources of the vitamin. Lean meats, eggs, legumes, nuts, green leafy vegetables, dairy products, and milk provide riboflavin in the diet. Breads and cereals are often fortified with riboflavin. Other than deficiency states, association with disease is unknown.

2.5 MINERALS

Approximately 15 inorganic elements are required in minute amounts. In humans, clinically symptomatic and reversible deficiency disease has been established for iron, iodine, copper, zinc, and selenium. Other elements, including chromium, manganese, molybdenum, and vanadium, have undoubted biological activity, but relationship to clinical practice is not as clear.

2.6 SUMMARY

The use of various dietary supplements, including vitamins, to prevent or delay disease or aging rests for the most part on epidemiological associations. It does appear from this data that a diet rich in vitamins is associated with a tendency to improved health. However, the results from controlled trials is dismal. The discrepancy between different types of studies is probably explained by the fact that dietary composition and supplement use are merely components in a cluster of healthy behaviors. An alternative hypothesis is that there are as yet unknown essential organic compounds in certain foods.

Much of the enthusiasm for the use of vitamin or mineral supplements to prevent disease or increase longevity results from the belief that supplementation is harmless. However, serious adverse events have been reported. Toxicity may result from excessive doses of vitamin A during early pregnancy and from other fat-soluble vitamins taken in high doses. There is increasing concern from randomized controlled trials that beta-carotene and vitamin E may be associated with a higher mortality risk.

The most prudent approach is to recommend a daily intake of fruits and vegetables as a likely source of essential nutrients. Failing compliance with a natural source of essential nutrients, and in populations at high risk of vitamin deficiency, vitamin supplements should be encouraged.

REFERENCES

1. Thomas DR. Vitamins in health, aging, and longevity. 2006. *Clin. Intervent. Aging.* 1(1):81–91.
2. Fairfield KM and Fletcher RH. 2002. Vitamins for chronic disease prevention in adults—scientific review. *JAMA.* 287(23):3116–3126.
3. Anonymous. 2000. Review: High levels of homocysteine are associated with an increased risk for cardiovascular disease. *ACP Journal Club.* 132:73.
4. Muntwyler J, Hennekens CH, Manson JE, Buring JE, and Gaziano JM. 2002. Vitamin supplement use in a low-risk population of US male physicians and subsequent cardiovascular mortality. *Arch. Int. Med.* 162:1472–1476.
5. Tabak C, Smit HA, Rasanen L, Fidanza F, Menotti A, Nissinen A, Feskens EJM, Heederik D, and Kromhout D. 1999. Dietary factors and pulmonary function: A cross sectional study in middle aged men from three European countries. *Thorax.* 54:1021–1026.
6. Nomura AM, Lee J, Stemmermann GN. Franke AA. 2003. Serum vitamins and the subsequent risk of bladder cancer. *J. Urol.* 170(4 Part 1):1146–1150.
7. Luchsinger JA, Tang MX, Shea S, and Mayeux R. 2003. Antioxidant vitamin intake and risk of Alzheimer disease. *Arch. Neurol.* 60:203–208.
8. Morris CD and Carson S. 2003. Routine vitamin supplementation to prevent cardiovascular disease: A summary of the evidence for the US Preventive Services Task Force. *Ann. Int. Med.* 139:56–70.
9. Asplund K. 2002. Antioxidant vitamins in the prevention of cardiovascular disease: A systematic review. *J. Int. Med.* 251:372–92.
10. Kumana CR, Cheung BM, Lauder IJ. 2003. Antioxidant vitamins did not reduce death, vascular events, or cancer in high-risk patients. *ACP J. Club.* 138:3.
11. Caraballoso M, Sacristan M, Serra C, and Bonfill X. 2003. Drugs for preventing lung cancer in healthy people. Cochrane Database of Systematic Reviews. Issue 2.
12. Ram FSF, Rowe BH, and Kaur B. 2001. Vitamin C supplementation for asthma. Cochrane Database of Systematic Reviews. Issue 4.
13. Trivedi DP, Doll R, Khaw KT. 2003. Effect of four monthly oral vitamin D3 (cholecalciferol) supplementation on fractures and mortality in men and women living in the community: randomised double blind controlled trial. *BMJ* 326:469.

14. Meyer HE, Smedshaug GB, Kvaavik E, Falch JA, Tverdal A, Pedersen JI. 2002. Can vitamin D supplementation reduce the risk of fracture in the elderly? A randomized controlled trial. *J. Bone Miner. Res.* 17:709–715.

15. Lips P, Graafmans WC, Ooms ME, Bezemer PD, Bouter LM. 1996. Vitamin D supplementation and fracture incidence in elderly persons: A randomized placebo-controlled clinical trial. *Ann. Intern. Med.* 124:400–406.

16. Dawson-Hughes B, Harris SS, Krall EA, and Dallal GE. 1997. Effect of calcium and vitamin D supplementation on bone density in men and women 65 years of age or older. *N. Engl. J. Med.* 337:670–676.

17. Chapuy MC, Arlot ME, Duboeuf F, et al. 1992. Vitamin D3 and calcium to prevent hip fractures in the elderly women. *N. Engl. J. Med.* 327:1637–1642.

18. Trivedi DP, Doll R, Khaw KT. 2003. Effect of four monthly oral vitamin D3 (cholecalciferol) supplementation on fractures and mortality in men and women living in the community: randomised double blind controlled trial. *BMJ.* 326:469.

19. Bischoff-Ferrari HA, Dawson-Hughes B, Willett WC, Staehelin HB, Bazemore MG, Zee RY, and Wong JB. 2004. Effect of vitamin D on falls: A meta-analysis. *JAMA.* 291:1999–2006.

20. Pfeifer M, Begerow B, Minne HW, Abrams C, Nachtigall D, Hansen C. 2000. Effects of a short-term vitamin D and calcium supplementation on body sway and secondary hyperparathyroidism in elderly women. *J. Bone Miner. Res.* 15:1113–1118.

21. Bischoff HA, Stahelin HB, Dick W, et al. 2003. Effects of vitamin D and calcium supplementation on falls: A randomized controlled trial. *J. Bone Miner. Res.* 18:343–351.

22. Gallagher JC, Fowler SE, Detter JR, Sherman SS. 2001.Combination treatment with estrogen and calcitriol in the prevention of age-related bone loss. *J. Clin. Endocrinol. Metab.* 86:3618–3628.

23. Dukas L, Bischoff HA, Lindpaintner LS, et al. Alfacalcidol reduces the number of fallers in a community-dwelling elderly population with a minimum calcium intake of more than 500 mg daily. *J. Am. Geriatr. Soc.* 2004. 52:230–236.

24. Graafmans WC, Ooms ME, Hofstee HM, Bezemer PD, Bouter LM, Lips P. 1996. Falls in the elderly: a prospective study of risk factors and risk profiles. *Am. J. Epidemiol.* 143:1129–1136.

25. Dhesi JK, Jackson SH, Bearne LM, Moniz C, Hurley MV, Swift CG, and Allain TJ. 2004. Vitamin D supplementation improves neuromuscular function in older people who fall. *Age & Ageing* 33:589–95.

26. Omenn GS, Goodman GE, Thornquist MD et al. 1996. Effects of a combination of β-carotene and vitamin A on lung cancer and cardiovascular disease. *N. Engl. J. Med.* 334, 1150–1155.

27. Miller ER 3rd, Pastor-Barriuso R, Dalal D, Riemersma RA, Appel LJ, Guallar E. 2005. Meta-analysis: High-dosage vitamin E supplementation may increase all-cause mortality. *Ann. Intern. Med.* 142, 37–46.

28. Sano M, Ernesto C, Thomas RG et al. 1997. A controlled trial of selegiline, α–tocopherol, or both as treatment for Alzheimer's disease. The Alzheimer's Disease Cooperative Study. *N. Engl. J. Med.* 336, 1216–1222.

29. Brown BG, Cheung MC, Lee AC, Zhao XQ, Chait A. 2002. Antioxidant vitamins and lipid therapy— End of a long romance? *Arterio. Thromb. Vasc. Biol.* 22:1535–1546.

30. Wakimoto P. Block G. 2001.Dietary intake, dietary patterns, and changes with age: An epidemiological perspective. *J. Gerontol. Series A–Biol. Sci. Med. Sci.* 56:65–80.

31. Thomas DR. 2002. Distinguishing starvation from cachexia. *Geriat. Clin. N.Am.* 18:883–892.

32. Drewnowski A, Shultz JM. 2001. Impact of aging on eating behaviors, food choices, nutrition, and health status. *J. Nutr. Hlth. Ag.* 5:75–9.

33. Andres E, Loukili NH, Noel E, Kaltenbach G, Abdelgheni MB, Perrin AE, Noblet-Dick M, Maloisel F, Schlienger JL, Blickle JF. 2004. Vitamin B12 (cobalamin) deficiency in elderly patients. *Can. Med. Assoc. J.* 171:251–259.

34. Thomas DR. 2004. Anemia and quality of life: Unrecognized and undertreated. *J. Gerontol. Series A–Biol. Sci. Med. Sci.* 59(3):238–241.

35. Paulozzi LJ, Mathews TJ, Erickson JD, Wong LC. 2001. Impact of folic acid fortification on the US food supply on the occurrence of neural tube defects. *JAMA.* 285:2981–6.

36. Giovannucci E, Stampfer MJ, Colditz GA, Hunter DJ, Fuchs C, Rosner BA, Speizer FE, Willett WC. 1998. Multivitamin use, folate, and colon cancer in women in the Nurses' Health Study. *Ann. Intern. Med.* 129:517–24.

3 Undernutrition and Refeeding in Elderly Subjects

Patrice Brocker and Stéphane M. Schneider

CONTENTS

The elderly subject is at risk for undernutrition for several reasons that make him or her all the more vulnerable to disease. Malnutrition in the elderly is mainly protein-energy undernutrition, but it can involve only micronutrient deficiencies. It is important to screen for undernutrition in all free-living elderly subjects, but even more so when hospitalized or institutionalized. There are several therapeutic approaches to undernutrition centered on dietary advice and enteral nutrition.

3.1 CAUSES OF UNDERNUTRITION

Numerous situations induce undernutrition in the elderly. Causes are often interrelated, particularly in hospitals or nursing homes (Table 3.1) [1]. Usually, undernutrition in an elderly subject is facilitated by the presence of hypermetabolism or hypercatabolism, exacerbated if he or she had insufficient food contribution before. The speed at which undernutrition takes over during hypercatabolism depends only partially on age-related metabolic changes.

3.1.1 PHYSIOLOGICAL CHANGES RELATED TO AGE

Physiological changes affect every step from food breakdown to nutrient metabolism.

3.1.1.1 Changes in the Digestive Tract

Taste threshold increases with age. Flavors need to be intensified for an elderly subject to savor their taste. Furthermore, numerous drugs affect taste (often by modifying the level of humidity in the mouth). This sensorial alteration with age could contribute to the increased selection of sweet foods [2].

Dentition alterations or poor gingival condition are frequent in elderly people, a condition often added to because dental care is expensive. Only painless chewing permits a correct diet. Degradation of oral conditions is responsible for a masticatory insufficiency, imposing a monotonous, poorly balanced and unappetizing diet [3].

Gastric mucous membrane shrinks with age. As a result, there is a decrease in the hydrochloric secretion, which delays gastric evacuation. In the small intestine, the decrease in secretion of enzymes is responsible for a delay in nutrient digestion. The delaying of the intestinal transit with age is responsible for intestinal stasis, constipation, and microbial overgrowth.

3.1.1.2 Metabolic Changes

Fat-free mass diminishes in sedentary subjects losing their mobility. Muscle mass is especially affected (there is a 50% decrease between ages 20 and 70). Protein metabolism (anabolism as well as catabolism) at the whole-body level is only slightly affected. Fatty acid requirements are the same in elderly subjects. Both men and women lose bone calcium with age, but this loss is greater in postmenopausal women. Furthermore, the active absorption of calcium decreases in elderly people. Consequently, a high supply of calcium is essential to satisfy the needs.

Total body water diminishes with age (20% loss about age 60). This is all the more serious as the water regulating mechanisms are impaired; the threshold for the perception of thirst is higher and the amount of urine decreases. The consequence is worsening dehydration, which can be prevented only by a regular and systematic fluid supply.

However, aging is not by itself a cause of undernutrition.

3.1.2 LOW FOOD INTAKE

Numerous factors induce a lack of interest in the diet for the elderly subject. If this lack of interests persists, insufficient food intake leads to the use of the nutritional stores of the body.

TABLE 3.1
Causes of Undernutrition

Environmental Factors	Social isolation
	Widowhood
	Economic difficulties, poverty
	Abuse
	Hospitalization
	Confusion due to change in environment
Oral problems	Difficulty in chewing
	Bad oral health
	Dentures
	Xerostomia, decreased salivary flow
	Oral candidiasis
	Taste impairment, glossodynia
Swallowing problems	Dysphagia
	Cerebrovascular accident, neurological disorders
Psychiatric disorders	Depression
	Behavioral disorders
Dementia	Alzheimer disease
	Other dementia
Neurological problems	Delirium
	Attention disorders
	Parkinson's disease
Drugs	Polymedication
	Adverse drug effects
	Prolonged corticosteroid treatment
Acute physical malady	PainInfectious diseases
	Fractures with impaired mobility
	Surgical procedure
	Constipation
	Pressure sore
Functional impairment	Assistance needed with feeding
	Impaired mobility and activities of daily living
Long-term dietary restrictions	Strict salt-free diet
	Low calorie diet for weight loss
	Diabetic, particularly in nursing home
	Fat-free diet
	Fiber-free diet

Source: From HAS 2007. Stratégie de prise en charge en cas de dénutrition protéino-énergétique chez la personne âgée. Paris

3.1.2.1 Social Causes

Social isolation is frequent in elderly subjects, especially in urban areas. This isolation worsens with age and the deaths of spouse and friends. To reinsert an elderly person into a circle of social activity is one of the ways to prevent undernutrition [4].

The diminution in resources mainly affects the widowed and subjects who are outcasts of the social system. Exclusion originates most often from the lack of knowledge of the existing social help. On the other hand, despite sufficient financial income, some elderly subjects are left short of funds because they spend a large part of their income on their families.

3.1.2.2 Diminished Capacities

Insufficient physical capacities that have the most important effects on food intake are:

- Reduced chewing capacity, whether related to dentition, jaw, or unfit dentures
- Dysphagia, mainly due to strokes and degenerative cerebral pathologies [5]
- Walking difficulties, responsible for a making shopping or visiting a restaurant more challenging

In institutions, autonomy losses make the elderly subject totally dependent on the quality and quantity of nursing care. The lack of dietitians, the lack of nutritional knowledge, the excessive standardization of menus, the short duration of mealtime, the lack of conviviality and non-adapted timetables all contribute to undernutrition.

Cognitive deteriorations may lead to insufficient food or the substitution of "junk food" instead of healthy meals [6]. Such deterioration can worsen self-prescribed diets, which are often responsible for unbalanced intake. Subjects with dementia rarely have insufficient food, except when their needs have considerably increased, as with patients who wander ceaselessly, thus using more calories but finding it impossible to sit down to a meal. Restoration of lunch as a social activity (by involving the elder in helping in its preparation, by setting the table, or by increasing the length of time allotted to meal time) increases food intake in demented subjects by restoring memories of more convivial mealtimes [7].

3.1.2.3 Preconceived Ideas

Preconceived ideas about food and ignorance of nutritional needs are widespread, and elderly people or their circles of friends and family or the nursing care of an institution often enhance this ignorance [1].

3.1.2.4 Digestive Diseases

Digestive diseases, as in younger adults, can cause undernutrition. Oral and esophageal candidiasis, which occurs more frequent in the elderly because of the reduction in salivary outflow, may cause burns during food ingestion [8]. First among various digestive diseases (cancers, atrophic gastritis, etc.), are gastric ulcers, which are often responsible for symptoms such as anorexia, distaste for meat, or dyspepsia, but these symptoms' lack of specificity sometimes leads to delayed diagnosis and treatment.

3.1.2.5 Dietary and Therapeutic Mistakes

Long-term weight-loss diets are dangerous because their effect can be multiplied when elderly subjects are very respectful of their medical prescriptions. A diet, if necessary, must always be limited in the length of time it is observed. Examples of abusive diets are numerous [9,10]:

- A low-calorie diet aiming for weight loss before the installation of a prosthesis can worsen sarcopenia.
- A strict salt-free diet can worsen anorexia when its duration goes beyond the necessary, i.e., a phase of acute heart failure.
- Fiber-free diet for irritable bowel syndrome.
- When the diet is not prescribed by a doctor, the subject may impose it on himself.

Hospitalization is itself often a cause of undernutrition; apart from the illness that caused the admission, the hospital's food is too rarely appetizing.

Abundant consumption of medications at the beginning of meals is a cause of anorexia, as is alcohol consumption. Many drugs modify either the taste or the moisture inside the mouth.

3.1.2.6 Depression

Depression is frequent in geriatric patients and is almost constant in institutions. Causes of depression are very numerous: a sense of uselessness, difficulty in accepting the diminution of capacities (physical or intellectual), isolation, loss of a spouse, etc. Food consumption can be regulated only when the depression is cured.

3.1.3 HYPERMETABOLISM/HYPERCATABOLISM

An increase in nutritional needs constitutes the other part of the causes of undernutrition. Diseases in subjects weakened by low food intake induce a state of true undernutrition. Hypermetabolism is activated for every illness, whether it is an infection (lymphocytes), tissue destruction as in a myocardial infarction or a stroke (phagocytes) or tissue mending as it happens for fractures or pressure sores. The intensity and the duration of this hypermetabolism and hypercatabolism depend upon the size of tissue lesions and the speed of healing. Whatever the mechanisms of activation, there will be hyperstimulation of the macrophages and monocytes. Causes of hypermetabolism and hypercatabolism are infections, cancers and, in a more general way, every chronic or acute inflammatory condition (rheumatisms, pressure sores, etc.). Some organ deficiencies (heart or respiratory failures) increase energy expenditure.

3.2 CONSEQUENCES OF UNDERNUTRITION

Undernutrition has multiple and varied consequences, which makes it a very serious condition. It is important to recognize and prevent these, as they are not always foreseeable [10].

3.2.1 INCREASE IN MORBIDITY AND MORTALITY

Undernutrition increases the infectious morbidity in institutionalized elderly subjects from two to six times, multiplying the risk of mortality over 1 year by 4-fold during a hospitalization after the age of 80 [11]. In elderly subjects who are apparently in good condition otherwise, 5-year death probability is ten times higher if they are undernourished (albumin < 35 g/L).

3.2.2 ALTERATIONS IN THE GENERAL CONDITION

Undernutrition leads to an alteration of the general condition, which causes the following symptoms:

- Constant weight loss [12] resulting from a loss of body fat mass and lean mass, especially of the muscle mass (sarcopenia). Muscular hypercatabolism due to undernutrition creates in the elderly subject a very quick depletion of the protein stores already diminished because of aging and the more sedentary lifestyle.
- Asthenia and anorexia, the norm during undernutrition [13,14], contribute to a worsening of the nutritional status.
- During hypercatabolism (acute pathology), if not properly treated in a short time by adding a nutritional support, the patient then enters a vicious cycle [1] :
  - Hypercatabolism → undernutrition → immune deficiencies → new disease = new, more extended hypercatabolism → more serious undernutrition → immune deficiencies → new pathology → new, more extended hypercatabolism → even more serious undernutrition → etc. The consequence of this sequence is quite often the death of the patient.

Psychological disorders, ranging from simple apathy to depressive syndromes are frequent. At any level, they can be serious, and they can also simulate authentic dementia [1, 9].

Body protein (muscles) and fat stores are already diminished in elderly subjects. During an acute episode, in order to provide an appropriate response, the elderly subject must draw upon already diminished stores. The patient thus enters a negative spiral likely to jeopardize vital prognosis if he or she is not fed—the longer the sickness, the greater the consequences to the nutritional stores. Furthermore, after an acute episode, the body never completely reconstitutes the lost stores; the elderly subject will not completely recover his or her previous weight, contrary to what a younger adult can do. The convalescence period, which permits one to reconstitute the lost stores, is longer (three to four times the duration of the acute illness) and less effective for the elderly subject.

3.2.2 Immune Deficiency

Undernutrition induces a dysfunction of the immune system, with consequences such as lymphopenia ($<1,200/mm^3$). Every aspect of immunity is affected—cellular immunity, function of T lymphocytes, humoral immunity, function of B lymphocytes, and nonspecific immunity.

Undernutrition worsens the physiological immune deficiency due to aging and leads to a true acquired immune deficiency in the undernourished elderly, which weakens defense mechanisms and induces infections [15]. If an infection occurs, it worsens undernutrition by the anorexia it brings on and by hypermetabolism and hypercatabolism. The elderly subject affected by undernutrition will hence draw upon muscular protein stores to fight against the infection. If infection occurs, it will have, in most cases, a nosocomial origin—originating while under medical care—and will be more difficult to cure [16].

3.2.3 Digestive Disorders

The slowing down of intestinal peristalsis induces a digestive stasis that results in the creation of a fecal impaction that increases the risks of infection through microbial overgrowth. Diarrhea is frequent and can coexist with the fecal impaction (fake diarrhea). This is a serious symptom that can also appear during the first stages of refeeding. Undernutrition also contributes to the onset of pressure sores and their persistence [17,18].

3.2.4 Food–Drug Interactions and Toxicity

Drugs often influence nutrient metabolism through their effects on nutrient intake, absorption, metabolism, and excretion. In addition to these effects, food itself or specific constituents in food and beverages, as well as vitamins, minerals, and other dietary supplements, can influence drug kinetics. Worsening of sarcopenia promotes falls and can have effects on general mobility, thus lessening one's autonomy.

3.2.4 Consequences of Micronutrient Deficiencies

The deficiency in micronutrients (vitamins and trace elements) may be isolated, but undernutrition always accompanies a micronutrient deficiency. The deficiencies in B vitamins (especially folate) can be the source of asthenia, of psychological disorders—even encephalopathy—neurological disorders (polyneuritis), anemia, and immune deficiency (folate, B6, vitamin D, etc.). Such deficiencies increase the risk for an earlier onset (or relapse) of cardiovascular diseases or cognitive disorders such as Alzheimer-like dementia.

Deficiencies in vitamin D and calcium worsen osteoporosis, which can be made more complex by fractures. Deficiency in zinc leads to a loss of taste and thus contributes to the maintenance of anorexia. The deficiency in zinc also induces an immune deficiency and some skin disorders, as well as delayed wound healing.

Economic and social consequences are quite significant. For a given disease, the length of hospitalization is multiplied by a factor of two to four in an undernourished subject. Undernutrition brings higher morbidity and death rates, with an increase in drug consumption and with an evolution toward loss of autonomy, which can be the reason for institutionalization [19].

3.3 DIAGNOSIS OF UNDERNUTRITION

3.3.1 MEDICAL HISTORY

The single most important clinical aspect is weight loss, which should be expressed in actual weight or in percent of the patient's usual weight. Furthermore, the interval since the weight loss started should be explored. The patient should be asked whether a loss of appetite is present, but, with regard to prognosis, it is not relevant whether the patient declares the weight loss to be voluntary or involuntary. Often it is helpful to question the patient about restrictive diets and consumption of alcohol or tobacco. Concomitant illnesses and the accompanying medications, including possible side effects, have to be taken into account. Here special attention should be paid to depression, dementia and dysphagia.

Since functionality in the elderly is closely correlated with nutritional status, it is usually advisable to determine their basic and instrumental activities of daily living (ADLs and IADLs) [20]. Finally, as isolation and poverty often become more frequent as one ages, some information about the living conditions and the social relationships of the patient have to be obtained.

3.3.2 CLINICAL SIGNS OF UNDERNUTRITION

The attending nurse or physician must pay attention to physical signs of overt undernutrition. The most prominent are muscle atrophy, loss of subcutaneous fat, and peripheral edema as a consequence of hypoprotidemia. Micronutrient deficiencies can cause a wide range of symptoms that may affect the skin, the mucous membranes, the central and peripheral nervous system, the eyes, and other organs as well.

Low intake of energy and different nutrients is an important aid to find out which patient is at risk of undernutrition [14]. The 7-day diary and the 24-hour recall strongly depend upon the cooperation of the patient and often are inappropriate when memory loss is present. It seems therefore to be more appropriate, especially in institutions, to use eating protocols where intake is documented by estimating it via meals served. These eating protocols should be filled in for at least three days in a row.

Anthropometric measurements are an essential part of the nutritional assessment in the elderly [21]. They comprise the determination of body height, body weight, circumference of upper arm and calf, and the measurement of the triceps skinfold.

A mobile patient should be weighed post-voiding, standing on a well-calibrated scale wearing light clothing and without shoes. If the patient is immobile, a chair scale or a lifting scale, depending on the amount of his or her disability, has to be used. When assessing the body weight, special conditions like edema and ascites have to be taken into account. The significance of an individual's weight course always exceeds that of a single measurement.

With regard to height, the measurement of the knee height and the calculation of the original body height are helpful in immobile patients and in those with kyphosis [22].

Generally, the body-mass index reflects body composition in the elderly with regard to body fat and lean body mass to a lesser degree than in a younger population. The cut-off for undernutrition for adults below age 65 has been set at 18.5 kg/m², while for prognostic reasons in the elderly the threshold is usually set between 20 and 22 kg/m² [10,23]. For example, French societies have set the cut-off for undernutrition at 21 and for severe malnutrition at 18 [9].

Because of its relevance with regard to functionality, a parameter reflecting muscle status in the aged will be particularly useful. Calf circumference proved to be superior to upper arm circumference. The former shows a good correlation with other nutritional anthropometric markers (BMI, free fat mass, triceps skin fold) and mobility [24,25]. The cut-off for calf circumference is set at 31 cm.

3.3.3 BIOLOGICAL SIGNS OF UNDERNUTRITION

The most widely used laboratory parameter to assess the nutritional status is serum albumin. Its strong association with prognosis has been documented in different populations [26]. However, its serum level may be influenced by a wide variety of acute and chronic inflammatory conditions. In addition, aging *per se* as well as hepatic and renal dysfunction can cause decreases of the serum level. Another disadvantage is its long half-life of 21 days. As a result, low serum albumin levels in hospital patients are rarely the consequence of a poor nutritional status. On the whole, serum albumin shows a low specificity with regard to undernutrition.

Alternative parameters are transferrin, transthyretin, retinol-binding protein, and insulin growth factor-1. Their half-lives are shorter, but their specificity is only marginally improved. Furthermore, their routine use will clearly increase laboratory costs.

Additional examinations such as measurement of micronutrients should not be part of routine practice and should be ordered only when suspicion of specific deficits exists.

On the whole, laboratory examinations are not an essential component of the diagnostic instruments with regard to undernutrition in the elderly. Furthermore, a recent study showed that weight loss and anthropometric data exhibited a stronger correlation with live threatening complications of geriatric hospital patients than albumin and transthyretin [27].

Bioelectrical impedance analysis and dual-energy x-ray analysis measurements are interesting fields of ongoing research in body composition in the elderly but at present they don't have to be part of the daily routine.

3.3.4 SCREENING AND ASSESSMENT TOOLS

Effective tools for screening and assessing the nutritional status of the elderly are certainly needed. In addition, an intervention plan should be based on the results of the screening tool. All elderly above age 65 should be screened routinely once a year [10]. Because of limited financial and personal resources within all European health care systems the screening procedure has to be quick with acceptable sensitivity and specificity. The amount of time necessary for screening should not exceed 5 minutes. Along with existing indexes (MUST, NRS, NRI) used in adults, there are few geriatric indexes available. The one worth mentioning is the Mini Nutritional Assessment.

The short form of the Mini Nutritional Assessment (MNA-SF) fulfils at least some of these expectations. It was derived from the original version of the MNA by identifying six items that strongly correlated with the conventional nutritional assessment of experienced physicians [28] (Table 3.2). If the score is 11 or less the patient is classified as at risk of undernutrition and the full MNA has to be done (see http://mna-elderly.com). The sensitivity of the MNA short form with regard to overt undernutrition has been successfully tested [29]. It has been designed especially for the nutritional screening in the community setting, while an nutritional assessment using the original "long" MNA should be the first step in nursing and hospital patients because of the high prevalence of undernutrition in these institutions.

According to the result of the assessment the patient is categorized as well nourished, at risk, or overt undernutrition. In a multitude of studies it has been shown that the MNA correlates well with nutritional intake, anthropometry, laboratory data, functionality, morbidity, length of hospital stay, and mortality [30,31] (Figure 3.1).

TABLE 3.2

Mini Nutritional Assessment—Short Form

A   Has food intake declined over the past 3 months, due to loss of appetite, digestive problems, chewing or swallowing difficulties?

    0. = severe loss of appetite

    1. = moderate loss of appetite

    2. = no loss of appetite

B   Weight loss during last 3 months?

    0. = weight loss greater than 3 kg

    1. = does not know

    2. = weight loss between 1 and 3 kg

    3. = no weight loss

C   Mobility

    0. = bed or chair bound

    1. = able to get out of bed/chair but does not go out

    2. = goes out

D   Has suffered psychological distress or acute disease in the past 3 months?

    0. = yes

    2. = no

E   Neuropsychological problems?

    0. = severe dementia or depression

    1. = mild dementia

    2. = no psychological problems

F   BMI

    0. = BMI less than 19

    1. = BMI 19 to less than 21

    2. = BMI 21 to less than 23

    3. = BMI 23 or greater

Source: Adapted with permission from Société des Produits Nestlé, Vevey, Switzerland.

3.4 TREATMENT OF UNDERNUTRITION

In most instances a symptomatic therapy concentrating on nutritional intake will not be successful if treatable pathologic causes are ignored. This may apply to oral problems, depression, gastrointestinal disorders, or endocrinology abnormalities. In every patient where undernutrition is diagnosed or where a person is considered to be at risk, the treating physician must start a diagnostic work-up that searches for organic or psychological causes. In addition, this may be paralleled by the introduction of a nutritional intervention, as the sooner it is introduced, the better the outcome.

3.4.1 STRATEGY

Nutritional support will mostly depend on two factors: spontaneous food intake and nutritional status (Table 3.3). In all cases, nutritional support aims at providing 30–40 kcal/kg/day and 1.2–1.5 g protein/kg/day [9].

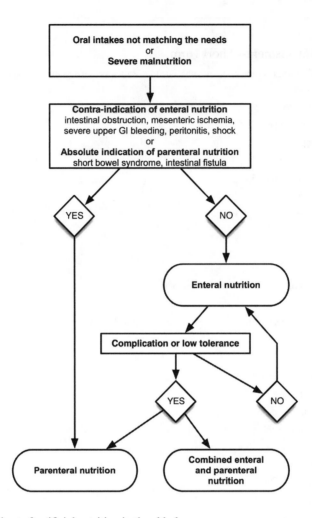

FIGURE 3.1 Flow chart of artificial nutrition in the elderly.

3.4.2 DIETARY COUNSELING

The first measure to start treatment of undernutrition, especially in the outpatient setting, may be dietary counseling, which will be most effective if undertaken by a qualified dietitian, whose involvement certainly depends on the local resources and the possibility of reimbursement. Unfortunately, no studies have addressed the isolated effects of dietary counseling in the elderly. Nevertheless, the positive impact of individualized care by a dietitian was shown by a recent study for patients with dementia in a long-term care facility [32]. In this population weight loss could be prevented or weight could be increased in the intervention group.

3.4.3 FOOD FORTIFICATION

After counseling a patient about optimizing his or her diet, the next step may be dietary fortification, which usually concentrates on increasing energy and protein intake. This may be achieved by increasing the use of energy- and protein-rich food by including oil, cream, butter, sugar, high-fat milk, powdered milk and cheese in the daily diet. As an alternative, there is the option to add carbohydrates, lipids, or protein via commercial powders or liquids to the diet. A wide range of products is available. Most are without a specific recognizable flavor and can be stirred into milk, yogurt, soups, or sauces. The very few controlled trials available show that the oral intake of energy but not

TABLE 3.3
Nutritional Support Strategy in the Elderly

	Nutritional Status		
	Normal	**Undernutrition**	**Severe Undernutrition**
	Spontaneous Oral Intake		
Normal	Follow-up	Dietary advice Food fortification 1-month reassessment	Dietary advice Food fortification + ONS 2-week reassessment
Decreased, but > 50% of normal intake	Dietary advice Food fortification 1-month reassessment	Dietary advice Food fortification 2-week reassessment, and if failure: ONS	Dietary advice Food fortification + ONS 1-week reassessment, and if failure: EN
Decreased, < 50% of normal intake	Dietary advice Food fortification 1-week reassessment, and if failure: ONS	Dietary advice Food fortification + ONS 1-week reassessment, and if failure: EN	Dietary advice EN 1-week reassessment

EN = enteral nutrition; ONS = oral nutritional supplements
Source: Adapted with permission from Société des Produits Nestlé, Vevey, Switzerland.

of protein may be increased [33]. Dietary fortification is one useful means of treating undernutrition but its effectiveness has not yet been sufficiently proven.

Snacks, sweet or spicy, may occasionally be practical adjuncts to conventional nutritional therapy [34]. In particular, finger food is reportedly well accepted by the demented.

3.4.4 ORAL NUTRITIONAL SUPPLEMENTS

A recent meta-analysis [35] showed reduced mortality and fewer complications for hospital patients who were undernourished and who were treated with supplements. The best results with regard to mortality were obtained for those above age 75, those provided with a supplemental intake over 400 kcal/day, those in poor general condition, and those who were undernourished. There also was a trend toward a reduced length of stay in hospital for the intervention group. Results with regard to functional parameters were so diverse that no clear statement could be made, but several studies showed improvements.

According to the recently published European Society for Clinical Nutrition and Metabolism (ESPEN) guidelines for enteral nutrition in geriatric patients, oral supplementation increases energy and nutrient intake [36], and can maintain or improve nutritional status. Oral nutritional supplements are indicated for elderly patients with undernutrition and for those who are at risk. They should be given early when there is proof of insufficient intake, of weight loss above 5% in 3 months or above 10% in 6 months, or when the body mass index (BMI) is calculated below 22 kg/m². They are also indicated for the frail elderly to maintain their nutritional status.

For most patients, supplementation will be prescribed for 1 or 2 months, and prescription will be extended after a positive effect has been documented. Acceptance of supplementation by the patient may become a problem, therefore the intervention has to be explained and the patient motivated if possible. Supplements should be given between meals and occasionally before bedtime. Otherwise, they can reduce intake during regular meals. The consumption of each supplement should not take more than 30 minutes and it should ideally be controlled and documented by the nursing staff. To improve acceptance it may be advisable to change the consistency of the product—ice in the summer, foam if found attractive—and to respect the preferences of the patients with regard to available flavors.

For most supplements, one ml equals one kcal. Hypercaloric drinks (1.5–2 kcal/ml) are available and may prove useful under certain circumstances. Furthermore, supplements with high protein content may be indicated for severely hypoprotidemic patients. A realistic goal for the amount of calories consumed via nutritional supplements could be set at 400 kcal/day. If the acceptance is good this may be adapted to 600 kcal/day. Enteral nutrition (EN) should always be considered first in a patient with a functioning gastrointestinal tract [37], and parenteral nutrition should be considered only when PN is contraindicated or not tolerated (Figure 3.1). As enteral nutrition is often prolonged due to persistent anorexia or dysphagia, percutaneous endoscopic gastrostomy will often be the route of choice for artificial nutrition in the elderly. Percutaneous endoscopic gastrostomy (PEG) tubes will not be needed in house-ridden or institutionalized elderly patients. EN may be delivered as continuous or cyclical, with similar nutritional results [38,39]. However, only cyclical nocturnal nutrition may allow the patient to have physical activity during the daytime and to eat normally at meal times.

There is no evidence in favor of a specific formula in the elderly. Elemental or semi-elemental formulas are not preferable to polymeric ones. Last, fiber supplementation can improve bowel function with reduced stool frequency and more solid stool consistency without affecting the nutritional efficiency of enteral feeding in hospitalized geriatric patients [40].

3.4.5 Outcomes

Life expectancy under nutritional support is lower in elderly patients than in younger ones [41]. This is true for survival in home EN patients [42] and after percutaneous endoscopic gastrostomy, where age is an independent factor associated with complications and mortality [43].

There is a resistance to refeeding in the elderly because, for the same amount of nitrogen and energy provided by EN, the increase in weight, fat-free mass, and chronic phase proteins is lower in elderly patients than in younger adults [38, 44]. When an extra 7,500 kcal are needed to gain one kg of body weight in young undernourished patients, 8,800 to 22,600 kcal are needed in elderly patients [45]. Chronic inflammation [46] as well as a higher splanchnic extraction [47] of proteins might be responsible. Many tube-fed patients are bedridden, and the consequent immobility further enhances muscle wasting and prevents gain in lean mass. Health-related quality of life is lower in elderly home enteral patients compared with younger patients [48]. The former achieve a lower rehabilitation than their younger counterparts [49].

3.4.6 Clinical Conditions

Even though the same diseases leading to nutritional support can be found throughout the lifespan, there are differences in indications in elderly patients [49]. For example, hip fracture is a common condition in the elderly. A Cochrane analysis that includes four trials testing supplementary overnight enteral nutrition failed to show benefits on survival, but these studies were heterogeneous [50]. Bastow et al. have shown a benefit of EN on anthropometric measurements and on a reduction of rehabilitation time and hospital stay in the most undernourished patients [51] .

In neurological dysphagia, nutritional therapy depends on the type and extent of the swallowing disorder. Nutritional therapy may range from normal food to mushy meals (modified consistency), thickened liquids of different consistencies, or total EN delivered via nasogastric or gastrostomy tube. In a Cochrane analysis of interventions for dysphagia in acute stroke, enteral nutrition delivered via gastrostomy tube was associated with a greater improvement of nutritional status when compared with that delivered via nasogastric tube [52]. As dysphagia will rarely improve after 2 weeks, if severe dysphagia persists longer than 14 days after the acute event, a gastrostomy tube should be placed immediately [36].

An indequate intake of energy and nutrients is a common problem in demented patients. Under-nutrition may be caused by several factors including anorexia (common cause: polypharmaco therapy), insufficient oral intake (forgetting to eat), depression, apraxia of eating or, less often, enhanced energy requirement due to hyperactivity (constant pacing) [36]. In advanced stages of dementia, dysphagia may develop and might be an indication for EN in a few cases. Most studies, with a small level of evidence, have showed a worse outcome in enterally fed demented patients or demented patients receiving gastrostomy, compared with either the absence of intervention in demented patients [42] or the same interventions in non-demented patients [43,53]. Enteral nutrition may be recommended at early stages of the disease, or after an acute weight loss in patients with Alzheimer's disease [7]. However, for patients with terminal dementia (irreversible, immobile, unable to communicate, completely dependent, lack of physical resources) EN is not recommended (grade of recommendation C) [36].

3.4.6.1 Pressure Sores

Pressure ulcers are associated with an increased risk of morbidity and mortality. A systematic review by Stratton et al. shows that enteral nutritional support, particularly high protein supplements, can significantly reduce the risk of developing pressure ulcers (by 25%). However, available studies on the effect of EN do not show improved healing of decubitus ulcers [18]. The importance of protein in pressure sore healing was suggested in an 8-week non-randomized study in 28 undernourished nursing home residents with decubitus ulcers [54]. The administration of a formula with 61 g protein per liter (24 energy percent) was more successful in decreasing total pressure ulcer surface area than a TF formula with 37 g protein per liter (14 energy percent).

3.4.7 ETHICAL ISSUES

Ethical issues are crucial when deciding whether to start an elderly patient on artificial nutrition. Public controversy about life-sustaining technologies for elderly people now focuses on decisions about withholding or withdrawal of tube feeding, but debate about the legal and ethical issues involved in these decisions tends to obscure the relevant clinical considerations [55]. The patient's informed consent needs to be obtained, with family or a caregiver as possible surrogates. Sedation of the patient for acceptance of the nutritional treatment is never justified. Proposing percutaneous endoscopic gastrostomy because the patient takes too long to feed is also unacceptable.

REFERENCES

1. Ferry, M., Alix, E., Brocker, P., Constans, T., Lesourd, B., Mischlich, D., Pfitzenmeyer, P. and Vellas, B. 2007. *Nutrition de la personne agée*. [Malnutrition in the elderly]. Masson, Paris.
2. Bellisle, F. 1996. The "taste of" and "the taste for" in the elderly subjects. *Cah Nutr Diet* 31, 171–176.
3. Dormenval, V., Mojon, P. and Budtz-Jorgensen, E. 1999. Associations between self-assessed masticatory ability, nutritional status, prosthetic status and salivary flow rate in hospitalized elders. *Oral Dis* 5, 32–38.
4. Hendy, H. M., Nelson, G. K. and Greco, M. E. 1998. Social cognitive predictors of nutritional risk in rural elderly adults. *Int J Aging Hum Dev* 47, 299–327.
5. Finiels, H., Strubel, D. and Jacquot, J. M. 2001. Deglutition disorders in the elderly. Epidemiological aspects. *Presse Med* 30, 1623–1634.
6. Faxen-Irving, G., Basun, H. and Cederholm, T. 2005. Nutritional and cognitive relationships and long–term mortality in patients with various dementia disorders. *Age Ageing* 34, 136–141.
7. Guérin, O., Andrieu, S., Schneider, S. M., Milano, M., Boulahssass, R., Brocker, P. and Vellas, B. 2005. Different modes of weight loss in Alzheimer disease: A prospective study of 395 patients. *Am J Clin Nutr* 82, 435–441.
8. Brocker, P., Bourée, P., de Rekeneire, N., Maugourd, M. F., Périllat, A. and Moulias, R. 2000. Prevalence of oropharyngeal candidiasis in the elderly: A French multicentric study. In *Année Gérontologique*, pp. 133–150, Serdi, Paris.
9. HAS 2007. Stratégie de prise en charge en cas de dénutrition protéino-énergétique chez la personne âgée. Paris.

10. Raynaud, A., Revel-Delhom, C., Alexandre, D., Alix, E., Ancellin, R., Bouteloup, C., Brocker, P., Cha-piro, S., Dumarcet, N., Haslé, A., Lecocq, J. M., Lefèvre, M. P., l'Hermine, A., Lurcel, J., Ménivard, N., Perette, M. A., Perrin, A. M. and Hébuterne, X. 2007. Management strategies of protein-energy malnutrition in the elderly. *Nutr Clin Metabol* 21, 120–133.
11. Vetta, F., Ronzoni, S., Taglieri, G. and Bollea, M. R. 1999. The impact of malnutrition on the quality of life in the elderly. *Clin Nutr* 18, 259–267.
12. Blaum, C. S., Fries, B. E. and Fiatarone, M. A. 1995. Factors associated with low body mass index and weight loss in nursing home residents. *J Gerontol A Biol Sci Med Sci* 50, M162–168.
13. Brocker, P. 1998. Anorexia in elderly subjects. *Rev Geriatrie* 23, 165–169.
14. Morley, J. E. 1997. Anorexia of aging: Physiologic and pathologic. *Am J Clin Nutr* 66, 760–773.
15. Moulias, S. 2002. Nutrition and immunity in the elderly. *Ann Med Interne Paris*. 153, 446–449
16. Paillaud, E., Herbaud, S., Caillet, P., Lejonc, J. L., Campillo, B. and Bories, P. N. 2005. Relations between undernutrition and nosocomial infections in elderly patients. *Age Ageing* 34, 619–625.
17. Bonnefoy, M., Coulon, L., Bienvenu, J., Boisson, R. C. and Rys, L. 1995. Implication of cytokines in the aggravation of malnutrition and hypercatabolism in elderly patients with severe pressure sores. *Age Ageing* 24, 37–42.
18. Stratton, R. J., Ek, A. C., Engfer, M., Moore, Z., Rigby, P., Wolfe, R. and Elia, M. 2005. Enteral nutri-tional support in prevention and treatment of pressure ulcers: A systematic review and meta-analysis. *Ageing Res Rev* 4, 422–450.
19. Amarantos, E., Martinez, A. and Dwyer, J. 2001. Nutrition and quality of life in older adults. *J Gerontol A Biol Sci Med Sci* 56 Spec No 2, 54–64.
20. Katz, S., Ford, A. B., Moskowitz, R. W., Jackson, B. A. and Jaffe, M. W. 1963. Studies of illness in the aged. The index of ADL: A standardized measure of biological and psychosocial function. *JAMA* 185, 914–919.
21. Omran, M. L. and Salem, P. 2002. Diagnosing undernutrition. *Clin Geriatr Med* 18, 719–736.
22. Chumlea, W. C. and Guo, S. 1992. Equations for predicting stature in white and black elderly individu-als. *J Gerontol* 47, M197–203.
23. Flodin, L., Svensson, S. and Cederholm, T. 2000. Body mass index as a predictor of 1 year mortality in geriatric patients. *Clin Nutr* 19, 121–125.
24. Bonnefoy, M., Jauffret, M., Kostka, T. and Jusot, J. F. 2002. Usefulness of calf circumference measure-ment in assessing the nutritional state of hospitalized elderly people. *Gerontology* 48, 162–169.
25. Rolland, Y., Lauwers-Cances, V., Cournot, M., Nourhashemi, F., Reynish, W., Riviere, D., Vellas, B. and Grandjean, H. 2003. Sarcopenia, calf circumference, and physical function of elderly women: A cross-sectional study. *J Am Geriatr Soc* 51, 1120–1124.
26. Corti, M. C., Guralnik, J. M., Salive, M. E. and Sorkin, J. D. 1994. Serum albumin level and physical disability as predictors of mortality in older persons. *JAMA* 272, 1036–1042.
27. Sullivan, D. H., Bopp, M. M. and Roberson, P. K. 2002. Protein-energy undernutrition and life-threat-ening complications among the hospitalized elderly. *J Gen Intern Med* 17, 923–932.
28. Rubenstein, L. Z., Harker, J. O., Salva, A., Guigoz, Y. and Vellas, B. 2001. Screening for undernutrition in geriatric practice: Developing the short-form mini-nutritional assessment MNA-SF. *J Gerontol A Biol Sci Med Sci* 56, M366–372.
29. Cohendy, R., Rubenstein, L. Z. and Eledjam, J. J. 2001. The Mini Nutritional Assessment-Short Form for preoperative nutritional evaluation of elderly patients. *Aging Milano.* 13, 293–297.
30. Bauer, J. M., Vogl, T., Wicklein, S., Trogner, J., Muhlberg, W. and Sieber, C. C. 2005. Comparison of the Mini Nutritional Assessment, Subjective Global Assessment, and Nutritional Risk Screening NRS 2002. for nutritional screening and assessment in geriatric hospital patients. *Z Gerontol Geriatr* 38, 322–327.
31. Guigoz, Y., Lauque, S. and Vellas, B. J. 2002. Identifying the elderly at risk for malnutrition. The Mini Nutritional Assessment. *Clin Geriatr Med* 18, 737–757.
32. Keller, H. H., Gibbs, A. J., Boudreau, L. D., Goy, R. E., Pattillo, M. S. and Brown, H. M. 2003. Pre-vention of weight loss in dementia with comprehensive nutritional treatment. *J Am Geriatr Soc* 51, 945–952.
33. Odlund Olin, A., Armyr, I., Soop, M., Jerstrom, S., Classon, I., Cederholm, T., Ljungren, G. and Ljungqvist, O. 2003. Energy-dense meals improve energy intake in elderly residents in a nursing home. *Clin Nutr* 22, 125–131.

34. Turic, A., Gordon, K. L., Craig, L. D., Ataya, D. G. and Voss, A. C. 1998. Nutrition supplementation enables elderly residents of long-term-care facilities to meet or exceed RDAs without displacing energy or nutrient intakes from meals. *J Am Diet Assoc* 98, 1457–1459.
35. Milne, A. C., Avenell, A. and Potter, J. 2006. Meta-analysis: Protein and energy supplementation in older people. *Ann Intern Med* 144, 37–48.
36. Volkert, D., Berner, Y. N., Berry, E., Cederholm, T., Coti Bertrand, P., Milne, A., Palmblad, J., Schneider, S., Sobotka, L., Stanga, Z., Lenzen-Grossimlinghaus, R., Krys, U., Pirlich, M., Herbst, B., Schutz, T., Schroer, W., Weinrebe, W., Ockenga, J. and Lochs, H. 2006. ESPEN Guidelines on Enteral Nutrition: Geriatrics. *Clin Nutr* 25, 330–359.
37. Zaloga, G. P. 2006. Parenteral nutrition in adult inpatients with functioning gastrointestinal tracts: assessment of outcomes. *Lancet* 367, 1101–1111.
38. Hébuterne, X., Broussard, J. F. and Rampal, P. 1995. Acute renutrition by cyclic enteral nutrition in elderly and younger patients. *JAMA* 273, 638–643.
39. Ciocon, J. O., Galindo-Ciocon, D. J., Tiessen, C. and Galindo, D. 1992. Continuous compared with intermittent tube feeding in the elderly. *JPEN* 16, 525–528.
40. Vandewoude, M. F., Paridaens, K. M., Suy, R. A., Boone, M. A. and Strobbe, H. 2005. Fibre-supplemented tube feeding in the hospitalised elderly. *Age Ageing* 34, 120–124.
41. Mitchell, S. L. and Tetroe, J. M. 2000. Survival after percutaneous endoscopic gastrostomy placement in older persons. *J Gerontol A Biol Sci Med Sci* 55, M735–739.
42. Schneider, S. M., Raina, C., Pugliese, P., Pouget, I., Rampal, P. and Hébuterne, X. 2001. Outcome of patients treated with home enteral nutrition. *JPEN* 25, 203–209.
43. Shah, P. M., Sen, S., Perlmuter, L. C. and Feller, A. 2005. Survival after percutaneous endoscopic gastrostomy: The role of dementia. *J Nutr Health Aging* 9, 255–259.
44. Hébuterne, X., Schneider, S., Péroux, J. and Rampal, P. 1997. Effects of refeeding by cyclic enteral nutrition on body composition: Comparative study of elderly and younger patients. *Clin Nutr* 16, 283–289.
45. Hébuterne, X., Bermon, S. and Schneider, S. M. 2001. Ageing and muscle: The effects of malnutrition, re–nutrition, and physical exercise. *Curr Opin Clin Nutr Metab Care* 4, 295–300.
46. Roubenoff, R., Harris, T. B., Abad, L. W., Wilson, P. W., Dallal, G. E. and Dinarello, C. A. 1998. Monocyte cytokine production in an elderly population: Effect of age and inflammation. *J Gerontol A Biol Sci Med Sci* 53, M20–26.
47. Boirie, Y., Gachon, P. and Beaufrere, B. 1997. Splanchnic and whole-body leucine kinetics in young and elderly men. *Am J Clin Nutr* 65, 489–495.
48. Schneider, S. M., Pouget, I., Staccini, P., Rampal, P. and Hébuterne, X. 2000. Quality of life in long-term home enteral nutrition patients. *Clin Nutr* 19, 23–28.
49. Howard, L. and Malone, M. 1997. Clinical outcome of geriatric patients in the United States receiving home parenteral and enteral nutrition. *Am J Clin Nutr* 66, 1364–1370.
50. Avery, A. J., Groom, L. M., Brown, K. P., Thornhill, K. and Boot, D. 1999. The impact of nursing home patients on prescribing costs in general practice. *J Clin Pharm Ther* 24, 357–363.
51. Bastow, M. D., Rawlings, J. and Allison, S. P. 1983. Benefits of supplementary tube feeding after fractured neck of femur: A randomised controlled trial. *Br Med J Clin Res Ed.* 287, 1589–1592.
52. Bath, P. M., Bath, F. J. and Smithard, D. G. 2000. Interventions for dysphagia in acute stroke. *Cochrane Database Syst Rev*, CD000323.
53. Mitchell, S. L., Kiely, D. K. and Lipsitz, L. A. 1997. The risk factors and impact on survival of feeding tube placement in nursing home residents with severe cognitive impairment. *Arch Intern Med* 157, 327–332.
54. Breslow, R. A., Hallfrisch, J., Guy, D. G., Crawley, B. and Goldberg, A. P. 1993. The importance of dietary protein in healing pressure ulcers. *J Am Geriatr Soc* 41, 357–362.
55. Maslow, K. 1988. Total parenteral nutrition and tube feeding for elderly patients: Findings of an OTA study. *JPEN* 12, 425–432.

Section II

Nutrition and Promotion of Health

4 Nutrition and the Geriatric Surgery Patient

Sheldon Winkler, Meredith C. Bogert, and Charles K. Herman

CONTENTS

4.1   INTRODUCTION

The geriatric patient who requires surgical treatment presents a number of problems not encountered in younger patients, the majority of which are the result of the changes that occur with aging
or with poor nutrition. Surgical morbidity, postoperative healing, and the patient's return to function
may be improved through the application of knowledge of the physical, metabolic, and endocrine
changes associated with aging, as well as of the nutritional deficiencies common among this cohort
of patients [1].

4.2   EFFECTS OF SURGERY ON THE BODY

Any stress, including that from a surgical procedure, causes a dramatic release of ACTH from the
anterior pituitary that, in turn, directs the release of cortisol from the adrenal cortex. The circulating
cortisol level remains elevated by a factor of 2 to 5 times normal for about 24 hours after the procedure [2] and acts upon skeletal tissue to bring about breakdown of skeletal muscle tissue proteins
into amino acids for localized wound healing and for glucose production by the liver.

Concomitantly, epinephrine and norepinephrine are released and remain elevated for up to 48
hours, stimulating breakdown of liver glycogen with release of glucose for cellular energy needs
during the immediate postoperative period [3]. The increase in epinephrine suppresses release of
insulin [4], glucagon concentrations rise [5], and the liver is stimulated to begin gluconeogenesis to
return to preoperative levels and to support the energy requirements of the healing process.

Additional reactions to surgery include alterations in water regulation mediated by release of
antidiuretic hormone and aldosterone, which increases water reabsorption in the renal collecting
ducts and increases sodium retention in the renal tubules, respectively [6,7]. It is believed that the
release of these hormones is stimulated by signals from blood pressure- and osmolarity-sensitive
receptors [3]. This diminished ability to excrete water in the early postoperative period results in
temporary weight gain and a return to normal blood volume [8].

After the above events, the patient enters a metabolic transition period of 1 or 2 days in which
the body begins to turn from corticosteroid and epinephrine-initiated breakdown to rebuilding and
healing. During this time, shedding of the retained water is effected, while conserving nitrogen
and potassium. The slow process of healing and regaining weight can now begin, and is marked by
protein synthesis, wound healing, buildup of muscle tissue, and increasing strength [3].

All of these processes occur with a fair degree of predictability in the adequately nourished
adult patient. The process is imperiled, as is the prognosis for full recovery, if the adult is elderly
or malnourished.

4.3   GENERAL NUTRITIONAL NEEDS OF THE ELDERLY

4.3.1   PROTEIN

Muscle accounts for 45% of body weight in young adults. This drops to 27% in the very old, who
clinically show a marked decrease in the size and strength of all skeletal muscle [9]. In the elderly,
protein depletion of body stores is seen primarily as a decrease of skeletal muscle mass. Muscle
changes are conspicuous in the small muscles of the hands and face and in the muscles of mastication. Chronic dietary protein inadequacy may be involved in depressed immune function, decreasing muscle strength, and poor wound healing in older adults [10]. Until recently, it was thought

that adults over 50 years of age should ingest 0.8 g of protein per kilogram of weight daily [11], but recent guidelines have suggested from 1 to 1.25 g of high-quality protein per kilogram of weight daily [12,13].

The best sources of protein for the elderly diet are meat and fish. These foods should be boiled [poached or braised], not fried; boiling prepares meats and fish for the elderly gastrointestinal tract by breaking down the complex proteins into the more easily digested proteoses, whereas frying denatures and coagulates the proteins and makes them difficult to digest [9].

4.3.2 CARBOHYDRATES

It is generally believed that carbohydrate absorption is somewhat impaired in the elderly, although decreased renal function may contribute to carbohydrate loss as well. The increase in lactose intolerance that can occur over time is due to a decrease in lactase activity in the gut lining, but may not be as severe as is often believed. Ausman and Russell [14] reported a double-blind study of healthy elderly subjects who were divided into two groups: the first received lactose-containing products, the second received lactose-free products. Approximately 30% of both groups reported bloating and gastrointestinal discomfort, leading to the conclusion that the true prevalence of lactose intolerance in the elderly is difficult to define.

Current dietary guidelines from the USDA (United States Department of Agriculture) [15] suggest that carbohydrates should compose from 45% to 65% of daily calories, and the complex carbohydrates (starches) are preferred over simple carbohydrates (sugars). More recently, carbohydrate intake of 130g/day has been suggested for adults over 70 years of age, with a recommendation that "added sugars" (soft drinks, candy, desserts, etc.) make up no more than 25% of total energy intake [16].

4.3.3 FAT

Generally, the elderly are able to digest and absorb fats in a diet containing 100 g of fat per day; at higher levels [120 g/day], there may be a slightly reduced ability to absorb them [17]. A rare problem with fat absorption can occur with a bacterial overgrowth in the small intestine that interferes with normal bile salt structure and function, but fat malabsorption was not found even in elderly hypochlorhydric individuals [18]. The U.S. FDA (Food and Drug Administration) guidelines recommend a diet with 25 to 35% of its daily caloric intake in the form of fat. In addition, it advises that saturated fat intake be reduced to less than 10% of daily calories, and that cholesterol be limited to less than 300 mg daily [15,19]. These recommendations are for all adults, with no differentiation for the elderly.

4.3.4 WATER

Water, the most important nutrient in the diet, is essential to all body functions. Water loss must be balanced every day by an adequate intake from drinking water, beverages, soups, and other foods, especially vegetables. If this balance is not maintained, and if water loss exceeds intake, chronic dehydration results. Geriatric patients are particularly susceptible to negative water balance, often caused by excessive water loss through insufficient or damaged kidneys.

Mucosal surfaces become dry and easily irritated in the dehydrated patient. Insufficient fluid consumption in general [and water consumption in particular] can have a deleterious effect on salivary gland function and on overall health in the elderly.

The average sedentary adult male must consume at least 2,900 ml of fluid daily, and the average sedentary adult female at least 2,200 ml per day, in the form of noncaffeine, nonalcoholic beverages, soups, and foods. Solid foods contribute approximately 1,000 ml of water, with an additional 250 ml derived from the water of oxidation [20].

4.3.5   FIBER

There is no definite requirement for dietary fiber in the daily diet of adults or the elderly. Different kinds of dietary fiber contribute to the motility of the gastrointestinal tract. In studies of different populations, a diet rich in fiber seems to be correlated with decreased rates of cancer and cardiac disease. An increase in dietary fiber is prescribed in the treatment of several diseases common in elderly persons, namely constipation, hemorrhoids, diverticulosis, hiatal hernia, varicose veins, diabetes mellitus, hyperlipidemia, and obesity [14,21]. The current recommendation is 14 g of fiber for every 1000 calories consumed per day [15] and the U.S. FDA requires that dietary fiber be listed on the nutrition facts panel on food labels [22].

4.4   MALNUTRITION IN THE ELDERLY

Malnutrition is a common finding in elderly patients, especially when they are hospitalized. In those patients whose nutritional status is borderline, the stress of illness may bring about deficiencies, and failure to correct malnutrition delays recovery and prolongs the hospital stay [23]. The elderly are a more diverse population than any other age group, with individuals having widely varying capabilities and levels of functioning [14]; they are at particular risk for marginal deficiencies of vitamins and trace elements. Diagnosis of malnutrition must rely on several methods, for each elderly adult has his or her own energy and intake requirements that must be based on health status, life situation (whether living independently or institutionalized), activity level, amount of lean muscle mass, and overall frame size.

Preoperative serum albumin level is considered the best predictor of postoperative complications (including mortality) after general surgery [24,25]. The albumin level reflects the patient's nutritional status over the previous 1 to 2 months due to its 21-day half-life; prealbumin levels are reflective only of the prior week period due to the much shorter half-life of 3 days. Individuals who exist in a state of marginal nutritional health may have the balance tipped by illness or other forms of stress. The early recognition of malnutrition is a challenge to healthcare providers and caregivers. A recent study found that nurses in a long-term care facility considered only 15.2% of the patients to be malnourished, while the Mini Nutritional Assessment [26] they used identified 56.7% as malnourished [27]. Prevention of malnutrition can forestall disease development or exacerbation by bolstering immune competence [28].

4.4.1   FACTORS CONTRIBUTING TO MALNUTRITION IN THE ELDERLY

Balanced nutrition is a major component of the general well-being of individuals throughout their lives. A vicious cycle exists in that the aging process compromises the body's ability to obtain nutrients from food, and the quality of an individual's nutrition influences how he or she ages [29]. Inadequate intake is only one of many causes of nutritional deficiency in the elderly [23].

4.4.1.1   Loss of Appetite and Diminished Taste and Smell

When asked why they don't eat, many elderly patients will say that food doesn't taste good or they are just not hungry. Diminished appetite has many causes, physical, psychological, and social, that can interact to interfere with the ability or desire to purchase, prepare, or eat food [30].

Depressed taste and smell contribute to loss of appetite. Forty percent of U.S. adults with chronic chemosensory problems (1.5 million persons) are 65 years of age or older [31]. In addition to aging, a decline in taste and smell can be caused by medications [32], radiotherapy [33], dental conditions or prostheses, and disease. Those diseases that can affect the senses of taste and smell include nervous system disorders (particularly Alzheimer's and Parkinson's diseases), chronic renal problems, endocrine disorders (diabetes mellitus, hypothyroidism, Cushing's syndrome), local ENT ailments, and viral infections [34,35]. Specific nutritional deficiencies (zinc and vitamins B3 and B12) and the nutritional problems relating to cancer can also be involved.

The dimming of taste can result from the degeneration or reduction in the total number of taste buds. It is now believed that every taste bud has some degree of sensitivity to all of the primary taste sensations, and that the brain detects the type of taste by the ratio of stimulation of the different taste buds [36]. Taste buds normally reproduce themselves approximately every 10 days in a healthy adult; renewal is slowed in the elderly, especially in postmenopausal women suffering from estrogen deficiency. Shortages of protein or zinc also retard taste bud renewal [34].

Olfactory acuity declines with age. The number of olfactory nuclei in the brain decline, and the olfactory receptors in the roof of the nasal cavity regress. Older patients generally have greater difficulty in differentiating among food odors, but are best at discriminating fruits from other stimuli [37]. Most studies suggest that the sense of smell is more impaired by aging than the sense of taste [34].

Appetite is also influenced by food palatability. As taste and smell are amalgamated in the determination of palatability and acceptance, the loss of flavor can make foods tasteless with a resultant decline in appetite. Thus, decreased gustatory or olfactory ability can have an adverse effect on diet and nutrition.

Psychological and social factors have a significant impact on appetite. Decreased appetite is one of the DSM-IV (Diagnostic and Statistical Manual, Fourth Edition) diagnostic criteria for depression. The prevalence of depression in the community-resident elderly population is estimated to be almost 20% [38]. The symptoms of depression in the surgical patient must be differentiated from physical illness, as nearly 20% of older adults with depression present with physical complaints [39]. In the elderly, social activities that involve food consumption may also be limited. Absence of these social cues may result in a decrease in appetite.

4.4.1.2 Edentulism and Oral Health Status

Both partial and complete edentulism, with a reduction in the number and occlusion of teeth, can impact negatively on the patient's ability to masticate food. Decreased masticatory efficiency can contribute to indigestion and a reduction in food intake, with concomitant reduction in lower nutrient intake [40].

4.4.1.3 Gastrointestinal Malfunction

The gastrointestinal tract of the elderly undergoes changes that contribute to a reduced ability to extract the full nutritional benefits from ingested foods. A reduction in gastric secretion of hydrochloric acid, intrinsic factor, and pepsin occurs in 20% of healthy adults over 60 years of age. The rate of gastric emptying of liquids increases with age, raising the pH in the ileum and negatively affecting the digestion of proteins and fats. If food is improperly digested, the constituent nutrients (proteins, vitamins, minerals, etc.) will not be available to be absorbed and utilized. In addition, a diminution of hepatic size and blood flow results in reduced ability to synthesize albumin and several other plasma proteins, and to metabolize certain medications [41].

4.4.1.4 Loss of Lean Body Mass

A loss of lean body mass accompanies the natural aging process, but the dramatically reduced level of physical activity seen in many of the elderly causes a marked reduction in muscle tissue. The weakness that accompanies this reduction in muscle volume and tone can contribute to difficulties in carrying out daily life activities, including mastication. The vicious cycle of declining energy (anergy), activity, muscle mass, and food intake impacts negatively on quality of life and on overall health and longevity.

4.4.2 Malnutrition in the Elderly Surgical Patient

As the geriatric population is projected to increase dramatically over the course of the next 20 years, a growing number of elderly patients will require both elective and emergency surgery. The risk of malnutrition and subclinical deficiencies [42] of this age group can have a direct impact on postoperative healing ability. The importance of nutrition in the treatment of the elderly hospital patient has frequently been underestimated. The older patient is more likely to be admitted to a hospital with some degree of malnutrition and the metabolic response to surgery is likely to be more severe [43].

The development of in-patient malnutrition often begins long before hospital admission. It may be partially a result of the lengthy time period from onset of symptoms to first presentation at the doctor's office through presentation at the referred surgeon's office, and finally to the hospital for the surgery. Bowling and Silk [44] conducted a study to assess this time period, and concluded that it could cause many patients to become malnourished prior to admission, which could have implications on the incidence of complications and the length of hospital stay.

4.5   NUTRITION AND WOUND HEALING

The role of nutrition in wound healing became more clearly defined with the development of intravenous feeding, known as total parenteral nutrition (TPN), in the 1960s. This major advance enabled physicians to provide the patient with a nutritionally complete diet, even if the patient could not eat. In addition, researchers were able to document the adverse effects of nutritional deficiencies on the success of surgical procedures, and how correction of nutritional deficits could alter the surgical/healing outcome for the better [45].

4.5.1   THE PROCESS OF WOUND HEALING

Several mechanisms are involved in wound healing, including inflammation, epithelialization, collagen synthesis, angiogenesis, collagen remodeling, and fibronectin-mediated wound contraction. This complex process occurs optimally when there is a sufficient supply of the raw materials—protein, carbohydrate, fat, vitamins, and minerals—that are needed to rebuild the damaged tissues. The lack of any of these important building blocks will adversely affect healing.

4.5.1.1   Protein

Protein deficiency is a major factor in poor wound healing, primarily as a result of depression of fibroblast proliferation and, thus, of the syntheses of connective tissue ground substance (proteoglycans), collagen, new blood vessels, and remodeling of the healing site [46]. For surgical patients, the recommended daily intake for protein rises to 2 to 4 g protein per kilogram of body weight per day [47]. The essential amino acids are those that cannot be synthesized via transamination; they must be ingested in food. One of these, methionine, has been shown to accelerate the rate of fibroplasia by its conversion to cystine. The mechanism is unclear, but formation of protein-strengthening disulfide bonds in collagen protein synthesis and self-assembly are critical to the stability of this complex molecule, which is essential in scar formation and healing [45]. Another essential amino acid, histidine, influences the tensile strength of wounds. Deficiency of histidine in experimental animals reduced the strength of wounds; addition of histidine to the diet restored wound strength to normal levels [48].

In protein deficiency, there is a protraction of the inflammatory phase of wound healing [49] in which proteolytic enzymes are secreted by macrophages and granulocytes, with a resulting 30 to 50% increase in proteolysis of the tissues around the wound site [50]. Protein malnutrition is characterized by dry, flaking skin, and by peripheral edema [51], that can mask malnutrition by concealing the amount of muscle wasting that has occurred in the patient [52]. In addition, the tissue edema can impair nutrient diffusion to the wound [53]. Hair appears dull, lacking normal color, and demonstrates increased pluckability. Muscle cramping and wasting also can be seen [54].

4.5.1.2 Carbohydrates and Fat

The precise role of carbohydrates and fat in wound healing is less well known than that of proteins. Glucose is utilized as an energy source for cellular metabolism, including metabolism by those cells involved in wound healing. Leukocytes participate in phagocytosis and inflammatory activities, influencing growth factor release that stimulates the proliferation of fibroblasts needed for initial healing activities. Fats are essential components of cell membranes and are needed for synthesis of new cells. However, no known impairment of wound healing has been associated with a deficiency of essential fatty acids [55].

4.5.1.3 Iron and Trace Minerals

Minerals play critical and interrelated roles in wound healing, especially in the processes involved in the synthesis of collagen. The enzymes essential to the synthetic process require cofactors to be present to catalyze the steps in the synthesis. These cofactors include magnesium [55], iron, manganese, copper, and calcium [47]. Studies to date have not implicated nutritional deficiencies of manganese or copper in impairment of wound healing in patients with good oral intake, primarily because these elements are present in enough different foods that deficiency usually does not occur. A significant exception has been documented, however, in patients who received long-term total parenteral nutrition (TPN) without additional supplementation of these minerals [56]. Copper is important in erythropoesis and in collagen stability [46].

Severe iron deficiency anemia may reduce the bactericidal competence of leukocytes; this may be offset by a concomitant reduction in rate of bacterial growth [46]. Iron is essential for the restoration of normal red blood cell numbers following blood loss from surgery. The serum level of transferrin, a protein used to transport iron, will be higher than normal in the iron-deficient patient, and its level of saturation with iron will be low. Iron is also used as a cofactor in the hydroxylation of proline in the collagen synthetic pathway. A deficiency of iron will decrease the structural integrity of collagen and, hence, decrease wound strength.

4.5.1.4 Zinc

In contrast to the trace minerals, a deficiency of zinc will have markedly adverse effects on wound healing by decreasing the rate of epithelialization, reducing the rate of increase in wound strength, and reducing collagen strength. Zinc has been found to be a cofactor of enzymes responsible for cellular proliferation and protein synthesis (DNA polymerase, RNA polymerase, reverse transcriptase, and ribosomes) [57]. A deficiency would interfere with the cellular proliferation required in the wound healing process, including that of inflammatory cells, epithelial cells, and fibroblasts. In addition, zinc acts to stabilize cell membranes by inhibiting lipid peroxidases, and may play a role in the storage of vitamin A in the liver [46]. Zinc deficiency also has a negative effect on the immune system by decreasing cellular and humoral immune function; the patient can become more susceptible to infections that may interfere with healing.

Experiments with high levels of zinc supplementation have been tried in the unsuccessful attempt to accelerate the healing process. It is known that insufficient zinc impairs wound healing, and that a return to normal blood levels will result in a return to the normal rate of healing [58,59]. Excessive zinc interferes with copper metabolism and with wound healing by affecting lysyl oxidase, the enzyme crucial to collagen cross-linking [46]. The recommended daily allowance (RDA) for zinc is 15 mg for healthy adults.

Topical zinc oxide as a wound dressing has been found to enhance the re-epithelialization of partial-thickness wounds [60] and to decrease inflammation [61].

4.5.1.5 Vitamins

Vitamins are essential cofactors in many functions of the body, including wound healing. Vitamin C [ascorbic acid] is essential in the synthesis of collagen. Vitamin C deficiency will produce a marked alteration in the healing process: without it, the primary sequence of amino acids in the collagen protein is improperly elaborated, the procollagen protein cannot be secreted from the fibroblast, and self-assembly of the collagen polymer cannot occur, as Vitamin C is required for the hydroxylation of proline residues.

Consequences of vitamin C deficiency are incomplete wound healing and an increased risk for wound dehiscence [45]. Scurvy is the clinical disease resulting from vitamin C deficiency, manifested as decreased integrity of bone, soft tissue, and small blood vessels. Since vitamin C is water-soluble, it is excreted renally and must be replenished frequently. The RDA for vitamin C is 60 mg per day. It has been suggested that adequate supplementation of vitamin C be given both pre- and postoperatively, in view of the possibility that surgical patients require more ascorbic acid than healthy persons [62].

Vitamin A can influence the course of patients who receive systemic steroids by reversing the impaired healing effect that steroids have on lysosomal membranes [63–65], and may be a cofactor in collagen synthesis and cross-linking [55]. Vitamin A plays a role in cellular differentiation of epithelial cells; deficiency can lead to hyperkeratosis. Like zinc, it has been used as a topical agent to mitigate delayed epithelialization and closure of wounds. Deficiency of vitamin A also plays a role in the increase in the incidence of infections [66]. Vitamin A appears to improve host defenses by enhancing cell-mediated immune function [67–71]. It increases the number of antibody-producing cells, thus fostering antibody production, and can increase the phagocytic and tumoricidal ability of macrophages [72–75]. In a well-nourished patient, vitamin A is stored in the liver in adequate amounts (since it is a fat-soluble vitamin). In a malnourished patient, 25,000 IU of supplemental vitamin A should be taken daily before and after elective surgery. If surgery will interfere with normal eating for a long period, or if the patient develops gastrointestinal complications postoperatively, vitamin A supplementation should be given to the well-nourished patient as well [46].

An excess of vitamin E will delay wound healing and will interfere with the beneficial effects of vitamin A. Excessive vitamin E is similar to steroids in the inhibition of collagen synthesis and wound healing [76,77]. It has been tried as a topical agent for reduction of hypertrophic scar and keloid formation, but has not been found to be particularly effective.

Vitamin K is utilized in the synthesis of prothrombin and clotting factors, and plays a role in bone healing, where it is required for the synthesis of calcium-binding protein [78]. Vitamin K deficiency results in excessive bleeding into the wound area during healing, and can predispose the area to the development of infection [46]. Other vitamins that contribute on a minor scale by aiding cross-linking of collagen are riboflavin, pyridoxine, and thiamine [79].

4.6   CLINICAL STUDIES OF NUTRITION AND WOUND HEALING

Biochemical understanding of the roles of nutrients in wound healing has been gained through the use of animal models. The measurement of wound healing usually requires direct sampling of the wound site by punch biopsy, or manipulation of the wound borders by tugging at them until they begin to pull apart to measure the tensile strength of the wound. Since neither of these procedures is possible in the postoperative patient, indirect measurements have been used. One study, however, examined the rates of epithelialization of study-induced anterior thigh wounds in healthy young [18 to 55 years] and elderly [over 65 years] subjects and found that the elderly subjects had a 1.9-day delay in epithelialization [80].

Current nutritional assessment methods (measurements of stored fat, arm muscle circumference, serum albumin, serum prealbumin, transferrin, total plasma protein, and immune status) can only roughly estimate the nutritional state of a patient [45,81], but should be used conjuctively in an attempt to gauge the patient's preoperative condition. The serum level of albumin is often used as an indicator of an individual's protein intake and of the status of the visceral protein pool [47,49]. In one study, it was found to be somewhat useful as a prognostic index for length of hospital stay following major surgery when corrected for patient age [82]. The normal concentration of serum albumin is 4.0 g/dl. A level of 3.5 to 3.9 g/dl indicates mild protein deficiency, 2.5 to 3.5 g/dl is moderately deficient, and less than 2.5 g/dl is considered to be severely protein deficient. However, the serum albumin concentration is not a specific indicator of malnutrition, as patients with hepatic disease and other chronic diseases prevalent in the elderly population commonly demonstrate low levels. Additionally, albumin has a relatively long half-life of 21 days and, therefore, is not reflective of short-term nutritional status. Prealbumin and transferrin have shorter half-lives, but are similarly nonspecific.

A group of 66 patients over 70 years of age who required emergency surgery were followed to determine the incidence of euthyroid sick syndrome (ESS), nutritional abnormalities, and postoperative outcome. The patients were assessed preoperatively for levels of thyroid hormone, catecholamines, cortisol, interleukin-6, interleukin-1, and C-reactive protein. Mortality rates and length of stay in the hospital were related. ESS was diagnosed in 34 patients, and was associated with low serum albumin levels, low triceps skinfold thickness, high cortisol and norepinephrine levels, high death rate, and longer hospital stay. A serum albumin level less than 3.5g/dl was virtually always associated with ESS [83].

Mullen et al. [84] found that surgical complications doubled in patients with a serum albumin concentration of less than 3.0 mg/dl, as compared with levels above 3.0. Patients whose serum transferrin was less than 220 g/dl had a complication rate five times higher than that of patients whose levels were greater than 220 g/dl. Mullen et al. [85] found that preoperative nutritional supplementation in cancer patients reduced surgical complications; Muller et al. [86] showed that preoperative TPN used in malnourished patients with gastrointestinal cancer significantly reduced major complications such as wound dehiscence.

Vaxman et al. [87] studied the effects of high doses of ascorbic acid and pantothenic acid on the wound healing process of human skin. They found that these supplements influenced the levels of trace elements in human skin and scars (Mg, Cu, and Mn levels increased, while Fe levels decreased), and acted to increase the resistance of scars to tensional forces.

The role of nutrition in the development of postoperative orthopedic infections was reviewed by Smith [88], who reported that nutritional deficiencies significantly increased the morbidity and mortality of orthopedic patients [89–91]. In addition, poor nutritional status in patients undergoing orthopedic surgery contributed to wound problems [45,92–94], to difficulties with fracture healing [95,96] to development of sepsis [97], and to multiple organ system failure [98,99].

Another study of 414 very old [≥75 yrs] hospitalized patients showed that malnutrition was predictive for long hospital stay and high mortality [100]. Nutritional support yielded a clinical benefit especially reducing infectious complications in high-risk or malnourished patients following gastrointestinal cancer surgery [101]. In a study of gastrectomy patients, those receiving early postoperative enteral nutritional support exhibited improved surgical wound healing [102].

A study of 90 surgical patients receiving intravenous nutrition found that the group who received intravenous (IV) nutrition before and after the procedure had better wound healing than those who received IV nutrition only after the procedure [103]. The same investigators also studied a group of 66 surgical patients with three degrees of malnutrition: normal nutritional status, mild protein energy malnutrition, and moderate to severe protein energy malnutrition. Patients with normal nutritional status demonstrated higher amounts of normal collagen (measured by hydroxyproline content) after 7 days, while those with malnutrition had significantly lowered collagen formation. Of interest was the finding that the two protein energy malnourished groups did not differ significantly from each other. This study demonstrated that even mild to moderate protein energy deficiencies will adversely affect healing [104].

A study involving transtibial amputees for occlusive arterial disease found that those patients who received a nutritional supplement had improved wound healing [105]. Similarly, a study using nutrition as a prognostic indicator in 47 amputations found that the malnourished patients had a higher frequency of impaired wound healing and an increased risk of postoperative cardiopulmonary and septic complications. All six deaths in the study occurred in the malnourished group [106].

4.7 THE HEALTH PROFESSIONALS FOLLOW-UP STUDY

The Health Professionals Follow-Up Study (HPFS) was initiated in 1986 to evaluate a series of hypotheses about men's health, relating nutritional factors to the incidence of serious illnesses such as cancer and heart disease. Initially, Walter Willett and his colleagues enlisted 51,529 men in health professions to participate in the study. The investigators believed that health professionals would be motivated and committed to participating in a long-term project and would appreciate the necessity of answering the survey questions accurately. The study group included dentists, optometrists, osteopathic physicians, pharmacists, podiatrists, and veterinarians.

Members of the study group receive questionnaires every 2 years with questions about diseases and health-related topics such as smoking, physical activity, and medications. Questionnaires that ask detailed dietary information are administered at 4-year intervals.

The study is sponsored by the Harvard School of Public Health and funded by the National Heart, Lung, and Blood Institute and the National Cancer Institute. Since its inception, over 100 published research articles have resulted from study data. Study participants receive a newsletter every 2 years with research highlights. Following are significant findings related to nutrition and disease from the newsletter [107].

4.7.1 BLADDER CANCER

A diet high in cruciferous vegetables, especially broccoli and cabbage, may reduce the risk of developing bladder cancer. Other vegetables and fruits are not especially protective against this particular cancer.

4.7.2 COLORECTAL CANCER

A dietary pattern characterized by high intakes of red and processed meats, sweets and desserts, French fries, and refined grains, is associated with an increased risk of colon cancer. Men who ate beef, pork, or lamb as a main dish 5 or more days per week had 3.5 times the incidence of colorectal cancer as compared with men eating these foods less than once per month. A reduction of animal fat intake and increase in the consumption of vegetables and fruit is recommended. Increasing folic acid intake may be beneficial. Current evidence suggests moderate intakes of calcium (approximately in the range of 800 to 1000 mg/day) may be most prudent.

4.7.3 CORONARY HEART DISEASE

Higher intakes of vitamin C from foods or supplements were not associated with a reduction in risk of heart disease. Men who consumed more carotene, vitamin E supplements, and drank alcohol moderately, and were lean, had a lower risk of developing coronary heart disease.

Men who did not gain weight after age 21 were at the lowest risk of subsequent heart disease, while men who gained 25 to 40 pounds after age 21 were at a 60% increase in risk. As men age beyond 65 years, the size of their waist is a better predictor of risk of coronary heart disease than overall weight.

Men who consumed the most saturated fat had a 22% increased risk of myocardial infarction, as compared with men who consumed the least. However, this risk was largely attributable to the lack of fiber in their diets and not to the saturated fat.

Men in the top 20% of potassium intake had a 40% reduction in risk of stroke compared with men in the bottom 20%. A high potassium intake is best achieved by increasing consumption of fruit and vegetables and their juices. A high intake of magnesium and cereal fiber also appear to be beneficial. Fruits and vegetables that were found to offer the most protection against ischemic stroke were broccoli, green leafy vegetables, and citrus fruits and juices. In contrast, legumes and potatoes were not associated with a reduced risk for ischemic stroke.

A recommended heart healthy diet is high in vegetables, fruits, nuts, soy protein, cereal fiber, whole grains (due to bran content), chicken, fish, and polyunsaturated fat, and low in saturated and trans fat.

4.7.3 DIABETES

Men who were 20 to 40 pounds overweight were 10 times more likely to develop diabetes than men of ideal weight. Men who can control their drinking at a moderate level (1 to 2 drinks per day) are at lowest risk of diabetes.

A dietary pattern (Western) characterized by higher intakes of red and processed meats, refined grain products, potatoes, French fries, and sweets, coupled with obesity and physical inactivity, dramatically elevated the risk of type 2 diabetes. In particular, high consumption of processed meats including hot dogs, bacon, and sausages, was significantly associated with diabetes risk.

It was also found that participants who regularly drank coffee had significantly lower risk of type 2 diabetes than non-coffee-drinking study participants. While this is good news for coffee drinkers, it is not known why coffee is beneficial for diabetes.

4.7.4 HYPERTENSION

Adequate amounts of dietary fiber, potassium, and magnesium were each significantly associated with lower risk of hypertension when considered individually and after adjustment for age, relative weight, alcohol, and energy intake.

4.7.5 KIDNEY STONES AND GALLSTONES

A high animal protein diet was associated with a 33% higher risk of kidney stone formation, while a high potassium diet (fruits and vegetables) was related with a 50% lower risk.

Diet is a risk factor for gallstone disease. Specifically, high intake of polyunsaturated and monounsaturated fats in the context of an energy-balanced diet was associated with a reduced risk for gallstone disease in men. Nuts are a particularly good source of these fats. However, trans fat from partially hydrogenated oil appeared to be harmful. Highly refined carbohydrates with a high glycemic index increased risk relative to less processed, high-fiber carbohydrate sources. A frequent moderate intake of alcohol decreased the risk for symptomatic gallstone disease, in contrast to infrequent or episodic alcohol intake.

Previously, obesity was the only accepted modifiable risk factor for gallstone disease. The HPFS suggests that the key is abdominal obesity, as measured by waist-to-hip ratio or simply waist circumference. Men with a waist circumference of 40 inches or more had 2.3 times the risk of gallstone disease as compared with those whose waists measured approximately 34 inches or less.

4.7.6 PARKINSON'S DISEASE

Higher coffee consumption was associated with a lower risk of Parkinson's disease, while Parkinson's disease was more common among men with higher consumption of dairy products. Preliminary findings suggest that vitamin E from food, but not from vitamin supplements, may reduce risk.

4.7.7 PROSTATE CANCER

Men who were the highest consumers of fat were at 80% higher risk for being diagnosed with advanced prostate cancer. This elevated risk was entirely due to fat from animal sources, particularly red meat, but not vegetable oils. Findings from the study also suggest that a diet high in animal fat may promote the growth of existing prostate cancers.

The only carotenoid related to a lower risk was lycopene, an antioxidant, which is found almost exclusively in tomato products. Men with higher levels of blood lycopene have a reduced risk of prostate cancer. Tomato sauce is an excellent source of lycopene. Both dietary and supplemental sources of calcium were associated with higher risk, which suggests that calcium, rather than some other component of dairy foods, contributed to the elevation in risk.

Higher intakes of red meat, processed meats, and dairy products were associated with a moderately increased risk of metastatic prostate cancer. Men who regularly consume fatty fish, such as salmon, have a lower risk of metastatic prostate cancer, by a protective association with omega-3 fatty acids.

The study strongly supports recommendations for men to reduce intake of red and processed meats, and instead rely more on fish, poultry, and plant sources as their main sources of protein. Greater tomato sauce and fish consumption, especially fatty fish such as salmon, also reduces the progression risk of prostate cancer. Eating cruciferous vegetables (broccoli, cabbage, Brussels sprouts) frequently, about 3 to 5 servings per week, may reduce prostate cancer risk by 20 to 30%.

4.8 NUTRITION, DIETING, AND SURGERY

A multiplicity of diets have been introduced and many subsequently withdrawn from the market over the past three decades. Methods of caloric restriction have become popular (Weight Watchers), as well as diets that focus on restriction of individual food groups (Atkins and Ornish). A feature common to all diets is their inconsistent success in long-term weight loss, which may be attributable not only to the diets themselves, but also to associated patient noncompliance and attrition.

There is limited scientific evidence on overall nutrition and metabolism and the related effects on health maintenance, disease prevention, and convalescence, including recovery from surgery, for popular well-publicized diets. Three of the most popular diets in recent years will be discussed, including the scientific studies investigating their effectiveness and their physiologic basis and effects on metabolism.

4.8.1 ATKINS DIET

The Atkins Diet was developed by Dr. Robert Atkins in the 1960s and became widely known in the 1970s with the release of a series of books describing his theories. In recent years, the Atkins franchise and the Atkins symbol have been used on a variety of products. The theory is based on the concepts that the main cause of obesity is the consumption of refined carbohydrates, such as sugar, flour, and corn syrups, and that the consumption of dietary fat does not necessarily contribute to obesity. In this diet, the restriction of carbohydrates induces a state of ketosis in which the body begins to break down fat stores in lieu of using glucose supply for energy.

Atkins described four phases of his diet: induction, ongoing weight loss, premaintenance, and lifetime maintenance. In the induction phase, carbohydrate intake is strictly restricted to 20 net grams per day ("net" carbohydrates are described as those that contribute to glucose levels, which excludes fiber and sugar alcohols). In the ongoing weight loss phase, an increase in carbohydrate intake is allowed, but still below a level that allows continued weight loss. Carbohydrate intake is further increased in the premaintenance phase, which may be above a level that induces ketosis. The lifetime maintenance phase stresses long-term adherence to these principles of carbohydrate restriction and a return to earlier, more restrictive phases if weight gain occurs.

One of the largest randomized trials, conducted by Gardner et al. at Stanford University, has found the diet to result in a greater weight loss over a period of 12 months than other popular diets [108]. Low-carbohydrate ketogenic diets, such as the Atkins diet, have been shown to have a greater improvement on subjective symptoms, including mood changes and the sensation of hunger, than low-fat diets [109]. A recent study conducted by the Centers for Disease Control and Prevention suggests that the diet is relatively well tolerated, with approximately 40% of male users and 30% of female users reporting long-term use of the diet (greater than 12 months) [110]. A study by Dansinger et al. at Tufts-New England Medical Center showed a mean weight loss of 2.1 kg in patients adhering to the Atkins diet over a 1-year period, with 53% of patients remaining compliant during that time [111]. Animal studies have demonstrated significant changes in metabolism caused by a ketogenic diet, correlating changes in gene expression to weight loss, improved glucose tolerance, and increased energy expenditure [112].

Concerns have been raised over possible detrimental consequences of the diet on overall nutritional balance and health with prolonged use. Some studies have suggested an increase in mortality in patients adhering to this diet [113–115]. Particular concern has been expressed over increases in cardiovascular risk and mortality that may be attributable to the fat intake and carbohydrate restriction [113,114]. Studies by Rankin and Turpyn have described a positive correlation between increasing C-reactive protein levels and a low-carbohydrate, high-fat diet, which is indicative of a systemic inflammatory state [116]. Effects on neurotransmitter metabolism have been postulated, as a ketogenic diet has been shown to be beneficial in seizure prophylaxis in epileptic children [117]. Despite such metabolic changes, there remains a paucity of data to support maintenance of weight loss for greater than 12 months from a low-carbohydrate, ketogenic diet.

4.8.2 WEIGHT WATCHERS DIET

The Weight Watchers diet, philosophically different from the Atkins diet, is based on caloric restriction. A "points" system is used that incorporates the total number of calories, grams of fat, and grams of dietary fiber. Patients are not restricted to any specific food intake, but must consume a quantity per week that is less than the total points allowed. Exercise can be figured into the formula, allowing for a higher caloric intake.

Patients on the Weight Watchers diet were found to have a mean weight loss of 3.0 kg at 1 year, with 65% remaining compliant during that period. In addition, the low-density to high-density lipoprotein ratio (LDL/HDL ratio) was reduced approximately 10% with statistical significance [111]. Long-term weight loss has been demonstrated in patients continuing to follow the Weight Watchers diet. One study of over 1000 patients investigated weight loss maintenance at 5 years: 19% of patients were within 5 lbs. of goal weight; 43% maintained a loss of 5% or greater; and 70% remained below initial weight [118].

4.8.3 ORNISH DIET

The Ornish diet was developed by Dean Ornish as a cardioprotective diet, but recently has become popular in weight-loss regimens as well. The diet is vegetarian and places strict restrictions on food group intake. Foods containing significant amounts of cholesterol and saturated fats are prohibited, including all meat and fish; nonfat dairy products and egg whites are allowed to a limited extent. Complex carbohydrates, such as fruit and grains, are favored over simple carbohydrates, such as sugars and alcohol. The Ornish diet is composed of 70% carbohydrates, 20% proteins, and 10% fats. According to Ornish, the typical American diet is 40% carbohydrates, 20% proteins, and 40% fats [119].

The majority of studies into the Ornish diet relate to coronary heart disease prevention and treatment. Using coronary angiography, Ornish et al. demonstrated a regression in coronary artery stenosis using his low-fat vegetarian diet when combined with smoking cessation, stress management, and exercise, but without the use of lipid-lowering medications. In this study, 82% of experimental patients showed a reduction in coronary artery diameter stenosis, while control group patients showed a progression at 1 year [120]. Short-term improvements in exercise tolerance and left ventricular motion have also been demonstrated, as well as a decrease in plasma cholesterol levels of 20.5% over a period of 24 days of dietary changes and stress management training [14].

The Dansinger et al. study reported an average weight loss of 3.3 kg at 1 year for patients on the Ornish diet [111]. As with the Atkins and Weight Watchers diets, a reduction in the LDL/HDL ratio was also seen. Adherence to the Ornish diet over 1 year was 50% [111].

The nutritional adequacy of a low-fat vegan diet has been questioned and investigated. In addition, recent data suggesting cardioprotective benefits of some nuts and fish oils have also questioned the Ornish diet's restrictions. Recent research has shown the diet to be nutritionally adequate if nutrient-fortified plant foods are included (i.e., fortified soy protein beverages), except for a deficiency in vitamin D [121]. Hence, vitamin D supplementation is recommended for patients following the Ornish diet, especially for those with limited sun exposure.

4.9   DISCUSSION

As approximately 50% of hospital patients are malnourished [122], patients admitted to an acute care hospital should undergo a nutritional screening to determine their nutritional intakes. Older patients are more likely to be admitted to the hospital suffering some degree of malnutrition, and the nutritional consequences of their metabolic responses to trauma may be more severe. It is the insidious nature of malnutrition in the elderly that makes the recognition of early warning signs of malnutrition so important. Research is needed to provide more practical age, sex, and culturally specific nutrition parameters. Early detection of malnutrition and appropriate interventions could produce a shift toward prevention [123,124]. Nutritional assessment should be undertaken when evaluating patients before surgery, as well as throughout the entire postoperative period, to improve outcomes [125].

Careful planning before surgery can avoid common cognitive, affective, or functional complications in elderly patients. The elimination of medications that cause cognitive dysfunction could help avoid or lessen postoperative confusion. The assessment of preoperative nutritional status could identify patients with significant malnutrition who would be at higher risk for postoperative complications [126], including infection, delay or failure to heal, or excessive scarring. Essential to a good surgical outcome is the rapid synthesis of new tissue in the wound area, minimization of contamination, maximization of the patient's immune status, and protection of the wound site. When blood supply, oxygen, and nutrients are available, healing can proceed [127].

A high-carbohydrate, low-fat diet containing adequate sources of protein will promote good wound healing by providing sufficient calories to rebuild and heal, while sparing the patient's own muscle mass as an energy source [128]. The use of preoperative nutritional supplementation has been more effective for treating protein malnutrition than postoperative supplementation [103]. As little as 1 week of preoperative protein supplementation can improve wound healing. Recent protein intake is more important than protein or fat stores [129].

Supplements of amino acids have been found to be beneficial. Methionine and cysteine decrease the length of the inflammatory stage [46] and may protect against oxidative damage [47]. Arginine supplementation stimulates development of cytotoxic T-cells and proliferation of lymphocytes and increases resistance to infection [130–134].

Nusbaum [135] found that support services such as nutrition, nursing, and physical therapy are very important components in the postoperative care of geriatric patients. In general, advanced age per se is not a contraindication to surgery, but it does require careful preoperative evaluation and vigorous postoperative support. An important parameter of postoperative recovery is the regaining of the patient's preoperative lean body mass. Jensen and Hessov [136] investigated whether a 4-month dietary intervention with dietary advice and home supplementation would impact the speed of regaining muscle in the convalescing patient. They found that patients who received the intervention had a gain of lean body mass after 2 months. After an additional 2 months, both lean body mass and fat were gained. The investigators concluded that, after discharge from the hospital, patients should increase protein intake by taking protein-rich liquid supplements.

A recent weight loss of greater than 10% of lean body mass increases the chances for wound complications [137]. Recent preoperative intake of nutrients is most important [103,138]; not eating food for a week before surgery is worse than eating a limited regular diet for a longer period because nutritional depletion is correlated with wound complications [82,92,104,127].

If the patient has not eaten during the few days before surgery, or if the patient is not expected to eat much postoperatively, nutritional supplementation should be undertaken. Rapid replenishment of depleted nutrients is surprisingly effective, and a few days of parenteral nutrition can return the patient to relatively normal reparative capacity [103], although enteral nutrition is preferred if at all possible.

Surgery should be delayed significantly only if malnutrition is severe [85,103,127,139]. If the level of malnutrition is not severe, 2 to 3 days of supplementation should suffice. In all cases, nutritional supplementation begun preoperatively should be carried into the postoperative period [127]. Diabetes, if present, must be kept under strict control, for hyperglycemia will decrease vitamin C cellular uptake [140]. Increasing the level of vitamin C to 500 to 2000 mg per day can partially overcome this problem.

4.10 SUMMARY

The elderly surgical patient should be evaluated for malnutrition and monitored by the patient's primary physician and surgeon. Preoperative assessment of nutritional status should be the standard of care for the aged. The serum albumin level and the total lymphocyte count can be used to identify patients suffering from malnutrition. Surgery on a malnourished patient should be postponed, if possible, until the nutritional status has been restored to normal levels. A medical evaluation that focuses on the elderly patient's cardiopulmonary and nutritional status should be performed up to 8 weeks before the patient undergoes surgery. Following this evaluation, appropriate dietary, therapeutic, and prophylactic measures to reduce surgical morbidity and mortality can be implemented. The identification and management of nutritional deficiencies in the elderly can be a useful adjunct to successful surgery.

REFERENCES

1. Winkler S. 1992. Oral Aspects of Aging. In: Calkins E, Ford AB, Katz PR, eds. *Practice of Geriatrics.* 8th ed. Philadelphia: WB Saunders, 502–512.
2. Birke G, Franksson C, Plantin LO. 1955. The excretion pattern of 17-ketosteroids and corticosteroids in surgical stress. *Acta Endocrinol* 18:201–209.
3. Souba WW, Wilmore D. 1999. Diet and Nutrition in the Care of the Patient with Surgery, Trauma, and Sepsis. In: Goodheart RS, Shils ME, eds. *Modern Nutrition in Health and Disease*. Philadelphia: Lea and Febiger, 1589–1618.
4. Porte D, Graber AL, Kuzuwa T, et al. 1966. The effect of epinephrine on immunoreactive insulin levels in man. *J Clin Invest* 45:228–236.
5. Russell RC, Walker, CJ, Bloom SR. 1975. Hyperglucagonaemia in the surgical patient. *Br Med J* 1(5948):10–12.
6. Traynor C, Hall GM. 1981. Endocrine and metabolic changes during surgery: Anaesthetic implications. *Br J Anaesth* 53(2):153–160.
7. Deutsch S. 1975. Effects of anesthetics on the kidney. *Surg Clin North Am* 55(4):775–786.
8. Philbin DM, Coggins CH. 1978. Plasma antidiuretic hormone levels in cardiac surgical patients during morphine and halothane anesthesia. *Anesthesiology* 49(2):95–98.
9. Massler M. 1994. Nutrition and the denture-bearing tissues. In: Winkler S, ed. *Essentials of Complete Denture Prosthodontics*. 2nd ed. St. Louis: Ishiyaku EuroAmerica, Inc. 15–21.
10. Chernoff R. 1995. Effects of age on nutrient requirements. *Clin Geriatr Med* 11:641–651.
11. Munro HN, Young VR. 1978. Protein metabolism is the elderly: Observations relating to dietary needs. *Postgrad Med* 63:143–148.

12. Campbell WW, Crim MC, Dallal GE, et al. 1994. Increased protein requirements in elderly people: New data and retrospective assessments. *Am J Clin Nutr*, 60:501–509.

13. Castaneda C, Charnley JM, Evans WJ, Crim MC. 1995. Elderly women accommodate to a low-protein diet with losses of body cell mass, muscle function, and immune response. *Am J Clin Nutr*, 62:30–39.

14. Ausman LM, Russell RM. 1999. Nutrition in the Elderly. In: *Modern Nutrition in Health and Disease*. Goodheart RS , Shils ME, eds. Philadelphia: Lea and Febiger. 869–880.

15. US Department of Agriculture. 2005. Dietary Guidelines for Americans, Home and Garden Bulletin #232, Washington, DC, US Government Printing Office.

16. Dietary Reference Intakes for Energy, Carbohydrates, Fiber, Fat, Fatty Acids, Cholesterol, Protein, and Amino Acids (Macronutrients). 2005. The National Academies Press Food and Nutrition Board of the Institute of Medicine of the National Academies. 265–338.

17. Sawaya AL, Saltzman E, Fuss P, et al. 1995. Dietary energy requirements of young and older women determined by using the doubly labeled water method, *Am J Clin Nutr* 62:338–344.

18. Saltzman JR, Kowdley KV, Pedrosa MC et al. 1994. Bacterial overgrowth without clinical malabsorption in elderly hypochlorhydric subjects, *Gastroenterology* 106(3): 615–623.

19. Mayfield E. 1999. A Consumer's Guide to Fats, in *The FDA Consumer*, US Food and Drug Administration, Washington, DC, US Government Printing Office.

20. Kleiner SM. 1999. Water: An essential but overlooked nutrient, *J Am Diet Assoc* 99:200–206.

21. Gray DS. 1995. The clinical use of dietary fiber. *Am Fam Physician* 51(2):419–425.

22. Papazian R. 1997. Bulking up fiber's healthful reputation. *FDA Consumer*, US Food and Drug Administration Bulletin FDA 97–2313, Washington, DC, US Government Printing Office, revised 1998.

23. Zawada ET, Jr. 1996. Malnutrition in the elderly. Is it simply a matter of not eating enough? *Postgrad Med* 100(1):207–208, 211–214, 220–222.

24. Kudsk KA, Sacks GS. 2006. Nutrition in the Care of the Patient with Surgery, Trauma and Sepsis. In: Shils ME, ed. *Modern Nutrition in Health and Disease*. Philadelphia: Lippincott Williams and Wilkins, 1415.

25. Khuri SF, Daley J, Henderson W, Hur K, et al. 1997. Risk adjustment of the postoperative mortality rate for the comparative assessment of the quality of surgical care: Results of the National Veterans Affairs Surgical Risk Study. *J Am Coll Surg*, 185(4):315–327.

26. Guigoz Y, Vellas B, Garry P. 1996. Assessing the nutritional status of the elderly: The Mini Nutritional Assessment as part of the geriatric evaluation. *Nutr Rev*, 54 (Suppl 2), 59–65.

27. Suominen MH, Sandelin E, Soini H, Pitkala KH. How well do nurses recognize malnutrition in elderly patients? *Eur J Clin Nutr*, advance online publication, 19 September 2007, doi:10.1038/sj. 1602916.

28. Schlienger JL, Pradignac A, Grunenberger F. 1995. Nutrition of the elderly: a challenge between facts and needs. *Horm Res*, 43(1–3):46–51.

29. Mirie W. 1997. Aging and nutritional needs. *East Afr Med J*, 74(10):622–624.

30. Russell RM, Sahyoun NR. 1988. The Elderly. In: *Clinical Nutrition, 2nd ed.* Paige EM, ed. Washington, DC: C.V. Mosby, 110–116.

31. Hoffman HJ, Ishii EK, Macturk RH. 1998. Age-related changes in the prevalence of smell/taste problems among the United States adult population. Results of the 1994 Disability Supplement to the National Health Interview Survey (NHIS). *Ann NY Acad Sci*, 855:716–722.

32. Schiffman SS. 1991. Drugs influencing taste and smell perception. In: *Smell and Taste in Health and Disease*. Getchell TV, Doty RL, Bartoshuk LM, Snow JB, eds. New York: Raven Press, 845–850.

33. Beaven DW, Brooks SE. 1988. *Color Atlas of the Tongue in Clinical Diagnosis*, Ipswich, England: Wolfe Medical Publishers Ltd., 16.

34. Schiffman SS. 1997. Taste and smell losses in normal aging and disease. *JAMA*, 16:1357–1362.

35. Mowe M, Bohmer T. 1996. Nutritional problems among home–living elderly people may lead to disease and hospitalization. *Nutr Revs*, 54:S22–S24.

36. Hess MA. 1997. Taste: the neglected nutritional factor. *J Am Diet Assoc* 97(10 Suppl 2):S205–207.

37. Schiffman S, Pasternak M. 1979. Decreased discrimination of food odors in the elderly. *J Gerontol*, 34:73–79.

38. Murrell SA, Himmelfarb S, Wright K. 1983. Prevalence of depression and its correlates in older adults. *Am J Epidemio*, 117:173.

39. Busse EW, Simpson D. 1983. Depression and antidepressants and the elderly. *J Clin Psych*, 44:5(Sec 2):35.

40. Marshall, TA, Warren JJ, Hand JS, Xie X–J, Stumbo PJ. 2002. Oral health, nutrient intake and dietary quality in the very old. *JADA*, 133(10):1369–1379.

41. Rosenberg IH, Russell RM, Bowman BB. 1989. 1997. Aging and the digestive system. In: *Nutrition, aging and the elderly.* Munro HN, Danford DE, eds. New York: Plenum Press, 43–60.
42. Blumberg J. Nutritional needs of seniors. 1997. *J Am Coll Nutr,* 16(6):517–523.
43. Williams CM, Driver LT, Lumbers M. 1990. Nutrition in the older hospital patient. *J R Soc Health,* 110(2):41–2,44.
44. Bowling TE, Silk BA. 1996. How long does it take to operate? The implications for inpatient malnutrition. *Acta Gastroenterol Latinoam,* 26(2): 101–104.
45. Ruberg RL. 1984. Role of nutrition in wound healing. *Surg Clin N Am,* 64(4):705–714.
46. Levenson SM, Demetriou AA. 1992. Metabolic Factors. In: Cohen IK, Diegmann RF, Lindblad WJ, eds. *Wound Healing: Biochemical and Clinical Aspects.* Philadelphia, W.B. Saunders, 248–273.
47. Mazzotta MY. 1994. Nutrition and Wound Healing. *J Am Podiat Assoc,* 84(9):456–462.
48. Fitzpatrick DW, Fisher H. 1982. Carnosine, histidine, and wound healing. *Surgery,* 91:56–60.
49. Keller U, Clerc D, Kranzlin M, et al. 1986. Protein sparing therapy in the postoperative period. *World J Surg,* 10(1):12–19.
50. Erlichman RJ, Seckel BR, Bryan DJ, et al. 1991. Common complications of wound healing: Prevention and management. *Surg Clin North Am,* 71(6):1323–1351.
51. Gilder H. 1986. Parenteral nourishment of patients undergoing surgical or traumatic stress. *J Parenter Enter Nutr,* 10(1):88–91.
52. Wolfe RR. 1991. Current thoughts on the assessment of protein metabolism in humans. *J Burn Care Rehabil,* 12(3):211–213.
53. Bobel LM. 1982. Nutritional implications in the patient with pressure sores. *Nurs Clin North Am,* 22(2):379–390.
54. Welch PK, Dowson M, Endres JM. 1991. The effects of nutrient supplements on high risk long term patients receiving pureed diets. *J Nutr Eld,* 10(3):49–62.
55. Pollack SV. 1979. Wound Healing: A review. III. Nutritional factors affecting wound healing. *J Dermatol Surg Oncol,* 5(8):615–619.
56. Ruberg RL, Mirtallo J. 1981. Vitamin and trace element requirements in parenteral nutrition: An update. *Ohio State Med J,* 77(12):725–729.
57. Solomons NW. 1988. Zinc and copper. In: Shils ME, Young VR, eds. *Modern Nutrition in Health and Disease.* Philadelphia: Lea and Febiger, 238–262.
58. Chvapil M. 1980. Zinc and other factors of the pharmacology of wound healing. In: Hunt TK, ed. *Wound Healing and Wound Infection: Theory and Surgical Practice.* New York: Appleton-Century Crofts, 135–149.
59. Liszewski RF. The effect of zinc on wound healing: A collective review. *J Am Osteopath Assoc,* 1981.81(2):104–106.
60. Ågren MA, Chvapil M, Franzén L. 1991. Enhancement of re-epithelialization with topical zinc oxide in porcine partial-thickness wounds. *J Surg Res,* 50:101–105.
61. Guillard O, Masson P, Piriou A, Brugier J-C, Courtois P. 1987. Comparison of the anti-inflammatory activity of sodium acexamate and zinc acexamate in healing skin wounds in rabbits. *Pharmacology,* 34(5):296–300.
62. Schwartz PL. 1970. Ascorbic acid in wound healing—a review. *J Am Diet Assoc,* 56(6):497–503.
63. Erlich HP, Hunt TK. 1968. Effects of cortisone and vitamin A on wound healing. *Ann Surg,* 167:324–328.
64. Erlich HP, Tarvet H, Hunt TK. 1973. Effects of vitamin A and glucocorticoids upon inflammation and collagen synthesis. *Ann Surg,* 177:222–227.
65. Hunt TK. 1976. Control of wound healing with cortisone and vitamin A. In: Longacre JJ, ed. *The Ultrastructure of Collagen.* Springfield, IL: Charles C. Thomas, 497–503.
66. Atukorala TMS, Basu TK, Dickerson JWT. 1981. Effect of corticosterone on the plasma and tissue concentrations of vitamin A in rats. *Ann Nutr Metab,* 25:234–238.
67. Barbul A, Thysen B, Rettura G, et al. 1978. White cell involvement in the inflammatory wound healing and immune actions of vitamin A. *J Parent Enter Nutr,* 2:129–138.
68. Jurin M, Tannock JF. 1972. Influence of vitamin A on immunologic response. *Immunology,* 23:283–287.
69. Medawar PB, Hunt R. 1981. Anti-cancer action of retinoids. *Immunology,* 42:349–353.
70. Malkovsky M, Medawar PB, Hunt R, et al. 1984. A diet enriched in vitamin A acetate or *in vivo* administration of interleukin-2 can counteract a toleragenic stimulus. *Proc R Soc Lond Biol,* 220:439–445.

71. Seifter E, Rettura G, Levenson SM, et al. 1978. A mechanism of action of vitamin A in immunogenic tumor systems. *Curr Chemother Proc*, 10th Int. Cong Chemother, vol II, 1290–1291.

72. Cohen BE, Cohen IK. 1973. Vitamin A: Adjuvant and steroid antagonist in the immune response. *J Immunol*, 111:1376–1380.

73. Athanassiades TJ. 1981. Adjuvant effect of vitamin A palmitate and analogs on cell-mediated immunity. *J Natl Cancer Inst*, 67:1153–1156.

74. Pletsityvi KD, Askerov MA. 1982. Effect of vitamin A on immunogenesis. *Vopr Pitan* (English abstract), 11:38–40.

75. Tachibana K, Sone S, Tsubura E, et al. 1984. Stimulatory effect of vitamin A on tumoricidal activity of rat alveolar macrophages. *Br J Cancer*, 49:343–348.

76. Greenwald DP, Sharzer LA, Padawer J, et al. 1990. Zone II flexor tendon repair: Effects of vitamin A, E, beta-carotene. *J Surg Res*. 49:98–102.

77. Erlich HP, Tarver H, Hunt TK. 1972. Inhibitory effects of vitamin E on collagen synthesis and wound repair. *Ann Surg*, 175:235–240.

78. Gallop PM, Lian JB, Hawschka PV. 1980. Carboxylated and calcium-binding protein and vitamin K. *N Eng J Med*, 302:1460–1466.

79. Alvarez OM, Gilbreath RL. 1982. Effect of dietary thiamine on intermolecular collagen cross-linking during wound repair: Mechanical and biochemical assessment. *J Trauma*, 22(1):20–24.

80. Holt DR, Kirk SJ, Regan MC, Hurson M, Lindblad WJ, Barbul A. 1992. Effect of age on wound healing in healthy human beings. *Surgery*, 112(2):293–297.

81. Stotts NA, Whitney JD. 1990. Nutritional intake and status of clients in the home with open surgical wounds. *J Community Health Nurs*, 7(2): 77–86.

82. Warnold I, Lundholm K. 1984. Clinical Significance of preoperative nutritional status in 215 noncancer patients. *Ann Surg*, 3:299–305.

83. Girvent M, Maestro S, Hernandez R, et al. 1998. Euthyroid sick syndrome, associated endocrine abnormalities, and outcome in elderly patients undergoing emergency operation. *Surgery*, 123(5):560–567.

84. Mullen JL, Gertner MH, Buzby GP, et al. 1979. Implications of malnutrition in the surgical patient. *Arch Surg*, 114(2):121–125.

85. Mullen JL, Buzby GP, Matthews DC, et al. 1980. Reduction of operative morbidity and mortality by combined preoperative and postoperative nutrition support. *Ann Surg*, 192(5):604–613.

86. Muller JM, Brenner U, Denst C, et al. 1982. Preoperative parenteral feeding in patients with gastrointestinal carcinoma. *Lancet*, 1(8263):68–71.

87. Vaxman F, Olender S, Lambert A, et al. 1996. Can the wound healing process be improved by vitamin supplementation? *Eur Surg Res*, 28:306–314.

88. Smith TK. 1991. Nutrition: Its relationship to orthopedic infections. *Orthoped Clin N Am*, 22(3):373–377.

89. Foster MR, Heppenstall RB, Friedenberg ZB, et al. 1990. A prospective assessment of nutritional status and complications in patients with fractures of the hip. *J Orthop Trauma*, 4(1):49–57.

90. Jensen JE, Jensen TG, Smith TK, et al. 1982. Nutrition in orthopaedic surgery. *J Bone Joint Surg Am*, 64(9):1263–1272.

91. Mandelbaum BR, Tolo VT, McAfee PC, et al. 1988. Nutritional deficiencies after staged anterior and posterior spinal reconstructive surgery. *Clin Orthop*, 234:5.

92. Dickhaut SC, DeLee JC, Page CP. 1984. Nutritional status: importance in predicting wound healing in amputations. *J Bone Joint Surg Am*, 66(1):71–75.

93. Kay SP, Moreland JR. 1988. The effect of malnutrition on below-knee amputations. Scientific Program, American Academy of Orthopedic Surgeons Meeting, New Orleans, LA, 1986.

94. Young ME. Malnutrition and wound healing. 1988. *Heart Lung*, 17(1):60–67.

95. Cuthbertson DP. 1978. Post-traumatic metabolism: A multidisciplinary challenge. *Surg Clin N Am*, 58(5):1045–1054.

96. Einhorn TA, Levine B, Michel P. 1990. Nutrition and bone. *Orthop Clin North Am*, 21(1):43–50.

97. Keusch GT, Farthing MJG. 1986. Nutrition and infection. *Annu Rev Nutr*, 6:131–154.

98. Smith TK. 1987. Prevention of complications in orthopedic surgery secondary to nutritional depletion. *Clin Orthop*, 222:91–97.

99. Smith TK. 1984. Recognition and treatment of nutritional deficits in the multiply-injured patient. In: Meyers MH, ed. *The Multiply-Injured Patient with Complex Fractures*. Philadelphia: Lea and Febiger.

100. Kagansky N, Berner Y, Koren-Morag N, Perelman L, Knobler H, Levy S. 2005. Poor nutritional habits are predictors of poor outcome in very old hospitalized patients. *Am J Clin Nutr*, 82:784–791.

101. Bozzetti f, Gianotti L, Braga M, Di Carlo v, Mariani L. Postoperative complications in gastrointestinal cancer patients: The joint role of the nutritional status and the nutritional support. *J Clin Nutr*, 2007, doi:10.1016/j.clnu.2007.06.009.

102. Farreras N, Artigas V, Cardona D, Rius X, Trias M, Gonzalez JA. 2005. Effect of early postoperative entral immunonutrition on wound healing in patients undergoing surgery for gastric cancer. *Clin Nutr*, 24(1):55–65.

103. Haydock DA, Hill GL. 1987. Improved wound healing response in surgical patients receiving intravenous nutrition. *Brit J Surg*, 74(4):320–323.

104. Haydock DA, Hill GL. 1986. Impaired wound healing in surgical patients with varying degrees of malnutrition. *J Parent Enter Nutr*, 10(6):550–554.

105. Eneroth M, Apelqvist J, Larsson J, Persson BM. 1997. Improved wound healing in transtibial amputees receiving supplementary nutrition. *Int Orthop*, 21(2):104–108.

106. Pedersen NW, Pedersen D. 1992. Nutrition as a prognostic indicator in amputations. A prospective study of forty-seven cases. *Acta Orthop Scand*, 63(6):675–678.

107. *Health Professionals Follow-Up Study Newsletter*. Boston, MA: Harvard School of Public Health. 1991–2007.

108. Gardner CD, Kiazand A, Alhassan S, Kim S, Stafford RS, Balise RR, Kraemer HC, King AC. 2007 Comparison of the Atkins, Zone, Ornish, and LEARN diets for change in weight and related risk factors among overweight premenopausal women: The A to Z Weight Loss Study: A Randomized Trial. *JAMA*, Mar 7.297(9):969–77.

109. McClernon FJ, Yancy WS, Eberstein JA, Atkins RC, Westman EC. 2007. The effects of a low-carbohydrate ketogenic diet and a low-fat diet on mood, hunger, and other self-reported symptoms. *Obesity,* Jan. 15(1):182–87.

110. Blanck HM, Gillespie C, Serdula MK, Khan LK, Galusk DA, Ainsworth BE. 2006. Use of low-carbohydrate, high-protein diets among americans: Correlates, duration, and weight loss. *Med Gen Med*, Apr 5.8(2):5.

111. Dansinger ML, Gleason JA, Griffith JL, Seiker HP, Schaefer EJ. 2005. Comparison of the Atkins, Ornish, Weight Watchers, and Zone Diets for weight loss and heart disease risk reduction: A randomized trial. *JAMA,* Jan 5.293(1):43–53.

112. Kennedy AR, Pissios P, Otu H, Xue B, Asakura K, Furukawa N, Marino FE, Liu FF, Kahn BB, Libermann TA, Maratos-Flier E. 2007. A high-fat, ketogenic diet induces a unique metabolic state in mice. *Am J Physiol Endocrinol Metab*, Jun. 292(6):E1724–39.

113. Lagiou P, Sandin S, Weiderpass E, Lagiou A, Mucci L, Trichopoulos D, Adami HO. 2007. Low carbohydrate-high protein diet and mortality in a cohort of Swedish women. *J Intern Med*, Apr.261(4):366–74.

114. Trichopoulou A, Psaltopoulou T, Orfanos P, Hsieh CC, Trichopoulos D. 2007. Low-carbohydrate-high-protein diet and long-term survival in a general population cohort. *Eur J Clin Nutr,* May.61(5):575–81.

115. Cunningham W, Hyson D. 2006. The skinny on high-protein, low-carbohydrate diets. *Prev Cardiol*, Summer.9(3):166–71.

116. Rankin JW, Turpyn AD. 2007. Low carbohydrate, high fat diet increases c-reactive protein during weight loss. *J Am Coll Nutr,* Apr.26(2):163–69.

117. Hartman AL, Gasior M, Vining EP, Rogawski MA. 2007. The Neuropharmocology of the ketogenic diet. *Pediatr Neurol,* May.36(5).281–92.

118. Lowe MR, Miller-Kovach K, Phelan S. 2001. Weight-loss maintenance in overweight individuals one to five years following successful completion of a commercial weight loss program. *Int J Obes Relat Metab Disord*, Mar.25(3):325–31.

119. Ornish, Dean. *Eat More, Weigh Less: Dr. Dean Ornish's Life Choice Program for Losing Weight Safely While Eating Abundantly.* New York: Quill, 2001.

120. Ornish D, Brown SE, Scherwitz LW, Billings JH, Armstrong WT, Ports TA, McLanahan SM, Kirkeeide RL, Brand RJ, and Gould KL. 1990. Can lifestyle changes reverse coronary heart disease? The Lifestyle Heart Trial. *Lancet,* Jul 21.336(8708):129–33.

121. Ornish D, Schwartz LW, Doody RS, Kesten D, McLanahan SM, Brown SE, DePuey E, Sonnemaker R, Haynes C, Lester J, McAllister GK, Hall RJ, Burdine JA, Gotto AM. 1983. Effects of stress management training and dietary changes in treating ischemic heart disease. *JAMA*, Jan 7.249(1):54–59.

122. Lipkin EW, Bell S. 1993. Assessment of nutritional status. The clinician's perspective. *Clin Lab Med*, 13(2):329–352.

123. Barrocas A, Belcher D, Champagne C, Jastram C. 1995. Nutrition assessment—practical approaches. *Clin Geriatr Med*, 11(4):675–713.

124. McWhirter JP, Pennington CR. 1994. Incidence and recognition of malnutrition in hospital. *Br Med J*, 308(6934):945–948.
125. Rapp-Kesek D. 2007. Nutrition in elderly patients undergoing cardiac surgery. Acta Universitatis Upsaliensis. *Digital Comprehensive Summaries of Uppsala Dissertations from the Faculty of Medicine*, 245:53pp. ISBN 978-91-554-6842-2.
126. Hirsch CH. 1995. When your patient needs surgery: How planning can avoid complications. *Geriatrics*, 50(2):39–44.
127. Hunt TK, Hopf, HW. 1997. Wound healing and wound infection—what surgeons and anesthesiologists can do. *Surg Clin N Am*, 77(3):587–606.
128. Nirgiotis JG, Hennesey PJ, Black CT, et al. 1991. Low fat, high carbohydrate diets improve wound healing and increase protein levels in surgically stressed rats. *J Pediatr Surg*, 26(8):925–928.
129. Windsor J, Knight G, Hill G. 1988. Wound healing response in surgical patients: Recent food intake is more important than nutritional status. *Br J Surg*, 75(2):135–137.
130. Reynolds JV, Daly JM, Zhang S, et al. 1988. Immunomodulatory mechanisms of arginine. *Surgery*, 104(2):142–151.
131. Reynolds JV, Daly JM, Shou J, et al. 1990. Immunologic effects of arginine supplementation in tumor-bearing and non-tumor-bearing hosts. *Ann Surg*, 211(2):202–210.
132. Efron DT, Kirk SJ, Regan MC, et al. 1991. Nitric oxide generation from L-arginine is required for optimal human peripheral blood lymphocyte DNA synthesis. *Surgery*, 110(2):327–334.
133. Daly JM, Reynolds J, Thom A, et al. 1988. Immune and metabolic effects of arginine in the surgical patient. *Ann Surg*, 208(4):512–523.
134. Daly JM, Reynolds J, Sigal RK, et al. 1990. Effect of dietary protein and amino acids on immune function. *Crit Care Med*, 18(2 Suppl):S86–93.
135. Nusbaum NJ. 1996. How do geriatric patients recover from surgery? *South Med J*, 89(10):950–957.
136. Jensen MB, Hessov I. 1997. Dietary supplementation at home improves the regain of lean body mass after surgery. *Nutrition*, 13(5):475–476.
137. Orgill D, Demling RH. 1988. Current concepts and approaches to wound healing. *Crit Care Med*, 16(9):899–908.
138. Goodson WH, Lopez SA, Jensen JA, et al. 1987. The influence of a brief preoperative illness on postoperative healing. *Ann Surg*, 205:250–255.
139. Delany HM, Demetriou AA, Teh E, et al. 1990. Effect of early postoperative nutritional support on skin wound and colon anastomosis healing. *J Parent Enter Nutr*, 14(4):357–361.
140. Marhoffer W, Stein M, Maeser D, et al. 1992. Impairment of polymorphonuclear leukocyte function and metabolic control of diabetes. *Diabetes Care*, 15:256–260.

5 The Role of Micronutrients in Preventing Infections in the Elderly

Alia El-Kadiki

CONTENTS

5.1   INTRODUCTION

Multivitamins and minerals are the most commonly used dietary supplements in the United States [1]. This is largely due to the belief that multivitamin supplements could improve health and prevents certain diseases, among which are infections [2]. Classical vitamin deficiency syndromes are uncommon in Western societies. However, certain groups, such as elderly people, are at higher risk for suboptimal vitamin status and vitamin deficiency [3]. Many factors can lead to micronutrient deficiency in the elderly such as poor dentition, social isolation, depression, and dementia. The presence of other diseases such as diabetes and intestinal ischemia cause malabsorption [4,5]. Also, it is well known that in the elderly zinc has low intestinal absorption [6] and older people often take many medications that could affect vitamin absorption or metabolism [7].

Infection is among the most common disorder in the elderly. Acute respiratory infections account for more than 50% of all types of infections in this age group, followed by genitourinary, skin and gastrointestinal infections [8]. Acute respiratory infections last longer and are associated with higher mortality and morbidity [9]. An age-related decline in immune response is believed to be an important cause of the increased risk of infections.

The number of Americans aged over 65 years was 35 million in 2000 and expected to reach 69 million by 2030, accounting for approximately one fifth of the total U.S. population [10]. Infection in such a large section of the population is of considerable importance to public health. It is worth investigating potential modifiable factors, such as micronutrient supplements, that may reduce susceptibility to infection in this population. In this chapter the effects of micronutrient supplements on infection risks in this age group will be discussed in the light of recent data.

5.2 MICRONUTRIENTS

Micronutrients (trace elements and vitamins) are required in microgram quantities for correct function of the human body. Most micronutrients or their derivatives have central roles in certain biochemical pathways. All the required micronutrients should be available from a balanced diet, which includes fruit and vegetables, dairy products, and meat or pulses. Trace elements can be defined as those elements that (individually) make up no more than 0.01% of the dry weight of the body. Some are nonessential (e.g., lead), but others are required for normal health, function and development [11].

Vitamins are conventionally divided into two groups according to their solubility characteristics. The B group of vitamins and vitamin C are water-soluble, while vitamins A, D, E and K are insoluble in water but soluble in lipid or lipid solvents and are classified as fat-soluble vitamins. Fat-soluble vitamins are stored in the liver and are not easily excreted, so toxic overload is possible from excessive intake. Toxicity with water-soluble vitamins is less likely. Among the fat-soluble vitamins, A and E are extensively studied in relation to infections and immune markers.

Vitamin A refers to retinol and the carotenoids that are converted to retinol [12]. Preformed vitamin A can be obtained mostly from dietary animal sources (liver, fish liver oils, eggs, and dairy products), whereas carotenoids that can be converted into retinol are obtained from vegetables (dark-green leafy vegetables and deep-orange fruits). Vitamin A plays an essential role in a large number of physiological functions that encompass vision, growth, reproduction, hematopoiesis, and immunity [13]. The association between vitamin A and immunity was noticed even before its structure was realized in 1931 [14].

Vitamin E consists of a family of eight related compounds, the tocopherols and the tocotrienols. The major chemical forms of vitamin E are the tocopherols α, β, ℓ, and Δ. Gamma-tocopherol is the most abundant form in foods and is usually the form used in supplements [12].

5.3 MICRONUTRIENTS AND IMMUNE FUNCTION

Many factors, including, among others, age, genetic predisposition, smoking, and nutrition status, can affect immune functions. An adequate intake of vitamins and trace elements is required for the efficient function of the immune system [15] and protection from reactive oxygen species. A variety of reactive oxygen species are formed continuously in tissues by endogenous and exogenous mechanisms [16]. These free radicals are immunosuppressive. Antioxidant vitamins and trace elements (vitamins C, E, selenium, copper, and zinc) are free-radical scavenging nutrients that protect cells from damage by pro-oxidants [17,18].

Some evidence suggests that micronutrients, such as zinc, selenium, and β-carotene play an important role in maintaining a balance between cell-mediated and humoral immunity by regulating patterns of cytokine secretion [19–20]. Studies have also shown that low-dose supplementation of zinc and selenium leads to significant improvement in the humoral response following vaccination in elderly patients [21]. Vitamin A deficiency impairs both innate immunity (mucosal epithelial regeneration) and adaptive immune response to infection, resulting in impaired ability to counteract extracellular pathogens [22]. It is also associated with pathological changes in the respiratory system [23], gastrointestinal tract [24], genitourinary [25] and ocular tissues [13]. Vitamin D deficiency is correlated with a higher susceptibility to infections due to impaired localized innate immunity and defects in antigen-specific cellular immune response [26].

Most cells of the immune system, with the exception of B cells, express vitamin D receptors. In recent years there have been efforts to understand possible noncalcemic roles of vitamin D, including its role in the immune system. Some results suggest an important role for vitamin D in autoimmune disorders, providing a fertile and interesting area of research that may herald important new therapies [27].

Vitamin B6 is essential for nucleic acid and protein synthesis. It is an essential coenzyme for more than 60 enzymes, many of which are involved in the metabolism of aminoacids. Antibodies and cytokines are built up of aminoacids and require vitamin B6 as a coenzyme in their metabolism.

Folate plays a crucial role in nucleic acid and protein synthesis by supplying, in concert with vitamins B6 and B12, one carbon unit. Inadequate folate intake significantly alters the immune response. The major function of vitamin C is to control the redox potential within cells, acting as an antioxidant and scavenger for free radicals. Vitamin E is a powerful antioxidant. Being fat soluble, it is particularly important in protecting lipids, including cell membranes, from oxidative damage. Selenium is essential for optimum immune response and influences the innate and acquired immune systems. It plays a key role in the redox regulation and antioxidant function through glutathione peroxidase that removes excess of potentially damaging free radicals produced during oxidative stress.

Zinc is required for many enzymes either structurally or as a cofactor. These include enzymes involved in nucleic acid synthesis. It is essential for highly proliferating cells such as those in the immune system and so influences both innate and acquired immune functions. Copper is required for the activity of several enzymes, including superoxide dismutase. This enzyme is responsible for the destruction of free radicals. Copper has been shown to have a role in the development and maintenance of the immune system. It is reasonable to conclude that micronutrients can influence the body's defense through various mechanisms including proliferation of immune system cells, synthesis of proteins such as antibodies and scavenging of free radicals.

5.4 EFFECT OF MICRONUTRIENT SUPPLEMENTS ON THE AGING IMMUNE SYSTEM

Aging, even in the absence of nutritional deficiencies, is associated with impaired immune response, particularly the cell-mediated arm of the system. On the other hand, effects of micronutrient supplements on different surrogate markers of immune response (e.g., antibody titers, delayed-type hypersensitivity responses and cytokine production) have been investigated in this age group, using a variety of study designs. Most of these studies reported an enhancement of at least one surrogate marker. Vitamins A, C, E, zinc, and selenium supplementation were shown to have beneficial effects on the immune system [28]. Vitamin A supplementation to preschool children is known to decrease the risks of mortality and morbidity from some forms of infections. These effects are likely to be the result of the actions of vitamin A on immunity. Some of the immunomodulatory mechanisms of vitamin A have been described [29]. Also, ß-carotene in high doses has been described as stimulating delayed-type hypersensitivity [30]. Vitamin C may enhance immune functions such as phagocytosis, neutrophil chemotaxis and lymphocyte proliferation [31,32]. But contrasting findings of vitamin C have also been published [33].

Meydani et al. [34], studied the effect of vitamin E supplementation on immune response *in vivo* in 88 healthy elderly subjects. They were randomized to a placebo group or groups receiving 60, 200, or 800 mg/d of vitamin E for 4 months. Their results indicate that a level of vitamin E greater than what is currently recommended enhances certain clinically relevant *in vivo* indexes of T-cell-mediated functions in healthy elderly persons. No adverse effects were observed with vitamin E supplementation. Another 3-month intervention trial among apparently healthy elderly subjects demonstrated no effect of 100 mg alpha-tocopheryl acetate on the overall immune responsiveness of this population [35]. This finding was consistent with that of Meydani et al.

Combined vitamin supplementation has been shown to enhance the immune response of elderly individuals. Penn et al. randomized 30 elderly subjects to receive either placebo or dietary supplementation with physiological doses of vitamins A, C, and E for 28 days [36]. Following vitamin supplementation, cell-mediated immune function improved. In contrast, no significant changes were noted in the immune function of the placebo group. Another study demonstrated improvement of immune function in elderly females after consumption of 1 g of vitamin C and 200 mg of vitamin E daily for 16 weeks [31]. Wolvers et al. [37] demonstrated, in a recent study, enhancement of delayed-type hypersensitivity in elderly subjects (average 57 +/– 10 y) who received a mix of micronutrient supplements (vitamin E, C, ß-carotene, and zinc) for 10 weeks, compared with a placebo group. Fortes et al. [38] found an improvement in the cell-mediated immune response following zinc supplementation (25mg zinc sulphate). However, vitamin A (800 ug retinol palmitate) had a negative effect on immune indicators in the older population in the same study.

Several studies reported some changes in the immune system following administration of micronutrients. The observed effect of these supplements on immune response does not necessarily imply a beneficial clinical outcome for the subjects receiving these supplements. Studying the clinical effects, such as frequency and severity of infectious episodes, has much greater relevance.

5.5   EFFECTS OF MICRONUTRIENT SUPPLEMENTS ON FREQUENCY AND SEVERITY OF INFECTIONS

One of the earliest clinical trials to investigate such clinical effects was conducted in France by Chavance et al. in 1989 [39]. This trial enrolled a total of 218 subjects over 60 years of age. The participants received either multivitamin supplements or placebo for 4 months. No significant difference was found between the two groups in the incidence of infections. In fact, the observed incidences were higher in the treatment group than in the placebo group.

Girodon et al. [40] reported results of a large trial in which 725 institutionalized elderly patients from 25 geriatric centers in France were separated into four groups and randomized to receive vitamins (ß-carotene, ascorbic acid, and vitamin E), minerals (zinc and selenium sulphide), both, or neither. The trial showed an enhanced antibody response to the influenza vaccine and a reduction in the incidence of respiratory infections in the minerals group (P = 0.06), but not in the vitamins group. Supplementation with either trace elements or vitamins significantly reduced the incidence of urogenital infections. Survival analysis for the 2 years, to exclude seasonal variation, did not show any differences among the 4 groups and any beneficial effects of mineral supplementation may be due to the correction of subclinical deficiencies in those who received such supplementations.

In another study from the Netherlands [41], a total of 652 non-institutionalized individuals aged 60 years or more were enrolled. Physiological doses of multivitamin and minerals, 200 mg of vitamin E, both, or placebo, were given for 15 months. Neither daily multivitamin and mineral supplementation at physiological doses nor 200 mg of vitamin E showed a favorable effect on incidence and severity of acute respiratory tract infections. Instead, adverse effects of vitamin E on illness severity were observed.

A study by Meydani et al. [42] reported that supplementation with 200 IU per day of vitamin E for 1 year, did not have a statistically significant effect on the incidence of lower respiratory tract infections in elderly nursing home residents. However, they observed a protective effect of vitamin E supplementation on upper respiratory tract infections, particularly the common cold. A U.S. study in primary care found that multivitamin and multimineral supplements had no significant clinical effects on infections in people aged 65 and over [43].

Barringer and colleagues assessed the effect of a typical 1-a-day multivitamin and mineral supplement for 1 year on infection rate among individuals aged 45 years or older. They demonstrated a reduction in incidence of infection. However, in subgroup analyses, persons with diabetes had the largest benefit in infection-related outcomes; this accounted for most of the overall observed effect. Correction of micronutrient deficiencies would be the most likely explanation for their results.

Merchant et al. evaluated the associations between intakes of antioxidants and B vitamins and the risk of community-acquired pneumonia in well-nourished middle-aged and older men [44]. This was a prospective study conducted among 38,378 male health professionals, aged 44 to 79. There were no associations between total intakes of antioxidants or B vitamins and the risk of pneumonia.

They concluded that vitamin supplements are unlikely to reduce the risk of pneumonia in well-nourished, middle-aged and elderly men.

A meta-analysis of randomized controlled trials found the evidence for multivitamin and mineral supplements on the risk of infections in older people to be weak and conflicting [45]. However, an updated review for this meta-analysis concluded there was no benefit for the use of multivitamins in preventing infections in the elderly [46]. A trial conducted by Avenell et al. [47] largely confirms previous research. They found that routine multivitamin and multimineral supplementation in older people (910 men and women aged 65 or over) living at home does not affect self-reported infection-related morbidity. Participants were recruited from six general practices in Grampian, Scotland. The limitation of this study was the low doses of multivitamins and multiminerals used. This trial provided good evidence against the efficiency of multivitamin supplementation in preventing symptoms of acute respiratory infection among healthy elderly subjects. While there is evidence linking micronutrient supplementation to changes in immune responses, their roles in reducing the risk of infections in well nourished elderly require careful consideration.

5.6   PROBLEMS WITH MICRONUTRIENT SUPPLEMENTS

There is no standard definition for multivitamins; any product containing two or more vitamins or trace elements can be listed as a multivitamin. The commonly used multivitamin supplement contains at least 10 vitamins and 10 minerals [48]. The potential for adverse effects from excessive lipid-soluble vitamins, such as vitamin A, is well documented [49]. Higher doses of zinc and vitamin A supplements impair cellular immunity and the health of bones among older people with vitamin D deficiency [50,51]. Recent studies have suggested that beta carotene may act as a co-carcinogen [52,53]. Also, supplementation with high doses of ß-carotene, five times the nutritional requirement, led to an increased incidence of lung cancers [54]. Bjelakovic et al. did a systematic review to analyze the effects of antioxidant supplements (beta carotene, vitamins A, E, C, and selenium) on all causes of mortality in adults [55]. They included antioxidant supplements at any dose, duration, and route of administration. Then they analyzed the antioxidants administered singly, in combination with other antioxidants, or with other vitamins or trace elements. They found that ß-carotene, vitamin A, and vitamin E given singly or combined with another antioxidant supplement significantly increased mortality. In another study, vitamin E seemed to worsen the severity of infections [56]. After exclusion of high-bias risk trials, however, vitamin E given singly or combined with other micronutrients significantly increased mortality. This is in agreement with a recent meta-analysis [57]. The possible harm of micronutrient supplements is another factor that requires consideration.

5.7   CONCLUSION

Aging is often associated with a decline in immunocompetence, particularly in T cell-mediated functions. Nutrient deficiencies can contribute to further impairments in immune function in the elderly and thus render them even more vulnerable to acute and chronic infections than they would be if they were nutrient sufficient. Although micronutrients may help normalize certain parameters in the immune system, in elderly subjects suffering from nutritional deficiencies several clinical studies argued that those changes have no demonstrable clinical benefits in terms of reduction of mortality and morbidity in adequately nourished elderly people. From the above studies it is clear that the healthy elderly population received no benefit from these supplements in terms of prevention of infections, although it is possible that nutritionally deprived individuals may have benefited. However, concerns about the potential side effects of micronutrients should make well-nourished persons cautious about taking such supplements.

REFERENCES

1. Huang H-Y, Caballero B, Chang S, Alberg A J, Semba R D et al. 2006. The efficiency and safety of multivitamin and mineral supplement use to prevent cancer and chronic disease in adults: A systematic review for a National Institute of Health State–of–the Science Conference. *Ann Intern Med.* 145, 372–385.

2. Sloan E. How and why do we use supplements? 2006. A National Institutes of Health State–of–the Science Conference on Multivitamin/Mineral Supplements and Chronic Disease Prevention. Bethesda, MD: U.S. Department of Health and Human Services. 25–28.

3. Fairfield K M and Fletcher R H. 2002. Vitamins for chronic disease prevention in adults. *JAMA* 287 (23), 3116–3126.

4. Johnson K A, Bernard M A and Funderburg K. 2002. Vitamin nutrition in older adults. *Clin Geriatr Med* 18, 773–799.

5. Hickson M. 2006. Malnutrition and aging. *Postgrad Med J.* 82, 2–8.

6. Bales C W, Steinman L C, Freeland-Graves J H et al. 1986. The effect of age on plasma zinc uptake and taste acuity. *Am J Clin Nutr.* 44, 664–669.

7. Roe D A. 1985. Drug effects on nutrient absorption, transport, and metabolism. *Drug Nutrient Interact* 4, 117–135.

8. Ory M G, Lipman P D, Karlen P L, Gerety M B, Stevens V J, Singh M A et al. 2002. Recruitment of older participants in frailty/injury prevention studies. *Prev Sci* 3, 1–22.

9. Nicholson K G, Kent J, Hammersley V, Cancio E. 1997. Acute viral infections of upper respiratory tract in elderly people living in the community: Comparative, prospective, population based study of disease burden. *BMJ* 315,1060–1064.

10. Curns A T, Holman R C, Sejvar J J, Owings M F, Schonberger L B. 2005. Infectious disease hospitalizations among older adults in the United States from 1990 through 2002. *Arch Intern Med.* 165, 2514–2520.

11. Taylor A. 1996. Detection and monitoring of disorders of essential trace elements. *Ann Clin Biochem* 33, 486–510.

12. Fairfield K M and Fletcher R H. 2002. Vitamins for chronic disease prevention in adults. *JAMA* 287 (23), 3116–3126.

13. Sommer, A. and West K P. 1996. Vitamin A deficiency: Health, survival, and vision. New York: Oxford University Press.

14. Karrer P, Morf R, Schöpp K. 1931. Zur kenntnis des vitamins-A aus fischtranen. Helv. *Chim. Acta* 14, 1036–1040.

15. Lesourd B M. 1995. Protein undernutrition as the major cause of decreased immune function in the elderly: Clinical and functional implications. *Nutr Rev.* 53. suppl, S86–S94.

16. Frei B. 1994. Reactive oxygen species and antioxidant vitamins: Mechanisms of action. *Am J Med.* 97:5S–13S.

17. Machlin L J, Bendich A. 1987. Free radical tissue damage: Protective role of antioxidant nutrients. *FASEB J* 1, 441–445.

18. Wintergerst E S, Maggini S, Hornig D H. 2007. Contribution of selected vitamins and trace elements to immune function. *Ann Nutr Metab.* 51. 4, 301–23.

19. Beck F W, Prasad A S, Kaplan J, Fitzgerald J T, Brewer G J. 1997. Changes in cytokine production and T cell subpopulations in experimentally induced zinc-deficient humans. *Am. J. Physiol.* 272, E1002–E1007.

20. Scott M E, Koski K G. 2000. Zinc impairs immune responses against parasitic nematode infections at intestinal and systemic sites. *J. Nutr.* 130, 1412S–1420S.

21. Girodon F, Galan P, Monget A-L, Boutron-Ruault M-C, Brunter-Lecomte P, Preziosi P et al. 1999. Impact of trace elements and vitamin supplementation on immunity and infections in institutionalized elderly patients. A randomized controlled trial. *Arch Intern Med* 159, 748–54.

22. Wintergerst E S, Maggini S, Hornig D H. 2007. Contribution of selected vitamins and trace elements to immune function. *Ann Nutr Metab.* 51(4), 301–23.

23. McDowell E M, Keenan K P, Huang M. 1984. Effects of vitamin A-deprivation on hamster tracheal epithelium. A quantitative morphologic study. *Virchows Arch B Cell Pathol Incl Mol Pathol.* 45(2), 197–219.

24. Warden R A, Strazzari M J, Dunkley P R and O'Loughlin E V. 1996. Vitamin A-deficient rats have only mild changes in jejunal structure and function. *J. Nutr.* 126, 1817–1826.

25. Molloy C J and Laskin J D. 1988. Effect of retinoid deficiency on keratin expression in mouse bladder. *Exp Mol Pathol.* 49, 128–140.

26. Wintergerst E S, Maggini S, Hornig D H. 2007. Contribution of selected vitamins and trace elements to immune function. *Ann Nutr Metab.* 51(4), 301–23.

27. Deluca HF, Cantorna MT. 2001. Vitamin D: Its role and uses in immunology. *FASEB J.* 15. 14, 2579–85.

28. Lesourd B M. 1997. Nutrition and immunity in the elderly. *Am J Clin Nutr* 66, 478s–84s.

29. Villamor E and Fawzi WW. Effects of Vitamin A supplementation on immune responses and correlation with clinical outcomes. 2005. *Clin Microbiol Rev.* 18(3), 446–464.

30. Herraiz L A, Hsieh W C, Parker R S, Swanson J E, Bendich A, Roe D A. 1998. Effect of UV exposure and beta-carotene supplementation on delayed-type hypersensitivity response in healthy older men. *J Am Coll Nutr* 17, 617–624.

31. de la Fuente M, Ferrandez M D, Burgos M S, Soler A, Prieto A, Miquel J. Immune function in aged women is improved by ingestion of vitamin C and E. 1998. *Can J Physiol Pharmacol.* 76, 373–380.

32. Jayachandran M, Rani P J A, Arivazhagan P. 2000. Neutrophil phagocytic function and humeral immune response with reference to ascorbate supplementation in aging humans. *J Anti-Aging Med* 3, 37.

33. Delafuente J C, Prendergast J M, Modigh A. 1986. Immunologic modulation by vitamin C in the elderly. *Int J Immunopharmacol.* 8, 205–211.

34. Meydani S N, Meydani M, Blumberg J B, Leka L S, Siber G, Loszewski R, Thompson C, Pedrosa M C, Diamond R D, Stollar B D. 1997. Vitamin E supplementation and *in vivo* immune response in healthy elderly subjects. A randomized controlled trial. *JAMA* 277(17), 1380–6.

35. De Waart B F, Portengen L, Doekes G, Verwaal C J, Kok F J. 1997. Effect of 3 months vitamin E supplementation on indices of the cellular and humoral immune response in elderly subjects. *Br J Nutr* 78, 761–774.

36. Penn N D, Purkins L, Kelleher J, Heatley R V, Mascie-Taylor B H, Belfield P W. 1991. The effect of dietary supplementation with vitamin A, C and E on cell=mediated immune function in elderly long=stay patients: A randomized control trial. *Age aging* 20, 169–74.

37. Wolvers D A, Herpen-Broekmans W M. 2006. Effect of a mixture of micronutrients, but not of bovine colostrums concentrate, on immune function parameters in healthy volunteers: A randomized placebo-controlled study. *Nutr J* 5, 28 doi:10. 1186/1475–2891–5–28.

38. Fortes C, Forastiere F, Agabiti N, Fano F, Pacifici R, Virgili F et al. 1998. The effect of zinc and vitamin A supplementation on immune response in an older population. *JAGS.* 46, 19–26.

39. Chavance M, Herbeth B, Lemoine A, Zhu B-P. 1993. Does multivitamin supplementation prevent infections in healthy elderly subjects? A controlled trial. *Int J Vit Nutr Res* 63, 11–6.

40. Girodon F, Galan P, Monget A-L, Boutron-Ruault M-C, Brunter-Lecomte P et al. 1999. Impact of trace elements and vitamin supplementation on immunity and infections in institutionalized elderly patients. A randomized controlled trial. *Arch Intern Med* 159, 748–54.

41. Graat J M, Schouten E G, Kok F J. 2002. Effect of daily vitamin E and multivitamin-mineral supplementation on acute respiratory tract infections in elderly persons: A randomized controlled trial. *JAMA* 288, 715–721.

42. Meydani S N, Leka L S, Fine B C, Dallal G E, Keusch G T, Singh M F, Hamer D H. 2004. Vitamin E and respiratory tract infections in elderly nursing home residents: A randomized controlled trial. *JAMA* 292, 828–836.

43. Barringer T A, Kirk J K, Santaniello A C, Foley K L, Michielutte R. 2003. Effect of a multivitamin and mineral supplement on infection and quality of life. A randomized, double-blind, placebo-controlled trial. *Ann Intern Med* 138, 365–71.

44. Merchant A T, Curhan G, Bendich A, Sing V N, Willett W C and Fawzi W W. 2004. Vitamin Intake Is not associated with community-acquired pneumonia in U.S. men. *J. Nutr.* 134, 439–444.

45. El-Kadiki A, Sutton A J. 2005. Role of multivitamins and mineral supplements in preventing infections in elderly people: Systematic review and meta-analysis of randomised controlled trials. *BMJ* 330, 871–4.

46. Sutton A, El-Kadiki A. Assessing concerns regarding the validity of three trials included in Role of multivitamins and mineral supplements in preventing infections in elderly people: Systematic review and meta-analysis of randomised controlled trials. http://bmj.bmjjournals. com/cgi/content/full/bmj. 38399. 495648. 8F/DC2. Accessed 30 Dec. 07.

47. Avenell A, Campbell M K, Cook J A, Hannaford P C, Kilonozo M M, McNeil G et al. 2005. Effect of multivitamin and multimineral supplements on morbidity from infections in older people. MAVIS trial: Pragmatic, randomised, double blind, placebo controlled trial. *BMJ* 331, 324–329.

48. Huang H-Y, Caballero B, Chang S, Alberg A J, Semba R D, Schenyer C R et al. 2006. The efficacy and safety of multivitamin and mineral supplement use to prevent cancer and chronic disease in adults: A systematic review for a National Institutes of Health State-of-the-Science Conference. July 31.

49. Hathcock J N. 1997. Vitamins and minerals: Efficacy and safety. *Am J Clin Nutr* 66, 427–437.

50. Gariballa S E, Sinclair A J. 1998. Nutrition, ageing and ill–health. *Br J Nutr* 80, 7–21.

51. Scientific Advisory Committee on Nutrition. Review on dietary advice on vitamin A. www. sacn. gov. uk/news/2005_04. html. accessed 1 Aug 2005.

52. Paolini M, Abdel-Rahman S Z, Sapone A et al. 2003. Beta-carotene: A cancer chemopreventive agent or a co-carcinogen? *Mutat Res.* 543:195–200.

53. Lee B M, Park K K. 2003. Beneficial and adverse effects of chemopreventive agents. *Mutat Res.* 523–524:265–278.

54. The Alpha-Tocopherol, Beta Carotene Cancer Prevention Study Group. 1994. The effect of vitamin E and beta carotene on the incidence of lung cancer and other cancers in male smokers. *N Eng J Med.* 330; 1029–1035.

55. Bjelakovic G, Nikolova D, Gluud L L, Simonetti R G, Gluud C. 2007. Mortality in randomized trials of antioxidant supplements for primary and secondary prevention. Systematic review and meta-analysis. *JAMA.* 297, 842–857.

56. Graat J M, Schouten E G, Kok F J. 2002. Effect of daily vitamin E and multivitamin-mineral supplementation on acute respiratory infections in elderly persons. A randomized controlled trial. *JAMA* 288, 715–21.

57. Miller E R III, Pastor-Barriuso R, Dalal D, Riemersma R A, Appel L J, Guallar E. 2005. Meta-analysis: High-dosage vitamin E supplementation may increase all-cause mortality. *Ann Intern Med.* 142, 37–46.

6 Antioxidants and Heart Disease

Vijaya Juturu and Vidyasagar Sriramoju

CONTENTS

6.1 ANTIOXIDANTS

Antioxidants, natural substances that exist as vitamins, minerals, and other compounds in foods, are classified into hydrophilic and hydrophobic. Water-soluble antioxidants react with oxidants in the cell cytoplasm and the blood/plasma. Lipid-soluble antioxidants protect cell membranes from lipid peroxidation and free radicals. The antioxidant defense of some of the compounds are by chelating transition metals such as selenium and zinc and enhancing the activity of antioxidant enzymes and preventing them from catalyzing the production of free radicals in the cell. Biological functions of antioxidants are reported in Table 6.1.

6.2 CELLULAR DAMAGE, OXIDATION, AND ANTIOXIDANTS

Oxidation is a chemical reaction that transfers electrons from a substance to an oxidizing agent. The oxidation reactions produce free radicals and damage cells. An imbalance between oxidants and antioxidants in favor of the oxidants, potentially leading to damage, is termed oxidative stress.

Oxidation of low-density lipoprotein (LDL) is believed to contribute to the development of atherosclerosis [1]. Macrophage cells preferentially take up oxidized LDL, become loaded with lipids, and convert into "foam cells" [2]. Foam cells accumulate in fatty streaks, early signs of atherosclerosis. Humans produce auto-antibodies against oxidized LDL, and the levels of such auto-antibodies are higher in patients with atherosclerosis [1].

The identification of LDL oxidation as a key event in atherosclerosis suggests that it may be possible to reduce the risk of atherosclerosis by antioxidant supplementation [2].

6.3 DIETARY INTAKE OF ANTIOXIDANTS

Antioxidants are present in foods as vitamins, minerals, carotenoids, and polyphenols, among others. Many antioxidants are often identified in food by their distinctive colors—the deep red of cherries and tomatoes; the orange of carrots; the yellow of corn, mangos, and saffron; and the blue-purple of blueberries, blackberries, and grapes. The best-known components of food with antioxidant activities are vitamins A, C, and E; β-carotene; the mineral selenium; and more recently, the compound lycopene. In the Iowa women's health study, the dietary intakes of flavanones, anthocyanidins, and certain foods rich in flavonoids were associated with reduced risk of death due to coronary heart disease (CHD), cardiovascular disease (CVD), and all causes [3].

In the NHANES survey (1999–2000), 52% of adults reported taking a dietary supplement; 35% took a multivitamin/multimineral and 12 to 13% were using vitamin E supplements [4]. In the Rotterdam study [5], the relationship of vitamin E with disease of the arteries was reported in 4,367 Netherland subjects, aged 55–94 years who had no previous CVD at baseline. In men, vitamin E intake was associated with lower arterial disease. Vitamin E intake was inversely associated with peripheral arterial disease.

In the SECURE trial, a total of 732 patients >/=55 years of age who had vascular disease or diabetes and at least one other risk factor and who did not have heart failure or a low left ventricular ejection fraction randomly received Ramipril 2.5 mg/d or 10 mg/d and vitamin E (RRR-alpha-tocopheryl acetate) 400 IU/d or their matching placebos [6]. There were no differences in atherosclerosis progression rates between the treatments after 4 years of follow-up. The relationship of vitamin E intake and change in tissue levels was associated with decreased risk of CVD in case-control and prospective cohort studies.

Overall, the studies support the conclusion that the association of vitamin E intake from food or supplements may reduce cardiac events. [7–19]. In two studies, no benefit from vitamin E supplementation on stroke [12] or MI [18] was observed. Low levels of α-tocopherol have been associated with increased risk for coronary artery disease. Higher serum concentrations of α-tocopherol (up to 13–14 mg/L, which is within the normal range) are associated with moderately lower total and cause-specific mortality in older male smokers [20]

6.4 ANTIOXIDANTS AND CARDIOVASCULAR DISEASE

In the women's antioxidant cardiovascular study [21], vitamin E (600 IU), beta carotene (50 mg) and vitamin C (500 mg) per day observed no significant changes in CVD morbidity and mortality or in the individual secondary outcomes of myocardial infarction, stroke, and coronary revascularization

TABLE 6.1
Biological Function of Antioxidants

Antioxidant	Biological Function
Carotenoids	
Beta-carotene	Neutralizes free radicals that may damage cells; bolsters cellular antioxidant defenses
Lutein, Zeaxanthin	May contribute to maintenance of healthy vision
Lycopene	May contribute to maintenance of prostate health
Flavonoids	
Anthocyanidins	Bolster cellular antioxidant defenses; may contribute to maintenance of brain function
Flavanols—Catechins, Epicatechins, Procyanidins	May contribute to maintenance of heart health; improves endothelial function and may reduce CVD risk
Flavanones	Neutralize free radicals that may damage cells; bolster cellular antioxidant defenses
Flavonols	Neutralize free radicals that may damage cells; bolster cellular antioxidant defenses
Proanthocyanidins	May contribute to maintenance of urinary tract health and heart health
Isothiocyanates	
Sulforaphane	May enhance detoxification of undesirable compounds and bolster cellular antioxidant defenses
Phenols	
Caffeic acid, Ferulic acid	May bolster cellular antioxidant defenses; may contribute to maintenance of healthy vision and heart health
Sulfides/Thiols	
Diallyl sulfide, Allyl methyl trisulfide	May enhance detoxification of undesirable compounds; may contribute to maintenance of heart health and healthy immune function
Dithiolthiones	Contribute to maintenance of healthy immune function
Resveretol	Protects cells from free radicals
Vitamins and minerals	
Vitamin A	Protects cells from free radicals
Vitamin E	Protects cells from free radicals, helps with immune function and DNA repair
Vitamin C	Protects cells from free radicals
Selenium	Protects cells from free radicals and enhances immune function
Other	
Carnosine	Attenuates cellular oxidative stress
Melatonin	Protects against cardiac ischemia/reperfusion
Carnitine	Increases cardiac output, improves heart muscle function, stimulates energy supply to the heart, increases endurance, enhances cardiac performance and regulates heart arrythmias; helps maintain blood lipid profile and promote fatty acid utilization within heart muscle
Lipoic acid	protect lipids against oxidation
Glutathione	neutralize free radicals which may damage cells

or CVD death. Vitamin E seems to have a marginal effect in the primary CVD outcome. In addition, the participants who received a combination of vitamin C and vitamin E seemed to have fewer strokes in the overall 9.4-year period of the study (Table 6.2).

In 2005, Tucker [22] reported that men consuming the combination of ≤5 servings of fruits and vegetables per day (FV/d) and ≤12% energy from saturated fat (SF) were 31% less likely to die of

TABLE 6.2

Summary of the Effects of Antioxidants on Cardiovascular Disease

Antioxidants	Observational Studies	Interventional Studies
Beta-carotene	Inverse association of intake and CHD mortality	Incidence of fatal CHD was significantly higher; significant increase in lung cancer mortality and a nonsignificant increase in CHD mortality
L-Carnitine	Heart muscle levels of L-carnitine are decreased in angina pectoris, myocardial infarction, and chronic coronary insufficiency	IncreaseS the heart's function or reduceS the side effects of drugs used to treat CHF.
Lutein, Zeaxanthin	Inverse association of intake and CHD mortality	No data available
Lycopene	Inverse association of intake and CHD mortality	No data available
Anthocyanidins	Inverse association of intake and CHD mortality	No data available
Flavonoids	Inverse association of intake and CHD mortality	Reduce platelet activation
Coenzyme Q10	Inverse association of intake and CHD mortality	Decreases LDL oxidation, but no event reduction data; may reduce symptoms and improve ejection fractions in patients with heart failure
Vitamin E	Inverse association of plasma vitamin E level and CHD mortality	Vitamin E significantly reduced the incidence of overall fatal and nonfatal CHD events by 47% and the incidence of nonfatal myocardial infarction by 77%; no significant effect on overall mortality (relative risk: 1.18). Event reduction was better with supplementation at 400 IU per day, but the study was not powered to assess dose–response significance; increased vitamin E levels are associated with decreased CHD mortality and inversely correlated with risk of angina; incidence of nonfatal myocardial infarction was lower
Vitamin C	Inverse association between plasma vitamin C and CHD mortality	Supports the antioxidant and endothelial effects of vitamin C; improves arterial vasoreactivity; no significant reduction in total or cerebrovascular mortality
Selenium	Inversely associated with CHD mortality	May help limit the oxidation of LDL

any cause ($P < 0.05$), and 76% less likely to die from CHD ($P < 0.001$), relative to those consuming <5 FV and >12% SF. Men consuming either low SF or high FV, but not both, did not have a significantly lower risk of total mortality; but did have 64–67% lower risk of CHD mortality ($P < 0.05$) relative to those doing neither. The Dietary Approaches to Stop Hypertension (DASH) Trial highlighted the role of higher FV intake in blood pressure control [23]. Based in large part on this trial, the recently released AHA Dietary Guidelines issued, for the first time, recommendations to choose ≥5 FV servings/d [24]. Data from the 1989–1991 USDA Continuing Survey of Food Intakes by Individuals revealed that only 12% of the U.S. adult population consumed the recommended two servings of fruit and three of vegetables per day [25]. Bazzano [26] reported that consuming fruit and vegetables ≥3 times/d compared with <1 time/d was associated with a 27% lower stroke incidence (relative risk [RR]: 0.73), a 42% lower stroke mortality (0.58), a 24% lower ischemic heart disease mortality (0.76), a 27% lower cardiovascular disease mortality (0.73), and a 15% lower all-cause mortality (0.85) after adjustment for established cardiovascular disease risk factors. Dauchet [27] reported that the risk of stroke was decreased by 11% (RR: 0.89) for each additional portion per day of fruit, by 5% (RR: 0.95) for fruit and vegetables, and by 3% (RR: 0.97) for vegetables.

This chapter summarizes different antioxidants and their effects on cardiovascular disease.

6.4.1 BETA-CAROTENE

Epidemiologic studies show an inverse association between serum/adipose β-carotene levels and coronary heart disease risk [8,15]. However, interventional trials have not shown any benefit, and perhaps even an adverse effect, of β-carotene supplementation [28]. The American Heart Association states that the evidence does not justify use of antioxidants such as beta-carotene for reducing the risk of cardiovascular disease.

6.4.2 CARNITINE

Acetyl l-carnitine enhances energy production by facilitating the transport of fatty acids into the energy-producing units in the cells. It increases cellular respiration, membrane potential and cardiolipin levels. Acetyl l-carnitine improves energy production within brain cells and is considered a neuro-protective agent because of its antioxidant action and membrane stabilizing effects [29]. The important functions of L-carnitine are increasing cardiac output, improving heart muscle function, stimulating energy supply to the heart, increasing endurance, enhancing cardiac performance, and regulating heart arrythmias. McMackin [30] reported that L cartinitine in combination with alpha lipoic acid treatment increased brachial artery diameter by 2.3% (P = .008), consistent with reduced arterial tone. The combined alpha-lipoic acid/acetyl-L-carnitine treatment tended to decrease systolic blood pressure for the whole group (P = .07) and had a significant effect in the subgroup with blood pressure above the median (151+/–20 to 142+/–18 mm Hg; P = .03) and in the subgroup with the metabolic syndrome (139+/–21 to 130+/–18 mm Hg; P = .03). This study suggests that mitochondrial dysfunction may contribute to the regulation of blood pressure and vascular tone. However, there is no substantial evidence to suggest a recommendation for reducing cardiac risk.

6.4.3 CARNOSINE

The amino acid carnosine is a natural antioxidant found in high concentrations in the brain, muscle tissue, and the lens of the human eye. It is also known to be an antioxidant capable of protecting cell membranes and other cell structures. Carnosine inhibits glycosylation and cross-linking of proteins induced by reactive aldehydes, and is effective in reducing advanced glycation end-products (AGE) formation by competing with proteins for binding with the sugars. The other additional functions of carnosine are as immunomodulator, neurotransmitter, metal ion chelator, and wound healing agent. It was demonstrated that carnosine was effective in overcoming muscle fatigue, lowering blood pressure, reducing stress and hyperactivity and inducing sleep. Carnosine has a protective effect, preserving nerve cells from damage and death, making it a promising treatment for patients with stroke. Carnosine attenuates cellular oxidative stress and can inhibit the intracellular formation of reactive oxygen species and reactive nitrogen species. Carnosine protects cardiomyocytes from damage and improves contractility of the heart [31]. Intervention trials are required to study its effects on cardiac events and risk.

6.4.4 FLAVONOIDS

A large number of epidemiological studies suggest that dietary factors, including increased intake of flavonoid-containing foods and beverages, reduce cardiovascular risk, and recent studies have shown that such beverages have favorable effects on endothelial function [32]. Consumption of epigallocatechin gallate (EGCG), or green tea extract, improves endothelial function and may reduce CVD risk. Dietary flavonoids (mainly quercetin) were inversely associated with stroke incidence after adjustment for potential confounders, including antioxidant vitamins. The relative risk (RR) of the highest vs. the lowest quartile of flavonoid intake (>or = 28.6 mg/d vs <18.3 mg/d) was 0.27 (95% confidence interval [CI], 0.11 to 0.70). Lekakis [33] reported that red grape polyphenol extract (600 mg, contained 4.32 mg epicatechin, 2.72 mg catechin, 2.07 mg gallic acid, 0.9 mg trans-resveratrol, 0.47 mg rutin, 0.42 mg epsilon-viniferin, 0.28 mg, p-coumaric acid, 0.14 mg ferulic acid and 0.04 mg quercetin per gram) caused an increase in flow-mediated dilatation, peaking at 60 min, which was significantly higher than the baseline values (4.52+/–1.34 versus 2.6+/–1.5%; P < 0.001) and the corresponding values at 60 min after the intake of placebo (4.52+/–1.34 vs. 2.64+/–1.8%, P < 0.001).

Epidemiological studies report that quercetin, an antioxidant flavonol found in apples, berries, and onions, is associated with reduced risk of coronary heart disease and stroke [34,35]. Quercetin supplementation also reduces blood pressure in hypertensive rodents. Quercetin is a flavonol that belongs to a group of polyphenolic compounds known as flavonoids. In a randomized, double-blind, placebo-controlled, crossover study, 730 mg quercetin for 28 d reduces systolic, diastolic, and mean arterial pressure in subjects with stage 1 hypertension. The quercetin-induced lowering of systolic blood pressure observed in stage 1 hypertensive subjects (–7.2 mm Hg) is clinically relevant because reductions of this magnitude are associated with a decrease in mortality of ~14% from stroke and ~9% from coronary heart disease [36]. These studies suggest that flavonoid compounds can be used as adjunct therapy in reducing coronary risk factors.

6.4.5 GLUTATHIONE

Glutathione is a cysteine-containing peptide. It has antioxidant properties, since the thiol group in its cysteine moiety is a reducing agent and can be reversibly oxidized and reduced. The reduced form of glutathione reduces other metabolites and enzyme systems as well as reacting directly with oxidants. The level of oxidized glutathione in serum serves as an index of myocardial oxidative stress during and after reperfusion [37]. Due to its high concentration and its central role in maintaining the cell's redox state, glutathione is one of the most important cellular antioxidants. The concentration of glutathione declines with age and in some age-related diseases [38].

6.4.6 LIPOIC ACID

Lipoic acid, needed for mitochondrial function, is also an antioxidant. It is made in our cells and participates as a co-factor in the conversion of carbohydrates to energy. It can eliminate free radicals in the water compartment of the cell, similar to vitamin C, and protect lipids against oxidation similar to vitamin E. Lipoic acid is the only antioxidant that can boost the level of intracellular glutathione, a cellular antioxidant of tremendous importance. Alpha-lipoic acid increases the ability of blood vessels to release nitric oxide and to relax blood vessels. This will help to improve the changes that take place in vascular disease [30].

6.4.7 LUTEIN

Increased dietary intake of lutein is protective against the development of early atherosclerosis. In the Los Angeles Atherosclerosis Study, participants with no history of heart disease or stroke observed the highest levels of lutein and averaged only a 0.004 mm increase in artery thickness over 18 months (whereas those with the lowest levels of lutein increased an average of 0.021 mm [39]).

6.4.8 LYCOPENE

Lycopene, an antioxidant carotenoid without provitamin A activity, has been shown to be a more potent antioxidant than other common dietary carotenoids, alpha-, or beta-carotene, found in tomatoes. In a cross-sectional analysis, low plasma levels (lower than the median) of lycopene were associated with an 18% increase in intima-media thickness in men, compared with men whose plasma levels of lycopene were higher. Low serum level of lycopene (the lowest quarter) had a greater than threefold risk of an acute coronary event or stroke as compared with others. Lycopene intake may have a protective role in prevention of CVD [40].

6.4.9 MELATONIN

Melatonin is a powerful antioxidant that can easily cross cell membranes and the blood–brain barrier. It does not undergo redox cycling, which is the ability of a molecule to undergo repeated reduction and oxidation. Melatonin, once oxidized, cannot be reduced to its former state because it forms several stable end-products upon reacting with free radicals. Melatonin protects against cardiac ischemia/reperfusion (I/R)-induced mitochondrial oxidative damage and is well documented as an antioxidant agent that prevents or modulates the production of reactive oxygen species (ROS) responsible for the reperfusion injury by upregulating cytochrome C [41].

6.4.10 PROANTHOCYANIDINS

Grape seeds are typically available as byproducts from wine manufacturing. Extracts from either grape seeds or pine bark yield compounds known as oligomeric procyanthocyanidins (OPCs). OPCs, a group of closely related compounds that are strong antioxidants, scavenge both water- and fat-soluble oxidants. Light to moderate alcohol consumption was found to be associated with an approximately 20% reduction in the risk for ischemic stroke and may even be beneficial in preventing subsequent strokes. The risk of CHD decreased by ~20% (RR = 0.80, 95% confidence interval [CI]: 0.78–0.83) when 0 to 2 drinks of alcohol were consumed per day. The consumption of alcohol 3 to 4 days per week decreased the risk of MI by 32% (RR = 0.68, 95% CI: 0.55–0.84), regardless of the type of alcoholic beverage consumed [42].

6.4.11 VITAMIN C

Vitamin C is one of the most popular and commonly used water-soluble antioxidant vitamins in the United States. Its administration enhances the contractile response to dobutamine and improves myocardial efficiency in patients with heart failure [43]. Some studies have reported no benefits of a daily dose of 700 mg or more, while other research reports that daily low-dose vitamin C (45 mg or more) may reduce the risk of death from stroke [44]. Vitamin C does not appear to lower cholesterol levels or reduce the risk of heart attacks. Effects on cholesterol plaques in heart arteries (atherosclerosis) remain unclear, and some studies suggest possible beneficial vasodilation (artery opening) properties [45]. Prospective cohort studies suggest that maximum reduction of CHD risk may require vitamin C intakes [46,47].

6.4.12 VITAMIN E

Vitamin E may inhibit the development and proliferation of LDL oxidation but no reduction in atheroma size [48]. In the Antioxidant Supplementation in Atherosclerosis Prevention (ASAP) study, a combined supplementation with reasonable doses of both vitamin E and slow-release vitamin C can retard the progression of common carotid atherosclerosis in men. Vitamin E supplementation improves the imbalance of oxidative stress and antioxidant status in plasma but not in plaque [49]. Marchioli [50] reported that vitamin E had a nonsignificant 20% (95% confidence intervals 0.92–1.56, P = 0.18) increased risk of developing congestive heart failure (CHF). Vitamin E treatment, however, was associated with a significant 50% increase (95% CI 1.03–2.20, P = 0.034) of CHF in patients with left ventricular dysfunction (ejection fraction < 50%). The Heart Outcomes Prevention Evaluation (HOPE) Study showed a neutral impact for vitamin E (400 IU/day with 5 years of follow-up) on a range of CVD outcomes [51]. Williams [52] showed benefits of vitamin E for intermittent claudication. In another small double-blind crossover study no relationship between 1600 IU/day of vitamin E and symptoms of angina were observed [53]. Overall, the evidence of tocopherol on secondary prevention is inconclusive.

The primary prevention studies [54–58], suggest that there is insufficient evidence to support a relationship between vitamin E and reduction of risk of CVD.

A vitamin E-supplemented group had lower mortality of ischemic heart disease (602/637) and ischemic stroke death rates (56,67) than a non-supplemented group [56]. In the secondary analyses, [54] a statistically significant beneficial effect for vitamin E on the incidence of angina pectoris and no beneficial effects were observed for incidence of major coronary events [58] or intermittent claudication [57]. Takamatsu [55], observed that the frequency of coronary disorders was higher in the control group than in the group receiving vitamin E. Some of these studies were not designed to measure the association between vitamin E and reduced risk of CVD. Further studies are required to focus on the effect of tocopherol on CVD mortality risk and the progression/regression of heart disease only (with no other chronic conditions) in long-term trials.

6.4.13 RESVERATOL

Resveratrol may reduce the risk of heart disease, cancer, blood clots, and stroke. Red grapes and their juice, and red wine contain resveratrol. Animal studies support the evidence that resveratol in combination with statin may be more effective or beneficial during the ischemic scenario than statin alone [59]. The heart weight/tibial length ratio of vehicle-treated myosin-immunized rats was increased by 1.8-fold compared with unimmunized rats, and resveratrol attenuated the heart weight increase [60]. Resveratrol significantly decreased cellular infiltration, fibrosis, and expression of inflammatory cytokines in the myocardium. Expressions of antioxidant genes were increased in myosin-immunized hearts, and resveratrol decreased those expressions. Resveratrol also attenuated myocarditis 21 days after immunization. SIRT1, a potential effector of resveratrol, was increased in the myocardium of myosin-immunized rats compared with unimmunized rats. The SIRT1 protein was localized mainly in infiltrating mononuclear cells. These studies suggest that resveratrol enhances immune function and protects cardiac injury. Controlled human clinical trials are required to study the effects of resveratrol on cardiac events and risk. Resveratrol may be a therapeutic modality for myocarditis.

6.4.14 ELLAGIC ACID

Ellagic acid is a phenolic compound that may decrease cholesterol levels. Ellagic acid is found in red grapes, kiwifruit, blueberries, raspberries, strawberries, blackberries, and currants. In doses of 0.5–1 mg/kg, ellagic acid causes a marked antioxidant effect in animals [61].

6.4.15 SELENIUM

Epidemiological studies have provided some evidence for the role of selenium deficiency in the etiology of atherosclerotic disease [62]. This mineral helps strengthen the heart's energy-producing system and protects the heart muscle from deterioration. The heart needs a selenium-containing protein called selenoproteins G. Selenium deficiency results in inadequate amounts of this selenoprotein in the heart, which causes structural damage. Cardiomyopathy associated with low selenium intake has been described in areas of exceptionally low selenium intake and in patients receiving total parenteral nutrition. An inverse association between the incidence of ischaemic heart disease and selenium intake has been described in population comparisons. Selenium deficiency causes myopathy as a result of the depletion of selenium-associated enzymes, which protect cell membranes from damage by free radicals [63]. Selenium supplementation increased selenium from 82 micrograms/l to 122 micrograms/l (p < 0.001 and remained unaltered in the placebo group (83 micrograms/l). During the 6-month follow-up period there were four cardiac deaths in the placebo group whereas no patients in the selenium group died during the follow-up period [64]. Further long-term studies are required on selenium supplementation effects on cardiac events.

6.4.16 COENZYME Q10

Coenzyme Q10, or ubiquinone, is a lipid-soluble vitamin found naturally within the mitochondria. Coenzyme Q10 is responsible for oxidative phosporylation in the myocardium and acts as a free radical scavenger in the event of lipid peroxidation.

A unique form of ubiquinone (UbiQGel) has FDA Orphan Drug status for the treatment of mitochondrial cytopathies. Supplementation with CoQ10 significantly affects endothelium-bound ecSOD activity. Mohr [65] reported that intake of a single oral dose of 100 or 200 mg CoQ increased the total plasma coenzyme content by 80 or 150%, respectively, within 6 h. Long-term supplementation (three times 100 mg CoQ/day) resulted in fourfold enrichment of CoQH2 in plasma and LDL with the latter containing 2.8 CoQH2 molecules per LDL particle (on day 11). Approximately 80% of the coenzyme was present as CoQH2 and the CoQH2/CoQ ratio was unaffected by supplementation, indicating that the redox state of coenzyme Q10 is tightly controlled in the blood. This study suggests that an oral supplementation of CoQ10 increases the resistance of LDL to radical oxidation.

6.5   HERBAL ANTIOXIDANT ACTIVITY

Several epidemiological studies reported that fruits and vegetables were found to be good sources of antioxidants. All health organizations are recommending and encouraging people to consume more fruits and vegetables [5,6,8,12,18,22,23,26,34].

6.5.1 GREEN TEA

Green tea, thea sinesis, has long been consumed in Asian cultures. It has recently surfaced in Western society as another herbal remedy demonstrating antioxidant activity. Polyphenols found in green tea are postulated to possess antioxidant properties. Lipophylic polyphenols act as scavengers of free radicals, they make up a hydroxyl group of rich substances capable of breaking chain reactions upon LDL particles. Studies have shown that drinking around three cups of tea each day can reduce the incidence of heart attack by 11% and the rate of death from heart disease by 11% [66,67]. Taubert [68] reported that tea consumption involving a total of 343 subjects with a median duration of 4 weeks reported no significant effects on blood pressure. The estimated pooled changes were 0.4 mm Hg (95% CI, –1.3 to 2.2 mm Hg; $P = .63$) in systolic and –0.6 mm Hg (95% CI, –1.5 to 0.4 mm Hg; $P = .38$) in diastolic blood pressure. The majority of the studies show beneficial effects of tea polyphenols on heart disease risk factors. Further long-term studies are required to see the association of tea with CHD events and risk factors.

6.5.2 COCOA

Cocoa is a natural source of flavanols. A 4-week study of both cocoa and dark chocolate found significant improvements in high density lipoprotein (HDL)-cholesterol [69], while another found that total cholesterol and LDL cholesterol levels were lowered following the consumption of 100g of dark chocolate (DC) for 15 days [70]. Ambulatory blood pressure (BP) decreased after DC (24-hour systolic BP –11.9+/-7.7 mm Hg, P < 0.0001; 24-hour diastolic BP –8.5+/-5.0 mm Hg, P < 0.0001) but not WC. DC but not WC decreased the homeostasis model assessment of insulin resistance (HOMA-IR) (P < 0.0001), but it improved the quantitative insulin-sensitivity check index (QUICKI), insulin sensitivity index (ISI), and flow mediated dilatation (FMD). DC also decreased serum LDL cholesterol (from 3.4+/–0.5 to 3.0+/–0.6 mmol/L; P<0.05).

Two studies reported blood pressure values for individuals with normal blood pressure fed cocoa or chocolate. Wang et al. showed a dose–response effect that speculated the greater amount of flavanols ingested, the greater the effect on reducing oxidized LDL formation [71]. The increase with cocoa was less than that seen with aspirin, indicating that cocoa may be associated with a short-term reduction in platelet reactivity, which in turn may reduce the risk for formation of clots [72]. Grassi et al. found similar results after 15 days of feeding 100g of DC and that that DC reduced blood pressure and WC had no effect [70]. Two studies testing dark chocolate or cocoa found significant improvement in overall function of the endothelium in healthy volunteers [73]. Another study investigated this effect in participants with high blood pressure and found 100g of DC fed for 15 days to produce significant improvements in endothelial function as well as other health factors related to insulin resistance and blood pressure [70]. In summary, DC decreased BP and serum LDL cholesterol, improved FMD, and ameliorated insulin sensitivity in hypertensives.

Fisher and colleagues were able to determine, via the use of nitric oxide inhibitors, that the endothelial improvements associated with cocoa flavanols were mediated via nitric oxide [74]. Four days of flavanol-rich cocoa induced consistent and striking peripheral vasodilation (P = 0.009). On day 5, pulse wave amplitude exhibited a large additional acute response to cocoa (P = 0.01). L-NAME completely reversed this vasodilation (P = 0.004). In addition, intake of flavanol-rich cocoa augmented the vasodilator response to ischemia. Flavanol-poor cocoa induced much smaller responses (P = 0.005), and none was induced in the time-control study. Flavanol-rich cocoa also amplified the systemic pressor effects of L-NAME (P = 0.005). These studies suggest that cocoa improves heart health by improving endothelial function and reducing the coronary risk factors.

6.6   SAFETY OF ANTIOXIDANTS

Antioxidants are available in most of the multivitamins and there are no adverse reports or deaths through using multivitamins. However, 10 to 15 cases of vitamin A toxic reactions are reported per year in the United States, usually at doses greater than 100,000 IU/d [75]. No adverse effects have been reported for beta-carotene. Ascorbic acid toxic reactions are rare at dosages less than 4 g/d. Selenium was associated with a 9% lower risk of death. Selenium is toxic if it is more than 6 mg/day. Other antioxidants have no reports of adverse events and studies are not well reported safety of antioxidants.

6.7   DIETARY GUIDELINE FOR AMERICANS

Health organizations have recognized the beneficial roles fruits and vegetables play in the reduced risk of disease and encourage consumers to eat more antioxidant-rich fruits and vegetables. Table 6.3 recommends fruits and vegetables to increase essential nutrients to protect against chronic diseases. In addition, the 2005 Dietary Guidelines for Americans stated [76], "Increased intakes of fruits, vegetables, whole grains and fat-free or low-fat milk and milk products are likely to have important health benefits for most Americans" [77].

6.8   CONCLUSIONS

Antioxidants are essential to protect the cells, to improve the immune function, and to maintain the integrity of cardiovascular system. The studies on antioxidants are controversial. The majority of observational studies, in which a scientist looks at a system from the outside, report their importance to reduce mortality and improve heart health. However, interventional studies, or clinical trials, have not provided enough significant evidence to recommend supplementation for daily use.

Interventional studies have a few limitations. Most are carried out in combination with one or two other nutrients on subjects having other risk factors. In the meta-analysis, the studies were reviewed for primary and secondary prevention of heart disease. However, the overall conclusions

TABLE 6.3
Recommendations for Antioxidants from Different Health Organizations

- Consume a varied diet that contains five to seven servings of fruits and vegetables each day.
- Receive lifestyle counseling and continue cholesterol treatment when indicated.
- Supplementation of ß-carotene for CHD prevention is not routinely recommended.

The American Heart Association (2002)	Eat a variety of fruits and vegetables. Choose five or more servings per day.
The American Cancer Society (2003)	Eat five or more servings of fruits and vegetables each day
Canadian Task Force on Preventive Health Care (2003)	Reviewing the role of vitamin E supplementation in the prevention of cardiovascular disease and cancer
The American Academy of Family Physicians states (2003)	Special dietary intervention or nutrient supplementation must be on an individual basis using the family physician's best judgment based on evidence and harmful effects
U.S. Department of Health and Human Services and U.S. Department of Agriculture : Dietary guidelines for Americans, 2005	Two to six and a half cups of fruits and vegetables a day or the equivalent of four to 13 servings
The World Cancer Research Fund and the American Institute for Cancer Research (2000)	Evidence of dietary protection against cancer is strongest and most consistent for diets high in vegetables and fruits
National Cancer Institute (NCI) (2006)	"5–A–Day for Better Health" Eat five or more servings of vegetables and fruit daily for better health
Food and Drug Administration (FDA) (2005)	A health claim for fruits and vegetables in relation to cancer. Diets low in fat and high in fruits and vegetables may reduce the risk of some cancers
FDA, in cooperation with National Cancer Institute (1997)	Diets rich in fruits and vegetables may reduce the risk of some types of cancer and other chronic diseases
Center for Disease Control	Fruits and vegetables are critical to promoting good health.

were drawn by combining these studies. They were not evaluated for oxidative stress markers in reducing the risk of heart disease, although antioxidants are primarily helpful in reducing oxidative stress and in improving the status of heart health.

Important vitamins and minerals are depleted from the tissues during acute and chronic inflammatory processes. Antioxidant studies need to be conducted in heart disease conditions such as in dilated cardiomyopathy and myocardial infarction, where there are active inflammatory processes and depletion of nutrients in blood and tissues. Well controlled long-term double-blind studies are required in healthy individuals, individuals with diagnosed heart disease and also in postcardiac-surgery patients in order to differentiate the effects of antioxidants.

REFERENCES

1. Frei, B. 1995. Cardiovascular disease and nutrient antioxidants: Role of low-density lipoprotein oxidation. *Crit Rev Food Sci Nutr.* 35(1–2):83–98.
2. Aviram, M. 1995. LDL-platelet interaction under oxidative stress induces macrophage foam cell formation. *Thromb Haemost.* 74(1):560–4.
2a. Ylä-Herttuala, S. 1991. Biochemistry of the arterial wall in developing atherosclerosis. *Ann NY Acad Sci*; 623:40–59.

3. Mink, P.J., Scrafford, C.G.,, Barraj L.M., Harnack, L., Hong, C.P., Nettleton, J.A., Jacobs, D.R. Jr. 2007. Flavonoid intake and cardiovascular disease mortality: A prospective study in postmenopausal women. *Am J Clin Nutr.* 85(3):895–909.

4. Radimer, K., Bindewald, B., Hughes, J., Ervin, B., Swanson, C., Picciano, M.F. 2004. Dietary supplement use by US adults: Data from the National Health and Nutrition Examination Survey, 1999–2000. *Am J Epidemiol.* 160(4):339–49.

5. Klipstein-Grobusch, K., den Breeijen, J.H., Grobbee, D.E., Boeing, H., Hofman, A., Witteman, J.C. 2001. Dietary antioxidants and peripheral arterial disease: The Rotterdam Study. *Am J Epidemiol.* 154(2):145–9.

6. Lonn, E. 2001. Do antioxidant vitamins protect against atherosclerosis? The proof is still lacking. *J Am Coll Cardiol.* 38(7):1795–8.

7. Kushi, L.H., Folsom A.R., Prineas, R.J., Mink, P.J., Wu, Y., Bostick R.M. 1996. Dietary antioxidant vitamins and death from coronary heart disease in postmenopausal women. *N Engl J Med.* 334:1156–1162.

8. Rimm, E.B., Stampfer, M.J., Ascherio, A., Giovannucci, E., Colditz, G.A., Willett, W.C. 1993. Vitamin E consumption and the risk of coronary heart disease in men. *N Engl J Med.* 328:1450–1456.

9. Stampfer, M.J., Hennekens, C.H., Manson, J.E., Colditz, G.A., Rosner, B., Willett, W.C. 1993. Vitamin E consumption and the risk of coronary disease in women. *N Engl J Med.* 328:1444–1449.

10. Knekt, P., Reunanen, A., Jarvinen, R., Seppanen R., Heliovaara, M., Aromaa, A. 1994. Antioxidant vitamin intake and coronary mortality in a longitudinal population study. *Am J Epidemiol.* 139:1180–1189.

11. Bolton-Smith, C., Casey, C.E., Gey, K.F., Smith, W.C., Tunstall-Pedoe, H. 1991. Antioxidant vitamin intakes assessed using a food-frequency questionnaire: Correlation with biochemical status in smokers and non-smokers. *Br J Nutr.* 65(3):337–46.

12. Keli, S.O., Hertog, M.G., Feskens E.J., Kromhout, D. 1996. Dietary flavonoids, antioxidant vitamins, and incidence of stroke: The Zutphen study. *Arch Intern Med.* 156:637–642.

13. Losonczy, K.G., Harris, T.B., Havlik, R.J. 1996. Vitamin E and vitamin C supplement use and risk of all-cause and coronary heart disease mortality in older persons: The Established Populations for Epidemiologic Studies of the Elderly. *Am J Clin Nutr.* 64(2):190–6.

14. Meyer, F., Bairati, I., Dagenais, G.R. 1996. Lower ischemic heart disease incidence and mortality among vitamin supplement users. *Can J Cardiol.* 12(10):930–4.

15. Sahyoun, N.R., Jacques, P.F., Russell, R.M. 1996. Carotenoids, vitamins C and E, and mortality in an elderly population. *Am J Epidemiol.* 144(5):501–11.

16. Ascherio, A., Rimm, E.B., Hernan, M.A., Giovannucci, E., Kawachi, I., Stampfer, M.J., Willett, W.C. 1999. Relation of consumption of vitamin E, vitamin C, and carotenoids to risk for stroke among men in the United States. *Ann Intern Med.* 130:963–970.

17. Donnan, P.T., Thomson, M., Fowkes, F.G., Prescott, R.J., Housley, E. 1993. Diet as a risk factor for peripheral arterial disease in the general population: The Edinburgh Artery Study. *Am J Clin Nutr.* 57(6):917–21.

18. Klipstein-Grobusch, K. J., Geleijnse, M., den Breeijen, J.H., Boeing, H., Hofman, A., Grobbee, D.E., Witteman, J.C. 1999. Dietary antioxidants and risk of myocardial infarction in the elderly: The Rotterdam Study. *Am J Clin Nutr.* 69:261–266.

19. Kritchevsky, S.B., Shimakawa, T., Tell, G.S., Dennis, B., Carpenter, M., Eckfeldt, J.H., Peacher–Ryan, H., Heiss, G. 1995. Dietary antioxidants and carotid artery wall thickness. The ARIC Study. Atherosclerosis Risk in Communities Study. *Circulation.* 92(8):2142–50.

20. Wright, M.E., Lawson, K.A., Weinstein, S.J., Pietinen, P., Taylor, P.R., Virtamo, J., Albanes, D. 2006. Higher baseline serum concentrations of vitamin E are associated with lower total and cause-specific mortality in the Alpha-Tocopherol, Beta-Carotene Cancer Prevention Study. *Am J Clin Nutr.* 84(5):1200–7.

21. Ohira, T., Hozawa, A., Iribarren, C., Daviglus, M.L., Matthews, K.A., Gross, M.D., Jacobs, D.R. Jr. 2007. Longitudinal Association of Serum Carotenoids and Tocopherols with Hostility: The CARDIA Study. *Am J Epidemiol.* Oct 10; E-pub ahead of print.

22. Tucker, K.L., Hallfrisch, J., Qiao, N., Muller, D., Andres, R., Fleg, J.L., Baltimore Longitudinal Study of Aging. 2005. The combination of high fruit and vegetable and low saturated fat intakes is more protective against mortality in aging men than is either alone: The Baltimore Longitudinal Study of Aging. *J Nutr.* 135(3):556–61.

23. Appel, L.J., Moore, T.J., Obarzanek, E., Vollmer, W.M., Svetkey, L.P., Sacks, F.M. et al. 1997. A clinical trial of the effects of dietary patterns on blood pressure. DASH Collaborative Research Group. *N Engl J Med.* 336(16):1117–24.

24. Krauss, R.M., Eckel, R.H., Howard, B., Appel, L.J., Daniels, S.R., Deckelbaum, R.J. 2000. AHA Dietary Guidelines: Revision 2000: A statement for healthcare professionals from the Nutrition Committee of the American Heart Association. *Circulation.* 102(18):2284–99.

25. Krebs-Smith, S.M., Cook, A., Subar,. AF., Cleveland, L., Friday, J. 1995. US adults' fruit and vegetable intakes, 1989 to 1991: A revised baseline for the Healthy People 2000 objective. *Am J Pub Hlth.* 85(12):1623–9.

26. Bazzano, L.A., He, J., Ogden, L.G., Loria, C.M., Vupputuri, S., Myers, L., Whelton, P.K. 2002. Fruit and vegetable intake and risk of cardiovascular disease in US adults: The first National Health and Nutrition Examination Survey Epidemiologic Follow-up Study. *Am J Clin Nutr.* 76(1):93–9.

27. Dauchet, L., Amouyel, P., Dallongeville, J. 2005. Fruit and vegetable consumption and risk of stroke: A meta-analysis of cohort studies. *Neurology.* 65(8):1193–7.

28. Kris-Etherton, P.M, Lichtenstein, A.H, Howard, B.V., Steinberg, D., Witztum, J.L. Nutrition Committee of the American Heart Association Council on Nutrition, Physical Activity, and Metabolism. 2004. Antioxidant Vitamin Supplements and Cardiovascular Disease. *Circulation.* 110:637–641.

29. Gülçin I. 2006. Antioxidant and antiradical activities of L-carnitine. *Life Sci.* 78(8):803–11.

30. McMackin, C.J., Widlansky, M.E., Hamburg, N.M., Huang, A.L., Weller, S., Holbrook, M. et al. 2007. Effect of combined treatment with alpha-Lipoic acid and acetyl-L-carnitine on vascular function and blood pressure in patients with coronary artery disease. *J Clin Hypertens (Greenwich).* 9(4):249–55.

31. Stvolinsky, S.L., Dobrota, D. 2000 Anti-ischemic activity of carnosine. *Biochemistry (Mosc).* Jul;65(7):849–55.

32. Shenouda, S.M., Vita, J.A. 2007. Effects of flavonoid-containing beverages and EGCG on endothelial function. *J Am Coll Nutr.* 26(4):366S–372S.

33. Lekakis, J., Rallidis, L.S., Andreadou, I., Vamvakou, G., Kazantzoglou, G., Magiatis, et al. 2005. Polyphenolic compounds from red grapes acutely improve endothelial function in patients with coronary heart disease. *Eur J Cardiovasc Prev Rehabil.* 12(6):596–600.

34. Hertog, M.G., Feskens, E.J., Hollman, P.C., Katan, M.B., Kromhout, D. 1993. Dietary antioxidant flavonoids and risk of coronary heart disease: The Zutphen Elderly Study. *Lancet.* 342(8878):1007–11.

35. Knekt, P, Kumpulainen, J., Järvinen, R., Rissanen, H., Heliövaara, M., Reunanen, A. et al. 2002. Flavonoid intake and risk of chronic diseases. *Am J Clin Nutr.* 76(3):560–8.

36. Edwards, R.L., Lyon, T., Litwin, S.E., Rabovsky, A., Symons, J.D., Jalili, T. 2007. Quercetin reduces blood pressure in hypertensive subjects. *J Nutr.* 137(11):2405–11.

37. Curello, S., Ceconi, C., Cargnoni, A., Cornacchiari, A., Ferrari, R., Albertini, A. 1987. Improved procedure for determining glutathione in plasma as an index of myocardial oxidative stress. *Clin Chem.* 33:1448–1449.

38. Morrison, J.A., Jacobsen, D.W., Sprecher, D.L., Robinson, K., Khoury, P., Daniels, S.R. 1999. Serum glutathione in adolescent males predicts parental coronary heart disease. *Circulation.* 100(22):2244–7.

39. Dwyer, J.H., Navab, M., Dwyer, K.M., Hassan, K., Sun, P., Shircore, A. et al. 2001. Oxygenated carotenoid lutein and progression of early atherosclerosis: The Los Angeles atherosclerosis study. *Circulation.* 103(24):2922–7.

40. Rissanen, T., Voutilainen ,S., Nyyssönen, K., Salonen, J.T. 2002. Lycopene, atherosclerosis, and coronary heart disease. *Exp Biol Med (Maywood).* 227(10):900–7.

41. Giacomo, C.G., Antonio, M. 2007. Melatonin in cardiac ischemia/reperfusion-induced mitochondrial adaptive changes. *Cardiovasc Hematol Disord Drug Targets.* 7(3):163–9.

42. Camargo, C.A. Jr, Stampfer, M.J., Glynn, R.J., Buring, J.E., and Hennekens C.H. 1997. Moderate alcohol consumption and risk for angina pectoris or myocardial infarction in US male physicians. *Ann Intern Med* 126:372–375.

43. Shinke, T., Shite, J., Takaoka, H., Hata, K., Inoue, N., Yoshikawa, R. et al. 2007. Vitamin C restores the contractile response to dobutamine and improves myocardial efficiency in patients with heart failure after anterior myocardial infarction. *Am Heart J.* 154(4):645.e1–8.

44. Yokoyama, T., Date, C., Kokubo, Y., Yoshiike, N., Matsumura, Y., Tanaka, H. 2000. Serum vitamin C concentration was inversely associated with subsequent 20-year incidence of stroke in a Japanese rural community. The Shibata study. *Stroke.* 31(10):2287–94.

45. Gokce, N., Keaney, J.F. Jr, Frei, B., Holbrook, M., Olesiak, M., Zachariah, B.J. et al. 1999. Long-term ascorbic acid administration reverses endothelial vasomotor dysfunction in patients with coronary artery disease. *Circulation*. 99(25):3234–40.
46. Osganian, S.K., Stampfer, M.J., Rimm, E., Spiegelman, D., Hu, F.B., Manson, J.E., Willett, W.C. 2003. Vitamin C and risk of coronary heart disease in women. *J Am Coll Cardiol*. 42(2):246–52.
47. Knekt, P., Ritz, J., Pereira, M.A., O'Reilly, E.J., Augustsson, K., Fraser, G.E., Goldbourt, U., Heitmann, B.L., Hallmans, G., Liu, S., Pietinen, P., Spiegelman, D., Stevens, J., Virtamo, J., Willett ,W.C., Rimm, E.B., Ascherio, A. 2004. Antioxidant vitamins and coronary heart disease risk: a pooled analysis of 9 cohorts. *Am J Clin Nutr*. 80(6):1508–20.
48. Kaikkonen, J., Nyyssönen, K., Tomasi, A., Iannone, A., Tuomainen, T.P., Porkkala-Sarataho, E., Salonen, J.T. 2000. Antioxidative efficacy of parallel and combined supplementation with coenzyme Q10 and d–alpha–tocopherol in mildly hypercholesterolemic subjects: a randomized placebo–controlled clinical study. *Free Radic Res*. 33(3):329–40.
49. Micheletta, F., Natoli, S., Misuraca, M., Sbarigia, E., Diczfalusy, U., Iuliano, L. 2004. Vitamin E supplementation in patients with carotid atherosclerosis: Reversal of altered oxidative stress status in plasma but not in plaque. *Arterioscler Thromb Vasc Biol*. 24(1):136–40.
50. Marchioli, R., Levantesi, G., Macchia, A., Marfisi, R.M., Nicolosi, G.L., Tavazzi, L. et al. GISSI-Prevenzione Investigators. 2006. Vitamin E increases the risk of developing heart failure after myocardial infarction: Results from the GISSI-Prevenzione trial. *J Cardiovasc Med (Hagerstown)*. 7(5):347–50.
51. Lonn, E. Yusuf, S., Hoogwerf, S., Pogue, J., Yi, Q., Zinman, B. et al. 2002. HOPE Study/MICRO-HOPE Study. Effects of vitamin E on cardiovascular and microvascular outcomes in high-risk patients with diabetes: Results of the HOPE study and MICRO-HOPE substudy. *Diabetes Care*. 25:1919–1927.
52. Williams, H.T.G., Fenna, D., Macbeth R.A. 1971. Alpha tocopherol in the treatment of intermittent claudication. *Surg Gynecol Obstet* 132:662–666.
53. Gillilan, R.E., Mondell, B., Warbasse, J.R. 1977. Quantitative evaluation of vitamin E in the treatment of angina pectoris. *Am Heart J*. 93(4):444–9.
54. Rapola, J.M., Jirtamo, V., Sipatti, R., Huttunen, J.K., Albanes, D., Taylor, P.R., Heinonen, O.P. 1997. Randomized trial of alpha-tocopherol and beta-carotene supplements on incidence of major coronary events in men with previous myocardial infarction. *Lancet*. 349, 1715–1720.
55. Takamatsu, S., Makamatsu, T., Satoh, K., Imaizumi, T., Yoshida, H., Hiramoto, M. et al. 1995. Effects on health of dietary supplementation with 100 mg d-alpha-tocopheryl acetate daily for 6 years. *J Int Med Res*. 23(5):342–57.
56. Alpha-Tocopherol, Beta-Carotene Cancer Prevention Study Group. 1994. The effect of vitamin E and beta-carotene on the incidence of lung cancer and other cancers in male smokers. *N Engl J Med*. 330, 1029–1035.
57. Tornwall, M.E., Virtamo, J.,.Haukka, J.K., Albanes, D., Huttunen, J.K. 2001. Alpha-tocopherol (vitamin E) and beta-carotene supplementation does not affect the risk for large abdominal aortic aneurysm in a controlled trial. *Atherosclerosis*. 157(1):167–73.
58. Virtamo, J., Rapola, J.M., Ripatti, S., Heinonen, O.P., Taylor, P.R., Albanes, D., Huttunen, J.K. 1998. Effect of vitamin E and beta carotene on the incidence of primary nonfatal myocardial infarction and fatal coronary heart disease. *Arch Intern Med*. 158(6):668–75.
59. Penumathsa, S.V., Thirunavukkarasu, M., Koneru, S., Juhasz, B., Zhan, L., Pant, R. et al. 2007. Statin and resveratrol in combination induces cardioprotection against myocardial infarction in hypercholesterolemic rat. *J Mol Cell Cardiol*. 42(3):508–16.
60. Yoshida, Y., Shioi, T., Izumi, T. 2007. Resveratrol ameliorates experimental autoimmune myocarditis. *Circ J*. 71(3):397–404.
61. Iakovleva, L.V., Ivakhnenko, A.K., Buniatian, N.D. 1998. The protective action of ellagic acid in experimental myocarditis. *Eksp Klin Farmakol*. 61(3):32–4.
62. Juturu V., Subramanyam, G., Jayaram, V., Latheef, S.A.A. 2000. Selenium levels in dilated cardiomyopathy. *J Indian Med Assoc*. 98(4):166–9.
63. Venardos, K.M, Kaye, D.M. 2007. Myocardial ischemia-reperfusion injury, antioxidant enzyme systems, and selenium: A review. *Curr Med Chem*; 14(14):1539–49.
64. Flores-Mateo, G., Navas-Acien, A., Pastor-Barriuso, R., Guallar, E. 2006. Selenium and coronary heart disease: A meta-analysis. *Am J Clin Nutr*. 84(4):762–73.
65. Mohr, D., Bowry, V.W., Stocker, R. 1992. Dietary supplementation with coenzyme Q10 results in increased levels of ubiquinol-10 within circulating lipoproteins and increased resistance of human low-density lipoprotein to the initiation of lipid peroxidation. *Biochim Biophys Acta*. 1126(3):247–54.

66. Peters, U., Poole, C., Arab, L. 2001. Does tea affect cardiovascular disease? A meta-analysis. *Am J Epidemiol.* 154(6): 495–503.
67. Rietveld, A., Wiseman, S. 2003 Antioxidant effects of tea: Evidence from human clinical trials. *J. Nutr.* 133(10): 3285S–3292.
68. Taubert, D., Roesen, R., and Schomig, E. 2007. Effect of cocoa and tea intake on blood pressure: A meta-analysis. *Arch Intern Med.* 167(7): 626–634.
69. Wan, Y., Vinson, J.A., Etherton, T.D., Proch, J., Lazarus, S.A., Kris-Etherton, P.M. 2001. Effects of cocoa powder and dark chocolate on LDL oxidative susceptibility and prostaglandin concentrations in humans. *Am J Clin Nutr.* 74(5):596–602.
70. Grassi, D., Necozione, S., Lippi, C., Croce, G., Valeri, L., Pasqualetti, P. et al. 2005. Cocoa reduces blood pressure and insulin resistance and improves endothelium-dependent vasodilation in hypertensives. *Hypertension.* 46(2):398–405.
71. Wang, J.F., Schramm, D.D., Holt, R.R., Ensunsa, J.L., Fraga, C.G., Schmitz, H.H., Keen, C.L. 2000. A dose–response effect from chocolate consumption on plasma epicatechin and oxidative damage. *J Nutr.* 130(8S Suppl):2115S–9S.
72. Pearson, D.A., Paglieroni, T.G., Rein, D., Wun, T., Schramm, D.D., Wang, J.F. et al. 2002. The effects of flavanol-rich cocoa and aspirin on *ex vivo* platelet function. *Thromb Res.* 106(4–5):191–7.
73. Engler, M.B., Engler, M.M., Chen, C.Y., Malloy, M.J., Browne, A., Chiu, E.Y. et al. 2004. Flavonoid-rich dark chocolate improves endothelial function and increases plasma epicatechin concentrations in healthy adults. *J Am Coll Nutr.* 23(3):197–204.
74. Fisher, N.D., Hughes, M., Gerhard-Herman, M., Hollenberg, N.K. 2003. Flavanol-rich cocoa induces nitric-oxide-dependent vasodilation in healthy humans. *J Hypertens.* 21(12):2281–6.
75. Meyers, D.G., Maloley, P.A., Weeks, D. 1996. Safety of antioxidant vitamins. *Arch Intern Med.* 156(9):925–35.
76. U.S. Department of Health and Human Services and U.S. Department of Agriculture. Dietary Guidelines for Americans, 2005. 6th ed., Washington, DC: U.S. Government Printing Office, January 2005. http://www.mypyramid.gov/guidelines/index.html.
77. Fogli-Cawley, J.J., Dwyer, J.T., Saltzman, E., McCullough, M.L., Troy, L.M., Meigs J.B., Jacques P.F. 2007. The 2005 Dietary Guidelines for Americans and risk of the metabolic syndrome. *Am J Clin Nutr.* 86(4):1193–201.
78. American Heart Association. 2002. Vitamins and mineral supplements: AHA scientific position. Accessed at http://216.185.112.5/presenter.jhtml?identifier=4788 on 27 March 2002.
79. American Cancer Society. Prevention and early detection: Food and fitness. 2003. http://www.cancer.org/docroot/PED/ped_3.asp?sitearea=PED&level=1. Accessed on 28 April 2003.
80. Canadian Task Force on Preventive Health Care. 2003. http://www.ctfphc.org/Whats New/reviews_in_progress.htm. Accessed on 28 April 2003.
81. American Academy of Family Physicians. AAFP clinical recommendations: Vitamins. Accessed at http://www.aafp.org/x2590.xml on 28 April 2003.
82. Ogimoto, I., Shibata, A., Fukuda, K. 2000. World Cancer Research Fund/American Institute of Cancer Research 1997 Recommendations: Applicability to digestive tract cancer in Japan. Cancer Causes Control. 11(1):9–23.
83. National Cancer Institute. 5 A Day for Better Health Program Evaluation Report: Recommendations. http://www.cancercontrol.cancer.gov/5ad_7_recs.html Last updated : March 1, 2006.
84. FDA/CFSAN /Office of Nutritional Products, Labeling, and Dietary Supplements November 8, 2005–Qualified Health Claim Petition–Tomato lycopene, tomatoes and tomato products, which contain lycopene, lycopene in tomatoes and tomato products, lycopene in fruits and vegetables, including tomatoes and tomato products and reduced risk of prostate cancer (Docket No. 2004Q–0201).
85. Food and Drug Administration, U. S. Department of Agriculture, U. S. Environmental Protection Agency, Centers for Disease Control and Prevention May 1997 http://vm.cfsan.fda.gov/~dms/fsreport.html updated by dms/ear 5/12/97.
86. Center for Disease Control and Prevention. http://www.fruitsandveggiesmatter.gov/.
87. Müller, K., Carpenter, K.L., Mitchinson, M.J. 1998. Cell-mediated oxidation of LDL: Comparison of different cell types of the atherosclerotic lesion. *Free Radic Res.* 29(3):207–20.
88. Kaliora, A.C., Dedoussis, G.V. 2007. Natural antioxidant compounds in risk factors for CVD. *Pharmacol Res.* 56(2):99–109.
89. Szmitko, P.E., Verma, S. 2005. Cardiology patient pages. Red wine and your heart. *Circulation.* 111(2): e10–1.

7 Cardiometabolic Syndrome, Diabetes and Oxidative Stress:
Focus on the Aging Population

Hussein Naji Yassine and Craig S. Stump

CONTENTS

7.1 INTRODUCTION

The elderly population is recognized as one of the fastest growing age groups in the United States, and it has been widely predicted that over the next two decades this segment of the population will place a progressively heavier demand on the health care system[1]. A recent analysis of the data set from the Third National Health and Nutrition Examination Survey (NHANES III) has shown that the age-adjusted prevalence of obesity has increased from 22.9% (1994–1998) to 30.5% (1999–2002). Based on data from the NHANES (1999–2002), 9.3% of persons aged ≥20 years have diabetes, representing an estimated 19.3 million people in 2002. The percentage with diabetes was highest in those aged ≥65 years (21.6%). Remarkably, approximately one third (30.1%) of people with diabetes remain undiagnosed. An additional 26.0% of adults had impaired fasting glucose (IFG), a condition that signals an increased risk for diabetes that is associated with other cardiovascular risk factors. Thus, in 2002, a combined total of 35.3% of the adult U.S. population (73.3 million persons) had diabetes or IFG [2].

Since the burden of cardiovascular and metabolic diseases increase with aging, particular attention is being focused on obese elderly, many of whom meet criteria for the metabolic syndrome. The National Cholesterol Education Program (NCEP) Adult Treatment Panel III (ATP III) defines the metabolic syndrome as the presence of any three or more of the following: blood pressure (BP) ≥130/85 mmHg, waist circumference >102 cm in men and >88 cm in women, triglycerides ≥150 mg/dL, high-density liproproteins (HDL) < 40 mg/dL in men and <50 mg/dL in women, fasting glucose ≥110 mg/d [3]. Since the syndrome is a clustering of maladaptive characteristics that confers

TABLE 7. 1

Cardiometabolic Syndrome Risk Factors

1. Hypertension
2. Central/Visceral obesity
3. Hyperinsulinemia/insulin resistance
4. Impaired glucose tolerance
5. Endothelial dysfunction
6. Microalbuminuria
7. Chronic kidney disease
8. Low HDL cholesterol levels
9. High triglyceride levels
10. Small, dense LDL cholesterol levels
11. Increased apolipoprotein B levels
12. Increased fibrinogen levels
13. Increased plasminogen activator inhibitort 1 and decreased plasminoghen activator levels
14. Increased CRP level and other inflammatory markers
15. Absent nocturnal dipping of blood pressure and heart rate
16. Salt sensitivity
17. Left ventricular hyperytrophy
18. Premature/excess coronary artery disease, stroke, and peripheral vascular disease

HDL = high density lipoprotein; LDL = low density lipoprotein; CRP = C-reactive protein.

an increased risk of cardiovascular disease (CVD) (Table 7.1), we prefer the term cardiometabolic syndrome (CMS). "Cardiometabolic risk" has also been suggested [4]. These risk factors are also strongly associated with the development of type 2 diabetes. NHANES III has suggested that 33% of US adults who are 50 years of age or older and have impaired glucose tolerance also have CMS [5]. Of interest, the age-specific prevalence of the CMS increases dramatically, from just over 12% among individuals in their 30s, to 20% among those in their 40s, 35% among those in their 50s, and 45% in those 60 years and older [6].

Cardiovascular disease is the major cause of premature mortality in patients with type 2 DM accounting for 55% of deaths. Overall, mortality related to heart disease is estimated to be 2 to 4 times higher in patients with diabetes mellitus (DM) compared with those without DM [5]. In the large (n = 347,978) cohort of men who were screened for the Multiple Risk Factor Intervention Trial (MR-FIT) and followed for an average of 12 years, DM was significantly associated with increased risk of CVD death in all age groups studied. In addition, mortality associated with conventional CVD risk factors other than DM, such as hypertension, dyslipidemia, family history, and cigarette smoking, was significantly higher in men with DM than in non-diabetic men [7].

7.2 AGING, OXIDATIVE STRESS, AND THE CARDIOMETABOLIC SYNDROME

Aging is an inherently complex process that is manifested within an organism at genetic, molecular, cellular, organ, and system levels. Although the fundamental mechanisms are still poorly understood, a growing body of evidence points toward reactive oxygen species (ROS) as one of the primary determinants of aging. The "oxidative stress theory" holds that a progressive and irreversible accumulation of oxidative damage caused by ROS impacts on critical aspects of the aging process and contributes to impaired physiological function, increased incidence of disease, and a reduction

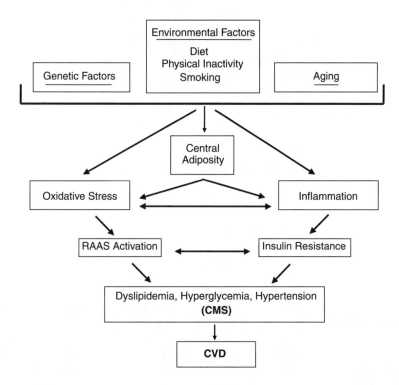

FIGURE 7.1 Factors linking oxidative stress, insulin resistance and cardiovascular disease. Note that aging per se has a limited and indirect effect on the development of CVD and that development of excessive intra-abdominal fat is central to the pathogenesis. CVD = cardiovascular disease; RAAS = renin-angiotensin-aldosterone system; CMS = Cardiometabolic Syndrome.

in life span. While compelling correlative data have been generated to support the oxidative stress theory, a direct cause-and-effect relationship between the accumulation of oxidative damage and aging has not been established [8].

Oxidative stress has clearly been shown to contribute to diabetic CVD, having implications in the development of hypertension, renal disease, and stroke [9,10]. Oxidative stress occurs when the production of oxidation products, particularly reactive oxygen species (ROS) and reactive nitrogen species, exceeds the neutralizing capacity of the antioxidant systems (Figure 7.1). In DM, the production of ROS is increased in vascular tissues [11]. Potential sources for ROS production include several enzymatic pathways (Table 7.2) including nicotinamide adenine dinucleotide phosphate-oxidase (NADPH) and xanthine oxidase, glucose autoxidation, and mitochondrial uncoupling [9].

Type 2 DM and CMS are characterized by several hemodynamic and metabolic abnormalities including vascular/endothelial dysfunction, increased sympathetic nervous system (SNS) activity and sodium retention, altered adipocyte differentiation and lipid storage, low-grade chronic inflammation, and an enhanced renin angiotensin aldosterone system (RAAS) [12]. Indeed, oxidative stress is instrumental in many of these maladaptive pathways, in part by antagonizing normal insulin signaling [13,14].

7.2.1 VASCULAR/ENDOTHELIAL DYSFUNCTION

An emerging area of research with important clinical ramifications in human aging is the role of ROS on vascular dysfunction [8]. Adequate blood vessel function is critically important to overall homeostasis due to the vessels' role in supplying cells with oxygen and nutrients. Thus, damage to them can have a profound impact on organ function and contribute to a myriad of diseases that

TABLE 7.2
Biochemical Sources of Reactive Oxygen Species (ROS)

- NADPH oxidase
- Xanthine oxidase
- Hemeoxygenase
- Cyclooxygenase
- Lipoxygenase
- Cytochrome P450 monooxygenases
- NOS uncoupling
- Mitochondrial oxidative phosphorylation

NOS = nitric oxide synthase

are typically associated with aging (e.g., diabetes, atherosclerosis, and hypertension). Endothelial cells that line blood vessels are especially vulnerable to potentially damaging circulatory factors, such as oxidized macromolecules and proinflammatory cytokines, and endogenous ROS generation. Insulin resistance and chronic hyperglycemia, which are associated with increased tissue ROS, also contribute to endothelial dysfunction leading to hypertension, microalbuminuria and diabetic nephropathy. Further, markers of endothelial dysfunction including E-Selectin, Intercellular Adhesion Molecule 1 (ICAM-1) and Vascular Cellular Adhesion Molecule 1 (VCAM-1) are associated with the development of type 2 DM [15]. In type 2 DM, nitric oxide (NO)-dependent vasodilation is impaired due to an imbalance in production and inactivation. Reduction of NO may also occur in hypertension associated with DM by way of increased plasma asymmetric dimethylarginine (ADMA) levels, an endogenous competitive inhibitor of NO synthase (NOS) [16,17], or suppression of superoxide dismutase (SOD), a free-radical scavenger [17]. It is important to note that many of these abnormalities become evident well before the development of clinical DM. The relationship of vascular endothelial dysfunction, microalbuminuria, and chronic kidney disease (CKD) to poor cardiovascular outcomes is increasingly recognized in epidemiological and clinical trials [18].

7.2.2 OXIDIZED LDL PARTICLES

Another important mechanism by which oxidative stress contributes to CVD is through the formation of oxidized low-density lipoprotein (LDL) particles, which are especially atherogenic. Circulating levels of oxidized LDL are increased in DM and prediabetic conditions [19]. Oxidized LDL particles originate in the arterial wall from cell-associated lipoxygenases or myeloperoxidases [20]. Pro-inflammatory oxidized LDL particles accumulate within the arterial wall, where they promote monocyte infiltration, and vascular smooth muscle cell (VSMC) migration and proliferation. They also contribute to endothelial dysfunction and atherothrombosis by inducing endothelial cell (EC) apoptosis, and by impairing the anticoagulant balance. This is particularly true in people with type 2 DM and CMS [21].

The susceptibility of LDL to oxidation increases with age [22]. In one study, LDL-derived hydroxy fatty acids were three- to fourfold higher in otherwise healthy persons between the ages of 56 and 66 years compared with younger individuals (22–54 years). Moreover, hydroxyl fatty acid levels were 10- to 20-fold higher in LDL particles from those between 68 to 74 years, and 30–40 fold higher in those 78–87 years of age [23]. While age may enhance LDL susceptibility to oxidation, hyperglycemia appears to have a potent but reversible effect on LDL oxidation [24].

7.2.3 THE RENIN-ANGIOTENSIN ALDOSTERONE SYSTEM

Hypertension in DM is characterized by reduced NO-mediated vasorelaxation, reduced barore-flex sensitivity, and enhanced SNS activity, abnormalities that are promoted by angiotensin II and aldosterone. Angiotensin II causes vascular and end organ dysfunction independent of its vasocon-strictive hemodynamic effects, in part by promoting oxidative stress and endothelial dysfunction [25]. Acting through its type 1 receptor (AT_1R), angiotensin II mediates ROS production through NADPH oxidase activation in a variety of tissues [26]. ROS, in turn, interferes with insulin signaling pathways, which in EC and VSMC decreases vascular NO [14]. Remarkably, ROS have been implicated in virtually every pathogenic stage of hypertension, vascular, and renal lesion formation [27]. RAAS activation is an important mediator of insulin resistance in other tissues including skeletal muscle, which offers a possible explanation for the relationship between DM, hypertension, and diabetic nephropathy [28]. Endothelial dysfunction exacerbates nephropathy, which becomes manifest as microalbuminuria, proteinuria, and CKD, important risk factors associated with CMS. Recent work in rodents suggests that NADPH oxidase-mediated oxidative stress contributes to diabetic nephropathy [29], and may be an important contributor to age-related cardiovascular dysfunction [30]. Likewise, there is evidence that AT_1R blockade attenuates age-related declines in renal and metabolic function [31].

7.3 FAT DISTRIBUTION, INFLAMMATION, AND ADIPOCYTOKINES

A chronic low-level inflammatory state often accompanies insulin resistance such that subclinical elevations of proinflammatory markers including interleukin-6 (IL-6), C-reactive protein (CRP), plasminogen activator inhibitor-1 (PA I-1), and fibrinogen are evident in CMS and often linked to the development of type 2 DM [32]. Chronic inflammation is also common to other related entities including obesity, arterial hypertension, and CMS that converge to increase the risk of cardiovascular and cerebrovascular disease.

Visceral fat accumulation is accompanied by progressive infiltration of macrophages [33], which secrete proinflammatory molecules such as tumor necrosis factor-α (TNF-α), IL-6, and IL-1β. These cytokines augment and perpetuate the proinflammatory diathesis and decrease insulin sensitivity [32]. Cytokines from adipocytes (adipocytokines) may also contribute to insulin resistance by increasing TNF-α, IL-6 or decreasing adiponectin as adipocyte volume expands. Inflammatory adipocytokines give rise to E-Selectin and ICAM-1 in the endothelium, which participate in the migration of inflammatory cells to the subendothelial space, promoting the development of unstable atherosclerotic plaques. These adipocytokines can also increase the risk of thrombosis by decreasing tissue plasminogen activator (tPA) and increasing PAI-1 [14], and can cause hypertension through direct pressor actions and interactions with the RAAS and the SNS [16,33]. Thus, visceral obesity contributes to the clustering of multiple risk factors for cardiovascular disease, particularly in the presence of DM.

Adiponectin is an insulin-sensitizing adipocytokine that is decreased with obesity, CMS and DM. Adiponectin administration has been shown to improve insulin action in animals, while inadequate levels of adiponectin are proposed to contribute to obesity-associated insulin resistance [34]. Indices of oxidative stress are significantly correlated with body mass index (BMI), and inversely related to plasma adiponectin. Furthermore, increased NADPH oxidase in adipose tissue may increase ROS production and dysregulate production of adipocytokines [35].

The observed insulin resistance of aging may be related more to changes in body composition than to aging per se [36,37]. Indeed, one study indicates that the surgical removal of selective intra-abdominal fat deposits prevents the age-related decrease in peripheral and hepatic insulin action and the onset of diabetes in a rat model of obesity and diabetes [38].

7.3.1 Age-Related Changes in the Pancreas and Tissue Sensitivity to Insulin

Glucose homeostasis, the maintenance of serum glucose concentration within a relatively narrow range, is dependent upon a highly regulated neural and hormonal system. A critical hormonal component of this homeostasis is insulin, which mediates the uptake of glucose in the peripheral tissues. The development of glucose intolerance has been well established to be a part of the human aging process [39–42]. This change in glucose metabolism has been shown to be due to diminished target tissue sensitivity to insulin [39,43,44] and to inadequate pancreatic β-cell function [39,45]. Both the prevalence and incidence rates of DM increase dramatically with age [2] and elderly subjects share the β-cell dysfunction and reduced insulin sensitivity that are characteristic of patients with type 2 DM, resulting in disturbed glucose metabolism [46], although to a lesser degree. The decrease in insulin sensitivity with age is thought in large part to be related to body fat redistribution, with increased intra-abdominal fat most strongly correlated with decreased insulin sensitivity [36,47]. However, the development of glucose intolerance and type 2 DM is not inevitable in the aged. Factors over which the individual has some control such as intra-abdominal obesity, physical inactivity, and diet play a major role in the development of glucose intolerance. Nevertheless, a small but significant decline in insulin secretion and tissue insulin sensitivity appears to be directly related to the aging process.

7.4 PREVENTION AND NON-PHARMACOLOGIC THERAPY

There is evidence from randomized controlled trials (RCT) that nutrition intervention as a part of a comprehensive diabetes education program improves blood glucose and HbA1c levels in persons with diabetes, including individuals over age 65 [48,49]. Although nutritional modifications are most effective when the patient is first diagnosed, it is beneficial at any time during the disease process and refresher therapy may be of value. Published data from the Diabetes Prevention Program showed greater benefit for the lifestyle intervention than drug therapy (metformin), and this benefit was greatest in those over 60 years of age [50].

Weight control is a cornerstone in the management of older obese adults with DM and CMS. However, mechanisms of energy balance are dysregulated in old age and the response to a negative energy balance is attenuated [51]. Consequently, older adults experience greater loss of muscle mass with intentional caloric restriction than younger adults [52]. Aging is already associated with an accelerated decline in lean tissue in men and women over the age of 60. This loss of muscle, which is clinically known as sarcopenia, is strongly related to impaired mobility, increased mortality and morbidity, and lower quality of life [53]. Adding to the controversy, no clinical trial data are available for the effects of tight glycemic control in the frail elderly population, where less stringent treatment goals may be appropriate given the possible issues of advanced disease, limited life expectancy, and multiple concomitant conditions. In younger subjects, improved glycemic control has been shown to sustain decreased rates of nephropathy, retinopathy, and neuropathy [48,49]. In the absence of clinical trial data in long-term care residents with diabetes, extrapolation of data in younger persons is generally accepted in order to reduce the burden of disease and improve the quality of remaining life. Treatment of frail older persons with diabetes requires a careful balance of American Diabetes Association and American Geriatric Society (ADA/AGS) treatment goals (Table 7.3) with an individualized approach to drug therapy to avoid potential adverse effects such as hypoglycemia [54,55].

7.4.1 Diet

Recently, there has been increased interest in the use of low-carbohydrate diets as potential therapy for obesity and glycemic control. The results of five RCTs in mostly middle-aged adults found that subjects randomized to a low-carbohydrate, high-protein/high-fat diet (approximately 25–40%

TABLE 7.3
Recommendations for Management of Diabetes in Adults

	ADA	AGS
Glycemic control A1c	<7%	<8%
Preprandial capillary plasma glucose (mg/dl)	80–120	90–130
Peak postprandial capillary plasma glucose (mg/dl)	<180	<180
Blood pressure (mm Hg)		
All diabetics	<130/80	<140/90
Overt proteinuria	<125/75	
Lipids (mg/dl)		
LDL cholesterol	<70–100	
Triglycerides	<150	
HDL cholesterol	<40	
Eye examinations	Yearly dilated exams	Every 2 years if low risk

HDL = high density lipoprotein; LDL = low density lipoprotein, ADA= American Diabetes Association; AGS= American Geriatric Society.

carbohydrate) achieved greater short-term (6 months), but not long-term (12 months), weight loss than those randomized to a low-fat diet (approximately 25–30% fat, 55–60% carbohydrate). A consistent difference in weight loss at 6 months was observed between groups across studies; subjects randomized to the low-carbohydrate diet lost 4–5 kg more weight than those randomized to the low-fat diet. In the low-carbohydrate group, the data from these studies also found greater improvements in serum triglyceride and HDL-cholesterol concentrations, but not in serum LDL-cholesterol concentration, than in the low-fat group. In addition, glycemic control was better with low-carbohydrate than a low-fat diet therapy in subjects who had type 2 DM [56–59]. It is important to note that these studies were short term.

However, a diet high in fiber and potassium and low in saturated fat, refined carbohydrates, and salt can improve glycemic control and the lipid profile, and significantly lower BP [60]. In the Dietary Approaches to Stop Hypertension (DASH) Study, a diet abundant in fruits and vegetables, as well as low-fat dairy products, with or without sodium restriction, substantially reduced BP in hypertensive patients [61]. Furthermore, epidemiologic and clinical investigations have identified three major dietary strategies that are particularly effective for preventing CVD:

1. Substitute nonhydrogenated unsaturated fats for saturated and trans-fats.
2. Increase consumption of omega-3 fatty acids from fish or plant sources.
3. Consume a diet high in fruits, vegetables, nuts, and whole grains and low in refined grain products [62].

Using data from the NHANES III (1988–1994), consumption of fruits and vegetables was found to be lower among people with CMS. Further, CMS was associated with suboptimal circulating concentrations of vitamin C, vitamin E, retinyl esters, and carotenoids [63]. The antioxidant properties of these substances may play an important role in the disease-risk reduction properties of fruits and vegetables and other plant-derived foods. However, studies evaluating the benefits of individual antioxidant vitamin supplements in preventing disease have to date been disappointing.

Alternatively, controlled intervention trials with fish oil supplements enriched in eicosapentaenoic acid (EPA) and docosahexaenoic acid (DHA) have shown a potential to reduce mortality in post-myocardial infarction patients with a substantial reduction in the risk of sudden cardiac death, which is markedly increased in CMS and DM. The cardioprotective effects of EPA/DHA appear to be related to anti-arrhythmic, blood triglyceride-lowering, anti-thrombotic, anti-inflammatory, and endothelial relaxation effects, but independent of changes in blood cholesterol or glucose [64]. Furthermore, one study suggested that the protective role of fish oil in atherosclerosis-prone mice (apoE –/–) may result from the induction of antioxidant enzymes [65].

7.4.2 PHYSICAL ACTIVITY

A sedentary lifestyle is associated with increased CVD, while physical activity lowers cardiovascular risk in part by lowering BP and improving insulin sensitivity. Data from longitudinal cohort studies from the Cooper Institute have shown that low cardiorespiratory fitness and physical inactivity are independent predictors of all-cause mortality in men with type 2 DM, and that unfit men have a higher risk of all-cause and CVD mortality than do fit men in all body fatness categories. Furthermore, although CVD and all-cause mortality were increased in men with CMS, this risk was no longer significant when cardiorespiratory fitness was considered [66]. Data on the amount and intensity of physical activity required for cardiovascular health is less clear. The most recent data show that high physical activity, defined as a combination of vigorous occupational activity more than 30 minutes daily and leisure-time physical activity more than 4 hours a week is associated with a lower risk of hypertension, independent of baseline BMI [67]. One author (HY) and colleagues have shown that frequent habitual exercise with its inherent mild weight loss has a significant beneficial impact on body composition and the risk factors associated with CMS, and cardiovascular and metabolic disease in an older obese population [68]. The addition of a diet-based weight loss program to an exercise intervention may be advantageous in younger age groups, but may be unnecessary in older obese adults who exercise habitually and consume a diet of approximate 2000 kcal. Given the relatively low aerobic fitness of these individuals with CMS, a walking program five times a week with each session lasting at least 30 minutes can bring about significant weight loss, and an improvement in clinical outcomes in as little as 12 weeks [68].

It is important to note that even with optimal physical activity and diet; some patients will still require pharmacologic treatment. Antiplatelet therapy with aspirin, RAAS inhibition with ACE inhibitors or angiotensin blockers, and HMG-CoA reductase (statin) lipid-lowering effects and pleiotropic benefits on inflammation have been shown to improve CVD survival for patients with DM and the CMS.

7.5 SUMMARY

Increasing numbers of older adults are being diagnosed with DM and CMS. It is of paramount importance that primary care providers recognize that DM is not solely a matter of blood sugar control. Physical activity with a healthy diet remains the cornerstone of treatment. Although weight loss through caloric restriction is widely accepted as the treatment of choice in younger populations, the elderly present additional challenges. A careful dietary approach that is low in fat and refined sugars together with regular daily activity as simple as brisk walking for at least 30 minutes have been shown to be highly effective. The importance of other dietary considerations, including the optimal amounts of monounsaturated and polyunsaturated fats, amount and sources of protein, and the effects of individual phytochemicals and antioxidants remains unsettled. Yet, the approach to treatment of these patients entails consideration of the underlying pathophysiologic mechanisms including oxidative stress, which may be impacted by pharmacologic therapy that includes antiplatelet therapy, RAAS inhibition, or statin use. Motivating patients to initiate and maintain lifestyle changes remains a challenge but is extraordinarily important for older patients at risk for diabetic CVD.

REFERENCES

1. Vita, A. J., Terry, R. B., Hubert, H. B., and Fries, J. F. 1998. Aging, health risks, and cumulative disability. *N Engl J Med* 338, 1035–1041.
2. Cowie, C. C., Rust, K. F., Byrd-Holt, D. D., Eberhardt, M. S., Flegal, K. M., Engelgau, et al. 2006. Prevalence of diabetes and impaired fasting glucose in adults in the U.S. population: National Health and Nutrition Examination Survey 1999–2002. *Diabetes Care* 29, 1263–1268.
3. Grundy, S. M., Brewer, H. B., Jr., Cleeman, J. I., Smith, S. C., Jr., and Lenfant, C. 2004. Definition of metabolic syndrome: Report of the National Heart, Lung, and Blood Institute/American Heart Association conference on scientific issues related to definition. *Circulation* 109, 433–438.
4. Stern, N. and Izkhakov, Y. 2006. The metabolic syndrome revisited: "cardiometabolic risk" emerges as common ground between differing views of the ADA and AHA. *J Cardiometab Syndr* 1, 362–363.
5. Ford, E. S., Giles, W. H., and Dietz, W. H. 2002. Prevalence of the metabolic syndrome among US adults: Findings from the third National Health and Nutrition Examination Survey. *JAMA* 287, 356–359.
6. Alexander, C. M., Landsman, P. B., Teutsch, S. M. and Haffner, S. M. 2003. NCEP-defined metabolic syndrome, diabetes, and prevalence of coronary heart disease among NHANES III participants age 50 years and older. *Diabetes* 52, 1210–1214.
7. Stamler, J., Vaccaro, O., Neaton, J. D. and Wentworth, D. 1993. Diabetes, other risk factors, and 12-yr cardiovascular mortality for men screened in the Multiple Risk Factor Intervention Trial. *Diabetes Care* 16, 434–444.
8. Kregel, K. C. and Zhang, H. J. 2007. An integrated view of oxidative stress in aging: Basic mechanisms, functional effects, and pathological considerations. *Am J Physiol Regul Integr Comp Physiol* 292, R18–36.
9. Yorek, M. A. 2003. The role of oxidative stress in diabetic vascular and neural disease. *Free Radic Res* 37, 471–480.
10. Onozato, M. L., Tojo, A., Goto, A., Fujita, T. and Wilcox, C. S. 2002. Oxidative stress and nitric oxide synthase in rat diabetic nephropathy: Effects of ACEI and ARB. *Kidney Int* 61, 186–194.
11. Sowers, J. R. 1990. Insulin resistance and hypertension. *Mol Cell Endocrinol* 74, C87–89.
12. Sowers, J. R. 2004. Treatment of hypertension in patients with diabetes. *Arch Intern Med* 164, 1850–1857.
13. Reaven, G. M., Lithell, H., and Landsberg, L. 1996. Hypertension and associated metabolic abnormalities—the role of insulin resistance and the sympathoadrenal system. *N Engl J Med* 334, 374–381.
14. McFarlane, S. I., Banerji, M., and Sowers, J. R. 2001. Insulin resistance and cardiovascular disease. *J Clin Endocrinol Metab* 86, 713–718.
15. Meigs, J. B., Hu, F. B., Rifai, N., and Manson, J. E. 2004. Biomarkers of endothelial dysfunction and risk of type 2 diabetes mellitus. *JAMA* 291, 1978–1986.
16. Williams, S. B., Cusco, J. A., Roddy, M. A., Johnstone, M. T., and Creager, M. A. 1996. Impaired nitric oxide-mediated vasodilation in patients with non-insulin-dependent diabetes mellitus. *J Am Coll Cardiol* 27, 567–574.
17. Fukai, T., Folz, R. J., Landmesser, U., and Harrison, D. G. 2002. Extracellular superoxide dismutase and cardiovascular disease. *Cardiovasc Res* 55, 239–249.
18. Sowers, J. R., Epstein, M., and Frohlich, E. D. 2001. Diabetes, hypertension, and cardiovascular disease: An update. *Hypertension* 37, 1053–1059.
19. Toshima, S., Hasegawa, A., Kurabayashi, M., Itabe, H., Takano, T., Sugano, J., et al. 2000. Circulating oxidized low density lipoprotein levels. A biochemical risk marker for coronary heart disease. *Arterioscler Thromb Vasc Biol* 20, 2243–2247.
20. Kopprasch, S., Pietzsch, J., Kuhlisch, E., Fuecker, K., Temelkova-Kurktschiev, T., Hanefeld, et al. 2002. In vivo evidence for increased oxidation of circulating LDL in impaired glucose tolerance. *Diabetes* 51, 3102–3106.
21. Mertens, A. and Holvoet, P. 2001. Oxidized LDL and HDL: Antagonists in atherothrombosis. *Faseb J* 15, 2073–2084.
22. Khalil, A., Wagner, J. R., Lacombe, G., Dangoisse, V., and Fulop, T., Jr. 1996. Increased susceptibility of low-density lipoprotein LDL to oxidation by gamma-radiolysis with age. *FEBS Lett* 392, 45–48.
23. Jira, W., Spiteller, G., and Schramm, A. 1996. Increase in hydroxy fatty acids in human low density lipoproteins with age. *Chem Phys Lipids* 84, 165–173.

24. Liguori, A., Abete, P., Hayden, J. M., Cacciatore, F., Rengo, F., Ambrosio, G., et al. 2001. Effect of glycaemic control and age on low-density lipoprotein susceptibility to oxidation in diabetes mellitus type 1. *Eur Heart J* 22, 2075–2084.

25. McFarlane, S. I. and Sowers, J. R. 2003. Cardiovascular endocrinology 1: aldosterone function in diabetes mellitus: Effects on cardiovascular and renal disease. *J Clin Endocrinol Metab* 88, 516–523.

26. Dzau, V. J. 2001. Theodore Cooper Lecture: Tissue angiotensin and pathobiology of vascular disease: a unifying hypothesis. *Hypertension* 37, 1047–1052.

27. Sowers, J. R. and Stump, C. S. 2004. Insights into the biology of diabetic vascular disease: what's new? *Am J Hypertens* 17, 2S–6S; quiz A2–4.

28. Henriksen, E. J. and Saengsirisuwan, V. 2003. Exercise training and antioxidants: Relief from oxidative stress and insulin resistance. *Exerc Sport Sci Rev* 31, 79–84.

29. Forbes, J. M., Cooper, M. E., Thallas, V., Burns, W. C., Thomas, M. C., Brammar, G. C., et al. 2002. Reduction of the accumulation of advanced glycation end products by ACE inhibition in experimental diabetic nephropathy. *Diabetes* 51, 3274–3282.

30. Oudot, A., Martin, C., Busseuil, D., Vergely, C., Demaison, L. and Rochette, L. 2006. NADPH oxidases are in part responsible for increased cardiovascular superoxide production during aging. *Free Radic Biol Med* 40, 2214–2222.

31. Gilliam-Davis, S., Payne, V. S., Kasper, S. O., Tommasi, E. N., Robbins, M. E. and Diz, D. I. 2007. Long-term AT1 receptor blockade improves metabolic function and provides renoprotection in Fischer-344 rats. *Am J Physiol Heart Circ Physiol* 293, H1327–1333.

32. Duncan, B. B., Schmidt, M. I., Pankow, J. S., Ballantyne, C. M., Couper, D., Vigo, A., et al. 2003. Low-grade systemic inflammation and the development of type 2 diabetes: the atherosclerosis risk in communities study. *Diabetes* 52, 1799–1805.

33. Weisberg, S. P., McCann, D., Desai, M., Rosenbaum, M., Leibel, R. L. and Ferrante, A. W., Jr. 2003. Obesity is associated with macrophage accumulation in adipose tissue. *J Clin Invest* 112, 1796–1808.

34. Havel, P. J. 2004. Update on adipocyte hormones: Regulation of energy balance and carbohydrate/lipid metabolism. *Diabetes* 53 Suppl 1, S143–151.

35. Furukawa, S., Fujita, T., Shimabukuro, M., Iwaki, M., Yamada, Y., Nakajima, Y., et al. 2004. Increased oxidative stress in obesity and its impact on metabolic syndrome. *J Clin Invest* 114, 1752–1761.

36. Cefalu, W. T., Wang, Z. Q., Werbel, S., Bell-Farrow, A., Crouse, J. R., 3rd, Hinson, W. H., et al. 1995. Contribution of visceral fat mass to the insulin resistance of aging. *Metabolism* 44, 954–959.

37. Coon, P. J., Rogus, E. M., Drinkwater, D., Muller, D. C., and Goldberg, A. P. 1992. Role of body fat distribution in the decline in insulin sensitivity and glucose tolerance with age. *J Clin Endocrinol Metab* 75, 1125–1132.

38. Gabriely, I., Ma, X. H., Yang, X. M., Atzmon, G., Rajala, M. W., Berg, A. H., et al. 2002. Removal of visceral fat prevents insulin resistance and glucose intolerance of aging: An adipokine-mediated process? *Diabetes* 51, 2951–2958.

39. Chen, M., Bergman, R. N., Pacini, G., and Porte, D., Jr. 1985. Pathogenesis of age-related glucose intolerance in man: Insulin resistance and decreased beta-cell function. *J Clin Endocrinol Metab* 60, 13–20.

40. Davidson, M. B. 1979. The effect of aging on carbohydrate metabolism: a review of the English literature and a practical approach to the diagnosis of diabetes mellitus in the elderly. *Metabolism* 28, 688–705.

41. Maneatis, T., Condie, R., and Reaven, G. 1982. Effect of age on plasma glucose and insulin responses to a test mixed meal. *J Am Geriatr Soc* 30, 178–182.

42. Shimokata, H., Muller, D. C., Fleg, J. L., Sorkin, J., Ziemba, A. W., and Andres, R. 1991. Age as independent determinant of glucose tolerance. *Diabetes* 40, 44–51.

43. Defronzo, R. A. 1979. Glucose intolerance and aging: Evidence for tissue insensitivity to insulin. *Diabetes* 28, 1095–1101.

44. Fink, R. I., Kolterman, O. G., Griffin, J., and Olefsky, J. M. 1983. Mechanisms of insulin resistance in aging. *J Clin Invest* 71, 1523–1535.

45. Kahn, S. E., Larson, V. G., Schwartz, R. S., Beard, J. C., Cain, K. C., Fellingham, G. W., et al. 1992. Exercise training delineates the importance of B-cell dysfunction to the glucose intolerance of human aging. *J Clin Endocrinol Metab* 74, 1336–1342.

46. DeFronzo, R. A., Bonadonna, R. C., and Ferrannini, E. 1992. Pathogenesis of NIDDM. A balanced overview. *Diabetes Care* 15, 318–368.

47. Basu, R., Breda, E., Oberg, A. L., Powell, C. C., Dalla Man, C., Basu, A., et al. 2003. Mechanisms of the age-associated deterioration in glucose tolerance: Contribution of alterations in insulin secretion, action, and clearance. *Diabetes* 52, 1738–1748.

48. The Diabetes Control and Complications Trial Research Group. 1993. The effect of intensive treatment of diabetes on the development and progression of long-term complications in insulin-dependent diabetes mellitus. *N Engl J Med* 329, 977–986.

49. UK Prospective Diabetes Study UKPDS. Group. 1998. Intensive blood-glucose control with sulphonylureas or insulin compared with conventional treatment and risk of complications in patients with type 2 diabetes UKPDS 33. *Lancet* 352, 837–853.

50. Knowler, W. C., Barrett-Connor, E., Fowler, S. E., Hamman, R. F., Lachin, J. M., Walker, E. A. and Nathan, D. M. 2002. Reduction in the incidence of type 2 diabetes with lifestyle intervention or metformin. *N Engl J Med* 346, 393–403.

51. Das, S. K., Moriguti, J. C., McCrory, M. A., Saltzman, E., Mosunic, C., Greenberg, A. S., and Roberts, S. B. 2001. An underfeeding study in healthy men and women provides further evidence of impaired regulation of energy expenditure in old age. *J Nutr* 131, 1833–1838.

52. Newman, A. B., Lee, J. S., Visser, M., Goodpaster, B. H., Kritchevsky, S. B., Tylavsky, F. A., et al. 2005. Weight change and the conservation of lean mass in old age: The Health, Aging and Body Composition Study. *Am J Clin Nutr* 82, 872–878; quiz 915–876.

53. Kyle, U. G., Genton, L., Hans, D., Karsegard, L., Slosman, D. O. and Pichard, C. 2001. Age-related differences in fat-free mass, skeletal muscle, body cell mass and fat mass between 18 and 94 years. *Eur J Clin Nutr* 55, 663–672.

54. Standards of medical care in diabetes. 2005. *Diabetes Care* 28 Suppl 1, S4–S36.

55. Brown, A. F., Mangione, C. M., Saliba, D., and Sarkisian, C. A. 2003. Guidelines for improving the care of the older person with diabetes mellitus. *J Am Geriatr Soc* 51, S265–280.

56. Samaha, F. F., Iqbal, N., Seshadri, P., Chicano, K. L., Daily, D. A., McGrory, J., et al. 2003. A low-carbohydrate as compared with a low-fat diet in severe obesity. *N Engl J Med* 348, 2074–2081.

57. Brehm, B. J., Seeley, R. J., Daniels, S. R., and D'Alessio, D. A. 2003. A randomized trial comparing a very low carbohydrate diet and a calorie-restricted low fat diet on body weight and cardiovascular risk factors in healthy women. *J Clin Endocrinol* Metab 88, 1617–1623.

58. Foster, G. D., Wyatt, H. R., Hill, J. O., McGuckin, B. G., Brill, C., Mohammed, B. S., et al. 2003. A randomized trial of a low-carbohydrate diet for obesity. *N Engl J Med* 348, 2082–2090.

59. Yancy, W. S., Jr., Olsen, M. K., Guyton, J. R., Bakst, R. P., and Westman, E. C. 2004. A low-carbohydrate, ketogenic diet versus a low-fat diet to treat obesity and hyperlipidemia: A randomized, controlled trial. *Ann Intern Med* 140, 769–777.

60. Lindstrom, J., Peltonen, M., Eriksson, J. G., Louheranta, A., Fogelholm, et al. 2006. High-fibre, low-fat diet predicts long-term weight loss and decreased type 2 diabetes risk: The Finnish Diabetes Prevention Study. *Diabetologia* 49, 912–920.

61. Sacks, F. M., Svetkey, L. P., Vollmer, W. M., Appel, L. J., Bray, G. A., et al. 2001. Effects on blood pressure of reduced dietary sodium and the Dietary Approaches to Stop Hypertension (DASH) diet. DASH-Sodium Collaborative Research Group. *N Engl J Med* 344, 3–10.

62. Hu, F. B. and Willett, W. C. 2002. Optimal diets for prevention of coronary heart disease. *JAMA* 288, 2569–2578.

63. Ford, E. S., Mokdad, A. H., Giles, W. H., and Brown, D. W. 2003. The metabolic syndrome and antioxidant concentrations: Findings from the Third National Health and Nutrition Examination Survey. *Diabetes* 52, 2346–2352.

64. Holub, D. J. and Holub, B. J. 2004. Omega-3 fatty acids from fish oils and cardiovascular disease. *Mol Cell Biochem* 263, 217–225.

65. Wang, H. H., Hung, T. M., Wei, J., and Chiang, A. N. 2004. Fish oil increases antioxidant enzyme activities in macrophages and reduces atherosclerotic lesions in apoE-knockout mice. *Cardiovasc Res* 61, 169–176.

66. Wei, M., Gibbons, L. W., Kampert, J. B., Nichaman, M. Z., and Blair, S. N. 2000. Low cardiorespiratory fitness and physical inactivity as predictors of mortality in men with type 2 diabetes. *Ann Intern Med* 132, 605–611.

67. Hu, G., Barengo, N. C., Tuomilehto, J., Lakka, T. A., Nissinen, A., and Jousilahti, P. 2004. Relationship of physical activity and body mass index to the risk of hypertension: A prospective study in Finland. *Hypertension* 43, 25–30.

68. Yassine, H. N., Marchetti, C. P., Brooks, L. M., Krishnan, R. K., Gonzalez, F., and Kirwan, J. P. 2008. Effects of exercise and weight loss on multiple cardiac risk factors associated with metabolic syndrome in an elderly population. *J. Gerontol.: Med. Sci.*, in press.

8 Calcium and Vitamin D in Aging Populations

Zhao Chen and Jeffrey Stanaway

CONTENTS

8.1 INTRODUCTION

In the past few decades, there have been major developments in understanding the role of nutrients in health and disease. Calcium and vitamin D are among the most interesting of these nutrients, having great relevance to public health, disease prevention, and clinical management in the elderly. Given the important role of vitamin D in calcium economy, these two nutrients are often studied and discussed together in the literature; however, it has increasingly been recognized that vitamin D has many functions other than regulating calcium absorption and metabolism in the human body. Similarly, calcium intake levels have been found to be associated with many health outcomes besides bone health. Although calcium and vitamin D levels needed to prevent nutrient deficiencies have long been established, the necessary amounts for optimal health among older men and women are still subjects of research and discussion. This chapter will review the basic metabolic processes of calcium and vitamin D in normal healthy populations, identify food and supplementary sources for them, discuss daily requirements and factors pertaining to their status in older people, and provide an updated summary of the associations between health and intake levels in optimal aging. We hope the information included will paint a comprehensive picture for individual consumers and health professionals regarding the impact of calcium and vitamin D on the overall health of elderly men and women.

8.2 METABOLISM OF CALCIUM AND VITAMIN D

8.2.1 CALCIUM METABOLISM

Calcium is usually absorbed in ionized form (Ca^{+2}) or bound to a soluble organic molecule. Absorption may occur through either active transport or passive diffusion. Active transport is the primary means of absorption at low to moderate intake levels, and occurs primarily in the duodenum and upper jejunum. This mechanism, which is dependent on 1,25-dihydroxyvitamin D, is regulated by dietary intake and needs, and is, therefore, saturable. This regulation alters fractional absorption so that it varies inversely with intake. Though fractional absorption does increase with decreased dietary intake, this increase is inadequate to compensate for the decreased calcium intake. Passive diffusion involves the movement of calcium between mucosal cells down an electrochemical gradient. Absorption by passive diffusion occurs mostly in the ileum. Passive diffusion is unregulated and unsaturable, and is, therefore, important when calcium intake is high [1,2].

About 99% of calcium is stored in bone and teeth. The remaining 1% occurs intracellularly, within organelles, and extracellularly, in blood, lymph, and other body fluids. Of the calcium in blood, about 50% occurs as free calcium; about 40% is bound to proteins, most commonly albumin; and the remaining 10% occurs in complexes with sulfate, phosphate, or citrate [1,2].

Calcium is excreted in urine, feces, and sweat. Urine is the primary means of calcium excretion, accounting for between 100 and 240 mg of daily calcium excretion; of this urinary calcium, about half occurs in ionized form (Ca^{+2}) while the remaining half occurs in calcium complexes. Fecal loss accounts for 45 to 100mg of calcium daily, and an average of 60mg of calcium is excreted with sweat through the skin each day. Excretion, primarily urinary excretion, is hormonally regulated [1,2].

Intracellular and extracellular calcium concentrations are tightly regulated, primarily by the actions of three hormones: parathyroid hormone (PTH), calcitonin, and calcitriol (1,25-dihydroxyvitamin D_3). PTH increases extracellular calcium concentration by stimulating calcium resorption from bone and increasing renal calcium reabsorption. Calcitonin lowers extracellular calcium concentrations by inhibiting bone resorption by osteoclasts. 1,25-dihydroxyvitamin D_3 acts by stimulating gastrointestinal calcium absorption [1,2].

8.2.2 VITAMIN D METABOLISM

Vitamin D may be consumed in the diet or produced endogenously through exposure of skin to sunlight. About 80% of dietary vitamin D is absorbed from micelles through passive diffusion into intestinal cells. Here, vitamin D integrates into chylomicrons and enters the lymphatic system and, subsequently, the blood. Most dietary vitamin D is absorbed in the distal small intestine, though absorption occurs most rapidly in the duodenum [1].

Though dietary intake is important for some individuals, especially those with limited sun exposure, that sun exposure is the primary source of vitamin D for people around the world. Endogenous production of vitamin D occurs in the skin, where exposure to ultraviolet B radiation (UVB; wavelength between 290 and 315nm) converts 7-dehydrocholesterol to previtamin D_3. Previtamin D_3 then undergoes thermal isomerization to vitamin D_3 (cholecalciferol). This vitamin D_3, and vitamin D_3 from the diet are activated to 1,25-dihydroxyvitamin D_3 in a two-step process: first, 25-hydroxylase, primarily in the liver, converts vitamin D_3 to 25-hydroxyvitamin D_3; then, in a reaction tightly regulated by PTH and serum calcium and phosphorus, 1α-hydroxylase in the kidney converts 25-hydroxyvitamin D_3 to 1,25-dihydroxyvitamin D_3 [3].

As a lipophilic molecule, more than 99% of circulating vitamin D is bound to plasma proteins for transportation in the blood. Vitamin D binding protein (DBP) is the most important of these proteins; however, albumin and lipoproteins may also bind vitamin D and its metabolites [3]. Vitamin D may be stored in adipose tissue for release during times of inadequate production and intake, typically during winter months when sun exposure is limited [4].

Vitamin D is excreted primarily in bile; some of this excreted vitamin D may be reabsorbed in the small intestine. Some vitamin D is metabolized to calcitroic acid, a more water-soluble molecule than vitamin D, and this calcitroic acid may be excreted in urine. Urinary excretion accounts for less than 5% of total vitamin D excretion [1].

Endogenous vitamin D production is influenced by length and intensity of sun exposure, skin pigmentation, and age. Variation in sunlight intensity by season, time of day, and latitude strongly affect vitamin D production. For those living more than 40° away from the equator, sun exposure is inadequate to sustain vitamin D synthesis for 3 to 4 months during the winter; synthesis may halt for up to 6 months among those living at extreme latitudes [5]. Skin melanin pigmentation may absorb UVB, thereby reducing vitamin D synthesis in the skin. Consequently, blacks may synthesize vitamin D less efficiently than whites, given the same level of sun exposure [6]. In addition to these factors, reduced levels of 7-dehydrocholesterol in the skin cause vitamin D synthesis to decrease with age: by age 70, vitamin D synthesis can be expected to decrease by approximately 75% [4].

Therefore, it is a great challenge to recommend a single daily intake of vitamin D to all people who may have different levels of sun exposure and skin synthesis [7].

8.3   FOOD SOURCES OF CALCIUM AND VITAMIN D

8.3.1   Calcium Sources

Dairy products are the primary source of dietary calcium in the United States, accounting for 71.7% of the calcium in the 2004 food supply. Other sources include vegetables (7.0%); grain products (4.9%); legumes, nuts, and soy (4.3%); meat, poultry, and fish (3.4%); fruits (2.6%); and eggs (1.8%) [8]. The relative contribution of calcium from each food group is shown in Figure 8.1.

Though dairy accounts for more than two-thirds of our calcium supply, other naturally calcium-rich foods are also important: bok choy, kale, broccoli, rhubarb, spinach, sweet potatoes, dried beans, and tofu are all rich in calcium. The low bioavailability of the calcium in some of these foods, however, limits their importance as sources of calcium. While spinach and milk contain similar amounts of calcium (135mg calcium/100g spinach, vs. 125mg calcium/100g milk), for example, the body will obtain nearly six times more calcium from milk than from spinach (6.90mg of absorbable calcium/100g spinach, vs. 40.13mg of absorbable calcium/100g milk). It is therefore critical to consider bioavailability and its affecting factors when evaluating the quality of calcium sources [9]. Table 8.1 shows the calcium content, fractional absorption, and absorbable calcium in different foods.

Certain dietary components, including phytates, oxalates, and tannins, can significantly reduce calcium absorption by binding calcium in insoluble complexes. Phytates are present in raw beans, seeds, nuts, grains, and soy isolates; oxalates are present in spinach, sweet potatoes, rhubarb, walnuts, and beans. Consequently, calcium in these foods is generally less absorbable. Similarly, excessive consumption of other dietary components, including sodium, protein, and caffeine, may modestly decrease calcium retention. Vitamin D deficiency can also impair calcium absorption. There is evidence to suggest that dietary fiber and lipids may hinder calcium absorption; however, the effect appears to be insignificant. [2,5,10].

Conversely, certain milk components are believed to improve calcium absorption. Phosphopeptides, derived from caseins, may sequester and protect calcium, thereby enhancing absorption in the distal intestine. Lactose may also enhance calcium absorption, possibly by increasing the permeability of intestinal mucosa. This effect appears to require doses as high as 50g of lactose per day, suggesting that the amount of lactose found in milk is insufficient to appreciably improve calcium absorption [2].

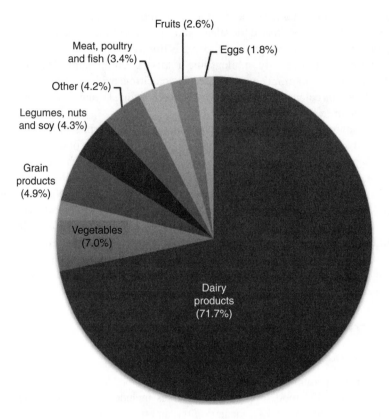

FIGURE 8.1   Sources of calcium in the U.S. food supply in 2004 [8].

Dairy products are the most widely recommended food sources of calcium [2,9]. Calcium-set tofu and low oxylate vegetables including kale, broccoli, and bok choy are especially good alternatives to dairy. Reducing sodium and caffeine intake and avoiding unusually high protein diets may also help to improve calcium status; limiting these factors, however, is likely to be a less practical and effective means of improving calcium status than increasing consumption of calcium-rich foods. Individuals choosing to avoid dairy should increase their consumption of low-oxylate vegetables and soy products, especially calcium-set tofu, and consider including fortified foods or calcium supplements [2,9].

8.3.2 VITAMIN D SOURCES

As stated earlier, dietary intake may be important (both vitamin D_3 and vitamin D_2—ergocalciferol) for people where sun exposure is limited. Since few foods are naturally rich in vitamin D, most dietary intake is from fortified foods such as milk products and fortified breakfast cereals. Though all milk in the United States and Canada is fortified with vitamin D, surveys suggest that actual vitamin D content is highly variable, with up to 70% of milk containing levels outside the allowable range of 8 to 12µg per quart [5].

Though vitamin D_2 may occur in plant products, vitamin D is found primarily in animal foods. Naturally rich foods include fatty fish, fish liver oils, and eggs from vitamin D-fed hens; mushrooms contain vitamin D_2 [4,5]. With fortification, however, vitamin D is now found in a wider range of food products. In the United States, nearly all fluid, concentrated, evaporated, and dried milks are fortified with vitamin D. Additionally, most ready-to-eat breakfast cereals and some yogurt, margarine, and fruit juices, are also fortified [11]. The vitamin D content of several natural and fortified vitamin D food sources is given in Table 8.2.

TABLE 8.1

Comparison of Calcium Content and Absorbable Calcium of Several Common Calcium Sources

Food	Calcium Content (mg Ca/100g food)[a]	Fractional Absorption[a]	Absorbable Calcium (mg Ca/100g food)[b]
Cheddar cheese	721.4	32.1%	231.6
Chinese mustard greens	249.4	40.2%	100.3
Tofu with calcium	204.8	31.0%	63.5
Bok choy	92.9	53.8%	50.0
Milk	125.0	32.1%	40.1
Yogurt	125.0	32.1%	40.1
Kale	71.8	49.3%	35.4
Broccoli	49.3	61.3%	30.2
White beans	102.7	21.8%	22.4
Pinto beans	52.0	26.7%	13.9
Rhubarb	145.0	8.5%	12.4
Spinach	135.3	5.1%	6.9
Sweet potatoes	26.8	22.2%	6.0
Red beans	23.6	24.4%	5.8

[a] Based on data from [9]
[b] Calculated as calcium content × fractional absorption

Attempts to assess bioavailability are complicated by endogenous production of vitamin D. Estimates suggest that between 55% and 99% of vitamin D from supplements given with oil or fat is absorbed. Absorption of vitamin D from food sources may be as much as 60% lower. Dietary fiber may reduce absorption and increase vitamin D elimination. Similarly, vitamin D absorption may be reduced by iron deficiency [12].

Healthy individuals with regular exposure to sunlight are unlikely to require dietary vitamin D. Sensible sun exposure is the best means of ensuring good vitamin D status for most people. Those who produce inadequate endogenous vitamin D due to limited sun exposure, aging or a vitamin D synthesis disorder, should increase consumption of foods with vitamin D and consider supplementation [4,12].

8.4 CALCIUM AND VITAMIN D SUPPLEMENTS

8.4.1 CALCIUM SUPPLEMENTS

Several different forms of calcium are used in calcium supplements. Calcium carbonate, the most common and least expensive form, contains the greatest percent elemental calcium of any of the commonly used calcium salts (40% calcium by weight). Calcium citrate is the second-most commonly used form. Estimates of the bioavailability of these and other forms of supplemental calcium vary by study and differing methodologies, and disagreement exists regarding the relative advantages and disadvantages of each form. Bioavailability estimates range from about 25% to nearly 40% and vary more with study design than with calcium form. Nevertheless, calcium citrate is generally regarded as being more absorbable for individuals with decreased stomach acid.

TABLE 8.2

Natural and Fortified Dietary Sources of Vitamin D

Food	Approximate Vitamin D Content[a]
Natural Sources	
Salmon	
Fresh, wild (3.5 oz)	600–1000 IU
Fresh, farmed (3.5 oz)	100–250 IU[c]
Canned (3.5 oz)	300–600 IU
Sardines, canned (3.5 oz)	300 IU
Mackerel, canned (3.5 oz)	250 IU
Tuna, canned (3.6 oz)	230 IU
Cod liver oil (1 tsp)	400–1000 IU
Shiitake mushrooms	
Fresh (3.5 oz)	100 IU[b]
Sun-dried (3.5 oz)	1600 IU[b]
Egg yolk	20 IU[c]
Fortified Sources	
Fortified milk (8 oz)	100 IU[c]
Fortified orange juice (8 oz)	100 IU
Infant formulas (8 oz)	100 IU
Fortified yogurts (8 oz)	100 IU[c]
Fortified butter (3.5oz)	50 IU[c]
Fortified margarine (3.5 oz)	430 IU[c]
Fortified cheeses (3 oz)	100 IU[c]
Fortified breakfast cereals (per serving)	100 IU[c]

[a] products contain vitamin D_3, unless otherwise indicated.
[b] product contains vitamin D_2.
[c] product may contain vitamin D_2 and/or vitamin D_3.

Source: Holick, M. F. 2007. *Nutrient content of the U.S. food supply, 1909–2004: A summary report.*

Regardless of calcium form, supplements are better absorbed when taken with food, and when taken in doses of 500mg or less [1,2,5].

Three primary safety concerns exist for calcium supplements: excessive calcium intake, medication interactions, and toxic metals found in certain supplements. Excessive calcium intake can cause kidney stones and hypercalcemia and interfere with iron, zinc, magnesium, and phosphorus absorption; consequently, all adults, plus children over the age of 1 year, should consume no more than 2,500mg of calcium per day from all sources (food and supplements combined) [5]. Calcium supplements may interfere with certain medications, including digoxin, fluoroquinolones, levothyroxine, tetracycline family antibiotics, tiludronate disodium, anticonvulsants, thiazide, glucocorticoids, mineral oil, stimulant laxatives, and certain antacids [13]. Calcium supplements containing calcium carbonate derived from fossilized oyster shell, dolomite, or bone meal may contain aluminum or lead, and are, therefore, not recommended [1].

8.4.2 VITAMIN D SUPPLEMENTS

The difficulty of obtaining adequate vitamin D from dietary sources as well as concerns regarding the health risks associated with excessive sun exposure indicate that supplementation may be an important means to obtain adequate vitamin D [4]. Supplemental vitamin D is typically synthesized through the irradiation of ergocalciferol or cholecalciferol, and can be in the either vitamin D_2 or D_3, in crystalline or resin form [11]. Evidence suggests that absorption of vitamin D from supplements ranges from 55 to 99%, and may be greater than absorption from food sources [12]. While vitamin D is potentially toxic at high levels, supplementation appears to be safe when total dietary intake from all sources (food and supplements) is limited to less than 50µg (2,000 IU) per day [5].

8.5 CALCIUM AND VITAMIN D IN DISEASE PREVENTION AND OPTIMAL HEALTH IN THE ELDERLY

Early nutritional science largely focused on short-latency deficiency diseases and would often link one nutrient with one specific disease, or so called index disease [14]. Calcium and vitamin D are both considered bone-related nutrients and have been studied extensively in that regard. Though the index disease for vitamin D is rickets (or osteomalacia), among the elderly, the major health outcome associated with both calcium and vitamin D is osteoporosis. Osteoporosis, the most common bone disease, is characterized by low bone density, deterioration of bone microstructures, compromised bone strength, and increased risk for bone fractures. The importance of calcium and vitamin D in preventing osteoporosis has been widely accepted only in the past 10 years. As recently as 1989, *British Medical Journal* published a two-part review suggesting no relationship between low calcium intake and the development of osteoporosis [15,16]. This slow understanding of the role of calcium and vitamin D in bone density and mass may result because osteoporosis is a latent disease [14] and people having certain potential to adjust their fractional absorption to adapt to a low-calcium diet. Cumulative evidence supports an association between low calcium intake [13] and vitamin D levels [14,4] and low bone density. Inadequate calcium intake may prevent growing children from reaching their genetic potential for peak bone mass. Low calcium levels in adults may not be able to offset the obligatory losses of calcium during late adult life. Both factors contribute to osteoporosis development. It has been demonstrated that supplementing calcium and vitamin D in older men and women may help them maintain their bone density and reduce nonvertebral fracture risk [17,23]. Studies have demonstrated that increasing serum 25-hydroxyvitamin D concentrations from 50nmol/L to 80 nmol/L can increase calcium absorption by more than 60% [10] and reduce bone fracture by 30% [18].

The most recent large Women's Health Initiative trial among U.S. postmenopausal women suggests that calcium and vitamin D supplementation may reduce hip fracture risk, clinical spinal fracture, and total fracture risk [19]. The borderline statistically significant reduction in fracture risk may have resulted from the sample's comprising healthy women with higher calcium and vitamin D intakes than the general population. In addition, the follow-up was not long enough to generate the number of fractures that would have achieved statistical significance.

Beside osteoporosis, calcium has also been found to play a role in colorectal cancer, other malignancies, hypertension, obesity, and autoimmune diseases [20]. The relationship between calcium intake and other health outcomes, such as obesity, hypertension and cancer, may be related to a second mechanism involving the functionality of calcium within the gut lumen. Unabsorbed calcium binds with substances such as food oxalate and unabsorbed fatty and bile acids [14].

It has been hypothesized that vitamin D may have two distinct functions in its effect on health. The first, the classic endocrine function with calcium metabolism, is regulated by parathyroid hormone (PTH). The major target tissues are gut and bone in this function. The second and more recently recognized function of vitamin D is related to autocrine (or perhaps paracrine) function. Many extrarenal human tissues and cells express 25-hydroxyvitamin D-1α-hydroxylase, which is needed to convert 25-hydroxyvitamin D to the active form, 1,25-hydroxyvitamin D [20]. Vitamin D receptors have been found in a variety of tissues besides bone and intestine. Hence, vitamin D may be made and degraded locally at these target cells or tissues for the purpose of regulating local cell proliferation and differentials [14]. Poor vitamin D status is associated with many adverse health outcomes including osteoporosis; fractures; falls; colon, breast, and prostate cancers; pain; multiple sclerosis; type I & II diabetes; poor glucose homeostasis; rheumatoid arthritis; hypertension; infections; inflammatory autoimmune diseases; and cardiovascular diseases. In addition, vitamin D deficiency has been linked to higher risk of schizophrenia and depression, lung function and wheezing illnesses [4].

Given the close link between vitamin D and calcium metabolism, it is often impossible to separate these two nutrients in their relationship to diseases and health conditions. For example, observational studies have shown that low vitamin D status, calcium, or diary intake are associated with a higher relative risk for type 2 diabetes and metabolic syndrome. Evidence from intervention trials is weaker, but also suggests that combined vitamin D and calcium supplementation may help prevent type 2 diabetes in high-risk populations. The evidence and potential mechanisms for calcium and vitamin D in the development of metabolic syndrome and type 2 diabetes are comprehensively reviewed in a European medical publication [21].

8.6 CALCIUM AND VITAMIN D REQUIREMENTS IN THE ELDERLY

8.6.1 Recommended Daily Intakes

8.6.1.1 Recommended Calcium Intakes

The Institute of Medicine set the adequate intake (AI) for calcium among men and women ages 51 years and older at 1,200mg (30mmol) per day. This recommendation is derived from a synthesis of the results of a myriad of studies on calcium, and aims to maintain calcium balance and reduce bone loss [5].

8.6.1.2 Recommended Vitamin D Intakes

As with calcium, the Institute of Medicine established AIs for vitamin D. The recommendations for vitamin D account for the reduction in endogenous vitamin D synthesis that accompanies aging, and the role of adequate vitamin D in reducing bone loss. The AI for vitamin D among men and women between the ages of 51 and 70 years is 10 μg (400 IU) per day; for men and women above the age of 70 years the AI increases to 15 μg (600 IU) per day [5]. However, 2005 Dietary Guidelines for Americans recommended an extra 25 μg (1000 IU) of vitamin D in populations at high risk for vitamin D deficiency, such as the elderly, people with darker skin, and people exposed to insufficient UV radiation. This amount aims to increase the circulating concentration of 25 (OH) D to 80 nmol/L. This is a substantial increase in the recommendation from the previous AI. It is expected that the recommended intake of vitamin D may increase further for certain populations and may even exceed the current upper level (UL) of 50 μg (2000 IU) [22].

8.6.2 Factors Contributing to Low Calcium and Vitamin D Levels in the Elderly

The elderly are prone to calcium deficiency for several reasons. Increased lactose intolerance with age may lead to reduced consumption of calcium-rich dairy, in turn reducing calcium intake. Moreover, calcium absorption via active transport can decrease with age. As 1,25-dihydroxyvitamin D_3 stimulates calcium absorption, much of the decrease in calcium absorption that accompanies age may result from vitamin D deficiency. Moreover, certain medications, such as glucocorticoids, can inhibit calcium absorption [2,5].

The ability to synthesize vitamin D decreases with age due to reduced levels of 7-dehydrocholesterol in the skin; by age 70, vitamin D synthesis can be expected to decrease by approximately

75% [4]. Improved skin protection to prevent sun damage, including increased clothing and sunscreen use, leads to reduced sun exposure among the elderly. Moreover, many chronic diseases can cause vitamin D deficiency, including malabsorption syndromes, chronic kidney disease, hyperparathyroidism, granulomatous disorders, and some lymphomas. Certain medications can also induce vitamin D deficiency by altering vitamin D absorption, synthesis, or metabolism [4,5].

8.7 SUMMARY

Calcium and vitamin D both play critical roles in maintaining health status for older adults. The physiological functions of these nutrients exceed our traditional understanding; hypotheses and theories regarding new mechanisms of these functions have been emerging. Given the growing evidence for relationships between different health outcomes and calcium and vitamin D, searching for adequate levels of calcium and vitamin D for optimal aging becomes a focus of research and discussion.

Since calcium and vitamin D deficiency continually exist in older populations, different strategies should be considered to improve their status. There are a number of foods naturally rich in vitamin D and calcium; incorporating these foods into the daily diet is important for the elderly to meet their nutrient needs. In the United States, dairy products are the major calcium sources. In addition, calcium has also been added into other food products, for example orange juice. Similarly, vitamin D-fortified orange juice and milk are also readily available. However, lactose deficiency is prevalent in older adults and prevents older people from consuming milk and other dairy products. Although having lactose-free milk or taking lactose supplements are possible solutions, these are not common practices in the elderly for convenience or economic reasons. Overall, for most of the elderly, it is difficult to reach the daily recommendation for vitamin D consumption of 1000 IU without supplementation. When taking supplements, vitamin D_3 is a preferred choice, given its better bioavailability relative to vitamin D_2. People should not consume the upper level of 50 μg daily for vitamin D without a physician's care and supervision. Overexposure to sun or artificial UV radiation to meet the vitamin D recommendation for the elderly is definitely not recommended at this time.

Similar to vitamin D, the recommended calcium intake of 1200 mg is difficult to achieve through dietary intake only. A variety of supplements are available on the market. Older people should consult with their physicians and health providers to avoid side effects when taking calcium and vitamin D supplements. In the next few years, new knowledge will evolve and improve our understanding of the health benefits of vitamin D and calcium. Keeping up with these new developments is important for health professionals who work with older people aiming for optimal aging.

REFERENCES

1. Groff, J. L., S. S. Gropper, and S. M. Hunt. 1995. *Advanced nutrition and human metabolism, 2nd ed.* St. Paul, Minnesota: West Publishing Company.
2. Gueguen, L., and A. Pointillart. 2000. The bioavailability of dietary calcium. *J Am Coll Nutr* 19 (2 Suppl):119S–136S.
3. Dusso, A. S., A. J. Brown, and E. Slatopolsky. 2005. Vitamin D. *Am J Physiol Renal Physiol* 289 (1): F8-28.
4. Holick, M. F. 2007. Vitamin D deficiency. *N Engl J Med* 357 (3):266-81.
5. Institute of Medicine (U.S.). Standing Committee on the Scientific Evaluation of Dietary Reference Intakes. 1997. *Dietary reference intakes: for calcium, phosphorus, magnesium, vitamin D, and fluoride.* Washington, D.C.: National Academy Press.
6. Dawson-Hughes, B. 2004. Racial/ethnic considerations in making recommendations for vitamin D for adult and elderly men and women. *Am J Clin Nutr* 80 (6 Suppl):1763S–6S.
7. Heaney, R. P. 2005. The Vitamin D requirement in health and disease. *J Steroid Biochem Mol Biol* 97 (1–2):13–9.
8. Hiza, H. A. B. and L. Bente. 2007. Nutrient content of the U.S. food supply, 1909–2004: A summary report. Washington, D.C.: U.S. Department of Agriculture, Center for Nutrition Policy and Promotion.

9. Weaver, C. M., W. R. Proulx, and R. Heaney. 1999. Choices for achieving adequate dietary calcium with a vegetarian diet. *Am J Clin Nutr* 70 (3 Suppl):543S–548S.
10. Heaney, R. P., M. S. Dowell, C. A. Hale, and A. Bendich. 2003. Calcium absorption varies within the reference range for serum 25-hydroxyvitamin D. *J Am Coll Nutr* 22 (2):142–6.
11. Calvo, M. S., S. J. Whiting, and C. N. Barton. 2004. Vitamin D fortification in the United States and Canada: Current status and data needs. *Am J Clin Nutr* 80 (6 Suppl):1710S–6S.
12. van den Berg, H. 1997. Bioavailability of vitamin D. *Eur J Clin Nutr* 51 Suppl 1:S76–9.
13. National Institutes of Health. 2007. Dietary supplement fact sheet: calcium 2005 [cited December 20 2007]. Available from http://dietary-supplements.info.nih.gov/factsheets/calcium.asp.
14. Heaney, R. P. 2003. Long-latency deficiency disease: insights from calcium and vitamin D. *Am J Clin Nutr* 78 (5):912–9.
15. Kanis, J. A. and R. Passmore. 1989. Calcium supplementation of the diet—I. *BMJ* 298 (6667):137–40.
16. Kanis, J. A. 1989. Calcium supplementation of the diet—II. *BMJ* 298 (6668):205–8.
17. Chapuy, M. C., M. E. Arlot, F. Duboeuf, J. Brun, B. Crouzet, S. Arnaud, P. D. et al. 1992. Vitamin D3 and calcium to prevent hip fractures in the elderly women. *N Engl J Med* 327 (23):1637–42.
18. Trivedi, D. P., R. Doll, and K. T. Khaw. 2003. Effect of four monthly oral vitamin D3 (cholecalciferol) supplementation on fractures and mortality in men and women living in the community: randomised double blind controlled trial. *BMJ* 326 (7387):469.
19. Jackson, R. D., A. Z. LaCroix, M. Gass, R. B. Wallace, J. Robbins, C. E. Lewis, et al. 2006. Calcium plus vitamin D supplementation and the risk of fractures. *N Engl J Med* 354 (7):669–83.
20. Peterlik, M. and H. S. Cross. 2005. Vitamin D and calcium deficits predispose for multiple chronic diseases. *Eur J Clin Invest* 35 (5):290–304.
21. Pittas, A. G., J. Lau, F. B. Hu, and B. Dawson-Hughes. 2007. The role of vitamin D and calcium in type 2 diabetes. A systematic review and meta-analysis. *J Clin Endocrinol Metab* 92 (6):2017–29.
22. Johnson, M. A., and M. G. Kimlin. 2006. Vitamin D, aging, and the 2005 Dietary Guidelines for Americans. *Nutr Rev* 64 (9):410–21.
23. Dawson-Hughes, B., S. S. Harris, E. A. Krall, and G. E. Dallal. 1997. Effect of calcium and vitamin D supplementation on bone density in men and women 65 years of age or older. *N Engl J Med* 337 (10):670–6.

9 Lipid Absorption in Aging

Laurie Drozdowski, Claudiu Iordache,
Trudy Woudstra, and Alan B. R. Thomson

CONTENTS

9.1 AGING

9.1.1 DEFINITIONS

Although each of us is familiar with inevitable age-related changes, the task of clearly defining the term aging. is challenging. Aging is a multifactorial process that includes both intrinsic and extrinsic factors. To further complicate matters, in humans the term can be considered from sociological, physiological, psychological, and molecular perspectives.

Lifespan is defined as the time spent living by any organism, and maximum lifespan is based on the lifespan of organisms living under favorable conditions determined by the longest-living member or of the top percentile [1]. Life expectancy is a summary statistic that estimates the average time yet to be lived by an individual at a given age [2]. Life expectancy is often expressed from birth. Unfortunately, the terms lifespan and life expectancy are often used interchangeably.

Significant changes in life expectancy have occurred through the ages [3]. Some two thousand years ago, life expectancy did not usually exceed 22 years. During the following centuries this number doubled to 45 years. Then, the 20th century witnessed the greatest increase in life expectancy, with an increase from 45 years to the current 75 years [1] and above. However, men and women do not have the same life expectancies. In Canada, life expectancy of males at birth is 77.8 years and for females it is 82.6 years [4]. The gap between life expectancies of the two genders has been narrowing over the past two decades, from a peak of 7.5 years in 1978 to its current difference of 5.6 years in 1997. Life expectancy in underdeveloped countries is much lower, and is the same for men and women. In the past century, women have benefited dramatically from improved prenatal and obstetrical care. Women in developed nations have thankfully also had enhanced access to food and education. As a result of these improvements for women, the gender longevity difference has grown in the United States. It is not clearly understood why women outlive men, but estrogen has been implicated in this phenomenon [3].

While we tend to use the term ontogeny. to describe development in early life, and aging. to describe later life, a better concept is the development over the lifetime of the animal. Thus, young. or old. are descriptive terms outlining a process over time. Aging then may be considered to be a continuum that begins at conception and proceeds until death. The definition of aging can be further refined as chronological age,. according to the passage of time. Although advancing age is associated with increases in morbidity and mortality in general, this approach fails to consider the health of the individual. Determining a specific age at which an individual becomes old. is arbitrary, and the concept of aging has changed over the centuries, with humans now experiencing increased longevity and quality of life.

When is a person old"? Who are the elderly"? While population statistics report occurrences of deaths and diseases by chronological age, it is far more difficult to delineate young and old by chronological age. Anecdotally, we are probably all able to think of people who are young. for their age; their health and lifestyle are major factors in their apparent youthfulness. Perhaps in considering the differences between these two arbitrary extremes (young versus old), it is more useful to consider biological age. and the processes. of aging.

The term old. is used to describe virtually all time-dependent changes in all life forms from molecules to ecosystems [5]. Aging is a biological process that limits the adaptive possibilities of an organism and thereby reduces lifespan. For example, the adaptive response of the intestine to dietary changes is altered in aging [6,7]. Masoro [8] proposed that aging refers to deteriorative changes that occur over time and reduce the ability of the organism to survive. However, Arking and Dudas [9] suggest that when we have reached a more sophisticated understanding of aging, we will be able to eliminate the word time. from our definition and instead use the physiological processes. Finch [10] stressed the importance of avoiding the implications associated with the word time. Use of the word aging is therefore limited, and instead changes observed over a lifespan are referred to as age-related. changes.

"Biological age reflects the presence or absence of disease. Because there is not always a direct relationship between age and disease, this definition is considered to be a better marker of health status. The term functional aging. has also been used to emphasize the limitations of defining health based on chronological age. This concept of biological age characterizes people based on what they can do in relation to others in society, but may also be used to characterize the level of functioning of organs and systems in the elderly.

The terms senescence is used interchangeably with aging by some authors, while others prefer to reserve its usage to describe changes that occur during the functional decline of an organism's life [10]. It is beyond the scope of this chapter to consider the implications associated with word usage. We will use the terms aging, age-related, and senescence interchangeably, and will use these terms to describe physiological changes that occur over the lifespan.

Finally, the concept of successful aging. takes this idea one step further and suggests that the aging process is variable and can be characterized as a balance between gains and loses [11]. The compression of morbidity and an enhanced quality of life are cornerstones of the concept of successful aging.

Rowe and Kahn [12] suggested that the effects of aging have been exaggerated, and that the modifying effects of diet, exercise, personal habits, and psychosocial factors were underestimated. For instance, Zavaroni and coworkers [13] evaluated the correlation between age and glucose intolerance, as well as extrinsic factors such as obesity, physical activity, and family history. They found that the contribution of age to glucose intolerance was relatively modest, as compared with other age-related environmental factors. Gerontological researchers may distinguish between pathological and non-pathological states in the aged, and perhaps researchers should also focus on the normal. or non-pathological aged, and on the differences between usual. and successful. aging [12]. This distinction emphasizes the link between intrinsic and extrinsic factors, including the relationship between the physiological and the psychosocial aspects of the individual. Because extrinsic factors play a major role in successful aging,. nutrition is an important modifiable factor in potentially enhancing the health of the aged.

9.1.2 THEORIES OF AGING

Nature or nurture, which one makes the greatest contribution to longevity? Twin studies have suggested that 25% of the variation in lifespan can be attributed to nature [14]. Studies of human progerias and the characterization of age genes in *Caenorhabditis elegans* suggest a possible larger contribution of genes. Several processes thought to contribute to the aging process include genetic programs, oxidative damage, genome instability, and cell death.

A number of theories have been proposed to describe the process of aging. Longevity genes have been identified in many species, suggesting that aging may be partially under genetic control. In yeast, overproduction of the enzyme Sir2 prolongs the life of yeast grown under normal nutrient conditions [15]. It has been suggested that increases in Sir2 (seen in response to CR or resveratrol, a polyphenol found in red wine) may increase gene silencing and thereby result in greater genomic stability [15]. Research undertaken in Drosophila identified single gene mutations that extend lifespan. These include the gene Methuselah, a secretion-type receptor that provides resistance to stress [16], and Indy (I'm not dead yet), whose gene product is homologous to Kreb's cycle intermediates [17,18]. Using *C. Elegans* as a model, the gene daf2, an insulin/insulin-like growth factor-1 (IGF-1) receptor homolog, has also been shown to affect lifespan [19]. In humans, a genetic component to aging has also been suggested: Werner's syndrome, a disorder characterized by an apparent accelerated senescence, has been associated with a single gene locus on chromosome 8 [20]. On the other hand, a genome-wide scan of elderly subjects suggested that there is a locus on chromosome 4 that influences a person's genetic susceptibility to age well and to achieve exceptional longevity [21].

Cellular theories emphasize that the environment, as well as intrinsic properties of the cell, often referred to as a cellular clock,. may limit survival. Pivitol research by Hayflick and Moorhead [22] found that normal human fetal cell strains were limited to 40–60 doublings before they entered senescence. These scientists developed the concept of the Hayflick limit. to explain the determination of longevity. From this early work, the concept of telomere shortening was then established as another mechanism of longevity determination. These repetitive deoxyribonucleic acid (DNA) sequences found at the end of chromosomes are progressively depleted with age, and may represent a method by which cells enter senescence. This theory has been challenged due to the lack of correlation between telomere length and lifespan in many animal species [23].

Aging may be the consequence of oxidative damage. Oxidative damage to DNA, protein, carbohydrates and lipids contributes to degenerative diseases in aging due to a disruption in cellular homeostasis. The activation of specific stress-signaling pathways results in alterations in gene expression mediated by a variety of transcription factors including nuclear factor-κβ (NF-κβ), p53, and heat shock transcription factor 1 [24]. While levels of antioxidants correlate with longevity in primates [25,26], it is not clear if antioxidant supplementation affects lifespan. It has been suggested, but not proven conclusively, that the success of calorie-restricted diets in extending the lifespan of rodents is related to a reduction in free radical formation [27–29]. The role of insulin/ IGF-1 signaling in the regulation of lifespan has been studied. The gene daf2, an insulin/IGF-1 receptor homolog, has been shown to affect the lifespan of *C. Elegans* [19]. Similarly, a related tyrosine kinase receptor, InR, regulates lifespan in Drosophila [30]. Holzenberger et al. [31] demonstrated the importance of this pathway in mammals. In this study, heterozygous knockout mice (*Igflr*$^{\pm}$) were used, as null mutants were not viable. These *Igflr*$^{\pm}$ mice had IGF-1 receptor levels that were half those seen in wild-type animals. These mice lived an average of 26% longer than did their wild-type littermates, without developing dwarfism or showing adverse changes in physical activity, fertility, or metabolism. This suggests that the link between insulin signaling and longevity seen in lower order organisms may also exist in mammals. Furthermore, the *Igflr*$^{\pm}$ mice showed a greater resistance to oxidative stress, a known determinant of aging [24]. This lends support to the theory that oxidative stress may play an important role in the aging process.

In addition to increased resistance to oxidative stress, insulin/IGF-1 signaling may affect aging via effects on Forkhead transcription factors of the FOXO class. Overexpression of FOXO extends lifespan [32]. Insulin/IGF-1 receptor binding, and subsequent activation of the P13K/Akt pathway, results in the phosphorylation of Akt, which inactivates FOXO by sequestering it in the cytoplasm [33]. This alters the effects of FOXO on resistance to stress, apoptosis, and longevity, and provides another potential link between insulin/IGF-1 and aging.

Other theories of aging focus on neuro-endocrine changes, including reductions in the levels of the steroid hormone dehydroepiandrosterone. Both animal and human studies have demonstrated that oral replacement of dehydroepiandrosterone may prevent or reduce age-associated events such as cancer and cardiovascular disease, and may stimulate immune function [34–36].

9.2 A SOCIETAL PERSPECTIVE

In Canada, seniors constitute the fastest growing segment of the population. In fact, the proportion of seniors has risen from 1 in 20 in 1921 to 1 in 8 in 2001. Within this group, the number of Canadians aged 85 or more is anticipated to increase substantially, up to 4% of the total population by the year 2041. Women make up the majority of seniors, with gender differences becoming more pronounced in the oldest age groups.

The aging of the population may be thought of as a modern day success story. For the first time in history, human beings have been afforded the opportunity to live an unprecedented number of years with a reasonable quality of life. This accomplishment is not without challenges, as society struggles to adapt to a changing demographic, with a unique set of physiological, psychological, and social needs of the elderly themselves, as well as their caregivers.

Several nongenetic factors may influence life expectancy, including improvements in sanitation and nutrition, as well as reductions in maternal mortality and the rates of infectious diseases. These changes, coupled with lower fertility rates, result in a changing demographic that presents society with the challenges of providing quality health care to an aging population, and facilitating the social, economic, and community involvement of seniors.

Although most rate their health as good. or very good,. seniors are more likely to visit health care professionals, to take medication, and to be hospitalized, when compared with their younger counterparts. Therefore, increases in this population and the associated increased health care utilization may place a burden on the system. Indeed, health expenditures for seniors in 2000–2001 represented 43% of the total health care expenditures. As they have contributed greatly to society, it is society's responsibility to provide ready access to quality health care for these special persons, who must be treated with respect and allowed to age with dignity.

The elderly are at high risk for malnutrition, yet unfortunately this is often under diagnosed [37]. Poor nutritional status is a key determinant of morbidity and mortality in the elderly [38–41]. Because nutrition is a modifiable risk factor, attempts should be made to design preventive nutritional strategies aimed at improving the quality of life, and consequently minimizing the use of health care resources.

Why are the elderly malnourished? A number of factors contribute, including: (1) inadequate intake, attributed to reduced appetite or difficulty in preparing food; (2) psychological factors, including depression; (3) social factors, including isolation and low income; and (4) physiological factors such as reduced sense of smell and taste, drug–nutrient interactions, and reductions in nutrient absorption [42]. Hospitalization is a risk factor for inadequate food intake in seniors [40], possibly due to the unattractive and monotonous food choices, or to the side effects of drug therapies. Reduced food intake is generally accepted as the main cause of undernutrition in the geriatric population, and as such, therapies should be aimed at increasing food intake. Malnutrition in the elderly may be indicative of prevailing social conditions, and therapies should be aimed at alleviating poverty, isolation, and depression in this age group.

Because one of the factors that may contribute to malnutrition relates to age-associated alterations in the physiology of the gastrointestinal tract, this topic will be reviewed in brief, and the topic of lipid absorption will be considered in detail.

9.3   NUTRITIONAL NEEDS OF THE ELDERLY

Nutritional needs vary throughout the lifespan of humans, and several age-related changes influence the nutritional needs and intakes of the elderly. First, there is a decrease in energy requirements. This is due partially to a decline in physical activity, and is also to a reduction in muscle mass. The loss of muscle mass, known as sarcopenia, is caused in part by reduced physical activity and also by biological changes, such as the loss of motor neurons and decreased hormonal influences associated with aging, as well as pathological states causing catabolic stress such as congestive heart failure [43]. There is a lifelong, age-related reduction in muscle mass and strength, with a more pronounced reduction in males than in females. The primary reduction in muscle mass is in the type II or fast twitch. fibers. The mass of type II fibers is selectively reduced by disuse, but their mass can be increased by strength-building exercise, specifically resistance training [44]. The fall in muscle mass reduces both the metabolic rate and the thermogenic effect, and reduces energy requirements by about 100 kilocalories per decade [43]. Sarcopenia may also reduce insulin sensitivity. Decreased muscle mass is often associated with a decrease in energy input, and with this there is often a reduction in micronutrient intake. With inadequate micronutrient intake, there may be an increased risk of infection and immune dysfunction [43].

The second factor influencing nutritional needs in the elderly is an increased protein requirement. The equilibrium between protein synthesis and degradation may be disrupted in aging [reviewed by 45]. Protein-calorie malnutrition is estimated to affect 11% to 22% of community-dwelling elderly outpatients [46]. The recommended daily allowance of protein is 0.8 g/kg of body weight [47]. Based on a nitrogen balance study, Campbell and colleagues recommend that protein intake should be increased to 0.91+/− 0.043 g/kg/day in healthy older men and women [48]. An increase in muscle was significantly enhanced in those elderly persons who were supplemented with protein during strength training, as compared with their non-supplemented counterparts [49]. However, protein supplementation without exercise has been shown to have little effect on improving muscle mass [50].

A third change to nutritional needs with aging is an increase in micronutrient requirements. Some physiological factors influencing the increased need for micronutrients include a reduction in the intestinal absorption of calcium, vitamin B12, iron, and folic acid; decreased metabolic utilization of vitamin B6; diminished synthesis of vitamin D; and a decline in immune function that may respond to vitamin E and other antioxidants [43,50]. In contrast to the increased need for micronutrients, there is a greater risk of micronutrient toxicity. This may be due to decreased metabolization of the micronutrients, particularly vitamin A, and to increases in adipose deposits, which store fat-soluble vitamins [43].

Finally, there is an overall decrease in nutrient intake by the elderly. Several factors may contribute to this reduction, such as decreased taste and olfactory perception, difficulty eating, anorexia, as well as difficulty in obtaining and preparing food. Anorexia presenting *de novo* in the older adult, called *anorexia tardive,* may be due to social factors, alcoholism, Alzheimer's disease and drugs [51]. Davis and coworkers [52], in a study of 4964 persons aged 55 years and older, found that those who lived alone consumed fewer calories than those living with others. Medications may cause the sensation of nausea, or they may reduce a person's ability to taste foods. Several medical illnesses are associated with weight loss and anorexia. Interleukins and tumor necrosis factor contribute to the anorexia experienced in some cancer patients, and some common gastrointestinal disorders such as gastroesophogeal reflux disease and peptic ulcer disease may also contribute to anorexia [51].

Difficulty in eating, despite a good appetite, may be caused by oral problems, functional impairments, or swallowing disorders. In the frail elderly, dental problems may be the best predictor of weight loss [51,53]. Presbyesophagus is a common cause of dysphagia and decreased food intake in the elderly. Dysphagia may result from neurological disorders such as stroke or Parkinson's disease. It may also represent structural lesions or central nervous system (CNS) disorders such as hypo/hyperthyroidism [54].

Obesity has clearly been shown to negatively influence health by increasing the risk of disease and by reducing lifespan. In a 32-year study of 1741 university alumni, smoking, higher body-mass index, and poor exercise patterns were associated with poorer health, as well as with decreased survival [55]. In keeping with these findings, CR is the most effective method to extend lifespan, and to reduce the deleterious effects of aging. In laboratory rodents as well as other mammalian and non-mammalian species, CR has repeatedly been shown to extend the lifespan by as much as 40% [56,57]. The mechanism for this extension is a reduction in the metabolic rate in the CR animal, and hence a reduction in oxidative stress [58]. Oxidative stress is the damage of DNA and proteins caused by highly reactive forms of oxygen. The reactive oxygen species are the consequence of aerobic metabolism [58,59]. In early reports of CR primates, there appeared to be a reduction in Type II diabetes and in cardiovascular disease, two diseases that are typically considered to be age-related [56]. In humans, CR may also contribute to lifespan extension. On the Japanese island of Okinawa, inhabitants consume 40% fewer calories than those on the mainland. This may contribute to the greater proportion of centenarians living on the island versus the mainland [60].

As well, there are benefits to increased weight in the elderly. Increased weight is associated with higher bone mineral density and a lower fracture rate [61]. Increased weight is also associated with higher lean muscle mass, with greater isometric strength and enhanced mobility. As well, excess weight may supply a reserve during periods of catabolic stress, such as illness. Some findings suggest that in the elderly, a more accurate predictor of mortality is weight change. rather than obesity. In a study of community-dwelling women, those with a change in weight status (either increase, decrease, or fluctuations) were at greater mortality risk than those women who maintained a steady weight [61].

9.4 AGING AND THE GASTROINTESTINAL TRACT

9.4.1 GENERAL CONSIDERATIONS

The aging of the population, coupled with the potential impact on the health care system, has focused attention on the physiological processes associated with aging. Only with an increased understand of the aging process can we work toward improving the quality of life for the elderly and reducing disease morbidity in this population.

There are age-related alterations in the gastrointestinal tract, but the challenge lies in excluding concomitant pathological factors as the cause of these changes. Certainly with aging, conditions such as diabetes, pancreatic or liver disease, cancer, or drug-induced enteropathy will have potential adverse effects on the form and function of the intestine. It is necessary to exclude these pathological factors, to consider the physiological changes that occur in the healthy elderly, and to understand how these factors influence the nutritional status of this older population.

9.4.1.1 Motility

Dysphagia is more common in the elderly than in younger persons [62]. Selective neurodegeneration may occur in the aging enteric nervous system [reviewed in 63], and may contribute to gastrointestinal symptoms such as dysphagia, gastrointestinal reflux, and constipation. Interestingly, CR in rodents can prevent the neuronal losses that occur with aging, suggesting that diet may influence gastrointestinal aging [64]. Alterations in esophageal motility may be due to reductions in the number of neurons in the myenteric plexus of elderly patients [65]. While gastric motility may be impaired with aging [66,67], small intestinal motility is unaffected [68–70]. Aging may affect the signal transduction pathways and cellular mechanisms controlling smooth muscle contraction, which may influence colonic motility and thereby contribute to the development of constipation [reviewed in 71].

9.4.1.2 Gastric Secretion

The data regarding aging and gastric acid secretion is inconclusive, as early studies were likely confounded by the presence of *Helicobacter pylori (H. pylori)* in some persons. Achlorhydria or hypochlorhydria may result from atropic gastritis as a result of medications such as proton pump inhibitors or as a result of gastric *H. pylori* infection [72, 73, 74]. This reduction in gastric acidity may increase the risk of small bowel bacterial overgrowth, potentially leading to malabsorption [75]. For example, McEvoy et al. [76] found that 71% of patients in a general geriatric ward had bacterial overgrowth of the small intestine, while 11% were found to be malnourished. Indeed, bacterial overgrowth in older adults is associated with reduced body weight, which is paralleled by reduced intake of several micronutrients [77].

9.4.1.3 Pancreatic Function

Although structural changes in the pancreas are seen with aging, no functional age-related alterations are seen, as assessed by using the fluorescein dilaurate test [78]. Some studies demonstrate reduced secretagogue-stimulated lipase, chymotrypsin, and bicarbonate concentrations in pancreatic juice with aging [79]. Other research suggests that there is little evidence of reduced pancreatic secretions with age, independent of other factors including the presence of disease and the effect of drugs [80].

9.4.1.4 Liver

There are age-related reductions in liver mass and blood flow, yet microscopic changes are subtle [81–83]. While structural and functional changes do not correlate well, there is evidence that liver function declines with age. For example, Cao et al. [84] used microarrays to show that aging in mice is accompanied by changes in the expression of genes in the liver involved in inflammation, cellular stress, and fibrosis, all of which are linked to age-related liver pathologies. Interestingly, CR in mice starting at weaning reversed the majority of the age-related hepatic changes, once again emphasizing the ability of the diet to influence the aging process.

9.4.1.5 Carbohydrates

Age-related alterations in the abundance of intestinal brush border membrane (BBM) enzymes may also impact upon the digestion and subsequent absorption of nutrients. In rats, BBM lactase phlorizin hydrolase (LPH) and sucrase-isomaltase (SI) activities fall with age [85]. Bacterial overgrowth, which is common in the elderly, may also negatively impact on disaccharidase activity and thereby possibly reduce carbohydrate absorption [86]. A study using breath hydrogen analysis following a 100 gm carbohydrate meal showed evidence of malabsorption with aging. Elderly patients (ranging from 65–89 years, mean age, 79 years) were compared with control subjects (ranging from 20–64 years, mean age, 35 years). Significantly more subjects in the elderly group (7 out of 21) excreted excess H_2 than controls (0 out of 19) [87]. This suggests that there may be malabsorption of carbohydrates in the elderly.

D-xylose absorption assessed from the urinary excretion of this sugar after oral intake decreases in aging humans. However, D-xylose excretion is dependent on renal function, and when that is taken into consideration, there is only a modest reduction in xylose absorption associated with aging [88].

In vitro transport experiments using BBM vesicles also demonstrated a reduction of Na^+-dependent glucose uptake in patients over the age of 70 [89]. In contrast, Wallis and coworkers [90] did not find changes in Na^+-dependent glucose transport in BBM vesicles isolated from duodenal biopsies from patients whose ages ranged from 55 to 91 years.

Experiments using rodent models of aging also demonstrate conflicting results. Several studies show reductions in D-glucose absorption in aged rats [91–93]. Depending upon the intestinal site studied, a normal or increased absorptive capacity was also found in a study using everted intestinal segments from old versus young rats [94]. Results from studies in mice also do not offer conclusive results on the effect of aging on nutrient absorption. Ferraris et al. [95] showed in aged mice a reduction in uptake and site density of the sodium dependent glucose transporter in the BBM, sodium glucose co-transporter 1 (SGLT1). This is in contrast to the findings of Thompson et al. [96], who showed an increase in intestinal glucose uptake in aged mice.

Our lab has recently investigated the effect of age on intestinal glucose uptake in Fischer 344 rats, using the *in vitro* intestinal sheet method [97,98]. Glucose uptake was reduced in 9-month-old and 24-month-old rats when compared with 1-month-old animals. When changes in mucosal surface area were taken into account, only ileal glucose uptake was reduced in the older animals. These age-associated changes in glucose uptake were not explained by alterations in the abundance of SGLT1, GLUT2, or sodium-potassium pump (Na^+K^+–ATPase) abundance.

The uptake of fructose has been studied in aging mice. Ferraris and Vinnekota [99] showed that D-fructose uptake per milligram of tissue was higher in the jejunum of young than in old animals. Adaptive increases in uptake, in response to increases in carbohydrate levels, were blunted in these mice, and were restricted to the more proximal regions of the small intestine.

The variations in the results from human, rat, and mouse studies may be due to the differences in the methodologies used. While some investigators studied uptake using BBM vesicles [89–93], others used everted intestinal rings [94,96,99] or intestinal sheets [97,98]. As well, the method of expressing results may contribute to the differences between studies. Uptake is often expressed on the basis of intestinal weight, and does not take into account any potential age-associated changes in mucosal weight or surface area. The strain and ages of the animals, and the site of the intestine used also differ between studies, and may explain the variability in the results.

9.4.1.6 Permeability

Hollander and colleagues demonstrated that intestinal permeability to medium-sized probes (mannitol, polyethylene glycol) increased in 28-month-old rats when compared with 3-month-old rats [100]. However, a study done in humans shows that the lactulose:mannitol ratio was not different between young and old subjects, indicating that intestinal permeability to these sugars does not change significantly with age [101].

9.4.1.7 Amino Acids, Vitamins, and Minerals

In *in vivo* perfusion studies with rats, vitamin A absorption increases in a linear fashion with age [102]. Reduced calcium absorption is reported in aging, and may result from attenuated vitamin D metabolites [103]. The pH microclimate of the rat jejunum is less acidic with aging, and this change may play a role in the reduced intestinal absorption of some nutrients, such as amino acids, lipids, and calcium [104]

When fed a meal containing 100g carbohydrate, one third of subjects over 65 years had excess breath hydrogen, suggesting malabsorption [87]. However, this is a large amount of carbohydrate for one meal, and this reduced absorptive capacity may have minimal nutritional impact for persons consuming lesser amounts of carbohydrate. In addition, breath hydrogen tests can be falsely positive in the presence of bacterial overgrowth of the small intestine. It should be recalled that bacterial overgrowth may occur more frequently among the elderly, and anerobic bacteria can produce proteases that interfere with disaccharidases in the BBM, thereby resulting in reduced carbohydrate absorption [86]. Thus, aging may be associated with a fall in carbohydrate absorption, but the mechanism of this decline remains unknown.

9.4.1.8   Lipid Absorption in Healthy Adults

Dietary lipids, a major source of energy, also provide structural support for many tissues. In adults in the West, lipids supply between 30–40% of total dietary energy. The dietary fat contains 95% triglycerides; the other 5% includes phospholipids, sterols, and small amounts of gangliosides, fatty alcohols, suphatides, vitamins, and carotenoids [105]. Dietary lipids must be hydrolyzed and solubilized before they are absorbed in the intestine. The hydrolysis is performed by lipases from saliva, stomach, pancreas, intestine, and liver. The solubilization of the lipids is carried out by the bile acids, which form micelles [106].

Lipid absorption is the sum of the mechanisms that transfer the dietary lipids from the lumen of the small intestine into the lymph and portal circulation [107]. This complex process includes the diffusion of lipids through the intestinal unstirred water layer (UWL), transport across the BBM, binding to cytosolic proteins, diffusion across the cytosol, metabolism of lipids and lipoprotein biosynthesis, and secretion of the lipids across the basolateral membrane (BLM) into the blood or lymph [108].

Most of the lipid transport across the BBM is the result of passive diffusion, and to a smaller extent, a component mediated by lipid binding proteins. The passive diffusion of lipids across the BBM has three steps: the adsorption in the outer leaflet of the BBM, the transmembrane movement, and the desorption from the cytosolic leaflet of the BBM [109]. The rate-limiting step in the diffusion of fatty acids across the enterocytes is the trans-membrane movement of fatty acids [110,111]. The permeability of the BBM is influenced by its fluidity and lipid composition. The fluidity of the BBM depends on the content of different lipids in the membrane [112]. There is an increased BBM fluidity during the suckling period as compared with adults, because the immature membranes contain a higher amount of cholesterol and phospholipids per milligram protein than do the mature BBM [113,114].

The postnatal maturation of the intestine is influenced by hormonal factors such as glucocorticosteroids (GC) and thyroid hormones. GC have an important role in membrane maturation in rat intestine. The administration of GC induces a precocious BBM maturation due to changes in the membrane fluidity, and also post-translational alterations of proteins in the BBM [115–117].

Intestinal uptake occurs predominantly in the upper third of the villus [118]. The lipids must first cross the UWL, and than permeate the BBM. In order to correctly assess the permeability characteristics of the BBM, the experimental values must be corrected for the effective resistance of the UWL. Failure to correct for UWL resistance leads to underestimation of the permeability properties of the BBM [119].

The passive diffusion of lipids can be explained by three possible models [120]:

1. The whole bile salt micelle is absorbed by the BBM. There is no experimental evidence to support this model [121].

2. The collision between micelle and BBM enables the lipids to be taken up directly from the micelle into the BBM. There is experimental evidence for supporting this model, as suggested by the linear relationship between cholesterol uptake and bile acid concentration [122, 123].

3. The lipids dissociate from the micelles into the aqueous phase of the UWL before being absorbed by BBM. The experiment that supports this latter possibility showed that fatty acid uptake decreases with an increase in the number of bile acid micelles when the concentration of fatty acids is held constant [124]. Thus, both models 2 and 3 may apply, depending upon the nature of the ingested lipids, the bile salts and phospholipids in the micelles, and the BBM lipid composition.

The UWL provides an acidic microclimate that is maintained by the BBM Na^+/H^+ exchanger [125,126]. This acidic microclimate enables the dissociation of fatty acids from the bile acid micelle [127,128] and the protonation of these fatty acids, thereby increasing their permeation across the BBM [129,130]. Other factors that could be involved in the rate of uptake of lipids are: the luminal lipid composition, the transposition of membrane lipids between the outer and the inner leaflet of the BBM [131], the membrane potential [132], and the lipid binding proteins in the enterocyte cytosol or BBM. The cytosolic lipid transfer proteins released from lysed cells may interact with dietary lipids, thus further influencing lipid uptake. It is unknown whether the normal enterocytes are permeable to cytosolic protein [107].

BBM proteins that have been identified to have a role in lipid binding include caveolin-1, scavenger receptor Class B Type 1 (SR-BI), fatty acid binding protein (FABP)$_{pm}$, fatty acid translocase (FAT)/CD36, fatty acid transport protein (FATP4), and cholesterol transport protein. Caveolin-1 is a 22 kDa integral protein found in an invagination of the BBM, which constitutes the caveolae. Caveolae have a unique structure, being composed of cholesterol and sphingolipids, as compared with plasma membranes that are composed largely by phospholipids. This composition enables caveolae and caveolae-related domains to form a liquid-order phase in membranes [133].

The caveolae membrane system is involved in endocytosis (which is the transcellular transport between the two surfaces of the cell), and in potocytosis (a mechanism for small molecule uptake independent of an endocytic process). A molecule binds to a receptor in a flat or open caveolae. The caveolae then invaginates, and may transiently form a sealed compartment independent of the extracellular space, but still remains contiguous with the plasma membrane. The formation of a sealed microenvironment facilitates the uptake of the molecules across the plasma membrane. The invaginated caveolae then flattens or opens, and the cycle is repeated [133–135].

Caveolin-1, the main constituent protein in caveolae, is necessary for the internalization and trafficking of the caveolae [134]. Caveolin-1 has binding affinity for long-chain fatty acids (LCFA) [136], and for cholesterol [137]. Caveolin-1 may act as a storage place for cholesterol, and may play a role in the sterol-sensing component of the BBM [137]. Also, caveolin-1 may participate in the intracellular targeting of cholesterol [138]. Furthermore, caveolin-1 may play a role in signal transduction, as suggested by the interaction of calveolin-1 with G-protein, Ras and Src kinases, or epidermal factor receptor [139].

SR-BI is a 57 kDa protein identified in both BBM and BLM, especially in the jejunum, and in negligible amounts in ileum [140]. SR-BI serves as a docking receptor, mediating the flux of lipid molecules. Interestingly, the flux of lipids is bidirectional: the lipid molecules move from the donor particle to the BBM, and back again [107].

The localization of SR-BI on the BBM of the jejunum is consistent with the hypothesis of its possible role in dietary cholesterol absorption, whereas SR-BI present on the BLM of the ileum suggests its possible involvement in intestinal lipoprotein uptake [140].

FABP$_{pm}$ is a 43 kDa protein located in the BBM and BLM [141]. FABP$_{pm}$ binds monoglycerides, LCFA, and cholesterol. The role of FABP$_{pm}$ in absorption of LCFA was demonstrated by the inhibition of [³H]-oleate uptake in jejunal explants or sheets of intestine using monospecific FABP$_{pm}$

antibody [125,126,142]. The uptake of oleic acid by FABP also involves the activation of Na^+/H^+ exchanger [125,126].

FAT is a 88 kDa glycoprotein found in tissues with high fatty acid metabolism such as adipocytes, cardiomyocytes, myocytes, mammary gland cells, and enterocytes [143]. FAT, first identified in rat adipocytes [144], has an 85% homology with human scavenger receptor CD36, which is found in platelets, monocytes, and endothelial cells. In the intestine, FAT/CD36 is located in BBM in the upper two thirds of the villi at the major sites of lipid absorption in the proximal small intestine [145]. FAT binds to negatively charged fatty acids; therefore, it might constitute a high-affinity, low-capacity transport system for ionized LCFA [146]. The effect of FAT/CD36 on transport seems to require as partner the cytosolic FABP [147]. Also, FAT/CD36 might be a lipid sensor in the intestine. Increases in both FAT messenger ribonucleic acid (mRNA) levels and cytosolic liver-fatty acid binding protein (L-FABP) are reported after mice are fed high lipid diets [148]. A diet rich in polyunsaturated fatty acids (PUFA) also increases the expression of FAT mRNA [145].

FATP is a 63 kDa protein found in different isoforms (five in rats and six in humans) [149]. FATP4 is the isoform expressed in the intestine of humans and FATP1 is found in murines. FATP4 is located in the BBM of the villi in the jejunum and ileum, with lower levels in the duodenum. FATP4 is involved in the transport of medium- and LCFA [150]. FATP from adipocytes is co-expressed in plasma membrane with long chain acyl-CoA synthetase (ACS); this system increases the efficiency of LCFA uptake [151]. It is not known whether the intestinal FATP has a similar system.

The cholesterol transport protein. is a 145 kDa integral protein present in BBM of rabbit enterocytes [152]. Another transporter that may also be involved in the intestinal uptake of cholesterol is the multidrug resistance protein (MDR) [153]. The existence of a transporter protein for cholesterol was suggested as early as 1990 by Thurnhofer and Hauser [154]. This conclusion resulted from the experiments in which the rate of cholesterol uptake was reduced by 80% after proteolytic treatments of the BBM [154]. Interestingly, the hydrolysis of cholesterol esters is not a prerequisite for cholesterol absorption by cholesterol transporters. The uptake of cholesteryl oleate by the BBM is as effective as that of free cholesterol. Moreover, the kinetics of cholesteryl oleate uptake was similar to the kinetics of an analog that is resistant to cholesterol esterases. Based on these experiments, it was concluded that the absorption of cholesterol and cholesterol esters in the BBM work side by side, depending on conditions in the lumen of the small intestine [155].

There is also efflux of cholesterol from cells [156]. Cholesterol absorption is reduced by plant sterols [157–160]. This action of plant sterols was initially explained by physicochemical effects of these compounds, which are in competition with cholesterol in their incorporation into bile salt micelles, and in the uptake from these micelles [159]. More recently, new transporters of cholesterol in BBM have been found, the ATP binding cassette (ABC) transporters: ABCA1 [156], ABCG5, ABCG8 [161], and NPC1L1 [162]. The hypocholestolemic effect of plant stanols has been explained by the presence of ATP binding cassette (ABCA1) transporters of cholesterol in BBM of intestingal mucosa cells [156]. ABCA1, as well as other ABC transporters, belong to the ABCG transporter family, which has been shown to be involved in the regulation of lipid traffic in macrophages, hepatocytes, and enterocytes [163]. There is some evidence that ABCA1 mediates the efflux of cholesterol back into the intestinal lumen. Interestingly, the ABCA1 expression is regulated by a nuclear receptor system formed by mandatory heterodimers between the liver X receptors (LXR) and retinoid X receptors (RXR). LXR binds cholesterol or plant sterols and RXR binds rexinoids [164]. Experiments with LXR/RXR heterodimers revealed that they regulate the expression of the ABCA1 transporter, and thus LXR/RXRs regulate the level of cholesterol in enterocytes [156].

The hypocholestolemic effect of plant stanols has been explained by the presence of those ABC transporters on intestinal mucosa cells, which appear to remove unwanted cholesterol and physterols from the enterocyte, mediating the efflux of cholesterol back into the intestinal lumen [165]. Discovery of those new transporters in lipids metabolism expands probability for developing new pharmaceutical agents to decrease cholesterol levels. The plasma cholesterol lowing effects of exetimibe may be due to its inhibition of the BBM cholesterol transporter, NPC1L1 [165, 166].

In enterocytes, the cytosolic lipid binding proteins bind and transport lipids and bile acids. Three of them have been identified in the intestine: intestinal-fatty acid binding protein (I-FABP); L-FABP, which is also found in the liver; and ILBP. I-FABP and L-FABP are expressed along the villi in both the jejunum and ileum [145]. I-FABP is a 15.1 kDa protein, found most abundantly in the distal ileum and at the villous tip [148,167]. L-FABP is a 14.1 kDa protein present mainly in the proximal jejunum at the crypt–villous junction. L-FABP is absent at the villous tips [168]. I-FABP has a greater affinity for saturated than for PUFA [169]. In contrast, L-FABP exhibits a greater affinity for PUFA than for saturated fatty acids (SFA) [169]. I-FABP binds protonated fatty acids, while L-FABP binds unprotonated fatty acids [169]. I-FABP transports fatty acids and releases them by a collisional interaction with membranes, which suggests a role in the uptake or targeting fatty acids. L-FABP transfers fatty acids in an aqueous diffusion mediated process, which suggests their having a role as a buffer for fatty acids in cytosol [170–172].

To study the role played by I-FABP in lipid absorption, several experiments have been performed with I-FABP knockout mice. Body weight gain was used as an indicator of dietary fat assimilation. The knockout male mice that were fed a low-fat diet or high-fat diet were consistently heavier than their normal counterparts. In contrast, the knockout female mice fed a low-fat diet were indistinguishable from normal mice. Only the knockout female mice fed a high-fat diet gained less weight than did the normal female mice. Measurements for lipid content in plasma and organs were also performed. Cholesterol, triacylglycerol (TG), glucose, and insulin were measured in the plasma. Samples of liver and epididymal fat pads were used to determine cholesterol and TG content in tissues, and their values were normalized to grams of organ weight. Although I-FABP has been suggested to be involved in the absorption of dietary fatty acids, the results of this study suggest that I-FABP is not imperative for fatty acid uptake. In fact, the higher concentrations of TG in the plasma of male knockout mice, which is consistent with their greater weight gain, implies that the rate of dietary fat transfer into the plasma compartment in male mice is actually increased in the absence of I-FABP [172,173].

The mRNA abundance for both I-FABP and L-FABP was enhanced by feeding rats with a PUFA-enriched diet [145]. The mRNA expression was also enhanced in starved rats [174]. It is possible that L-FABP influences growth and differentiation of enterocytes [108, 171]. L-FABP binds not only to fatty acids but also to growth factors, prostaglandins, and leukotrienes; L-FABP participates in the regulation of genes as a partner of the peroxisome proliferator-activated receptors (PPAR).

The mechanism and regulation of the uptake of extracellular LCFA into mammalian cells is not well understood. PPAR play unique roles in lipid homeostasis. PPARs are part of the nuclear hormone receptor superfamily, and three subtypes have been described, namely α, β, γ. They have unique tissue distribution patterns. Furthermore, the roles of PPAR in mediating changes in gene expression appear to be cell- and tissue-specific. Also, the type of agonist influences the magnitude of their responses. In the intestine for example, activation of PPARα by feeding rats with a diet containing Wy 14,643 (a hypolipidemic drug) resulted in a large induction of I-FABP mRNA, FAT mRNA, FATP mRNA, and peroxisomal Huntington's disease mRNA (the second enzyme of the peroxisomal beta-oxidation pathway) [175]. PPARα may be involved in up-regulating the expression of L-FABP and I-FABP genes in murine liver [176], in addition to the known induction of hepatic peroxisomal lipid-metabolizing enzymes [175]. The experiments with rats treated with bezafibrate, a PPAR hypolipidemic drug, showed an increased amount of L-FABP protein and mRNA in the liver of these rats [177], as well as an increase of the mRNA of FAT. These findings suggest a complementary role of FAT and FABP [145, 147]. PPARα activation increases the cytosolic transport and the oxidation of lipids. PPARα mediates fibrate and dietary PUFA induction of hepatic peroxisomal lipid-metabolizing enzymes, including acyl-CoA oxidase, a key enzyme in the regulation of peroxisomal lipid catabolism [175]. Interestingly, PUFA activate PPAR as potently as does the hypolipydemic drug Wy 14,643 [178]. In addition, the binding of PUFA to PPAR is increased as compared with other fatty acids [179].

ILBP is a 14 kDa protein expressed mainly in the cytosol of the enterocytes in the distal ileum. In rats, the ILBP amino acid sequence has a 25% homology with L-FABP and I-FABP, but they are immunologically distinct. The ileum is the only site of active bile acid absorption that is coincident with the localization of ILBP mRNA expression [180]. ILBP exhibits an increase in its affinity/capacity when stimulated by bile acids. Therefore, the ileal bile acid reabsorption system can be modulated by an intracellular increase of ILBP affinity/capacity which allows the maximal adaptation of transport activity to changing substrate loads [181].

The cytosolic acyl-CoA binding protein (ACBP) plays a role in the binding of LCFA [148,167,182]. ACBP is a 10 kDa protein that binds long chain acyl CoA esters (LCA). ACBP binds LCA with high affinity, and may play a role in LCFA transport and metabolism [182]. ABCP regulates the levels of LCA in the cell, and has a role in cellular signaling, and ACBP and LCA are involved in signal transduction and gene regulation [148,167,182].

The microsomal transport protein (MTP) is a heterodimer involved in the transfer of triglyceride, phospholipids, and cholesterol esters in apolipoprotein B (apo B) [183]. This heterodimer contains a 59 kDa multifunctional subunit, identical to protein disulfide isomerase, which is linked to the endoplasmic reticulum (ER), and a 97 kDa subunit with lipid transfer activity [184]. MTP also plays a key role in very light density lipoprotein (VLDL) synthesis. The absence of MTP in mutant MTP humans causes abetalipoproteinemia and the absence of VLDL in the plasma [185]. The major clinical consequence of this disorder is the deficiency of essential fatty acids and fat-soluble vitamins [184].

The rate-limiting step in lipid absorption may be the transport of TG from the ER to the Golgi. The intestine has two systems that enable it to traffic lipids between organelles. The first is the binding of lipids to cytosolic binding proteins, and the second is the chylomicron secretion after resynthesis of TG from absorbed fatty acids and monoacylglycerol. The capacity of the intestine to export chylomicrons is limited. The formation of the ER vesicle that transports the developing chylomicrons to the Golgi parallels the capacity of chylomicron secretion of the intestine. The rates of prechylomicron vesicle formation determine the rate of lipid absorption [130,186].

Lipid uptake is a dual process involving passive diffusion and protein-mediated transport. It is not known yet which system contributes more to lipid absorption [107,148,167]. The small intestine is subjected to large variations in lipid supply from the diet, bile, and sloughed intestinal cells. It is possible that passive diffusion may be a high-capacity, low-affinity system that operates during high lipid loads, and that the lipid binding proteins may constitute a low-capacity, high-affinity system that works at low lipid concentrations. Thus, the presence in the enterocyte of multiple lipid binding proteins raises the question of the physiological role of these proteins. Perhaps they may be involved in specific uptake or selection of fatty acids, or may play a role in fatty acid targeting as well as in cellular signaling.

9.4.1.9 Lipid Absorption in Aging

In aging there may be reduced gastric lipase and bile acid secretion, decreased lipid solubilization, and thus a decline in lipid absorption [187]. In a study of dietary fat intake and fecal fat output, the digestibility of fatty acids was reduced in old as compared with younger cats [188].

While a number of animal studies demonstrate reduced *in vitro* lipid absorption with aging [189,190], others have shown increases in lipid absorption in aged rats using an *in vivo* perfusion model [191]. However, *in vitro* uptake studies done with rabbit jejunal discs demonstrated a decline in the uptake of fatty acids and cholesterol with age when uptake was expressed on the basis of the weight of the intestine [189]. Radiolabeled fat breath tests have confirmed that lipid absorption is reduced in mature as compared with suckling rats [190].

The lipid composition of cell membranes alters the passive permeability properties and transporter activity across the membrane [192]. Enhanced fluidity of the BBM increases the transport of lipids and glucose, but decreases the activity of leucine aminopeptidase in the BBM [193,194].

TABLE 9.1
Effect of Age and Diet on Intestinal Weight

	1 Month			9 Months			24 Months		
	Chow	SFA	PUFA	Chow	SFA	PUFA	Chow	SFA	PUFA
	Tissue Weight (mg/cm)								
Jejunum	9.0 ± 0.7	8.8 ± 0.9	10.1 ± 1.4	12.3 ± 1.3	12.5 ± 0.5	11.2 ± 0.8	10.7 ± 1.5	13.6 ± 2.1	10.5 ± 1.1
Ileum	6.4 ± 0.7	$6.8 \pm 0.6^{\#}$	$9.4 \pm 0.8^{*}$	7.8 ± 0.8	10.4 ± 1.9	7.6 ± 1.1^{a}	11.1 ± 1.7^{a}	8.5 ± 0.9^{b}	$5.4 \pm 1.1^{*a}$
	Mucosal Weight (mg/cm)								
Jejunum	4.0 ± 0.5	4.6 ± 0.7	5.5 ± 0.9	6.3 ± 1.2	6.3 ± 0.6	5.9 ± 1.0	5.6 ± 1.1	7.2 ± 1.5	5.6 ± 0.8
Ileum	2.9 ± 0.6	3.1 ± 0.5	4.7 ± 0.7	3.5 ± 0.6	5.6 ± 1.1	3.9 ± 1.0	6.0 ± 1.1^{ab}	4.2 ± 0.7	2.9 ± 0.7
	Percentage of Intestinal Wall Composed of Mucosa								
Jejunum	44.5 ± 2.9	51.7 ± 3.7	55.0 ± 6.2	48.8 ± 5.2	50.6 ± 3.7	51.8 ± 6.2	48.7 ± 4.0	51.4 ± 3.6	51.2 ± 3.4
Ileum	38.3 ± 4.7	45.6 ± 5.0	49.9 ± 5.3	43.9 ± 3.1	51.4 ± 3.6	48.8 ± 5.4	50.1 ± 6.4	49.3 ± 4.0	42.8 ± 8.9

Values are Mean ± SEM

[a] Significantly different from 1-month-old rats $p \leq 0.05$
[b] Significantly different from 9-month-old rats $p \leq 0.05$
[*] Significantly different from chow fed animals $p \leq 0.05$
[#] Significantly different from PUFA $p \leq 0.05$

Source: Woudstra T. D., L. A. Drozdowski, G. E. Wild, M. T. Clandinin, L. B. Agellon, and A. B. R. Thomson. 2004. An isocaloric PUFA diet enhances lipid uptake and weight gain in aging rats. *Lipids* 39(4):343–54. With permission.

A decrease in intestinal BBM phospholipid composition and membrane fluidity have been reported in aging rats, and this may contribute to the reduced lipid absorption in the aged [194]. In contrast, aging is associated with a decrease in the thickness and resistance of the intestinal UWL [189], which would tend to increase the net absorption of nutrients, possibly to partially counteract the decreased permeability of the BBM to lipids with aging, but could partially explain the increased lipid absorption *in vivo*.

To answer whether the absorption of lipids altered by age or by dietary lipids, the jejunal and ileal uptake of fatty acids and cholesterol was first expressed on the basis of the weight of the entire wall of the intestine (nmol 100 mg^{-1} min^{-1}) (Table 9.1). In animals fed chow, the jejunal and ileal uptake of 18:0 fell between 1 and 9 months, the ileal uptake of 16:0 fell between 1 and 9, and 1 and 24 months. In animals fed SFA, there was reduced jejunal uptake of 18:0, 18:1 and 18:2 between 1 and 9 months and in 18:0 between 1 and 24 months. In animals fed PUFA, there was reduced jejunal uptake of 18:0 between 1 and 24 months. In 9-month-old animals fed a SFA diet there was increased ileal uptake of 18:2, and decreased uptake of 18:3 when compared with 9-month PUFA fed animals. At 24 months there was decreased ileal uptake of 18:0 in SFA fed animals when compared with PUFA fed animals.

The rate of uptake was also expressed on the basis of the weight of the mucosa (nmol 100 mg mucosal tissue^{-1}min^{-1}). In animals fed chow, there was reduced jejunal uptake of 18:0 between 1 and 9 months (Figure 9.1), reduced ileal uptake of 16:0 and 18:0 between 1 and 9 and between 1 and 24 months, and reduced ileal uptake of 18:2 between 1 and 24 months (Figure 9.2).

Woudstra et al. [195] showed changes in the rate of lipid uptake in the small intestine associated with aging. However, it depends on the method used to express the results as to whether there is an increase, decrease, or no alteration in the rate of uptake. For example, when results were expressed on the basis of serosal surface area, there was a decline in the jejunal rate of uptake of 18:3 between 9 and 24 months in chow fed animals. When using an *in vivo* perfusion technique and expressing

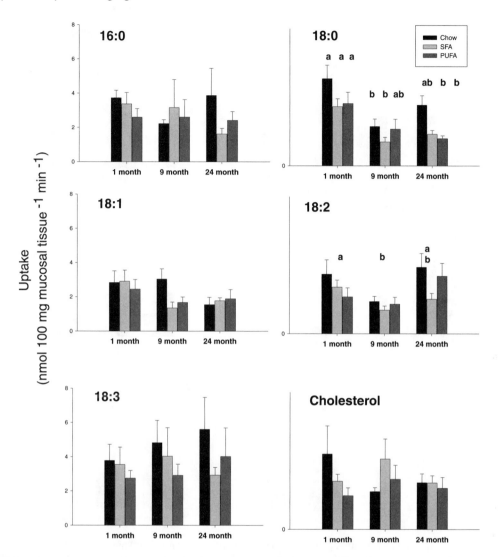

FIGURE 9.1 Jejunal uptake of fatty acids and cholesterol expressed as nmol 100 mg mucosal tissue –1min –1. Values are mean +/– SEM. Different letters denote a significant age effect; (p < 0.05) significant diet effect (SFA v.s. PUFA fed animals) (p < 0.05) (n = 8). (Woudstra T. D., L. A. Drozdowski, G. E. Wild, M. T. Clandinin, L. B. Agellon, and A. B. R. Thomson. 2004. An isocaloric PUFA diet enhances lipid uptake and weight gain in aging rats. *Lipids* 39(4):343–54. With permission.)

lipid uptake on the basis of the length of the intestine, the uptake of cholesterol and fatty acid was shown to increase in aging rats [102,191]. When the results of Woudstra et al. [195] were expressed on the basis of the weight of the entire wall of the intestine, there was an increase in the rate of jejunal uptake of 18:0 and 18:2 in the 24- as compared with 9-month-old chow fed animals. In contrast, in the ileum there was decreased uptake of 16:0 at 9 and 24 months when compared with 1 month. In an *in vivo* perfusion study, Holt and Dominguez [196] found a decrease in lipid uptake in 21- as compared with 4-month-old rats when uptake was expressed on the basis of intestinal weight. Methodology differences and the use of *in vitro* versus *in vivo* techniques may explain these contrasting findings. The jejunal and ileal uptake of 18:0 is lower in the 9-month as compared with the 1-month animals fed chow when results are expressed on the basis of intestinal weight. Thomson [189] also showed a decline in lipid uptake in the jejunum of 11- compared with 1-month-old rabbits. It is difficult to establish the pattern of changes in lipid uptake observed throughout the lifetime of

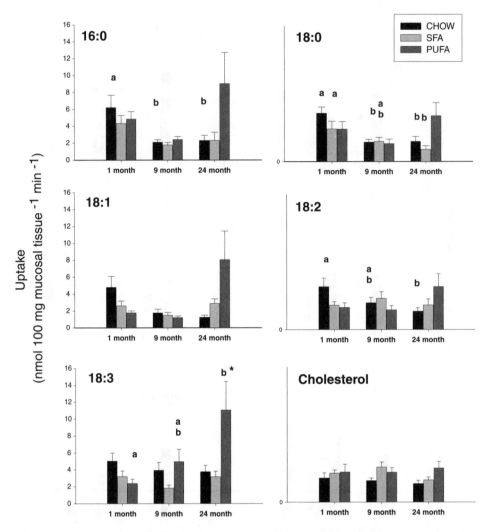

FIGURE 9.2 Ileal uptake of fatty acids and cholesterol expressed as nmol 100 mg mucosal tissue −1min −1. Values are Mean + SEM. Different letters denote a significant age effect; (p < 0.05), and * denotes a signifi-cant diet effect (SFA v.s. PUFA fed animals) (p < 0.05) (n = 8). (Woudstra T. D., L. A. Drozdowski, G. E. Wild, M. T. Clandinin, L. B. Agellon, and A. B. R. Thomson. 2004. An isocaloric PUFA diet enhances lipid uptake and weight gain in aging rats. *Lipids* 39(4):343–54. With permission.)

the animal based on current literature. Thus, differences in methodologies, units of expression, and ages of comparison clearly play a critical role in the conclusion of any findings.

It has been suggested that the ileum compensates for the loss of function of the jejunum in aging [197]; for example, an increased villous height and aminopeptidase activity was found in the ileum of rats refed a high-protein diet following a period of starvation [197]. In our study, chow fed ani-mals had no age-associated change in ileal villous height or in villous surface area of the 24-month animals compared to the 9- or 1-month animals (Figure 9.2), but age was associated with a decline in jejunal and ileal mucosal surface area in animals fed a SFA or PUFA diet (Figure 9.3). When lipid uptake was expressed on the basis of mucosal surface area (Figure 9.4), the uptake of some lipids actually increased between 1 and 9 or 24 months. Thus, the reduction in the surface area of these older animals did not result in a concomitant reduction in absorptive capacity. Therefore, changes in morphology or surface area of the small intestine may not accurately predict the ability of the aged intestine to absorb nutrients. While it has been suggested that increased ileal height may result

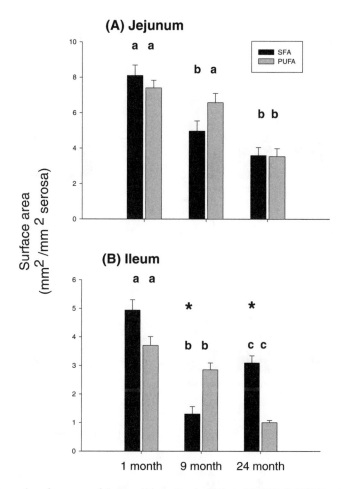

FIGURE 9.3   Mucosal surface area of the small intestine in SFA and PUFA fed F344 rats. Values are mean +/– SEM. Different letters indicate a significant difference between ages ($p < 0.05$), and * indicates a significant diet effect ($p < 0.05$) ($n = 4$). (Woudstra T. D., L. A. Drozdowski, G. E. Wild, M. T. Clandinin, L. B. Agellon, and A. B. R. Thomson. 2004. An isocaloric PUFA diet enhances lipid uptake and weight gain in aging rats. *Lipids* 39(4):343–54. With permission.)

in increased functional capacity of the ileum in aging [197], we show this may not be the case; i.e., increased intestinal surface area does not necessarily result in increased absorptive capacity.

9.4.1.10   The Effect of the Intestinal Unstirred Water Layer

The uptake of 12:0 is a reflection of the effective resistance of the intestinal UWL, with higher uptake reflecting lower resistance [189]. In chow fed animals, the jejunal uptake of 12:0 was increased between 9 and 24 months, suggesting lower effective resistance of the UWL in the 24-month rats. This lower resistance would help to increase uptake of diffusion-limited probes such as LCFA [124]. However, at 24 months, the jejunal uptake of lipids was unchanged when expressed as nmol 100 mg mucosal tissue^{-1} min^{-1}. Furthermore, in rats fed PUFA, the jejunal uptake of 12:0 increased between 1 and 24 months, reflecting lower unstirred layer resistance. The jejunal uptake of 18:0 fell between 1 and 24 months, indicating that the age-associated alterations in lipid uptake could not simply be explained by variations in the effective resistance of the intestinal UWL.

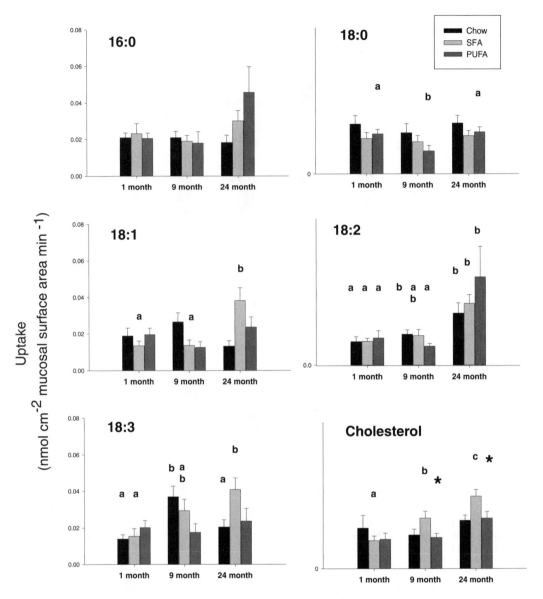

FIGURE 9.4 Jejunal uptake of fatty acids and cholesterol expressed on the basis of mucosal surface area. Values are Mean + SEM. Different letters denote a significant age effect; ($p < 0.05$), and * denotes a significant diet effect (SFA vs. PUFA fed animals) ($p < 0.05$) (n = 8). (Woudstra T. D., L. A. Drozdowski, G. E. Wild, M. T. Clandinin, L. B. Agellon, and A. B. R. Thomson. 2004. An isocaloric PUFA diet enhances lipid uptake and weight gain in aging rats. *Lipids* 39(4):343–54. With permission.)

9.4.1.11 Passive Lipid Uptake

Passive uptake of lipids across the BBM may be affected by membrane fluidity and by the pH microclimate of the UWL adjacent to the BBM [127–198]. The lipid composition of the BBM may contribute to alterations in lipid uptake [199]. In aging, there is an age-associated decrease in BBM fluidity [194], which could contribute to the decreased lipid absorption with aging. The low pH of the microclimate adjacent to the BBM increases the bile acid critical-micellar concentration, resulting in a dissociation of lipids from bile acid micelles [127,128]. In aging, there is an increase in the pH of the microclimate, which would contribute to reduced absorption in aging [104]. Measurements of the pH of the microclimate and the BBM composition were not analyzed in this study.

9.4.1.12 Intestinal Lipid Binding Proteins

There are many lipid binding proteins in the enterocyte cytosol and BBM [148,167]. It was speculated that some of these may be involved in lipid uptake. For example, using an antibody to the FABP in BBM reduced the lipid uptake [125,126,142]. Feeding animals a high-fat diet increases the intestinal lipid uptake and enhances the abundance of L-FABP [148,167]. The exposure of Caco-2 cells in culture to lipids increases both L-FABP and I-FABP in their cytosol [200]. However, the alterations in lipid uptake in diabetes, aging, or in response to intestinal resection are not correlated with variations in enterocyte abundance of I-/L-FABP [201]. Furthermore, in knockout mice lacking I-FABP, lipid uptake is normal under basal conditions [172].

The expression of L-FABP mRNA in the jejunum and ileum was not affected by the age of the animals fed chow or PUFA. In those fed SFA, the expression of L-FABP mRNA in the jejunum was higher at 24 as compared with 1 or 9 months (Figure 9.5). ILBP expression in the ileum was unaffected by age in animals fed SFA or PUFA, but in those fed chow the mRNA expression of ILBP was higher at 24 months as compared with 9 months. In contrast, the abundance of ILBP protein was unaffected by age or by diet and the abundance of I-FABP protein was also unaffected by age or by diet (Figure 9.5).

Thus, reduced lipid absorption in aging cannot be explained by alterations in the expression of the mRNA of the selected lipid binding proteins or in the abundance of these proteins. In I-FABP knockout mice, fatty acid uptake is maintained, demonstrating that the I-FABP protein is not required for intestinal lipid uptake [173]. In this study, in the ileum the rate of uptake of several fatty acids was reduced in the 24-month group as compared with the 1-month group, yet no difference was seen in the abundance of the binding proteins (ILBP, L-FABP, and I-FABP) or expression of their mRNAs. These findings, together with the observations in the knockout mice, suggest that lipid absorption is not dependent on the abundance of these lipid-binding proteins. It is possible that the distribution of transporters along the crypt–villous axis is altered in aging, without a change in the actual number of transporters. It may be that the increased rate of proliferation in the small intestine that is associated with aging results in fewer mature cells toward the villous tip [202]. It is also possible that the abundance of the lipid binding proteins is controlled post-transcriptionally or post-translationally. Finally, there are several other lipid binding proteins in the enterocyte, and these may play a role in lipid uptake. For example, the FATP4 [150], or the FAT in the BBM of enterocytes [144]. It has also been suggested that the rate-limiting step in lipid absorption is the formation of a prechylomicron transport vesicle in the ER [130,186]. Thus, we cannot dismiss the possibility that some lipid-binding proteins not assessed in this study play some role in the control of lipid uptake, and may have contributed to the change in lipid uptake observed with aging.

In total, these data suggest that lipid absorption is lower in the older than in the younger individual; but the extent depends on the method used to express the data. The mechanisms of this impairment remain unknown.

Older studies suggested that the lower serum chylomicron levels following a fatty meal indicate a reduced absorptive capacity among the aged [160]. In a study of only the healthy aged, there was no correlation between age and 72-hour fecal fat excretion [203]. However, the absorption of fat may take longer in the elderly, and this method of measuring serum chylomicron levels may not reflect total uptake of lipids [203]. There is also a reduction in postprandial serum bile acid levels in elderly humans, suggesting that bile acids are absorbed less effectively [204].

Early work using human subjects demonstrated reductions in lipid absorption with age [160]. There also appears to be reduced intestinal absorption of bile acids with age [204], although it is not clear if this negatively impacts lipid absorption in the elderly. When healthy elderly human subjects were studied, however, no correlation between age and 72-hour fecal fat excretion was found [203].

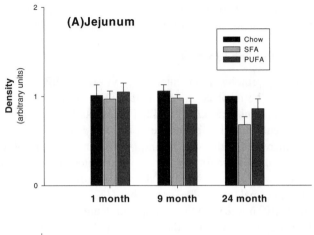

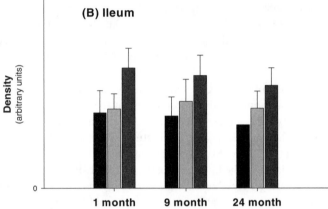

FIGURE 9.5 Abundance of I-FABP as determined by Western blot with values normalized to the 24 month chow fed group. Values are mean + SEM. No significant age or diet effect ($p < 0.05$) ($n = 4$). (Woudstra T. D., L. A. Drozdowski, G. E. Wild, M. T. Clandinin, L. B. Agellon, and A. B. R. Thomson. 2004. An isocaloric PUFA diet enhances lipid uptake and weight gain in aging rats. *Lipids* 39(4):343–54. With permission.)

After considering the results of all these studies, Holt [205] suggested that no important changes in lipid absorption with aging have been described.

9.5   POSSIBLE MECHANISMS OF ALTERED LIPID ABSORPTION WITH AGING

9.5.1   Faulty Adaptation

Intestinal adaptation is defined as the ability of the intestine to change functionally or morphologically in response to alterations in environmental stimuli. Generally, the adaptive changes are beneficial, such as increased nutrient absorption following small-intestinal resection, chronic alcohol ingestion, or sub-lethal abdominal radiation [206]. In contrast, the enhanced absorptive adaptation observed in diabetes contributes to the hyperglycemia, hyperlipidemia, and the obesity associated with this metabolic disorder.

The adaptive response of the gut is impaired in aging. Therefore, in times of stress such as injury or illness, malnutrition may result more readily [207]. For example, dietary restriction initiated in aged rats resulted in a dramatic weight loss, with no weight stabilization after 12 weeks of reintroduction of a normal diet. In addition, the intestines of the animals were atrophied and ileal hydrolase activity was decreased [7]. Following a period of underfeeding, elderly men continued to

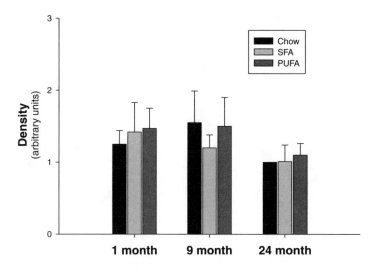

FIGURE 9.6 Abundance of ILBP in the ileum as determined by Western blot with values normalized to the 24-month chow-fed group. Values are mean + SEM. No significant age or diet effect ($p < 0.05$) ($n = 4$). (Woudstra T. D., L. A. Drozdowski, G. E. Wild, M. T. Clandinin, L. B. Agellon, and A. B. R. Thomson. 2004. An isocaloric PUFA diet enhances lipid uptake and weight gain in aging rats. *Lipids* 39(4):343–54. With permission.)

underfeed themselves for a period of 9–10 days, while their younger counterparts increased their energy intake [208]. This suggests that following a period of illness during which nutrient intake is reduced, the elderly may continue to underfeed themselves despite their recovery from the illness. Thus, the reduction in nutrient absorptive capacity of the small intestine that occurs with aging, plus the reduced adaptive response, will put the older patient at high risk for becoming malnourished.

Depending on the nutrients available, the intestine adapts to variations in dietary load and composition [209]. For example, increased dietary carbohydrates cause an increase in the Vmax for intestinal glucose uptake [210]. Nonessential and nontoxic amino acids are upregulated on high-protein diets, and this response may be impaired in aging [99]. Potentially toxic substances such as some essential amino acids, iron, and calcium may be downregulated by a dietary increase in these respective substrates [99,211]. Animals fed isocaloric diets enriched with SFA have greater glucose uptake than those animals fed PUFA diets [212]. In adult rats, a diet enriched with SFA results in increased intestinal sugar uptake when compared with an isocaloric diet enriched with PUFA [213–216]. Similarly, Vine et al. [217] studied the effect of various fatty acids on the passive and active transport properties of rat jejunum, and found that an SFA diet increased Na^+-dependent glucose uptake when compared with a diet enriched with n6 PUFA. Of importance, Woudstra et al. [195] showed that the intestinal response to dietary lipids may differ with age.

In mature animals, SFA increased the rate of uptake of fatty acids and cholesterol in the ileum when expressed on the basis of mucosal surface area (Figures 9.4 and 9.7). Previous work in mature rats has also shown an increase in the rate of uptake of lipids, cholesterol, and carbohydrates in animals fed a SFA-enriched diet [212]. The jejunal rate of cholesterol uptake was also increased in the mature and old SFA fed animals. In contrast, in the ileum of young and old animals, SFA reduced the rate of uptake of some lipids when calculated on the basis of mucosal surface area. The higher effective resistance of the UWL in the ileum of the young animals fed SFA may have contributed to the reduced uptake of lipids in the 1-month group. However, in the ileum of old animals fed SFA, the effective resistance of the UWL is reduced. This would increase the concentration of lipid at the membrane aqueous interface and increase lipid uptake [120]. Thus, the adaptive response to the composition of dietary lipid is age-dependent. In the ileum of 9-month-old animals, SFA increases the rate of lipid uptake, and yet in 24-month-old animals SFA decreases the rate of lipid uptake.

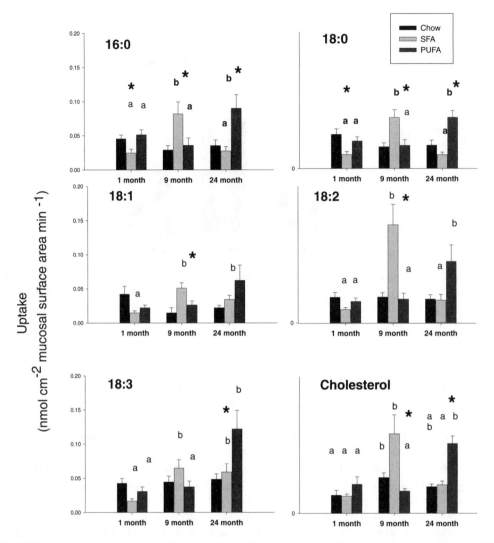

FIGURE 9.7 Ileal uptake of fatty acids and cholesterol expressed on the basis of mucosal surface area. Values are Mean + SEM. Different letters denote a significant age effect; ($p < 0.05$), and * denotes a significant diet effect (SFA vs. PUFA fed animals) ($p < 0.05$) (n = 8). (Woudstra T. D., L. A. Drozdowski, G. E. Wild, M. T. Clandinin, L. B. Agellon, and A. B. R. Thomson. 2004. An isocaloric PUFA diet enhances lipid uptake and weight gain in aging rats. *Lipids* 39(4):343–54. With permission.)

Investigators have previously shown an altered adaptive response associated with aging. In old F344 rats that are refed, following a period of starvation there is an exaggerated increase in enzyme activity when compared with same-aged controls and young refed animals [218]. This exaggerated response may suggest impairment in protein degradation in the old animal. In addition, villus cell proliferation rate is not controlled as tightly in older rats as compared with younger rats in response to refeeding [219]. It has also been shown that aging reduces the adaptive response of the small intestine to changes in dietary carbohydrates and amino acids [99]. By altering the type of dietary fat, Woudstra et al. [195] have shown that the old intestine is still capable of adapting to changes in dietary fat. However, this response is altered in the aging rats when compared with mature animals.

The mechanism responsible for this age-related alteration in adaptation to dietary lipids is not known. But clearly, the results of adaptive studies in young rats do not necessarily apply to older animals.

9.5.2 ANIMAL INTESTINAL MORPHOLOGY CHARACTERISTICS

In the jejunum, neither age nor diet had an effect on the weight of the intestine, the weight of the intestinal mucosa, or on the percentage of the intestinal wall composed of mucosa (Table 9.1). In contrast, in the ileum of rats fed chow, the weight of the intestine and the weight of the intestinal mucosa were approximately twice as high at 24 as compared with 1 month. In rats fed SFA, the ileal weight was lower at 24 than 9 months, but not as compared with 1 month. In rats fed PUFA, the mean ileal weight was lower at 24 than at 1 month. Therefore, the weight of the mucosa had to be taken into account when expressing the rate of uptake of the lipids.

The main function of the small intestine is nutrient absorption. In humans, the small intestine is approximately 6 meters in length [206] and 1.1 meters in mature Fischer 344 rats [6]. The most proximal region is the duodenum, followed by the jejunum, and most distally the ileum. The interior of the small intestine is the lumen, surrounded by the intestinal mucosa. Numerous mucosal villi increase the absorptive surface area by 7- to 14-fold. The height of the villi in humans ranges from 0.5 mm to 0.8 mm, and from approximately 0.3 mm to 0.5 mm in F344 rats [6]. The mucosa may be divided into three layers, (1) the muscularis mucosa, which is a thin layer of smooth muscle cells and separates the mucosa from the submucosa; (2) the lamina propria, which is a continuous sheet of connective tissue abundant in many immunologically important cells such as plasma cells, lymphocytes, and macrophages, and as well contains blood and lymph vessels; and (3) the epithelial layer, which can be further subdivided into two regions, the crypt and villous epithelium. The crypts of Lieberkühn are located at the base of the villi, and contain a number of cells such as mucus-secreting cells, endocrine cells, and immature and undifferentiated cells. The immature cells leave the crypt and migrate to the villous tip over a period of approximately 2–3 days in rats and 4–5 days in humans. During this time they differentiate into fully functional cells. The villous epithelium is a single cell layer that contains a large number of absorptive cells known as the enterocytes, which are highly polarized cells that facilitated vectorial transport of nutrients. The apical membrane is characterized by microvilli, and is known as the BBM. It is estimated that the BBM increases the absorptive surface area of the enterocyte by 14- to 40-fold.

Morphological changes are often associated with intestinal adaptation. Following bowel resection, hyperplasia of the remaining gut is associated with increased nutrient, water, and electrolyte absorption [220]. However, hyperplasia does not necessarily correlate with altered absorption [212]. For example, in the rat jejunum, the uptake of glucose is enhanced by dietary fats, but is not associated with increased mucosal surface area. Following small-bowel resection, the mass of the remnant intestine was increased to 50–70% of its pre-resection level, but glucose uptake was restored to only 33% [221]. These findings suggest that morphological changes do not necessarily accompany alterations in absorption, and vice versa.

Changes in the morphology of the small intestine may also contribute to age-associated alterations in nutrient absorption. In studies of F344 rats, there was no age-related change in the density of the villi in the small intestine, or in the size of the enterocytes [6]. However, with aging, there is an increase in the width of the villi throughout the intestine and an increase in duodenal and jejunal crypt depth, as well as increased ileal villous height, ileal mass, and ileal DNA content. The number of villi per unit area of intestine decreases in aged rats, suggesting that the overall surface area of the intestine may fall without an alteration in villous height or width [222]. The height, width, depth, and number of villi are incorporated into a measurement of surface area, and it may not be appropriate to predict changes in mucosal surface area based only on alterations in the height of the villi [223]. In fact, there would appear to be an age-related decline in mucosal surface area in rabbit jejunum [224]. In the jejunum of human subjects, no significant difference between young and old enterocyte height and jejunal surface-area-to-volume ratio was found [225].

Holt et al. [6] looked at age-related changes in the intestinal morphology of Fischer 344 rats. Increases in villous width were noted throughout the small intestine, while increases in villous height were limited to the ileum. Other studies in rats have shown age-related losses in villous and enterocyte heights [226]. Age-related declines in mucosal surface area have also been reported in rabbit jejunum [224]. Human studies generally show no changes in intestinal morphology, as determined from measurements of villous height, crypt depth, crypt-to-villous ratios, and enterocyte size [225,227,228]. In contrast, Warren et al. [229] showed a decrease in villous height with age. Martin et al. [230] described histological changes that occur in aging mice: when old mice were compared to young mice, there were larger villi, a reduced number of crypts, and fewer villi and crypts per mm along the small intestine. These changes were most pronounced in the distal, as opposed to the proximal small intestine. Research has failed to find a clear association between intestinal morphology and nutrient uptake with aging. For example, despite reductions in mucosal surface area, aged rats demonstrated increases in the jejunal uptake of SFA [224]. So, while it remains controversial as to whether aging is associated with morphological changes, even if such changes were to occur, the impact on nutrient uptake may not be clinically relevant.

Ciccocioppo et al. [231] suggested that intestinal architecture is maintained with aging by increases in proliferation and differentiation rates. This agrees with work done by Corazza et al. [232] that showed increased expression of proliferating cell nuclear antigen in older subjects when compared with their younger counterparts.

Morphological changes associated with aging fail to fully explain altered absorptive capacity in laboratory animals. For example, increased SFA uptake was observed in the jejunum of mature as compared with young rabbits, and yet surface area decreased [224]. These findings suggest that other factors may be responsible for the altered lipid uptake. For example, differentiation of the enterocytes as they migrate from crypt to villous tip is delayed in aging animals. There is a greater crypt cell proliferative rate, as well as a broadened zone of proliferation within the crypts of old rats [233]. The immunohistochemical expression of the proliferation cell nuclear antigen is markedly increased in the duodenal villi and crypts of humans over 65 years, as compared with younger persons [232]. This suggests that the abnormal proliferation pattern may explain the coexistence of normal morphology, and yet impaired absorptive function in the elderly [232]. In aged rats refed a high protein diet following 48 hours of starvation, there is a 35% increase in villous height in the ileum as well as an increased ileal aminopeptidase activity [197]. This suggests that the ileum may compensate for any age-associated loss of surface area of the jejunum. It is speculated that the ileum of aged rats may be exposed to a greater luminal load due to decreased uptake in the proximal small intestine, thereby causing hyperplasia of the ileum. Supporting this suggestion, ileal–jejunal transposed rats showed an increase in the mucosal mass of the transposed ileum in young, mature, and old animals [234]. Thus, there may be a modest decline in the surface area of the intestine in some species, but this by itself does not explain functional alterations.

Woudstra et al. [195] hypothesized that a diet enriched in SFA might help to correct the age-associated loss of function of the small intestine, but the current study suggests that a PUFA enriched diet may be more effective at reversing this loss in old F344 rats. This unexpected finding underscores the necessity of performing research in aging animals, because treatment effects found in young or mature animals may be altered by the aging process.

9.6   POSSIBLE SIGNALS OF INTESTINAL ADAPTATION

It has previously been shown that there is a higher rate of enterocyte proliferation in the aging intestine. In gastric mucosa increased expression in ornithine decarboxylase (ODC), epidermal growth factor (EGF) receptor, transforming growth factor-α (TGF-α), activator-protein 1 (AP-1) (c-fos/c-jun), and NF-κB may contribute to this hyperproliferation [235]. It has been suggested that NF-κB, AP-1 proteins (c-fos and c-jun) are activated in response to intrinsic factors such as oxidative stress and extrinsic factors such as dietary components [236]. In addition, AP-1 proteins may play an important role in the postnatal development of the intestine [237], and in models of intestinal adaptation [238,239]. EGF has also been shown to increase glucose uptake and surface area of the small intestine following small-bowel resection [240], possibly by activating the AP-1 proteins

[241]. ODC is the first enzyme of polyamine synthesis that is essential for nucleic acid and protein synthesis [242]. Control over polyamine synthesis may be less rigidly controlled in aging and ODC activity may increase in aging rats [243,244]. The role of these proteins in intestinal adaptation associated with aging and dietary lipids has not been investigated. Additional proteins of cell cycle regulation such as cyclin dependent-kinase inhibitor p16ink4α and transcription factor p53 may also play a role in age-associated and diet-induced changes in the small intestine. This speculation has not been examined experimentally [245,246].

It is possible that genes that signal the adaptive response to dietary lipids are also altered by the aging process. Some of the possible genes are (1) PPARs, which may contribute to dietary lipid-induced adaptation of the small intestine [247] and may increase in aging [248]; (2) ODC, which is required for protein and nucleic acid synthesis [242] may be less rigidly controlled in aging [243,244]; (3) EGF, as well as AP-1 proteins (c-jun/c-fos), which play a role in intestinal adaptation and development [237,240], and which may also be sensitive to oxidative stress such as that seen in aging [236] and; (4) cell cycle regulators such as the p53 and p16ink4a, which may also play a role in adaptation and may be altered in aging [245,246]. Further studies are needed to determine the role of these proteins in models of intestinal adaptation and aging.

ABBREVIATIONS

ABCA1 ATP binding cassette
ACBP acyl-CoA binding protein
ACS acyl-CoA synthetase
AP-1 activator-protein 1 (*c-fos/c-jun*)
Apo B apolipoprotein B
BBM brush border membrane
BLM basolateral membrane
CNS central nervous system
CR caloric restriction
DNA deoxyribonucleic acid
EGF epidermal growth factor
ER endoplasmic reticulum
FABP fatty acid binding protein
FAT fatty acid translocase
FATP fatty acid transport protein
GC glucocorticosteroids
I-FABP intestinal-fatty acid binding protein
IGF-1 insulin-like growth factor-1
Igflr⁺ heterozygous knockout mice
LCA acyl CoA esters
LCFA long-chain fatty acid
L-FABP liver-fatty acid binding protein
LPH lactase phlorizin hydrolase
LXR liver X receptors
MDR multidrug resistance protein
mRNA messenger ribonucleic acid
MTP microsomal transport protein
Na⁺K⁺-AT Pasesodium-potassium pump
NF-κB nuclear factor- κB
ODC ornithine decarboxylase
PPAR peroxisome proliferator-activated receptors
PUFA polyunsaturated fatty acid

RXR retinoid X receptors
SFA saturated fatty acid
SGLT sodium glucose co-transporters
SI sucrase-isomaltase
SR-BI scavenger receptor Class B Type I
TG triacylglycerol
TGF-α transforming growth factor-α
UWL unstirred water layer
VLDL very light density lipoproteins

REFERENCES

1. Smith, D. W. E. 1993. *Human Longevity*. Oxford University Press, New York.
2. Carnes, B. A., Olshansky, S. J., Gavrilov, L., Gavrilov, N., and Grahn, D. 1999. Human longevity: Nature versus nurture, fact or fiction. *Perspect. Biol. Med.* 42, 423–441.
3. Hazzard, W. R. 1999. The gender differential in longevity. In *Principles of Geriatric Medicine and Gerontology*. W. M. Hazzard, J. P. Blass, W. H. Ettinger Jr., J. B. Halter and J. G. Ouslander, Eds., pp. 69–80. McGraw-Hill Companies, Inc., New York.
4. Statistics Canada. 2006. Deaths http://www.statcan.ca.
5. Medawar, P. B. 1952. An *Unsolved Problem of Biology*. Lewis, London.
6. Holt, P. R., Pascal, R. R., and Kotler, D. P. 1984. Effect of aging upon small intestine structure in the Fischer rat. *J. Gerontol.* 39, 642–647.
7. Chambon-Sanovitch, C., Felgines, C., Farges, M. C., Pernet, P., Cézard, J. P., et al. 1999. Severe dietary restriction initiated in aged rats: Evidence for poor adaptation in terms of protein metabolism and intestinal functions. *Eur. J. Clin. Invest.* 29, 504–511.
8. Masoro, E. J. 1980. Rats as models for the study of obesity. *Exp. Aging Res.* 6, 261–270.
9. Arking, R. and Dudas, S. P. 1989. Review of genetic investigations into the aging process of Drosophila. *J. Am. Geriat. Soc.* 37, 757–773.
10. Finch, C. E. 1990. *Longevity, Senescence, and the Genome*. University of Chicago Press, Chicago.
11. Rowe, J. W. and Kahn, R. L. 1997. Successful aging. *Gerontologist* 37, 433–440.
12. Rowe, J. W. and Kahn, R. L. 1987. Human aging usual and successful. *Science* 237, 143–149.
13. Zavaroni, I., Dall'Aglio, E., Bruschi, F., Bonora, E., Alpi, O., Pezzarossa, A., and Butturini, U. 1986. Effect of age and environmental factors on glucose tolerance and insulin secretion in a worker population. *J. Am. Geriatr. Soc.* 34, 271–275.
14. Herskind, A. M., McGue, M., Holm, N. V., Sorensen, T. I., Harvald, B., and Vaupel, J. W. 1996. *The Heritability of Human Longevity: A Population-Based Study of 2872 Danish Twin Pairs Born 1870–1900. Human Genetics* 97, 319–323.
15. Lin, S. J., Defossez, P. A., and Guarente, L. 2000. Requirement of NAD and SIR2 for life-span extension by calorie restriction in *Saccharomyces cerevisiae*. *Science* 289, 2062–2063.
16. Lin, Y. J., Seroude, L., and Benzer, S. 1998. Extended life-span and stress resistance in the Drosophila mutant methuselah. *Science* 282, 943–946.
17. Helfand, S. L., and Rogina, B. 2003. Molecular genetics of aging in the fly: Is this the end of the beginning? *Bioessays* 25, 134–141.
18. Marden, J. K., Rogina, B., Montooth, K. L., and Helfand, S. L. 2003. Conditional tradeoffs between aging and organismal performance of Indy long-lived mutant flies. *Proc. Natl. Acad. Sci. USA* 100, 3369–3373.
19. Kenyon, C., Chang, J., Gensch, E., Rudner, A., and Tabliang, R. 1993. A *C. Elegans* mutant that lives twice as long as wild type. *Nature* 366, 461–464.
20. Yu, C. E., Oshima, J., Fu, Y. H., and Wisman, E. M. 1996. Positional cloning of Werner's syndrome gene. *Science* 272, 258–262.
21. Puca, A. A., Daly, M. J., Brewster, S. J., Matise, T. C., Barrett, J., Shea-Drinkwater, M., Kang, S., et al., T. 2001. A genome-wide scan for linkage to human exceptional longevity identifies a locus on chromosome 4. *Proc. Natl. Acad. Sci. USA* 98, 10505–10508.
22. Hayflick, L. and Moorehead, P. S. 1961. Serial cultivation of human diploid cell strains. *Exper. Cell Res.* 25, 585.

23. Campisi, J. 2001. From cells to organisms: Can we learn about aging from cells in culture? *Exp. Gerontol.* 36, 607–618.

24. Finkel, T. and Holbrook, N. J. 2000. Oxidants, oxidative stress and the biology of ageing. *Nature* 408, 239–247.

25. Talmasoff, J. M., Ono, T., and Cutler, R. G. 1980. Superoxide dismutase: Correlation with lifespan and specific metabolic rate in primate species. *Proc. Natl. Acad. Sci. USA* 77, 2777–2781.

26. Cutler, R. G. 1984. Carotenoids and retinol: Their possible importance in determining longevity of primate species. *Proc. Natl. Acad. Sci. USA* 81, 7627–7631.

27. Gredilla, R., Barja, G., and Lopez–Torres. M. 2001. Effect of short-term caloric restriction on H202 production and oxidative DNA damage in rat liver mitochondria and location of the free radical source. *J. Bioenerg. Biomembr.* 33, 279–287.

28. Lass, A., Sohal, B. H., Weindruch, R., Forster, M. J., and Sohal, R. S. 1998. Caloric restriction prevents age-associated accrual of oxidation damage to mouse skeletal muscle mitochondria. *Free Radic. Biol. Med.* 25, 1089–1097.

29. Feuers, R.J., Weindruch, R., and Hart, R. W. 1993. Caloric restriction, aging, and antioxidant enzymes. *Mutat. Res.* 295, 191–200.

30. Tatar, M., Kopelman, A., Epstein, D., Tu, M. P., Yin, C. M., and Garofalo, R. S. 2001. A mutant Drosophila insulin receptor homolog that extends life-span and impairs neuroendocrine function. *Science* 292, 107–110.

31. Holzenberger, M., Dupont, J., Ducos, B., Leneuve, P., Geloen, A., Even, P. C., et al. 2003. IGF-1 receptor regulates lifespan and resistance to oxidative stress in mice. *Nature* 421, 182–187.

32. Giannakou, M. E., Goss, M., Junger, M. A., Hafen, E., Leever, S. J., and Partridge, L. 2004. Long-lived Drosophila with over-expressed FOXO in adult fat body. *Science* 305, 361.

33. Nijhout, H. F. 2003. The control of growth. *Development* 130, 5863–5867.

34. Casson, P. R., Hornsby, P. J., and Buster, J. E. 1996. Adrenal androgens, insulin resistance and cardiovascular disease. *Semin. Repro. Endocrin.* 14, 29–34.

35. Majewska, M. D. 1995. Neuronal actions of dehydroepiandrosterone: Possible roles in brain development, ageing, memory and affect. *Ann. NY Acad. Sci.*774, 111–121.

36. Khorram, O., Vu, L., Yen, S. S. C. 1997. Activation of immune function by dehydroepiandrosterone DHEA in age-advanced men. *J. Gerontol., Biol. Sci. Med. Sci.* 52, 1–7.

37. Tierney, A. J. 1996. Undernutrition and elderly hospital patients: A review. *J. Adv. Nurs.* 23, 228–236.

38. Kerstetter, J. E., Holthausen, B. A., and Fitz, P. A. 1992. Malnutrition in the institutionalized older adult. *JAMA* 92, 1109–1116.

39. Mowe, M., Bohmer, T., and Kindt, E. 1994. Reduced nutritional status in an elderly population >70y is probable before disease and possibly contributes to the development of disease. *Am. J. Clin. Nutr.* 59, 317–324.

40. Sullivan, D. H., Sun, S., and Walls, R. C. 1999. Protein-energy undernutrition among elderly hospitalized patients. *JAMA* 281, 2013–2019.

41. Payette, H., Coulombe, C., Boutier, V., and Gray-Donald, K. 1999. Weight loss and mortality among the free-living frail elderly: A prospective study. *J. Gerontol.: Med. Sci.* 54A, M440–M445.

42. Payette, H., Boutier, V., Coulombe, C., and Gray-Donald, K. 2002. Benefits of nutritional supplementation in free-living, frail, undernourished elderly people: A prospective randomized community trial. *J. Am. Diet. Assoc.* 102, 1088–1095.

43. Fiatarone Singh, M. A. and Rosenberg, I. H. 1999. Nutrition and aging. In *Principles of Geriatric Medicine and Gerontology.* W. R. Hazzard, J. P. Blass, W. H. Ettinger Jr., J. B. Halter and J. G. Ouslander, Eds., pp. 81–96. McGraw-Hill Companies, Inc., New York.

44. Frontera, W. R., Hughe, V. A., Lutz, K. J., and Evans, W. J. 1991. A cross-sectional study of muscle strength and mass in 45- to 78-yr-old men and women. *J. Appl. Physiol.* 71, 644–650.

45. Gariballa, S. E. and Sinclair, A. J. 1998. Nutrition, ageing and ill health. *Br. J.Nutr.* 80, 7–23.

46. Miller, A. S., Furness, J. B. and Costa, M. 1989. The relationship between gastrin cells and bombesin-like immuno-reactive nerve fibers in the gastric antral mucosa of guinea-pig, rat, dog, and man. *Cell Tissue Res.* 257, 171–178.

47. National Academy of Science. 1989. Recommended dietary allowances. National Academy Press, Washington.

48. Campbell, W. W., Crim, M. C., Dallal, G. E., Young, V. R., and Evans, W. J. 1994. Increased protein requirements in the elderly: New data and retrospective reassessments. *Am. J. Clin. Nutr.* 60, 501–509.

49. Meredith, C. N., Frontera, W. R., O'Reilly, K. P., and Evans, W. J. 1992. Body composition in elderly men: Effects of dietary modification during strength training. *J. Am. Geriat. Soc.* 40, 155–162.

50. Blumberg, J. 1997. Nutritional needs of seniors. *J. Am Coll. Nutr.* 16, 517–523.

51. Gazewood, J. D., and Mehr, D. R. 1998. Diagnosis and management of weightloss in the elderly. *J Family Pract.* 47, 19–25.

52. Davis, M. A., Murphy, S. P., Neuhaus, J. M., and Lein, D. 1990. Living arrangements and dietary quality of older US adults. *J. Am Diet. Assoc.* 90, 1667–1672.

53. Sullivan, D. H., Martin, W., Flaxman, N., and Hagen, J. E. 1993. Oral health problems and involuntary weightloss in a population of frail elderly. *J. Am Geriat. Soc.* 41, 725–731.

54. Castell, D. O. 1994. Eating and swallowing disorders. In *Principles of Geriatric Medicine.* pp. 1259–1260. McGraw-Hill, New York.

55. Vita, A. J., Terry, R. B., Hubert, H. B., and Fries, J. F. 1998. Aging, health risks, and cumulative disability. *N. Engl. J. Med.* 338, 1035–1041.

56. Roth, G. S., Ingram, D. K., and Lane, M. A. 1999. Calorie restriction in primates: Will it work and how will we know? *J. Am Geriat. Soc* 47, 896–903.

57. Weindruch, R., and Walford, R. L. 1988. *The Retardation of Aging and Disease by Dietary Restriction.* Thomas, Springfield.

58. Sohal, R. S. and Weindruch, R. 1996. Oxidative stress, caloric restriction, and aging. *Science* 273, 59–63.

59. Beckman, K. B., and Ames, B. N. 1999. Mitochondrial aging: Open questions. *Ann. NY Acad. Sci.* 854, 118–127.

60. Kagawa, Y. 1978. Impact of Westernization on the nutrients of Japanese: Changes in physique, cancer, longevity and centenarians. *Prev. Med.* 7, 205–227.

61. Reynolds, M. W., Fredman, L., Langenberg, P., and Magaziner, J. 2000. Weight, weight change, and mortality in a random sample of older community-dwelling women. *J. Am Geriat. Soc* 47, 1409–1414.

62. Kawashima, K., Motohashi, Y., and Fujishima, I. 2004. Prevalence of dysphagia among community-dwelling elderly individuals as estimated using a questionnaire for dysphagia screening. *Dysphagia* 19, 266–71.

63. Saffrey, M. J. 2004. Ageing of the enteric nervous system. *Mech. Age. Dev.* 125, 899–906.

64. Cowen, T., Johnson, R. J., Soubeyre, V., and Santer, R. M. 2000. Restricted diet rescues rat enteric motor neurons from age related cell death. *Gut* 47, 653–660.

65. Santer, R. M. and Baker, D. M. 1988. Enteric neuron numbers and sizes in Auerbach's plexus in the small and large intestine of adult and aged rats. *J. Auton. Nerv. Syst.* 25, 59–67.

66. Moore, J. G., Tweedy, C., Christian, P. E., and Datz, F. L. 1983. Effect of age on gastric emptying of liquid–solid meals in man. *Dig. Dis. Sci.* 28, 340–344.

67. Wegener, M., Borsch, G., Schaffstein, J., Luth, I., Rickels, R., and Ricken, D. 1988. Effect of ageing on the gastrointestinal transit of a lactulose-supplemented mixed solid-liquid meal in humans. *Digestion* 39, 40–46.

68. Fich, A., Camilleri, M., and Phillips, S. F. 1989. Effect of age on human gastric and small bowel motility. *J. Clin. Gastroenterol.* 11, 416–420.

69. Altman, D. F. 1990. Changes in gastrointestinal, pancreatic, biliary, and hepatic function with aging. *Gastroenterol. Clin. North Am.* 19, 227–234.

70. Madsen, J. L. 1992. Effects of gender, age, and body mass index on gastrointestinal transit times. *Dig. Dis. Sci.* 37, 1548–1553.

71. Bitar, K. N. and Patil, S. B. 2004. Aging and gastrointestinal smooth muscle. *Mech. Age. Dev.* 125, 907–910.

72. Hurwitz, A., Brady, D. A., Schaal, S. E., Samloff, I. M., Dedon, J. and Ruhl, C. E. 1997. Gastric acidity in older adults. *JAMA* 278, 659–662.

73. Pereira, S. P., Gainsborough, N., and Dowling, R. H. 1998. Drug-induced hypochlorhydria causes high duodenal bacterial counts in the elderly. *Aliment. Pharmacol. Ther.* 12, 99–104.

74. Haruma, K., Kamada, T., Kawaguchi, H., Okamoto, S., Yoshihara, M., Sumii, K., et al. 2000. Effect of age and *Helicobacter pylori* infection on gastric acid secretion. *J. Gastroenterol. Hepatol.* 15, 277–283.

75. Saltzman, J. R. and Russell, R. M. 1998. The aging gut. Nutritional issues. *Gastroenterol. Clin. North Am.* 27, 309–324.

76. McEvoy, A., Dutton, J., and James, O.F. 1983. Bacterial contamination of the small intestine is an important cause of occult malabsorption in the elderly. *Br. Med. J.* 287, 789–793.

77. Parlesak, A., Klein, B., Schecher, K., Bode, J. C., and Bod, C. 2003. Prevalence of small bowel bacterial overgrowth and its association with nutrition intake in non-hospitalized older adults. *J. Am. Geriatr. Soc.* 51, 768–773.

78. Gullo, L., Ventrucci, M., Naldoni, P., and Pezzilli, R. 1986. Aging and exocrine pancreatic function. *J. Am. Geriatr. Soc.* 34, 790–792.

79. Laugier, R., Bernard, J. P., Berthezene, P., and Dupuy, P. 1991. Changes in pancreatic exocrine secretion with age: Pancreatic exocrine secretion does decrease in the elderly. *Digestion* 50, 202–11.

80. Dreiling, D. A., Triebling, A. T., and Koller, M. 1985. The effect of age on human exocrine pancreatic secretion. *Mt. Sinai. J. Med.* 52, 336–339.

81. Popper, H. 1986. Aging and the liver. *Prog. Liver Dis.* 8, 659–683.

82. Schmucker, K. L. 1998. Aging and the liver: An update. *J. Gerontol. A. Biol. Sci. Med. Sci.* 53, B315–B320.

83. Zoli, M., Magalotti, D., Bianchi, G., Gueli, C., Orlandini, C., Grimaldi, M., and Marchesini, G. 1999. Total and functional hepatic blood flow decrease in parallel with ageing. *Age Ageing* 28, 29–33.

84. Cao, S. X., Dhahbi, J. M., Mote, P. L., and Spindler, S. R. 2001. Genomic profiling of short- and long-term caloric restriction effects in the liver of aging mice. *Proc. Natl. Acad. Sci. USA* 98, 10630–10635.

85. Lee, M. F., Russell, R. M., Montgomery, R. K., and Krasinski, S. D. 1997. Total intestinal lactase and sucrase activities are reduced in aged rats. *J. Nutr.* 127, 1382–1387.

86. Riepe, S. P., Goldstein, J., and Alpers, D. H. 1980. Effect of secreted bacteroides proteases on human intestinal brush border hydrolases. *J. Clin. Invest.* 66, 314–322.

87. Feibusch, J. M. and Holt, P. R. 1982. Impaired absorptive capacity for carbohydrate in the aging human. *Dig. Dis. Sci.* 27, 1095–1100.

88. Hosoda, S. 1992. The gastrointestinal tract and nutrition in the aging process: An overview. *Nutr. Rev.* 50, 372–373.

89. Vincenzini, M. T., Iantomasi, T., Stio, M., Favilli, F., Vanni, P., Tonelli, F., and Treves, C. 1989. Glucose transport during ageing by human intestinal brush-border membrane vesicles. *Mech. Ageing Dev.* 48, 33–41.

90. Wallis, J. L., Lipski, P. S., Mathers, J. C., James, O. F. W., and Hirst, B. H. 1993. Duodenal brush-border mucosal glucose transport and enzyme activities in aging man and effect of bacterial contamination of the small intestine. *Dig. Dis. Sci.* 38, 403–409.

91. Doubek, W. G. and Armbrecht, H. J. 1987. Changes in intestinal glucose transport over the lifespan of the rat. *Mech. Ageing Dev.* 39, 91–102.

92. Freeman, H. J., and Quamme, G. A. 1986. Age-related changes in sodium-dependent glucose transport in rat small intestine. *Am. J. Physiol.* 251, G208–G217.

93. Lindi, C., Marciani, P., Faelli, A., and Esposito, G. 1985. Intestinal sugar transport during ageing. *Biochim. Biophys. Acta.* 816, 411–414.

94. Darmenton, P., Raul, F., Doffoel, M., and Wessely, J. Y. 1989. Age influence on sucrose hydrolysis and on monosaccharide absorption along the small intestine of rat. *Mech. Ageing Dev.* 50, 49–55.

95. Ferraris, R. P., Hsiao, J., Hernandez, R., and Hirayama, B. 1993. Site density of mouse intestinal glucose transporters declines with age. *Am. J. Physiol.* 264, G285–G293.

96. Thompson, J. S., Crouse, D. A., Mann, S. L., Saxena, S. K., and Sharp, J. G. 1988. Intestinal glucose uptake is increased in aged mice. *Mech. Ageing Dev.* 46, 135–143.

97. Drozdowski, L., Woudstra, T., Wild, G., Clandinin, M. T., and Thomson, A. B. 2003a. The age-associated decline in the intestinal uptake of glucose is not accompanied by changes in the mRNA or protein abundance of SGLT1. *Mech. Ageing Dev.* 124, 1035–1045.

98. Drozdowski, L., Woudstra, T., Wild, G., Clandinin, M. T., and Thomson, A. B. 2003b. Feeding a polyunsaturated fatty acid diet prevents the age-associated decline in glucose uptake observed in rats fed a saturated diet. *Mech. Ageing Dev.* 124, 641–652.

99. Ferraris, R. P. and Vinnakota, R. R. 1993. Regulation of intestinal nutrient transport is impaired in aged mice. *J. Nutr.* 123, 502–511.

100. Ma, T. Y., Hollander, D., Dadufalza, V., and Krugliak, P. 1992. Effect of aging and caloric restriction on intestinal permeability. *Exp. Gerontol.* 27, 321–333.

101. Saltzman, J. R., Kowdley, K. V., Perrone, G., and Russell, R. M. 1995. Changes in small-intestine permeability with aging. *J. Am. Geriatr. Soc.* 43, 160–164.

102. Hollander, D. and Morgan, D. 1979. Aging: Its influence on vitamin A intestinal absorption in vivo by the rat. *Exp. Gerontol.* 4, 301.

103. Morris, H. A., Nordin, B. E. C., Fraser, V., Hartley, T. F., Need, A. G., and Horowitz, M. 1985. Calcium absorption and serum 1,25 dihydroxy vitamin D levels in normal and osteoporotic women. *Gastroenterology* A1508.

104. Ikuma, M., Hanai, H., Kaneko, E., Hayashi, H., and Hoshi, T. 1996. Effects of aging on the microclimate pH of the rat jejunum. *Biochim. Biophys. Acta.* 1280, 19–26.

105. Mann, J., and Murray, S. 2002. Lipids. In *Essentials of Human Nutrition,* 2nd ed. J. Mann and A. S. Truswell, Eds., Ch. 3. Oxford University Press, Oxford.

106. Duan, R. D. 2000. Enzymatic aspects of fat digestion in the gastrointestinal tract. In *Fat Digestion and Absorption.* A. B. Cristophe and S. De Vriese, Eds., pp. 25–46. AOCS Press, Champaign.

107. Schulthess, G., Werder, M., and Hauser, H. 2000. Receptor mediated lipid uptake at the small intestinal brush border membrane. In *Fat Digestion and Absorption.* A. B. Cristophe, and S. De Vriese, Ed., pp. 60–95. AOCS Press, Champaign.

108. Thomson, A. B. R., Clandinin, M.T., Drozdowski, L., Woudstra, T., and Wild, G. 2004. Barrier function in lipid absorption. In *Encyclopedia of Gastroenterology.* L. R. Johnson, Ed., pp. 158–166. Elsevier, San Diego.

109. Hamilton, J. A. 1998. Fatty acid transport: Difficult or easy? *J. Lipid Res.* 39, 467–481.

110. Kleinfeld, A. M., Chu, P., and Romero, C. 1997. Transport of long-chain native fatty acids across lipid bilayer membranes indicates that transbilayer flip-flop is rate limiting. *Biochemistry* 36, 14146–14158.

111. Hamilton, J. A. and Kamp, F. 1999. How are free fatty acids transported in membranes? Is it by proteins or by free diffusion through the lipids? *Diabetes* 48, 2255–2269.

112. Meddings, J. B. 1988. Lipid permeability of rat jejunum and ileum: Correlation with physical properties of the microvillus membrane. *Biochim. Biophys. Acta.* 943, 305–314.

113. Schwarz, S. M., Hostetler, B., Ling, S., Mone, M., and Watkins, J. B. 1985. Intestinal membrane lipid composition and fluidity during development in the rat. *Am. J. Physiol.* 248, G200–G207.

114. Hubner, C., Lindner, S. G., Stern, M., Claussen, M., and Kohlschutter, A. 1988. Membrane fluidity and lipid composition of rat small intestinal brush-border membranes during postnatal maturation. *Biochim. Biophys. Acta.* 939, 145–150.

115. Neu, J., Ozaki, C. K., and Angelides, K. J. 1986. Glucocorticoid-mediated alteration of fluidity of brush border membrane in rat small intestine. *Pediatr. Res.* 20, 79–82.

116. Henning, S. J., Rubin, R. C., and Shulman, R. J. 1994. Ontogeny of the intestinal mucosa. In *Physiology of the Gastrointestinal Tract.* L.R. Johnson, Ed., pp. 571–610. Raven Press, New York.

117. Dai, D., Nanthakumar, N. N., Savidge, T. C., Newburg, D. S., and Walker, W. A. 2002. Region-specific ontogeny of alpha-2,6-sialyltransferase during normal and cortisone-induced maturation in mouse intestine. *Am. J. Physiol. Gastro. Liver Physiol.* 282, G480–G490.

118. Fingerote, R. J., Doring, K. A., and Thomson, A. B. 1994. Gradient for D-glucose and linoleic acid uptake along the crypt–villus axis of rabbit jejunal brush border membrane vesicles. *Lipids* 29, 117–27.

119. Thomson, A. B. R. and Wild, G. 2001. The influences of the intestinal unstirred water layer on the understanding of the mechanism of lipids absorption. In *Intestinal Lipid Metabolism.* C. M. Mansbach II, P. Tso, and A. Kuksis, Eds., Ch. 8. Kluwer Academic/Plenum Publishers, New York.

120. Thomson, A. B. R., and Dietschy, J. M. 1981. Intestinal lipid absorption: Major extrcellular and intracellular events. In *Physiology of the Gastrointestinal Tract.* L.R. Johnson, Ed., pp. 1147–1220. Raven Press, New York.

121. Wilson, F. A. and Dietschy, J. M. 1972. Characterization of bile acid absorption across the unstirred water layer and brush border of the rat jejunum. *J. Clin. Invest.* 51, 3015–3025.

122. Proulx, P., Aubry, H. J., Brglez, I., and Williamson, D. G. 1984. Studies on the uptake of fatty acid by brush border membranes of the rabbit intestine. *Can. J. Biochem.* 63, 249–256.

123. Burdick, S., Keelan, M., and Thomson, A. B. 1993. Different mechanisms of uptake of stearic acid and cholesterol into rabbit jejunal brush border membrane vesicles. *Lipids* 28, 1063–1067.

124. Westergaard, H. and Dietschy, J. M. 1976. The mechanism whereby bile acid micelle increase rate of fatty acid and cholesterol into mucosal cell. *J. Clin. Invest.* 58, 97–108.

125. Schoeller, C., Keelan, M., Mulvey, G., Stremmel, W., and Thomson, A. B. 1995. Oleic acid uptake into rat and rabbit jejunal brush border membrane. *Biochim. Biophys. Acta.* 1236, 51–64.

126. Schoeller, C., Keelan, M., Mulvey, G., Stremmel, W., and Thomson, A. B. 1995. Role of a brush border membrane fatty acid binding protein in oleic acid uptake into rat and rabbit jejunal brush border membrane. *Clin. Invest. Med.* 18, 380–388.

127. Shiau, Y. F. 1990. Mechanism of intestinal fatty acid uptake in the rat: The role of an acidic microclimate. *J. Physiol.* 421, 463–474.

128. Shiau, Y. F., Kelemen, R. J., and Reed, M. A. 1990. Acidic mucin layer facilitates micelle dissociation and fatty acid diffusion. *Am. J. Physiol.* 259, G671–G675.

129. Small, D. M., Cabral, D. J., Cistola, D. P., Parks, J. S., and Hamilton, J. A. 1984. The ionization behavior of fatty acids and bile acids in micelles and membranes. *Hepatology* 4, S77–S79.

130. Clandinin, M. T., and Thomson, A. B. R. 2000. Intestinal absorption of lipids: A view toward the millennium. In *Fat Digestion and Absorption*. A. B. Cristophe and S. De Vriese, Eds., pp. 298–324. AOCS Press, Champaign, IL.

131. Devaux, P. F. 1991. Static and dynamic lipid asymmetry in cell membranes. *Biochemistry* 30, 1163–1173.

132. Hollander, D. and Morgan, D. 1980. Effect of plant sterols, fatty acids and lecithin on cholesterol absorption in vivo in the rat. *Lipids* 15, 395–400.

133. Smart, E. J., Graf, G. A., McNiven, M. A., Sessa, W. C., Engelman, J. A., Scherer, P. E., et al. 1999. Caveolins, liquid-ordered domains, and signal transduction. *Mol. Cell Biol.* 19, 7289–7304.

134. Anderson, R. G. 1998. The caveolae membrane system. *Annu. Rev. Biochem.* 67, 199–225.

135. Liu, P., Rudick, M., and Anderson, R. G. 2002. Multiple functions of caveolin-1. *J. Biol. Chem.* 277, 41295–41298.

136. Trigatti, B. L., Anderson, R. G., and Gerber, G. E. 1999. Identification of caveolin-1 as a fatty acid binding protein. *Biochem. Biophys. Res. Commun.* 255, 34–39.

137. Field, F. J., Born, E., Murthy, S., and Mathur, S. N. 1998. Caveolin is present in intestinal cells: Role in cholesterol trafficking. *J. Lipid Res.* 39, 1938–5190.

138. Uittenbogaard, A. and Smart, E. J. 2000. Palmitoylation of caveolin-1 is required for cholesterol binding, chaperone complex formation, and rapid transport of cholesterol to caveolae. *J. Biol. Chem.* 275, 25595–15599.

139. Okamoto, T., Schlegel, A., Scherer, P. E., and Lisanti, M. P. 1998. Caveolins, a family of scaffolding proteins for organizing preassembled signaling complexes at the plasma membrane. *J. Biol. Chem.* 273, 5419–5422.

140. Cai, S. F., Kirby, R. J., Howles, P. N., and Hui, D. Y. 2001. Differentiation-dependent expression and localization of the class B type I scavenger receptor in intestine. *J. Lipid Res.* 42, 902–909.

141. Stremmel, W., Lotz, G., Strohmeyer, G., and Berk, P. D. 1985. Identification, isolation, and partial characterization of a fatty acid binding protein from rat jejunal microvillous membranes. *J. Clin. Invest.* 75, 1068–1076.

142. Stremmel, W. 1988. Uptake of fatty acids by jejunal mucosal cells is mediated by a fatty acid binding membrane protein. *J. Clin. Invest.* 82, 2001–2010.

143. Besnard, P., and Niot, I. 2004. Role of lipid binding protein in intestinal absorption of long chain fatty acids. In *Fat Digestion and Absorption*. A. B. Cristophe and S. De Vriese, Eds., pp. 96–118. AOCS Press, Champaign, IL.

144. Abumrad, N. A., Park, J. H., and Park, C. R. 1984. Permeation of long-chain fatty acid into adipocytes. Kinetics, specificity, and evidence for involvement of a membrane protein. *J. Biol. Chem.* 259, 8945–8953.

145. Poirier, H., Degrace, P., Niot, I., Bernard, A., and Besnard, P. 1996. Localization and regulation of the putative membrane fatty-acid transporter FAT in the small intestine. Comparison with fatty acid-binding proteins FABP. *Eur. J. Biochem.* 238, 368–373.

146. Baillie, A. G., Coburn, C. T., and Abumrad, N. A. 1996. Reversible binding of long-chain fatty acids to purified FAT, the adipose CD36 homolog. *J. Membr. Biol.* 153, 75–81.

147. Van Nieuwenhoven, F. A., Luiken, J. J., De Jong, Y. F., Grimaldi, P. A., Van der Vusse, G. J., and Glatz, J. F. 1998. Stable transfection of fatty acid translocase CD36 in a rat heart muscle cell line H9c2. *J. Lipid Res.* 39, 2039–2047.

148. Poirier, H., Niot, I., Degrace, P., Monnot, M. C., Bernard, A., and Besnard, P. 1997. Fatty acid regulation of fatty acid-binding protein expression in the small intestine. *Am. J. Physiol.* 273, G289–G295.

149. Hirsch, D., Stahl, A., and Lodish, H. F. 1998. A family of fatty acid transporters conserved from mycobacterium to man. *Proc. Natl. Acad. Sci. USA* 95, 8625–8629.

150. Stahl, A., Hirsch, D. J., Gimeno, R. E., Punreddy, S., Ge, P., Watson, N., et al. 1999. Identification of the major intestinal fatty acid transport protein *Mol. Cell* 4, 299–308.

151. Gargiulo, C. E., Stuhlsatz-Krouper, S. M., and Schaffer, J. E. 1999. Localization of adipocyte long-chain fatty acyl-CoA synthetase at the plasma membrane, *J. Lipid Res.* 40, 881–892.

152. Kramer, W., Glombik, H., Petry, S., Heuer, H., Schafer, H., Wendler, W., et al. 2000. Identification of binding proteins for cholesterol absorption inhibitors as components of the intestinal cholesterol transporter. *FEBS Lett.* 487, 293–297.

153. Tessner, T. G. and Stenson, W. F. 2000. Overexpression of MDR1 in an intestinal cell line results in increased cholesterol uptake from micelles. *Biochem. Biophys. Res. Commun.* 267, 565–571.

154. Thurnhofer, H. and Hauser, H. 1990. Uptake of cholesterol by small intestinal brush border membrane is protein-mediated. *Biochemistry* 29, 2142–2148.

155. Compassi, S., Werder, M., Boffelli, D., Weber, F. E., Hauser, H., and Schulthess, G. 1995. Cholesteryl ester absorption by small intestinal brush border membrane is protein-mediated. *Biochemistry* 34, 16473–16482.

156. Jogchum, P. and Mensink, R. P. 2002. Increased intestinal ABCA1 expression contributes to the decrease in cholesterol absorption after plant stanol consumption. *FASEB J.* 16, 1248–1253.

157. Subbiah, M. T. R. 1973. Dietary plant sterols: Current status in human and animal sterol metabolism. *Am. J. Clin. Nutr.* 26, 219–225.

158. Vahouny, G. V., and Kritchesvky, D. 1981. Plant and marine sterols and cholesterol metabolism. In *Nutritional Pharmacology.* G. Spiller, Ed., pp. 32–72. Alan Liss, New York.

159. Ikeda, I., Tanaka, K., Sugano, M., Vahouny, G. V., and Gallo, L. L. 1988. Inhibition of cholesterol absorption in rats by plant sterols. *J. Lipid Res.* 29, 1573–1582.

160. Becker, G. H., Meyer, J., and Necheles, H. 1950. Fat absorption in young and old age. *Gastroenterology* 14, 80–90.

161. Ostlund, R. 2002. Cholesterol absorption. *Curr. Opin. Gastroenterol.* 18, 254–258.

162. Altmann, S. W., Davis Jr., H. R., Zhu, L. J., Yao, X., Hoos, L. M., Tetzloff, G., et al. 2004. Niemann-Pick C1 Like 1 protein is critical for intestinal cholesterol absorption. *Science* 303, 1201–1204.

163. Schmitz, G., Langmann, T., and Heimerl, S. 2001. Role of ABCG1 and other ABCG family members in lipid metabolism. *J. Lipid Res.* 42, 1513–1520.

164. Repa, J. J., Turley, S. D., Lobaccaro, J. M. A., Medina, J., Li, L., Lustig, K., Shan, B., et al. 2000. Regulation of absorption and ABC1-mediated efflux of cholesterol by RXR heterodimers. *Science* 289, 1524–1529.

165. Sudhop, T. and Von Bergmann, K. 2002. Cholesterol absorption inhibitors for the treatment of hypercholesterolaemia. *Drugs* 62, 2333–2347.

166. Santosa, S., Varady, K. A., AbuMweis S., and Jones, P. J. 2007. Physiological and therapeutic factors affecting cholesterol metabolism: Does a reciprocal relationship between cholesterol absorption and synthesis really exist? *Life Sci.* 80, 505–514.

167. Wang, D. Q. Regulation of intestinal cholesterol absorption. *Annu. Rev. Physiol.* 69, 221–248.

168. Iseki ,S. and Kondo, H. 1990. An immunocytochemical study on the occurrence of liver fatty-acid-binding protein in the digestive organs of rats: Specific localization in the D cells and brush cells. *Acta. Anatomica.* 138, 15–23.

169. Cistola, D. P., Sacchettini, J. C., Banaszak, L, J., Walsh, M. T., and Gordon, J. I. 1989. Fatty acid interactions with rat intestinal and liver fatty acid-binding proteins expressed in *Escherichia coli*. A comparative 13C NMR study. *J. Biol. Chem.* 264, 2700–2710.

170. Hsu, K. T. and Storch, J. 1996. Fatty acid transfer from liver and intestinal fatty acid-binding proteins to membranes occurs by different mechanisms. *J. Biol. Chem.* 271, 13317–13323.

171. Besnard, P., Niot, I., Poirier, H., Clement, L., and Bernard, A. 2002. New insights into the fatty acid-binding protein FABP family in the small intestine. *Mol. Cell Biochem.* 239, 139–147.

172. Agellon, L. B., Toth, M. J., and Thomson, A. B. 2002. Intracellular lipid binding proteins of the small intestine. *Mol. Cell Biochem.* 239, 79–82.

173. Vassileva, G., Huwyler, L., Poirier, K., Agellon, L. B., and Toth, M. J. 2000. The intestinal fatty acid protein is not essential for dietary fat absorption in mice. *FASEB J.* 14, 2040–2046.

174. Besnard, P., Bernard, A., and Carlier, H. 1991. Quantification of mRNA coding for enterocyte fatty acid binding proteins FABP in rats: Effect of high lipid diet and starvation. *C. R. Acad. Sci. III* 312, 407–413.

175. Motojima, K., Passilly, P., Peters, J. M., Gonzalez, F. J., and Latruffe, N. 1998. Expression of putative fatty acid transporter genes are regulated by peroxisome proliferators-activated receptor alpha and gamma activators in a tissue- and inducer-specific manner. *J. Biol. Chem.* 273, 16710–16714.

176. Motojima, K. 2000. Differential effects of PPAR alpha activators on induction of ectopic expression of tissue-specific fatty acid binding protein genes in the mouse liver. *Int. J. Biochem. Cell Biol.* 32, 1085–1092.

177. Besnard, P., Mallordy, A., and Carlier, H. 1993. Transcriptional induction of the fatty acid binding protein gene in mouse liver by bezafibrate. *FEBS Lett.* 327, 219–223.

178. Keller, H., Dreyer, C., Medin, J., Mahfoudi, A., Ozato, K., and Wahli, W. 1993. Fatty acids and retinoids control lipid metabolism through activation of peroxisome proliferators-activated receptor-retinoid X receptor heterodimers. *Proc. Natl. Acad. Sci. USA* 90, 2160–2164.

179. Murakami, K., Ide, T., Suzuki, M., Mochizuki, T., and Kadowaki, T. 1999. Evidence for direct binding of fatty acids and eicosanoids to human peroxisome proliferators-activated receptor alpha. *Biochem. Biophys. Res. Commun.* 260, 609–613.

180. Gong, Y. Z., Everett, E. T., Schwartz, D. A., Norris, J. S., and Wilson, F. A. 1994. Molecular cloning, tissue distribution, and expression of a 14-kDa bile acid-binding protein from rat ileal cytosol. *Proc. Natl. Acad. Sci. USA* 91, 4741–4745.

181. Kramer, W., Corsiero, D., Friedrich, M., Girbig, F., Stengelin, S., and Weyland, C. 1998. Intestinal absorption of bile acids: Paradoxical behaviour of the 14 kDa ileal lipid-binding protein in differential photoaffinity labeling. *Biochem. J.* 333, 335–341.

182. Kragelund, B. B., Knudsen, J., and Poulsen, F. M. 1999. Acyl-coenzyme A binding protein ACBP. *Biochim. Biophys. Acta.* 1441, 150–161.

183. Lin, M. C., Arbeeny, C., Bergquist, K., Kienzle, B., Gordon, D. A., and Wetterau, J. R. 1994. Cloning and regulation of hamster microsomal triglyceride transfer protein. The regulation is independent from that of other hepatic and intestinal proteins which participate in the transport of fatty acids and triglycerides. *J. Biol. Chem.* 269, 29138–29145.

184. White, D. A., Bennett, A. J., Billett, M. A., and Salter, A. M. 1998. The assembly of triacylglycerol-rich lipoproteins: An essential role for the microsomal triacylglycerol transfer protein. *Br. J. Nutr.* 80, 219–229.

185. Wetterau, J. R., Aggerbeck, L. P., Bouma, M. E., Eisenberg, C., Munck, A., Hermier, M., et al. 1992. Absence of microsomal triglyceride transfer protein in individuals with abetalipoproteinemia. *Science* 258, 999–1001.

186. Mansbach, C. M. and Dowell, R. 2000. Effect of increasing lipid loads on the ability of the endoplasmic reticulum to transport lipid to the Golgi. *J. Lipid Res.* 41, 605–612.

187. Holt, P. R. and Balint, J. A. 1993. Effects of aging on intestinal lipid absorption. *Am J. Physiol.* 264, G1–G6.

188. Peachey, S. E., Dawson, J. M., and Harper, E. J. 1999. The effect of ageing on nutrient digestibility by cats fed beef tallow-, sunflower oil- or olive oil-enriched diets. *Growth Dev. Aging* 63, 61–70.

189. Thomson, A. B. 1980. Effect of age on uptake of homologous series of saturated fatty acids into rabbit jejunum. *Am. J. Physiol.* 239, G363–G371.

190. Flores, C. A., Hing, S. A., Wells, M. A., and Koldovsky, O. 1989. Rates of triolein absorption in suckling and adult rats. *Am. J. Physiol.* 257, G823–G829.

191. Hollander, D. and Dadufalza, V. D. 1983. Increased intestinal absorption of oleic acid with aging in the rat. *Exp. Gerontol.* 18, 287–292.

192. Spector, A. A. and Yorek, M. A. 1985. Membrane lipid composition and cellular function. *J. Lipid Res.* 26, 1015–1035.

193. Brasitus, T. A. and Dudeja, P. K. 1985. Alterations in the physical state and composition of brush border membrane lipids of rat enterocytes during differentiation. *Arch. Biochem. Biophys.* 240, 483–488.

194. Wahnon, R., Mokady, S., and Cogan, U. 1989. Age and membrane fluidity. *Mech. Ageing Dev.* 50, 249–255.

195. Woudstra, T. D., Drozdowski, L. A., Wild, G. E., Clandinin, M. T., Agellon, L. B., and Thomson, A. B. 2004. An isocaloric PUFA diet enhances lipid uptake and weight gain in aging rats. *Lipids* 39, 343–354.

196. Holt, P. R. and Dominguez, A. A. 1981. Intestinal absorption of triglyceride and vitamin D3 in aged and young rats. *Dig. Dis. Sci.* 26, 1109–1115.

197. Raul, F., Gosse, F., Doffoel, M., Darmenton, P., and Wessely, J. Y. 1988. Age related increase of brush border enzyme activities along the small intestine. *Gut* 29, 1557–1563.

198. Higgins, C. F. 1994. Flip-flop. The transmembrane translocation of lipids. *Cell* 79, 393–395.

199. Keelan, M., Cheeseman, C. I., Clandinin, M. T., and Thomson, A. B. R. 1996. Intestinal morphology and transport following ileal resection is modified by dietary fatty acids. *Clin. Invest. Med.* 19, 63–70.

200. Dube, N., Delvin, E., Yotov, W., Garofalo, C., Bendayan, M., Veerkamp, J. H., and Levy, E. 2001. Modulation of intestinal and liver fatty acid-binding proteins in Caco-2 cells by lipids, hormones and cytokines. *J. Cell Biochem.* 81, 613–620.

201. Thiesen, A. 2002. Steroids, Dietary lipids, Resection and Intestinal adaptation. PhD thesis, University of Alberta.
202. Jenkins, A. P., and Thompson, R. P. 1994. Mechanisms of small intestinal adaptation. *Digest. Dis.* 12, 27.
203. Arora, S., Kassarjian, Z., Krasinski, S. D., Croffey, B., Kaplan, M. M., and Russell, R. M. 1989. Effect of age on tests of intestinal and hepatic function in healthy humans. *Gastroenterology* 96, 1560–1565.
204. Salesman, J. M., Nagengast, F. M., and Tangerman, A. 1993. Effect of ageing on postprandial conjugated and unconjugated serum bile acid levels in healthy subjects. *Eur. J. Clin. Invest.* 23, 192–198.
205. Holt, P. R. 2001. Diarrhea and malabsorption in the elderly. *Gastro. Clin. North Am.* 30, 427–444.
206. Thomson, A. B. R. and Wild, G. 1997. Adaptation of intestinal nutrient transport in health and disease. *Digest. Dis. Sci.* 42, 453–488.
207. Hebuterne, X., Broussard, J. F., and Rampal, P. 1995. Acute renutrition by cyclic enteral nutrition in elderly and younger patients. *JAMA* 273, 638–643.
208. Roberts, S. B., Fuss, P., Heyman, M. B., Evans, W. J., Tsay, R., Rasmussen, et al. 1994. Control of food intake in older men. *JAMA* 272, 1601–6.
209. Diamond, J. M. 1991. Evolutionary design of intestinal nutrient absorption: Enough but not too much. *NIPS* 6, 92–96.
210. Ferraris, R. P. and Diamond, J. 1989. Specific regulation of intestinal nutrient transporters by their dietary substrates. *Ann. Rev. Physiol.* 51, 125–141.
211. Diamond, J. and Karasov, W. H. 1984. Effect of dietary carbohydrate on monosaccaride uptake by mouse small intestine in vitro. *J. Physiol.* 349, 419–440.
212. Thomson, A. B. R., Keelan, M., Clandinin, M. T., and Walker, K. 1986. Dietary fat selectively alters transport properties of rat jejunum. *J. Clin. Invest.* 77, 279–288.
213. Thomson, A. B. R., Keelan, M., Clandinin, M. T., and Walker, K. 1987b. A high linoleic acid diet diminishes enhanced intestinal uptake of sugars in diabetic rats. *Am. J. Physiol.* 252, G262–G271.
214. Thomson, A. B., Keelan, M., Clandinin, M. T., Rajotte, R. V., Cheeseman, C., and Walker, K. 1988. Use of polyunsaturated fatty acid diet to treat the enhanced intestinal uptake of lipids in streptozotocin diabetic rats. *Clin. Invest. Med.* 11, 57–61.
215. Thomson, A. B., Keelan, M., and Clandinin, M. T. 1991. Feeding rats a diet enriched with saturated fatty acids prevents the inhibitory effects of acute and chronic ethanol exposure on the in vitro uptake of hexoses and lipids. *Biochim. Biophys. Acta.* 1084, 122–128.
216. Thiesen, A., Tappenden, K. A., McBurney, M. I., Clandinin, M. T., Keelan, M., Thomson, B. K. A., et al. 2003d. Dietary lipids alter the effect of steroids on the uptake of lipids following intestinal resection in rats. Part I. Phenotypic changes and expression of transporters. *J. Pediatr. Surg.* 38, 150–160.
217. Vine, D. F., Charman, S. A., Gibson, P. R., Sinclair, A. J., and Porter, C. J. 2002. Effect of dietary fatty acids on the intestinal permeability of marker drug compounds in excised rat jejunum. *J. Pharm. Pharmacol.* 54, 809–819.
218. Holt, P. R., Kotler, D. P., and Yeh, K. Y. 1989. Age related increase of brush border enzyme activities along the small intestine. *Gut* 30, 887–888.
219. Holt, P. R., Yeh, K. Y., and Kolter, D. P. 1988. Altered controls of proliferation in small intestine in senescent rats. *Proc. Nat. Acad. Sci. USA* 95, 2771–2775.
220. Dowling, R. H. and Booth, C. C. 1967. Structural and functional changes following small intestinal resection in the rat. *Clin. Sci.* 32, 139–149.
221. O'Connor, T. P., Lam, M. M., and Diamond, J. 1999. Magnitude of functional adaptation after intestinal resection. *Am. J. Physiol.* 276, R1265–R1275.
222. Clarke, R. M. 1972. The effect of growth and of fasting on the number of villi and crypts in the small intestine of the albino rat. *J. Anat.* 112, 27–33.
223. Ecknauer, R., Vadakel, T., and Wepler, R. 1982. Intestinal morphology and cell production rate in aging rats. *J. Gerontol.* 37, 151–155.
224. Keelan, M., Walker, K., and Thomson, A. B. 1985. Intestinal morphology, marker enzymes and lipid content of brush border membranes from rabbit jejunum and ileum: Effect of aging. *Mech. Ageing Dev.* 31, 49–68.
225. Corazza, G. R., Frazzoni, M., Gatto, M. R. and Gasbarrini, G. 1986. Ageing and small-bowel mucosa: A morphometric study. *Gerontology* 32, 60–65.
226. Hohn, P., Gabbert, H., and Wagner, R. 1978. Differentiation and aging of the rat intestinal mucosa. II. Morphological, enzyme histochemical and disc electrophoretic aspects of the aging of the small intestinal mucosa. *Mech. Ageing Dev.* 7, 217–226.

227. Lipski, P. S., Bennett, M. K., Kelly, P. J., and James, O. F. 1992. Ageing and duodenal morphometry. *J. Clin. Pathol.* 45, 450–452.
228. Webster, S. G., and Leeming, J. T. 1975. The appearance of the small bowel mucosa in old age. *Age Ageing* 4, 168–174.
229. Warren, P. M., Pepperman, M. A., and Montgomery, R. D. 1978. Age changes in small-intestinal mucosa. *Lancet* 2, 849–850.
230. Martin, K., Kirkwood, T. B., and Potten, C. S. 1998. Age changes in stem cells of murine small intestinal crypts. *Exp. Cell Res.* 241, 316–323.
231. Ciccocioppo, R., Di Sabatino, A., Luinetti, O., Rossi, M., Cifone, M. G., and Corazza, G. R. 2002. Small bowel enterocyte apoptosis and proliferation are increased in the elderly. *Gerontology* 48, 204–208.
232. Corazza, G. R., Ginaldi, L., Quaglione, G., Ponzielli, F., Vecchio, L., Biagi, F., and Quaglino, D. 1998. Proliferation cell nuclear antigen expression is increased in small bowel epithelium in the elderly. *Mech. Aging Dev.* 104, 1–9.
233. Holt, P. R., Atillasoy, E. O., Gilman, J., Guss, J., Moss, S. F., Newmark, H., et al. 1998. Modulation of abnormal colonic epithelial cell proliferation and differentiation by low-fat dairy foods: A randomized controlled trial. *JAMA* 280, 1074–1079.
234. Tsuchiya, T., Ishizuka, J., Shimoda, I., Rajaraman, S., Uchida, T., Townsend, C. M., and Thompson, J. C. 1995. Effect of Ileo-jejunal transposition on the growth of the GI tract and pancreas in young and aged rats. *J. Gerontol.* 50A, M155–M161.
235. Xiao, Z. Q. and Majumdar, A. P. 2000. Induction of transcriptional activity of AP-1 and NF-kappaB in the gastric mucosa during aging. *Am. J. Physiol. Gastro. Liver Physiol.* 278, G855–G865.
236. Papaconstantinou, J. 1994. Unifying model of the programmed intrinsic and stochastic extrinsic theories of aging. The stress response genes, signal transduction-redox pathways and aging. *Ann. N. Y. Acad. Sci.* 719, 195–211.
237. Blais, S., Boudreau, F., Thorneloe, K., and Asselin, C. 1996. Differential expression of fos and jun family members during murine postnatal intestinal development. *Biol. Neonate* 69, 342–349.
238. Holt, P. R. and DuBois Jr., R. N. 1991. In vivo immediate early gene expression induced in intestinal and colonic mucosa by feeding. *FEBS Lett.* 287, 102–104.
239. Tappenden, K. A., Thomson, A. B., Wild, G. E., and McBurney, M. I. 1997. Short-chain fatty acid-supplemented total parenteral nutrition enhances functional adaptation to intestinal resection in rats. *Gastroenterology* 112, 792–802.
240. Hardin, J. A., Chung, B., O'loughlin, E. V., and Gall, D. G. 1999. The effect of epidermal growth factor on brush border surface area and function in the distal remnant following resection in the rabbit. *Gut* 44, 26–32.
241. Hodin, R.A., Saldinger, P., and Meng, S. 1995. Small bowel adaptation: Counterregulatory effects of epidermal growth factor and somatostatin on the program of early gene expression. *Surgery* 118, 206–210; discussion 210–211.
242. Heby, O. and Persson, L. 1990. Molecular genetics of polyamine synthesis in eukaryotic cells. *Trends Biochem. Sci.* 15, 153–158.
243. Yoshinaga, K., Ishizuka, J., Evers, B. M., Townsend Jr., C. M., and Thompson, J. C. 1993. Age-related changes in polyamine biosynthesis after fasting and refeeding. *Exp. Gerontol.* 28, 565–572.
244. Yoshinaga, K., Ishizuka, J., Townsend Jr., C. M., and Thompson, J. C. 1993. Age related changes in duodenal adaptation after distal small bowel resection in rat. *Dig. Dis. Sci.* 38, 410–416.
245. Thullberg, M., Bartkova, J., Khan, S., Hansen, K., Ronnstrand, L., Lukas, J., et al. 2000. Distinct versus redundant properties among members of the INK4 family of cyclin-dependent kinase inhibitors. *FEBS Lett.* 470, 161–166.
246. Shin, C. E., Falcone Jr., R. A., Kemp, C. J., Erwin, C. R., Litvak, D. A., Evers, B. M., and Warner, B. W. 1999. Intestinal adaptation and enterocyte apoptosis following small bowel resection is p53 independent. *Am. J. Physiol.* 277, G717–G724.
247. Poirier, H., Niot, I., Monnot, M. C., Braissant, O., Meunier–Durmort, C., Costet, P., Pineau, T., et al. 2001. Differential involvement of peroxisome-proliferator-activated receptors alpha and delta in fibrate and fatty-acid-mediated inductions of the gene encoding liver fatty-acid-binding protein in the liver and the small intestine. *Biochem. J.* 355, 481–488.
248. Tollet-Egnell, P., Flores-Morales, A., Stahlberg, N., Malek, R. L., Lee, N., and Norstedt, G. 2001. Gene expression profile of the aging process in rat liver: Normalizing effects of growth hormone replacement. *Mol. Endocrinol.* 15, 308–318.

10 Caffeine and the Older Person

Hilary A. Wynne

CONTENTS

Caffeine is the world's most ubiquitously used drug, with 87% of the U.S. population consuming food and beverages containing caffeine. Average intake is 193 mg per day [1]. As age increases, so does caffeine consumption, with men and women aged 35 to 64 years being the highest consumers. Estimated daily caffeine consumption increases with age in Britain, and is associated with smoking and greater alcohol consumption [2]. In an Australian community sample, age was positively associated with tea consumption but negatively associated with coffee preference. Women consumed more cups per day than men, but showed a low preference for coffee [3]. For adults in the United States, the main source of caffeine is coffee (71%) with soft drinks, tea, and chocolate products accounting for the rest, whereas soft drinks are the main source for children and teenagers [1]. Although coffee is the main source of caffeine, assessment of coffee alone underestimates total caffeine intake and, thus, studies of caffeine as a risk factor for disease must consider total caffeine intake to estimate risk with any degree of accuracy [4]. Caffeine absorption and subjective effects are not influenced by drink type, although coffee blends differ substantially in their proportion of caffeine.

Older people can make a purposeful decision to reduce coffee and caffeine intake, with 4% of those surveyed in one study having stopped altogether, mostly due to health concerns and unpleasant side effects such as palpitations [5]. In addition, some users describe unsuccessful attempts to stop use [6], indicating that there can be an element of dependence upon the drug. A study of a U.S. population, mean age 64 years (range 30–105 years) who had cut down on caffeinated coffee intake, showed respondents had begun drinking caffeinated coffee around age 20 and decaffeinated coffee around age 50. More women than men had decided to curtail caffeinated coffee. Women were more likely than men to do so because of sleep problems, while more men did so because their spouses stopped drinking it. Most people had done so on their own initiative, 80% for health concerns, with only 10% doing so on advice from a physician [7].

10.1 PHARMACOKINETICS

Caffeine is a methylxanthine which, along with other xanthines, theobromine, and theophylline, is widely distributed in food. Caffeine is rapidly and almost totally absorbed from the gastrointestinal tract, with a peak concentration at around 30 to 60 minutes, depending on the presence or absence of food. The main route of caffeine clearance is by cytochrome P4501A2 dependent 3-demethylation followed by N-acetyl transferase type 2 dependent acetylation. Therapeutic estrogen inhibits CYP1A2-mediated caffeine metabolism in postmenopausal women by some 30% [8], and clearance is also lower in people with cirrhosis, with measurement of clearance through plasma, saliva, or even breath testing, providing a useful method for measuring liver function in chronic liver disease [9]. Caffeine clearance has been reported to be reduced by 35% in healthy elderly subjects in comparison with young subjects [10], and caffeine metabolism can be induced by cigarette smoking by over 100% [9]. Intra-individual variability in CYP1A2 activity has been estimated as around 17% in both young and elderly healthy subjects and inter-individual variability around 48% and 43% in young and elderly respectively, with variability over time not being influenced by age nor, in people over 80 years of age, by malnutrition as indicated by low body mass index (BMI), hypoalbuminaemia, or weight loss of greater than 10% over the previous 6 months [11]. CYP1A2 activity is around half as great in healthy people in their 70s as in those in their 20s, and in non-smokers compared with smokers [12,13].

10.2 AGE-RELATED PHARMACODYNAMIC CHANGES

Long-term benefits from caffeine ingestion have been suggested, as higher lifetime and higher current exposure to caffeine have been associated with better performance by older women on some measures of cognitive performance, especially by those aged 80 or more years [14]. Recent evidence from a sample of adults in the community aged at least 65 years indicated that caffeine seems to reduce cognitive decline in women who do not have dementia, especially in older women [15]. No effect on the incidence of dementia was seen, but the study suggested that drinking more than three cups of coffee per day may be useful for prolonging the period of mild cognitive impairment in women before a formal diagnosis of dementia is made. In contrast, however, while cross-sectional studies have suggested an association between a high habitual caffeine intake and better verbal memory performance and psychomotor speed, the 6-year longitudinal follow-up of 1376 individuals aged between 24 and 81 years participating in the Maastricht Aging Study did not demonstrate such an association, suggesting that habitual caffeine intake will not promote a substantial reduction in age-related cognitive decline at a population level [16].

Evidence suggests that elderly people are more sensitive to the objectively measured effects of caffeine upon performance, but report fewer subjectively felt effects. While 250 mg caffeine improved search task performance in young and elderly, the slower ability of elderly to identify relevant information and evaluate it were also counteracted [17]. In a study of the effect of age on the effects of caffeine on a variety of psychomotor, cognitive, and subjective tests in moderate caffeine drinkers, young subjects (20–25 years) generally performed better than older subjects (50–65 years) at baseline, and caffeine induced small but significant improvements in both groups in vigilance and psychomotor performance as well as in alertness. Older subjects performed better earlier in the day, whereas young subjects' performance did not decline to as great an extent [18]. In adults over the age of 65 years who considered themselves to have better memory during the morning, caffeine ingestion prevented the decline in tested memory performance from morning to afternoon, whereas those given decaffeinated coffee showed a significant decline in performance from morning to afternoon, indicating that time-of-day effects may be mediated by non-specific changes in level of arousal [19].

In a dose–response study of the effects of doses of caffeine within the range contained in a typical serving of tea or cola, 0 to 50 mg, as well as 100 mg following caffeine abstinence, all doses affected cognitive performance, mood and thirst, and dose–response relationships for these effects were rather flat. Effects on performance were more marked in those with a higher level of habitual caffeine intake but they showed tolerance to the thirst-increasing properties, which were noted only in low caffeine consumers [20]. In contrast, however, 100 mg caffeine did not affect short-term memory span or speed, long-term memory retrieval functions or focused attention of middle aged (45–60 years) or older (60–75 years) people, suggesting that cognitive effects noted can depend on tests used or are dose related and occur at higher doses than studied here [21]. There is one piece of evidence that caffeine increases psychomotor performance measures of attention at low plasma concentrations (around 4.5 mg/l) in healthy volunteers, but the effect is not increased higher at (around 9 mg/l) plasma concentrations, with caffeine having little subjective effect in this study [22].

Although one explanation of the beneficial effects of caffeine on mood and performance is that caffeine removes the negative effects of caffeine withdrawal, this has been challenged by evidence of little effect of caffeine withdrawal on performance, and improvement in performance by caffeine not influenced by regular caffeine consumption patterns [23]. Caffeine withdrawal, overnight or longer term, can cause dysphoric symptoms, following which acute intake of 70 or 250 mg caffeine has various outcomes, increasing jitteriness and decreasing tiredness and headache, with hand steadiness decreasing as dose increased, with 70 mg but not 250 mg improving reaction time [24].

10.3   INSOMNIA

Research into insomnia has historically been hampered by lack of a standard definition or guidelines for assessment. Insomnia can be defined as difficulty falling asleep, difficulty remaining asleep, early morning awakening or non-restorative sleep, with secondary insomnia as difficulty initiating or maintaining sleep that occurs as a consequence of another primary medical or psychiatric disorder [25], although this can be co-morbid rather than causal. Primary insomnia and insomnia related to mental disorders are the two most common insomnia diagnoses, although distinguishing between them can be difficult in clinical practice. Insomnia is associated with increased activation of the arousal systems in the brain, including the ascending reticular activating or limbic arousal systems, or decreased activity in the sleep promoting areas, including those located in the pons. These are very sensitive to exogenous (e.g., noise, caffeine) and endogenous (e.g., depression) factors. This is the result of changes intrinsic to ageing and external environmental influences. Arousal such as by walking prior to trying to sleep increases sleep latency compared with resting by watching television in both those with normal sleep and with insomnia, supporting the contention that measured sleep tendency is a combination of sleep drive and level of central nervous system arousal [26].

10.3.1   Age Related Changes in Sleep Patterns

Sleep assessment can be done directly with polysomnography (EEG and EMG) as the gold standard, or alternatively by direct observation, which is time consuming, is not able to measure sleep architecture or latency, but can be clinically helpful. Prospective diaries or retrospective recall are easier to perform but less accurate.

Sleep phases have distinct brain wave patterns recognizable from electroencephalography(EEG). Normally, sleep begins with non-rapid eye movement (REM) stages, converting to REM over a 90-minute cycle and alternating during sleep. Synchronization of sleep patterns to day-night rhythm relies on melatonin release and is associated with phasic activities in other biological systems of metabolism, temperature, and endocrine activity. Normal aging is associated with intrinsic changes such as altered endogenous rhythms that have implications for sleep pattern [27], which is also affected by changes in external environmental influences. Poor nights of the deepest (EEG slow wave) sleep are associated with increasing age [28]. Alertness and cognitive function deteriorate with sleep deprivation. A history of chronic insomnia does not predict poor EEG sleep, but is linked with more pathological personality profiles, worse mood ratings, less subjective sleepiness, poorer memory performances, and longer midafternoon sleep latencies. Those with poor EEG sleep do have longer actual and perceived sleep latencies and lower ratings of sleep quality, which therefore are increasingly common with age. While women are more likely to report a subjective sleep problem, poor EEG sleep is actually associated with being male [28]. In a study exploring sleep satisfaction among 130 older adults living in a community, 20 (15.4%) were not satisfied with sleep, with depression negatively associated with sleep satisfaction after controlling for age and number of illnesses [29]. Best descriptors of sleep satisfaction were the total amount of sleep, number of awakenings, depth of sleep, and overall quality of sleep.

In a study of sleep disorders in a general population in Los Angeles, 42.5% reported insomnia, 11.2% nightmares, 7.1% excessive sleep, 5.3% sleep talking and 2.5% sleep walking. These conditions were often chronic and usually started early in life. Insomnia was more frequent in older people, particularly older women, and in people with lower educational socioeconomic status [30].

10.3.2 Caffeine and Insomnia

Caffeine antagonizes adenosine receptors: blockade of A1 adenosine receptors may prevent wake-active neurones in the basal forebrain from being silenced and A2A blockade prevents the sleep-active neurones in the preoptic area from becoming active. Caffeine thus increases the time it takes to fall asleep and to obtain deep sleep. Total sleep time is reduced, and there is a relative increase in the proportion of light sleep as opposed to REM and deep sleep [31]. Studies using electroencephalographic sleep recordings and wrist actigraphic measures have suggested that the effects of caffeine appear in a dose-related manner [32].

Normal young adults given caffeine 400 mg three times a day for a week as a means of increasing metabolic rate and physiological activity developed many symptoms consistent with those reported by patients with primary insomnia (poor sleep, increased latency, increasing fatigue despite physiological activation and increased anxiety). However, their sleep after physiological arousal by 400 mg caffeine was as restorative as without [33]. In an experimental approach to evaluate the effects of 200 mg caffeine on sleep in young (20–30 years) and middle-aged (40–60 years) moderate caffeine consumers (one to three cups of coffee per day), evening ingestion of caffeine lengthened sleep latency, reduced sleep efficiency and decreased sleep duration and amount of stage 2 sleep with generally similar effects in both age groups and indicating that sleep remains sensitive to effects of caffeine despite moderate consumption habits [34].

In a small study of six people declaring themselves as "suffering from caffeine-induced wakefulness," the caffeine-sensitive group had a prolonged elimination half life of caffeine when compared with the control group [35], but as no tests for pharmacodynamic response to caffeine were carried out, a contribution from a difference in sensitivity cannot be excluded.

Women with insomnia report greater night-to-night variation in sleep variables of time to fall asleep, awakening during sleep, feeling rested after sleep and overall sleep quality than do women with good quality sleep. Combinations of alcohol, caffeine, exercise, smoking, and history of physical disease explain only 9 to 19% of variance in perceived or somnographic sleep variables [36]. Compared with the women with good sleep, those with insomnia reported drinking less caffeine per day, being more abstinent from alcohol, having smaller variations in day-to-day alcohol intake and bedtimes [37]. Although some women with insomnia had limited or no caffeine and alcohol intake, many had not optimized behaviors contributing to insomnia.

An association between caffeine-containing beverage consumption and persistent complaints of poor sleep has been reported in elderly people in the United Kingdom [38]. One study of 181 elderly community-based subjects and 53 elderly patients receiving hospital care found a significant negative correlation between age and coffee, but not tea consumption. Sleep quality was negatively associated with age. For the 87 community dwelling people, in whom late afternoon caffeine concentrations were measured, caffeine concentrations were negatively correlated with sleep quality score, such that levels were lower in those with poorer sleep quality. In the hospital population, median caffeine concentration was higher in patients reporting sleep problems than those without [39]. Self-reported consumption of tea or coffee did not correlate with plasma caffeine concentrations. The findings may be the result of insomniacs residing in the community recognizing the adverse effects of caffeine upon sleep and restricting intake, whereas institutionalized individuals, who have less control over their environment, do not. A study of the effect of caffeine-free beverages on sleep profiles of elderly patients receiving continuing care revealed that, although caffeine levels fell as a result of a change from caffeine-containing to caffeine-free beverages, no change in sleep pattern was noted overall in the 28 patients studied [40].

Although reduced caffeine intake should ameliorate any causal or aggravating effect on insomnia, a survey of a representative national sample of benzodiazepine users in the United States, median age 54 years, indicated that 88% reported caffeine consumption in the 24 hours surveyed, with 26% of benzodiazepine users and 23% of non-users consuming greater than 250 mg, suggesting that avoidance or limitation of caffeine use is neglected as a strategy for symptom amelioration by benzodiazepine users at least [41].

Caffeine restriction can be an effective strategy for relieving urgency, frequency, and incontinence of urine. Self reports of caffeine-related urinary symptoms feature prominently in adults with urgency and frequency [42] and caffeine restriction can be effective in reducing incontinence severity in women over 60 years [43], relieving a common interferer with sleep in older women. In contrast, however, while a decrease in fluid intake improved symptoms of stress incontinence or detrusor overactivity for older women, changing from caffeine-containing to decaffeinated drinks did not [44].

10.4 CAFFEINE AND CARDIOVASCULAR DISEASE

A high total homocysteine concentration is associated with increased risk of cardiovascular disease. Consumption of coffee raises total homocysteine concentrations in healthy volunteers, partly through intake of caffeine, and partly through coffee (but not caffeine) affecting homocysteine metabolism [45]. In the Framingham Offspring Cohort of 1960 men and women aged 28–82 years, fasting total homocysteine concentrations were positively associated with caffeine intake [46] as well as being influenced by folate, B12, B6, flavin, alcohol, smoking, and hypertension. Caffeine serum concentrations are positively related to triglycerides in those taking caffeine-containing drugs and related to high-density lipoprotein (HDL) cholesterol in female nonusers. An association has been found between caffeine concentrations and total cholesterol and low-density lipoprotein (LDL) cholesterol levels [47].

In several short-term studies, coffee consumption has been associated with impairment of endothelial function. However, in the Nurses' Health Study cohort, neither caffeinated nor decaffeinated coffee had a detrimental effect upon endothelial function in healthy women or women with type 2 diabetes, aged 43 to 70 years. Indeed, the results suggested that coffee consumption was inversely associated with markers of inflammation and endothelial dysfunction [48].

There is extensive evidence that caffeine at dietary doses increases blood pressure, catecholamine, and plasma renin activity in normotensive individuals [49]. Tolerance to the cardiovascular effects develops but is not complete, and it has been estimated that dietary caffeine at a population level influences systolic blood pressure by 2.4 mmHg and diastolic blood pressure by 1.2 mg, the effect being more pronounced in younger people [50]. Evidence does suggest that coffee drinking just before or after a meal could be useful clinically by attenuating postprandial hypotension [51]. Evidence suggests that habitual coffee intake does not influence blood pressure of people taking antihypertensive medication [52].

In a study of age-related differences in blood pressure, heart rate, behavior, mood state, and norepinephrine kinetics after caffeine ingestion, systolic and diastolic blood pressure increased in older healthy men (65–80 years) by 9% and 3% respectively, while remaining unchanged in younger (19–26 years) men. Heart rate in both groups was unaltered. Self-reported feelings of tension and anger decreased in older men, while anger tended to increase in young men, suggesting that older people are more reactive to the pressor and less sensitive to the subjective effects of the drug. They were not mediated by changes in norepinephrine kinetics [53].

There are age-related differences in thermic response to caffeine with energy expenditure increasing less in response to caffeine ingestion in older women (50–67 years) than in younger women (21–31 years). Furthermore, the thermic response to caffeine is positively associated with the body weight and waist circumference in younger women, whereas a positive association with aerobic fitness is observed in older women [54]. Caffeine (6 mg/kg) increased exercise endurance, as measured by cycling and isometric arm flexion in men and women aged 70 years and over by 25% and 54% respectively, but not muscle strength, walking speed, reaction, and movement times, and it reduced postural stability by 25% [55]. Caffeine (6mg/kg) significantly increased the concentration of plasma epinephrine (by 42%, 39%, and 49%), serum-free fatty acids (by 53%, 44%, and 50%), and plasma lactate (by 46%, 36%, and 48%), and insulin resistance (by 21%, 26%, and 23%) during rest, after 5 minutes of cycling, and at exhaustion. At exhaustion, the concentration of plasma norepinephrine was elevated by 29%. Hence, caffeine ingestion elicits a metabolic response in elderly participants at 70 years old similar to that seen in younger subjects [56].

Although there is also caffeine in tea, its flavonoid components have been associated with a decreased risk of cardiovascular disease, perhaps through inhibition of lipoprotein oxidation by their antioxidant polyphenolic compounds and by their vasodilator effects. Nevertheless, an acute pressor effect, larger and more acute than with caffeine alone, has been reported in response to tea ingestion in men although this did not translate into significant alterations in ambulatory blood pressure during regular tea consumption [57] and the acute increase in systolic pressure found with tea in the fasting state is negated by co-consumption of food [58].

10.4.1 Caffeine and Coronary Heart Disease

Due to its haemodynamic and humoral effects, which suggested a mechanism whereby caffeine intake might prove a risk factor for coronary heart disease, this link has been assessed in several studies. On one hand, an epidemiological study of an Italian population suggested that, while alcohol intake was inversely associated with acute myocardial infarction, smoking and heavy (>6 cups expresso or mocha per day), but not moderate, coffee drinking increased the risk [57]. However, analysis of prospective cohort data from 8.8-year follow-up of 6594 participants aged 32 to 86 years with no history of cardiovascular disease (CVD) at baseline, but 426 cardiovascular deaths in the First National Health and Nutrition Examination Survey Epidemiological Follow-up Study (NHEFS) in the United States, found that participants aged >65 years with higher caffeinated beverage intake actually exhibited lower relative risk of cardiovascular disease and heart disease mortality than did participants with lower caffeinated beverage intake. In addition, there was a dose–response protective effect. The protective effect was found only in participants who were not severely hypertensive, however. No significant protective effect was found in participants aged <65 years, or for cerebrovascular disease mortality for those aged >65 years [58]. A meta-analysis of 13 case-control and 10 cohort studies incorporating data from almost half a million people showed that, while there was a significant association between high consumption of coffee (>4 cups per day) and coronary heart disease (CHD) reported among case-control studies, no association was found between consumption of coffee and CHD in long-term (up to 44 years) follow-up cohort studies, a consistent result across region of origin, fatal and non-fatal events, year of publication, and number of years of follow-up [59].

10.5 CAFFEINE AND DIABETES MELLITUS

Coffee consumption has been associated with improved glucose tolerance and a lower risk of type 2 diabetes in diverse populations. A prospective study of 910 adults aged >50 years without diabetes mellitus at baseline in 1984–7, and followed to 1992–1996 showed that, after controlling for sex, age, physical activity, BMI, smoking, alcohol intake, hypertension, and baseline fasting plasma glucose, past and current coffee drinkers had a reduced risk of incident diabetes (odds ratio 0.38 (95% CI 0.17–0.87) and 0.36 (0.19–0.68) respectively) compared with those who never drank coffee. The 317 participants with baseline impaired glucose who were past or current coffee drinkers were also at reduced risk for incident diabetes (0.31 (0.11–0.87) and 0.36 (0.16–0.83), respectively) [60]. The Nurses' Health Study and Health Professionals' Follow up Study of over 126,000 people also reported an inverse association between coffee intake and type 2 diabetes after adjustment for age, BMI, and other risk factors [61]. The negative relationship between diabetes risk and consumption of ground coffee and regular tea, observed for all NHEFS subjects, on closer investigation applied only to those of 60 years or less who had previously lost weight [62]. A retrospective cohort study of 17,413 people with 5-year follow-up also established a negative association between consumption of green tea, coffee, and total caffeine, and risk of type 2 diabetes in a Japanese population [63].

While physical activity and weight management are confirmed as important strategies for the prevention of type 2 diabetes, research to establish which constituents of coffee improve glucose tolerance and to produce practical advice or interventions with beneficial health outcomes is required.

10.6 CAFFEINE AND OSTEOPOROSIS

Caffeine consumption has been proposed as a risk factor for bone loss in postmenopausal women, and its association with risk of osteoporosis, breast cancer, endometrosis, and fibrocystic breast disease is possibly mediated through an effect on endogenous sex steroids. In postmenopausal women caffeine intake is inversely associated with bioavailable testosterone, and high caffeine intake is positively associated with plasma estrone and sex hormone-binding globulin [64]. A cross-sectional North American survey of 136 Caucasian women, average age 68 years, established that caffeine (average 200–300 mg caffeine intake per day in this cohort) had a negative association with bone mineral density at multiple skeletal regions, which was attenuated with higher calcium intake of a median of 750 mg per day [65].

A 2-year longitudinal study of 138 postmenopausal women with little or no exposure to the confounders of tobacco, alcohol, or drugs, which are known to affect bone status, indicated no association between dietary caffeine intake and total body or femoral neck bone density or bone mass, and no association between caffeine consumption and longitudinal changes in total body or femoral neck bone measurements, with or without adjustment for calcium intake [66]. However, cross-sectional measurements of bone mineral density in 489 elderly women (aged 65–77 years), and longitudinal measurements made in 96 of these women who were treated with a placebo for 3 years, indicated that women with high caffeine intakes had significantly higher rates of bone loss at the spine than did those with low intakes (–1.90 +/– 0.97% compared with 1.19 +/–1.08%; P = 0.038). When the data were analyzed according to vitamin D receptor (VDR) genotype and caffeine intake, women with the tt genotype had significantly higher rates of bone loss at the spine than did women with the TT genotype when their caffeine intake was >300 mg/d (approximately 514 g, or 18 oz, brewed coffee) [67].

Although establishing the extent of any relationship between caffeine and osteoporosis, which is a risk factor for low-trauma fractures, is important, establishment of the extent of any association between caffeine and fractures in postmenopausal women offers clinically more relevant information. In a cross-sectional survey of 34,703 postmenopausal Iowan women aged 55–69 years who reported alcoholic and caffeinated beverage intake and then were followed for 6.5 years for fracture occurrence, the adjusted relative risk for highest versus lowest caffeine intake quintiles was 1.09 (95% CI 0.99–1.21) for combined fracture sites. Wrist fractures were associated positively (relative risk (RR) for extreme quintiles 1.37, 95% CI 1.11–1.69) and upper arm fractures were negatively (RR 0.67 95% CI 0.48–0.94) associated with caffeine intake [68]. A cohort study of 31,527 Swedish women aged 40–76 years at baseline did establish a link between caffeine intake and fracture risk [69]. During a mean follow-up of 10.3 years, there were 3279 cases with osteoporotic fractures. The highest (>330 mg/d) compared with the lowest (<200 mg/d) quintile of caffeine intake was associated with a modestly increased risk of fracture: RR 1.2 (95% CI: 1.07–1.35). A high coffee consumption significantly increased the risk of fracture, whereas tea drinking was not associated with risk. The increased risk of fracture with both a high caffeine intake and coffee consumption was confined to women with a low calcium intake (<700 mg/d): RR 1.33 (95% CI: 1.07–1.65) with > four cups (600 ml/d) of coffee compared with fewer than one cup (150 ml/d). The same comparison estimated for women with a high propensity for fractures (more than two fracture types) revealed a RR of 1.88 (95% CI: 1.17–3.00). Thus, a daily intake of 330 mg of caffeine, equivalent to four cups (600 ml) of coffee, or more, may be associated with modestly increased risk of osteoporotic fractures, especially in women with a low intake of calcium.

If they know they have a low bone mass, postmenopausal women can be influenced to alter health behavior, while those with severe or moderate low bone mass, established by bone densitometry, are more likely to decrease caffeine intake than those with normal measurements [70].

10.7 NEUROLOGY

10.7.1 HEADACHE

People with chronic daily headache, in comparison with episodic headache controls, are more likely to have been high caffeine consumers before onset of chronic daily headache (OR 1.50, P0.05). No association was found for current caffeine consumption and, when analyzed for age, the association was confined to women under 40 years [71].

10.7.2 PARKINSON'S DISEASE

A possible protective effect of moderate doses of caffeine upon risk of Parkinson's disease was suggested by the Health Professionals' Follow up Study and the Nurses' Health Study where, in some 136,000 people followed up for at least 10 years, the relative risk of Parkinson's disease was lowest at moderate intake (1–3 cups coffee/day) in women and lowest at higher intake in men [72]. A 30-year follow-up of 804 Japanese-American men aged 45–68 years showed that increasing coffee and caffeine consumption was associated with lower risk of Parkinson's disease, independent of smoking [73], results consistent with those of a case-control study with prospective follow-up of residents of a retirement community in southern California [74]. The protective effect of coffee and tea intake and smoking has also been reported in an ethnic Chinese population [75]. In contrast, in a case-control study in Washington State, while smoking, either past or present, was associated with a reduced risk of Parkinson's disease, no associations were detected for caffeine intake, coffee or alcohol consumption, although reduced risks were observed for consumption of two cups/day or more of tea or cola drinks [76].

The mechanism of the hypothetical protective effect of cigarette smoking and caffeine consumption on Parkinson's disease has not been established. The possibility that it is explained in part by a neurological link with low sensation seeking, a personality trait believed to characterize Parkinson's disease, has been suggested in one case-control study [77].

10.8 CANCER

Since incidence of cancer at most sites increases with age, most data assessing the relationship between coffee consumption and cancer risk refers to the adult and elderly population. Several case-control studies have been published that have compared risk of various cancers in coffee drinkers and nondrinkers although, even when an association has been demonstrated, a causal rather than a nonspecific link is difficult to establish. Conclusions about the separate role of coffee are, in addition, difficult to make, as cigarette smoking and alcohol intake are commonly taken alongside. Information contained in the major review of data by the International Agency for Research of Cancer (IARC) in 1990 remains relevant [78].

10.8.1 CANCER OF THE STOMACH, OESOPHAGUS, PHARYNX, AND MOUTH

A recent review of the literature and meta-analysis of published cohort and case-control studies has concluded that there is no association between coffee consumption and gastric cancer risk [79]. Most studies have failed to establish a link between coffee consumption and oral cavity, pharynx, and oesophagus cancer [78], although a trend to increased risk with increasing temperature of the drink has been suggested [80].

10.8.2 CANCER OF THE PANCREAS

Although some case-control studies did suggest a positive association between coffee consumption and pancreatic cancer and engendered active research into this area, later work found no association [81]. A large prospective cohort study of nearly 2 million person-years of follow-up showed that neither coffee nor alcohol intake increased risk of pancreatic cancer nor did tea, decaffeinated coffee, or total caffeine intake [82]. While there is no strong association between coffee intake and risk of pancreatic cancer, the study of Porta et al. [83] established that mutations in the K-ras gene in exocrine pancreatic cancer were more common among regular coffee drinkers than among nonregular coffee drinkers, and that the coffee intake was higher among patients with a mutated tumor than a wild-type tumor. Pancreatic cancer cases without activating mutations in the K-ras gene drank significantly less coffee than cases with a mutation, with a dose–response relation indicating that caffeine, or coffee, may modulate K-ras activation [83]. Thus, it is possible that coffee may have a different impact on the etiology of distinct types of clinically similar pancreatic cancer. Although there may be a minor increased risk of pancreatic cancer among drinkers of large amounts of coffee, this increase is small and of limited practical importance.

10.8.3 HEPATOCELLULAR CANCER

The publication of results from four large Japanese cohort studies in which coffee was reported to have a preventive role has been supported by a meta-analysis of epidemiologic studies that indicated that an increase of two cups of coffee per day in consumption was associated with a 45% reduced risk of liver cancer (RR 0.57; 95% CI 0.49–0.67) [84].

10.8.4 CANCER OF THE COLON AND RECTUM

Evidence suggests an inverse association between coffee intake and colorectal cancer, perhaps through reduction in bile acids and neutral sterol secretion in the colon. There are over 1000 constituents of coffee, several of which are chemoprotective through induction of glutathione-S-transferase and inhibition of N-acetyl transferase, reducing mutagenesis. There is an inverse association between folate intake and risk of colorectal, but not rectal, cancer that is not modified by caffeine intake [85].

Frequent coffee consumption has been associated with a reduced risk of colorectal cancer in a number of case-control studies. A meta-analysis combining the results of 12 such case-control studies suggested a relative risk of 0.72 (95% CI 0.61–0.84) for high versus low coffee consumption [86]. Analysis of cohort studies did not reveal such an association (RR 0.97), but it included a relatively small number of cases. Using data from the Nurses' Health Study for women and the Health Professionals' Follow Up Study for men of almost 2 million person-years of follow-up, 1438 cases of colorectal cancer were observed. Caffeinated coffee, tea with caffeine, or caffeine intake were not associated with colon or rectal cancer risk. Regular consumers of two or more cups of decaffeinated coffee had a 52% (95% CI 19–71) lower incidence of rectal cancer than nonconsumers, although the mechanism of this link, which could have a number of biological or social explanations, is not known [87].

Lifestyle and dietary patterns differ markedly among populations and influence the relationship between caffeine and cancer risk. A Japanese study involving almost half a million person-years of follow-up, in which 457 cases of colorectal cancer were identified, established no association between self-reported coffee consumption at baseline and incidence of either proximal or distal colon cancer [88]. Similarly, a prospective analysis of coffee consumption and colorectal cancer in two Swedish population-based cohort studies of 61,433 women and 45,306 men, in whom there were 1279 incidence cases of colorectal cancer, found no association between these two factors [89].

10.8.5 BREAST CANCER

Several cohort and case-control studies, including a large Swedish cohort study of 59036 women and over half a million years of follow-up [90], and a large case-control study of an Italian population of nearly 6000 women with breast cancer [91], indicate that consumption of coffee, tea, and caffeine is not associated with breast cancer risk. A North American case-control study of 1932 women with breast cancer noted a 40% risk reduction in consumers of more than four cups of coffee per day in premenopausal women, with no association between breast cancer risk overall and intake of black tea or decaffeinated coffee, but breast cancer risk among postmenopausal women was not associated with coffee or tea consumption [92]. Further studies are required to assess the consistency of these findings. Caffeine consumption, as evidenced from an international case-control analysis, suggested that, among women with the germline mutations in the breast cancer susceptibility genes BRCA1 and BRCA2, coffee consumption is unlikely to be harmful and that there was a trend to reduced breast cancer risk with higher levels of consumption [93].

10.8.6 CANCER OF THE OVARY OR ENDOMETRIUM

Caffeine has been proposed to have a modulating effect on circulating estrogen levels, thereby influencing the development of hormone-related cancers. Coffee and caffeine consumption have been associated with higher ovarian cancer risk in several case-control studies [78].

Non-significant reduced epithelial ovarian cancer (EOC) risk has been noted among coffee users reporting drinking more than six cups daily compared with nonusers (OR 0.68, 95% CI 0.42–1.10) [94]. In an Australian population-based case-control study, increasing coffee consumption was associated with a decreased risk of EOC (p trend = 0.0009) with an OR of 0.51 (95% CI 0.32–0.80) for consumption of more than four cups of coffee per day compared with nondrinkers [95]. The association was significant only for serous and endometrioid/clear cell histological subtypes. Tea consumption, which contributed to caffeine intake, was not related to EOC, indicating that the association with coffee may not be due to caffeine but to other components within it.

As tea consumption was not related to EOC, in spite of its significant contribution to caffeine intake in this population, the authors concluded that the association observed with coffee is not due to caffeine, but to other components within coffee. In contrast, a North American case-control study suggested that black tea or decaffeinated coffee consumption was associated with a linear decline in ovarian cancer risk, with individuals consuming two or more cups daily experiencing a 30% decline in risk. However, no association was noted between any level of regular coffee consumption and risk of ovarian cancer. The chemoprotective effects of phytochemicals in black tea and decaffeinated coffee may be important, although the effects of phytochemicals in regular coffee may be counteracted by the elevated risk associated with its higher caffeine content [96].

Results have been inconsistent and inconclusive, as other case-control studies indicate that coffee intake is not associated with ovarian cancer risk [97]. In an attempt to explain such inconsistent findings, a North American case-control study sought to determine whether there was any association between coffee intake and histological subtype of ovarian cancer or menopausal status at diagnosis and suggested that caffeine was associated with increase in risk only among premenopausal women [98]. CYP1A2 is a key enzyme in the metabolism of coffee and in the activation of heterocyclic aromatic compounds that may be carcinogenic. The AA genotype is highly inducible, whereas the enzyme associated with the C allele is less so. One study reported no difference in risk of cancer between the CYP1A2 genotypes [99]. An interaction between CYP1A1 polymorphic variants and ovarian cancer risk has been reported in a North American case-control study, with elevated risk found in those carrying the Ile/Val variant and who consumed more than median levels of caffeine (risk ratio 2.69, 95% CI 1.18–6.18). No variation by histological type of ovarian cancer was observed [100]. The interactions between polymorphic variants such as described above could explain the weak or inconsistent associations between caffeine and ovarian cancer when genotype has not been considered.

No association with coffee intake has been found in a cohort [101] and case-control study of endometrial cancer [102]. A case-control study of 2122 breast, 220 endometrial and 166 ovarian cancer cases and 12,425 noncancer controls established a statistically significant inverse association between risk of endometrial cancer and coffee consumption, with no clear association evident for breast and ovarian cancer risk. However, there was no statistically significant association between caffeine intake and endometrial cancer [103].

10.8.7 CANCER OF THE PROSTATE

Cohort [104] and case-control studies [105–107] have established no evidence of a link between drinking coffee and prostate cancer and, although a decreased risk was observed with tea intake (OR 0.70) in one study [107], these results were not supported by results of others [105,106].

10.8.8 BLADDER CANCER

Considering the results from the published studies overall, one can conclude that coffee drinking is a weak risk factor for bladder cancer, although whether the link is nonspecific or causal, and the relative contribution of caffeine and the other chemicals in coffee, has not been established. A systematic review has suggested that coffee consumption versus nondrinking increases risk of urinary tract cancer by approximately 20%, with tea consumption having no effect [108]. When data from six case-control studies including 2729 cases and 5150 controls were pooled, increased bladder cancer risk was observed for intake of more than five cups of coffee per day and for tritialomethane exposure through water pollution, and an increased risk was noted with tap water intake, OR 1.46 (95% CI 1.20-1.78) for > 2 litre per day versus < 0.5 litre per day, but not with nontap water fluids, suggesting that carcinogenic chemicals in tap water may contribute to the increased risk [109].

10.8.9 LUNG CANCER

There is no consistent evidence of an effect of coffee intake upon lung cancer risk, although a Czech case-control study suggested an inverse association between coffee drinking and lung cancer risk [110]. An elevated risk was noted with increased caffeinated coffee intake, whereas decaffeinated coffee drinking was associated with decreased risk. No influence of tea consumption upon risk was shown, suggesting that any chemoprotective effects of phytochemicals in coffee and tea may be overshadowed by the elevated risk associated with caffeine in these beverages [111].

10.8.10 THYROID CANCER

A pooled analysis of 14 case-control studies conducted in the United States, Europe, and Asia, consisting of 2725 thyroid cancer cases and 4776 controls has concluded that thyroid cancer risk is not associated with consumption of coffee or tea [112].

10.9 SUMMARY

Overall, coffee drinking can be considered a risk indicator of bladder cancer and possibly for pancreatic cancer and inversely associated with colorectal cancer. Data for other cancer sites are limited and generally inconsistent, but, reassuringly, no strong associations have been confirmed.

Caffeine intake is almost ubiquitous. It has beneficial effects in terms of alertness and concentration, which is welcomed at times, and attenuates postprandial hypotension, of clinical benefit to some. The alertness it produces does contribute to insomnia and, as the metabolism of caffeine becomes slower with aging, avoidance several hours before bedtime may be required by some people to avoid this. While it has no association with most common cancers, a modest positive association with pancreatic cancer and bladder cancer and an inverse association with colon cancer risk is plausible, although associations may be due to residual confounding factors. Balancing the above and recognizing the importance of its social aspects to older people, the population in general can be reassured that, overall, caffeine intake can be considered beneficial, with specific advice to avoid or reduce being tailored to those with contraindications.

REFERENCES

1. Frary CD, Johnson RK, Wang MQ. 2005. Food sources and intakes of caffeine in the diets of persons in the United States. *Journal of the American Dietetic Association.* 105: 110–3.
2. Hewlett P, Smith P. 2006. Correlates of daily coffee consumption. *Appetite.* 46: 97–9.
3. Luciano M, Kirk KM, Heath AC, Martin NG. 2005. The genetics of tea and coffee drinking and preference for source of caffeine in a large community sample of Australian twins. *Addiction.* 100: 1510–7.
4. Brown J, Kreiger N, Darlington GA, Sloan M. 2001. Misclassification of exposure: Coffee as a surrogate for caffeine intake. *American Journal of Epidemiology.* 153: 815–20.
5. Hughes JR, Oliveto AH. 1997. A systematic study of caffeine intake in Vermont. *Experimental and Clinical Psychopharmacology.* 5: 393–8.
6. Hughes JR, Oliveto AH, Ligouri A, Carpenter J, Howard T. 1998. Endorsement of DSM-IV dependence criteria among caffeine users. *Drug and Alcohol Dependence.* 52: 98–107.
7. Soroko S, Chang J, Barrett-Connor E. 1996. Reasons for changing caffeinated coffee consumption: The Rancho Bernardo Study. *Journal of the American College of Nutrition.* 15: 97–101.
8. Pollock BG, Wylie M, Stack JA, Sorisio DA, Thompson DS, Kirshner MA, et al. 1999. Inhibition of caffeine metabolism by estrogen replacement therapy in post menopausal women. *Journal of Clinical Pharmacology.* 39: 936–40.
9. Park GJ, Katelaris PH, Jones DB, Seow F, Le Couteur DG, Ngu MC. 2003. Validity of the 13C-caffeine breath as a noninvasive, quantitative test of liver function. *Hepatology.* 38: 1227–36.
10. Schnegg M, Lauterburg BH. 1986. Quantitative liver function in the elderly assessed by galactose elimination capacity, aminopyrine demethylation and caffeine clearance. *Journal of Hepatology.* 3: 164–171.
11. Hamon-Vilcot B, Simon T, Becquemont L, Poirier JM, Piette F, Jaillon P. 2004. Effects of malnutrition on cytochrome P450 1A2 activity in elderly patients. *Therapie.* 59: 247–51.
12. Simon T, Bequemont L, Hamon B, Nouyrigat E, Chodjania Y, Poirier JM, et al. 2001. Variability of cytochrome P450 1A2 activity over time in young and elderly healthy volunteers. *British Journal of Clinical Pharmacology.* 52: 601–4.

13. Chung WG, Kang JH, Park CS, Cho MH, Cha YN. 2000. Effect of age and smoking on in vivo CYP1A2 flavin-containing mono-oxygenase, and xanthine oxidase activities in Koreans: Determination by caffeine metabolism. *Clinical Pharmacology and Therapeutics.* 67: 258–66.

14. Johnson-Kozlow M, Kvitz-Silverstein D, Barrett-Connor E, Morton D. 2002. Caffeine consumption and cognitive function among older adults. *American Journal of Epidemiology.* 156: 842–50.

15. Ritchie K, Carriere I, deMendonca A, Portet F, Dartigues JF, Rouaud O, et al. 2007. The neuroprotective effects of caffeine: A prospective population study (the Three City Study). *Neurology.* 69: 536–45.

16. van Boxtel MP, Schmitt JA, Bosma H, Jolles J. 2003. The effects of habitual caffeine use on cognitive change: A longitudinal perspective. *Pharmacology, Biochemistry and Behaviour.* 75: 921–7.

17. Lorist MM, Snel J, Mulder G, Kok A. 1995. Aging, caffeine and information processing: An event-related potential analysis. *Electroencephalography and Clinical Neurophysiology.* 96: 453–67.

18. Rees K, Allen D, Lader M. 1999. The influence of age and caffeine on psychomotor and cognitive function. *Psychopharmacology.* 145: 181–8.

19. Ryan L, Hatfield C, Hofstetter M. 2002. Caffeine reduces time-of-day effects on memory performance in older adults. *Psychological Science.* 13: 68–71.

20. Smit HJ, Rogers PJ. 2004. Effects of low doses of caffeine on cognitive performance, mood and thirst in low and moderate caffeine consumers. *Psychopharmacology.* 152: 167–73.

21. Schmitt JAJ, Hogenvorst E, Vuurman EFPM, Jolles J, Riedel WJ. 2003. Memory functions and focussed attention in middle-aged and elderly subjects are unaffected by a low, acute dose of caffeine. *Journal of Nutrition, Health and Aging.* 7: 301–3.

22. Bryant CA, Farmer A, Tiplady B, Keating J, Sherwood R, Swift CG, Jackson SH. 1998. Psychomotor performance: Investigating the dose–response relationships for caffeine and theophylline in elderly volunteers. *European Journal of Clinical Pharmacology.* 54: 309–13.

23. Hewlett P, Smith A. 2006. Acute effects of caffeine in volunteers with different patterns of regular consumption. *Human Psychopharmacology.* 21: 167–80.

24. Richardson NJ, Rogers PJ, Elliman NA, Russell J, O'Dell. Mood and performance effects of caffeine in relation to acute and chronic caffeine deprivation. *Pharmacology, Biochemistry and Behaviour* 1995. 52: 313–20.

25. Edinger JD, Bonnet MH, Bootzin RR, Dorsey CM, Espie CA, et al. 2004. Deviation of research diagnostic criteria for insomnia: Report of an American Academy of Sleep Medicine Work Group. *Sleep.* 27: 1567–96.

26. Bonnet MH, Arand DL. 2000. Activity, arousal, and the MSLT in patients with insomnia. *Sleep.* 23. 205–12.

27. Sack RL. Human melatonin production decreases with age. 1986. *Journal of Pineal Research.* 3: 379–88.

28. Rosa RR, Bonnet MH. 2000. Reported chronic insomnia is independent of poor sleep as measured by electroencephalography. *Psychosomatic Medicine.* 62: 474–82.

29. Ouellet N, Morris DL. 2006. Sleep satisfaction of older adults living in the community: Identifying associated behavioural and health factors. *Journal of Gerontological Nursing.* 32: 5–11.

30. Bixler EO, Kales A, Sladatos CR, Kales JD, Healey S. 1979. Prevalence of sleep disorders in the Los Angeles Metropolitan area. *American Journal of Psychiatry.* 136: 1257–62.

31. Karacans I, Thornby JI, Anch M, Booth GH, Williams RL, Salis PJ. 1976. Dose related sleep disturbances induced by coffee and caffeine. *Clinical Pharmacological Therapy.* 20: 682–9.

32. Hindmarch I, Rigney U, Stanby N, Quinlan P, Rycroft J, Lane JA. 2000. A naturalistic investigation of the effects of day-long consumption of tea, coffee and water on alertness, sleep onset and sleep quality. *Psychopharmacology* (Berl). 149: 203–16.

33. Bonnet MH, Arand DL. 2003. Insomnia, metabolic rate and sleep restoration. *Journal of Internal Medicine.* 254: 23–31.

34. Drapeau C, Hamel-Hebert I, Robillard R, Selmaoui B, Filipini D, Carrier J. 2006. Challenging sleep in aging: The effects of 200 mg of caffeine during the evening in young and middle-aged moderate caffeine consumers. *Journal of Sleep Research.* 15: 133–41.

35. Levy M, Zylber-Katz E. 1983. Caffeine metabolism and coffee attributed sleep disturbances. *Clinical Pharmacology Therapy.* 33: 770–5.

36. Cheek RE, Shaver JL, Lentz MJ. 2004. Lifestyle practices and nocturnal sleep in midlife women with and without insomnia. *Biological Research for Nursing.* 6: 46–58.

37. Cheek RE, Shaver JL, Lentz MJ. 2004. Variations in sleep hygiene practices of women with and without insomnia. *Research in Nursing and Health.* 27: 225–36.

38. Morgan K, Healey DW, Healey DJ. 1989. Factors influencing persistent subjective insomnia in old age: A follow-up study of good and poor sleepers aged 65–74. *Age Ageing*. 18: 117–22.

39. Curless R, French JM, James OFW, Wynne HA. 1993. Is caffeine a factor in subjective insomnia of elderly people? *Age Ageing*. 22: 41–5.

40. Stephens CM, Hankey C, Wynne HA. 1995. Effect of caffeine-free beverages on elderly hospitalised patients. *International Journal of Pharmacological Practice*. 3: 245–8.

41. Cooper M, Safran M, Eberhardt M. 2004. Caffeine consumption among adults on benzodiazepine therapy: United States 1988–1994. *Psychological Reports*. 95: 183–91.

42. Bryant CM, Dowell CJ, Fairbrother G. 2002. Caffeine reduction education to improve urinary symptoms. *British Journal of Nursing*. 11: 560–5.

43. Weinberger MW, Goodman BM, Carnes M. 1999. Long term efficacy of non-surgical urinary incontinence treatment in elderly women. *Journals of Gerontology Series A—Biological Sciences and Medical Sciences*. 54: 117–21.

44. Swithinbank L, Hashim H, Abrams P. 2005. The effect of fluid intake on urinary symptoms in women. *Journal of Urology*. 174: 187–9.

45. Verhoef P, Pasman WJ, Van Vliet T, Urgert R, Katan MB. 2002. Contribution of caffeine to the homocysteine-raising effect of coffee: A randomized controlled trial in humans. *American Journal of Clinical Nutrition*. 76: 1244–8.

46. Jacques PF, Bostom AG, Wilson PW, Rich S, Rosenberg IH, Selhub J. 2001. Determinants of plasma total homocysteine concentrations in the Framingham Offspring Cohort. *American Journal of Nutrition*. 73: 613–21.

47. Du Y, Malchert HU, Knopf H, Braemer–Hauth M, Gerding B, Pabel E. Association of serum caffeine concentrations with blood lipids in caffeine—drug users and nonusers—results of German National Health Surveys from1984 to 1999. *European Journal of Epidemiology* 2005. 20: 311–6.

48. Lopez–Garcia E, van Dam RM, Qi L, Hu FB. 2006. Coffee consumption and markers of inflammation and endothelial dysfunction in healthy and diabetic women. *American Journal of Clinical Nutrition*. 84: 888–93.

49. Robertson D, Frolich J, Carr K, Watson J, Hollifield J, Shand D, Oates J. 1978. Effects of caffeine on plasma renin activity, catecholamines and blood pressure. *New England Journal of Medicine*. 298: 181–6.

50. Jee SH, He J, Whelton PK, Suh I, Klag MJ. 1999. The effect of chronic coffee drinking on blood pressure. A meta-analysis of controlled clinical trials. *Hypertension*. 33: 647–52.

51. Rakic V, Beilin LJ, Burke V. 1996. Effect of coffee and tea drinking on post-prandial hypotension in older men and women. *Clinical Experiments in Pharmacological Physiology*. 23: 559–63

52. Eggertsen R, Andreasson A, Hedner T, Karlberg BE, Hansson L. 1993. Effect of coffee on ambulatory blood pressure in patients with treated hypertension. *Journal of Internal Medicine*. 233: 351–5.

53. Arciero PJ, Gardner AW, Benowitz NL, Poehlman ET. 1998. Relationship of blood pressure, heart rate and behavioural mood state to norepinephrine kinetics in younger and older men following caffeine ingestion. *European Journal of Clinical Nutrition*. 52: 805–12.

54. Arciero PJ, Bougopoulos CL, Windl BC, Benowitz NL. 2000. Influence of age on the thermic response to caffeine in women. *Metabolism, Clinical and Experimental*. 49: 101–7.

55. Norager CB, Jenson MB, Madsen MR, Laurberg S. 2005. Caffeine improved endurance in 75 year old citizens: A randomized, double-blind, placebo controlled, crossover study. *Journal of Applied Physiology*. 99: 2302–6.

56. Norager CB, Jensen MB, Weimann A, Madsen MR. 2006. Metabolic effects of caffeine ingestion and physical work in 75 year old citizens. A randomized, double-blind, placebo-controlled, cross-over study. *Clinical Endocrinology*. 65: 223–8.

57. Hodgson JM, Puddey IB, Burke V, Beilin LJ, Jordan N. 1999. Effects on blood pressure of drinking green and black tea. *Journal of Hypertension*. 17: 457–63.

58. Hodgson JM, Burke V, Puddey IB. 2005. Acute effects of tea on fasting and postprandial vascular function and blood pressure in humans. *Journal of Hypertension*. 23: 47–54.

59. Tavani A, Burtuzzi M, Negri E, Sorbara L, LaVecchia C. 2001. Alcohol, smoking, coffee and risk of non–fatal acute myocardial infarction in Italy. *European Journal of Epidemiology*. 17: 1131–7.

60. Greenberg JA, Dunbar CC, Schnoll R, Kokolis R, Kokolis S, Kassotis J. 2007. Caffeinated beverage intake and the risk of heart disease mortality in the elderly: A prospective analysis. *American Journal of Clinical Nutrition*. 85: 392–8.

61. Sofi F, Conti AA, Gori AM, Eliana Luisi ML, Casini A, Abbate R, Gensini GF. 2007. Coffee consumption and risk of coronary heart disease: A meta-analysis. *Nutrition Metabolism and Cardiovascular Disease*. 17: 209–23.

62. Smith B, Wingard DL, Smith TC, Kritz-Silverstein D, Barrett-Connor E. 2006. Does coffee consumption reduce the risk of type 2 diabetes in individuals with impaired glucose? *Diabetes Care*. 29: 2385–90.

63. Salazar-Martinez E, Willett WC, Ascherio A, Manson JE, Leitzmann MF, Stampfer MJ, Hu FB. 2004. Coffee consumption and risk for type 2 diabetes mellitus. *Annals of Internal Medicine*. 140: 1–8.

64. Greenberg JA, Axen KV, Schnoll R, Boozer CN. 2005. Coffee, tea and diabetes: The role of weight loss and caffeine. *International Journal of Obesity*. 29: 1121–9.

65. Iso H, Date C, Wakai K, Fukui M, Tamakoshi A. 2006. The relationship between green tea and total caffeine intake and risk for self-reported type 2 diabetes among Japanese adults. *Annals of Internal Medicine*. 144: 554–62.

66. Ferrini RL, Barrett-Connor E. 1996. Caffeine intake and endogenous sex steroid levels in post menopausal women. The Rancho Bernardo Study. *American Journal of Epidemiology*.. 144: 642–4.

67. Ilich JZ, Brownbill RA, Tamborini L, Crncevic-Orlic Z. 2002. To drink or not to drink: How are alcohol, caffeine and past smoking related to bone mineral density in elderly women? *Journal of the American College of Nutrition*. 21: 536–44.

68. Lloyd T, Johnson-Rollings N, Eggli DF, Kieselhorst K, Mauger ES, Cusatis DC. 2000. Bone status among post menopausal women with different habitual caffeine intakes: A longitudinal investigation. *Journal of the American College of Nutrition*. 19: 256–61.

69. Rapuri PB, Gallagher JC, Kinyamu HK, Ryschon KL. 2001. Caffeine intake increases the rate of bone loss in elderly women and interacts with vitamin D receptor genotypes. *American Journal of Clinical Nutrition*. 74: 694–700.

70. Hansen SA, Folsom AR, Kushi LH, Sellers TA. 2000. Association of fractures with caffeine and alcohol in post menopausal women: The Iowa Women's Health Study. *Public Health Nutrition*. 3: 253–61.

71. Hallstrom H, Wolk A, Glynn A, Michaelsson K. 2006. Coffee, tea and caffeine consumption in relation to osteoporotic fracture risk in a cohort of Swedish women. *Osteoporosis International*. 17: 1055–64.

72. Marcia CD, Anderson WB, Viechnicki MB, Greenspan SL. 2000. Bone mineral densitometry substantially influences health-related behaviours of post menopausal women. *Calcified Tissue International*. 66: 113–8.

73. Scher AI, Steward WF, Lipton RB. 2004. Caffeine as a risk factor for chronic daily headache: A population based study. *Neurology*. 63: 2022–7.

74. Asherio A, Zhang SM, Hernan MA, Kawachi I, Colditz GA, Speizer FE, Willett WC. 2001. Prospective study of caffeine consumption and risk of Parkinson's disease in men and women. *Annals of Neurology*. 50: 56–63.

75. Ross GA, Abbott RD, Petrovitch H, Morens DM, Grandinetti A, Tung KH, et al. 2000. Association of coffee and caffeine intake with risk of Parkinson's disease. *Journal of the American Medical Association*. 283: 2674–9.

76. Paganini-Hill A. 2001. Risk factors for Parkinson's disease: The Leisure World cohort study. *Neuroepidemiology*. 20: 118–24.

77. Tan EC, Tan C, Fook-Chong SM, Lum SY, Chasi A, et al. 2003. Dose-dependent protective effect of coffee, tea and smoking in Parkinson's disease: A study in ethnic Chinese. *Journal of the Neurological Sciences*. 3216: 163–7.

78. Checkoway H, Powers K, Smith-Weller T, Franklin GM, Longstreth WT Jr, Swanson PD. 2002. Parkinson's disease risks associated with cigarette smoking, alcohol consumption and caffeine intake. *American Journal of Epidemiology*. 155: 732–8.

79. Evans AH, Lawrence AD, Potts J, MacGregor L, Katzenschlager R, et al. 2006. Relationship between impulsive sensation seeking traits, smoking, alcohol and caffeine intake and Parkinson's disease. *Journal of Neurology, Neurosurgery and Psychiatry*. 77: 317–21.

80. World Health Organisation, International Agency for Research on Cancer (IARC) monographs evaluation of carcinogenic risks to humans. 51: 41–206, 1991.

81. Botelho F, Lunet N, Barros H. 2006. Coffee and gastric cancer: A systematic review and meta-analysis. *Cadernos de Saude Publica*. 22: 889–900.

82. Sharp L, Chilvers CE, Cheng KK, McKinney PA, Logan RF, Cook-Mozaffari P, et al. 2001. Risk factors for squamous cell carcinoma of the oesophagus in women: A case-control study. *British Journal of Cancer*. 85: 1667–70.

83. Villeneuve PJ, Johnson KC, Hanley AJ, Mao Y. 2000. Alcohol, tobacco and coffee consumption and the risk of pancreatic cancer: results from the Canadian Enhanced Surveillance System case-control project. Canadian Cancer Registries Epidemiology Research Group. *European Journal of Cancer Prevention.* 9: 49–58.

84. Michaud DS, Giovannucci E, Willett WC, Colditz GA, Fuchs CS. 2001. Coffee and alcohol consumption and the risk of pancreatic cancer in two prospective United States cohorts. *Cancer Epidemiology, Biomarkers and Prevention.* 10: 429–37.

85. Porta M, Malats N, Guarner L, Carrato A, Rifa J, Salas A, et al. 1999. Association between coffee drinking and K-ras mutations in exocrine pancreatic cancer. PANKRAS II Study Group. *Journal of Epidemiology and Community Health.* 53: 702–9.

86. Larsson SC, Wolk A. 2007. Coffee consumption and risk of liver cancer: A meta–analysis. *Gastroenterology.* 132: 1740–5.

87. Larsson SC, Giovannucci E, Wolk A. 2005. A prospective study of dietary folate intake and risk of colorectal cancer: Modification by caffeine intake and cigarette smoking. *Cancer Epidemiology, Biomarkers and Prevention.* 14: 740–3.

88. Giovannucci E. 1998. Meta-analysis of coffee consumption and risk of colorectal cancer. *American Journal of Epidemiology.* 147: 1043–1052 .

89. Michels KB, Willett WC, Fuchs CS, Giovannucci E. 2005. Coffee, tea and caffeine consumption and incidence of colon and rectal cancer. *Journal of the National Cancer Institute.* 97: 282–92.

90. Naganuma T, Kuriyama S, Akhter M, Kakizaki M, Nakaya N, Matsuda–Ohmori K, et al. 2007. Coffee consumption and risk of colorectal cancer: a prospective cohort study in Japan. *International Journal of Cancer.* 120: 1542–7.

91. Larsson SC, Bergkvist L, Giovannucci E. Wolk A. 2006. Coffee consumption and incidence of colorectal cancer in two prospective cohort studies of Swedish women and men. *American Journal of Epidemiology.* 163: 638–44.

92. Michels KB, Holmberg L, Bergkvist L, Wolk A. 2002. Coffee, tea and caffeine consumption and breast cancer incidence in a cohort of Swedish women. *Annals of Epidemiology.* 12: 21–6.

93. Tavani A, Pregnolato A, La Vecchia C, Favero A, Franceschi S. 1998. Coffee consumption and the risk of breast cancer. *European Journal of Cancer Prevention.* 7: 77–82.

94. Baker JA, Beehler GP, Sawant AC, Jayaprakash V, McCann SE, Moysich KB. 2006. Consumption of coffee, but not black tea, is associated with decreased risk of premenopausal breast cancer. *Journal of Nutrition.* 136: 166–71.

95. Nkondjock A, Ghadirian P, Kotsopoulas J, Lubinski J, Lynch H, et al. 2006. Coffee consumption and breast cancer risk among BRCA1 and BRCA2 mutation carriers. *International Journal of Cancer.* 118: 103–7.

96. Riman T, Dickman PW, Nilsson S, Nordlinder H, Magnusson CM, Persoon IR. 2004. Some life-style factors and the risk of invasive epithelial ovarian cancer in Swedish women. *European Journal of Epidemiology.* 19: 1011–9.

97. Jordan SJ, Purdie DM, Green AC, Webb PM. 2004 Coffee, tea and caffeine and risk of epithelial ovarian cancer. *Cancer Causes and Control*: 14: 359–65.

98. Baker JA, Boakye K, McCann SE, Beehler GP, Rodabaugh KJ, Villella JA, Moysich KB. 2007. Consumption of black tea or coffee and risk of ovarian cancer. *International Journal of Gynecological Cancer.* 17: 50–4.

99. Tavani A, Gallus S, Dal Maso L, Franceschi S, Montella M, Conti E, La Vecchia C. 2001. Coffee and alcohol intake and risk of ovarian cancer: an Italian case-control study. *Nutrition and Cancer.* 39: 29–34.

100. Kuper H, Titus–Ernstoff L, Harlow BL, Cramer DW. 2000. Population based study of coffee, alcohol and tobacco use and risk of ovarian cancer. *International Journal of Cancer.* 88: 313–8.

101. Goodman MT, Tung KH, McDuffie K, Wilkens LR, Donlon TA. 2003. Association of caffeine intake and CYP1A2 genotype with ovarian cancer. *Nutrition and Cancer.* 46: 23–9.

102. Terry KL, Titus-Ernstoff L, Garner EO, Vitonis AF, Cramer DW. 2003. Interaction between CYP1A1 polymorphic variants and dietary exposures influencing ovarian cancer risk. *Cancer Epidemiology, Biomarkers and Prevention.* 12: 187–90.

103. Stensvold I, Jacobsen BK. 1994. Coffee and cancer: A prospective study of 43000 Norwegian men and women. *Cancer Causes and Control.* 5: 401–408.

104. Levi F, Franceschi S, Negri E, La Vecchia C. 1993. Dietary factors and the risk of endometrial cancer. *Cancer.* 71: 3575–3581.

105. Hirose K, Niwa Y, Wakai K, Matsuo K, Nakanishi T, Tajima K. 2007. Coffee consumption and the risk of endometrial cancer: Evidence from a case-control study of female hormone-related cancers in Japan. *Cancer Science.* 98: 411–5.
106. Ellison LF. 2000. Tea and other beverage consumption and prostate cancer risk: A Canadian retrospective cohort study. *European Journal of Cancer Prevention.* 9: 125–30.
107. Hsieh CC, Thanos A, Mitropoulos D, Deliveliotis C, Mantzoros CS, Trichopoulos D. 1999. Risk factors for prostate cancer: A case-control study in Greece. *International Journal of Cancer.* 80: 699–703.
108. Sharpe CR, Siemiatychi J. 2002. Consumption of non-alcoholic beverages and prostate cancer risk. *European Journal of Cancer Prevention.* 11: 497–501.
109. Jain MG, Hislop GT, Howe GR, Burch JD, Ghadirian P. 1998. Alcohol and other beverage use and prostate cancer risk among Canadian men. *International Journal of Cancer.* 78: 707–11.
110. Zeegers MP, Tan FE, Goldbohm RA, van den Brandt PA. 2001. Are coffee and tea consumption associated with urinary tract cancer risk? A systematic review and meta-analysis. *International Journal of Epidemiology.* 30: 353–62.
111. Villanueva CM, Cantor KP, King WD, Jaakkola JJ, Cordier S, Lynch CF, et al. 2006. Total and specific fluid consumption as determinants of bladder cancer risk. *International Journal of Cancer.* 118: 2040–7.
112. Kubik A, Zatloukal P, Tomasek L, Kriz J, Petruzelka L, Piesko I. 2001. Diet and risk of lung cancer among women. A hospital based case control study. *Neoplasma.* 48: 262–6.
113. Baker JA, McCann SE, Reid ME, Nowell S, Beehler GP, Moysich KB. 2005. Associations between black tea and coffee consumption and risk of lung cancer among current and former smokers. *Nutrition and Cancer.* 52: 15–21.
114. Mack WJ, Preston-Martin S, Dal Maso L, Galanti R, Xiang M, et al. 2003. A pooled-analysis of case-control studies of thyroid cancer: Cigarette smoking and consumption of alcohol, coffee and tea. *Cancer Causes and Control.* 14: 773–85.

11 Vitamin K and Health in the Aged

Jennifer Truong and Sarah L. Booth[*]

CONTENTS

11.1 INTRODUCTION

Vitamin K is a fat-soluble vitamin named for its role in coagulation. The "K" comes from the Scandinavian word "koagulation" as the 1939 discovery of the vitamin is credited to Henrik Dam, a Danish scientist. In contrast to the other fat-soluble vitamins, scientific knowledge on the physiological benefits of increased vitamin K consumption is modest. Technological advances in the late 1970s facilitated the routine measurement of vitamin K concentrations in circulation and, over the next two decades, a battery of biochemical functional measures were developed and validated

[*] In part supported by USDA agreement no. 58-1950-7-707. Any opinions, findings, conclusion, or recommendations expressed in this publication are those of the authors and do not necessarily reflect the view of the U.S. Department of Agriculture.

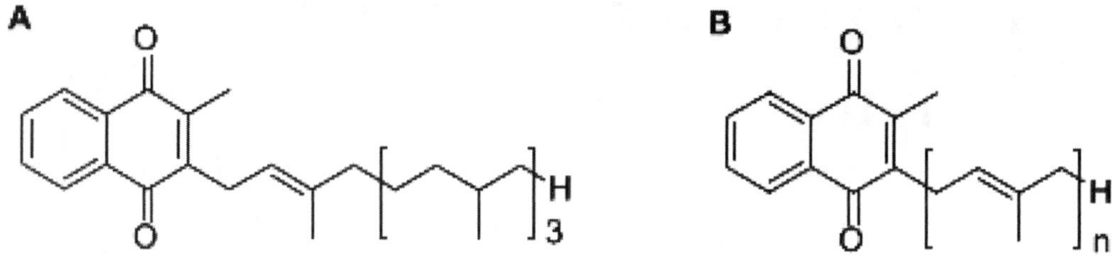

FIGURE 11.1   Dietary forms of vitamin K: Phylloquinone (A) and Menaquinones (B).

to assess vitamin K nutritional status. Collectively, these measures have provided the capacity to identify subgroups of the population that are at risk for subclinical vitamin K deficiency. Discovery of physiological roles for vitamin K beyond that of coagulation has had impact on our understanding of the role of vitamin K nutrition in the elderly.

This chapter will focus on the dietary and nondietary determinants of vitamin K status in the elderly, including potential drug and nutrient interactions with vitamin K. The current state of knowledge regarding its role in bone health, osteoarthritis, and cardiovascular disease will be reviewed.

11.2 BIOCHEMICAL ROLES

Vitamin K is found in two natural forms: phylloquinone and menaquinones. All forms share the common structure, 2-methyl-1,4-napthoquinone (Figure 11.1). Phylloquinone (vitamin K_1) is present in dark green vegetables, such as broccoli and spinach, and certain plant oils, such as soybean and canola. During commercial hydrogenation of phylloquinone-rich plant oils, 2′,3′-dihydrophylloquinone is formed from phylloquinone, and is found in foods made with partially hydrogenated fat. The synthetic water-soluble form of phylloquinone is called phytonadione.

Menaquinones (vitamin K_2) belong to a group of compounds that are present in modest amounts in the diet exclusively from animal sources, but, to a greater extent, derived from endogenous bacterial synthesis. The menaquinones differ in structure from phylloquinone in their 3-substituted lipophilic side chain. The major menaquinones contain 4–10 repeating isoprenoid units, indicated by MK-4 to MK-10 (Figure 11.1). Menaquinone-4 (MK-4) is alkylated from menadione (vitamin K_3), a synthetic form of vitamin K that is present in animal feeds, or is the product of tissue-specific conversion directly from dietary phylloquinone [1].

The only known biochemical role for vitamin K is as the cofactor for the vitamin K-dependent carboxylase that catalyzes the amino acid glutamic acid (Glu) to γ-carboxyglutamic acid (Gla) [2]. This carboxylation reaction is critical to the calcium-binding function of these vitamin K-dependent proteins. The hepatic vitamin K-dependent proteins involved in coagulation are factors II (prothrombin), VII, IX, X and proteins C, S and Z, all of which require vitamin K for physiologic activation [2].

Additional vitamin K-dependent proteins are present in extra-hepatic tissues; however, their physiologic functions are still an area of active research. (Table 11.1) Three vitamin K-dependent proteins isolated in bone and cartilage are osteocalcin (bone Gla protein), matrix Gla protein (MGP) and protein S, and these are implicated in bone, joint, and heart health.

TABLE 11.1
Vitamin K-Dependent Proteins and Their Functions

Proteins	Physiologic Function
Hepatic	
Factor II (prothrombin)	Procoagulant
Factor VII	Procoagulant
Factor IX	Procoagulant
Factor X	Procoagulant
Protein C	Anticoagulant
Protein S	Anticoagulant
Protein Z	Unknown
Bone	
Osteocalcin	Regulation of bone mineral maturation
Matrix Gla Protein	Calcification inhibitor
Protein S	Regulation of osteoclast activity
Cartilage	
Gas6	Regulation of osteoclast activity
Matrix Gla Protein	Calcification inhibitor
Vascular Smooth Muscle Cells	
Matrix Gla Protein	Calcification inhibitior
Non–Specific	
Proline-rich Gla proteins 1,2	Unknown
Transmembrane Gla proteins	Unknown

11.3 MEASUREMENT OF VITAMIN K STATUS

11.3.1 COAGULATION TIME

Measurement of blood clotting times has classically been used as a measure of vitamin K deficiency, but is insensitive and nonspecific for the assessment of vitamin K nutritional status. Prothrombin time (PT), usually reported as an International Normalized Ratio (INR), and activated partial thromboplastin time (aPTT) are routine clinical tests that may reflect frank vitamin K deficiency. As there are multiple etiologies of prolonged INR/PTT, such as hepatic dysfunction, hematologic disease, or several other acute or chronic conditions that are unrelated to vitamin K deficiency, these tests are nonspecific. Healthy adults are able to maintain normal coagulation times despite sustained intakes of low amounts of dietary phylloquinone [3], whereas other, more sensitive measures of vitamin K status indicate subclinical vitamin K deficiency following dietary restriction. Therefore, INR and PTT are more appropriately used as clinical tools to monitor stability of the use of oral anticoagulant such as warfarin. More sensitive and specific measures are available to measure vitamin K nutritional status.

11.3.2 PLASMA OR SERUM PHYLLOQUINONE

The primary circulating form of vitamin K is phylloquinone, which generally reflects recent intake over the previous 24 hours. Large variability, in part related to the interrelationship between circulating vitamin K and lipid concentrations, is seen with circulating concentrations of vitamin K. The inter- and intra-individual variability in dietary intakes of vitamin K are also much wider compared with other fat-soluble vitamins [4]. In a metabolic study involving older women (60–80 years), 3-hour and 6-hour postprandial increases in plasma phylloquinone reflected the administered dose of dietary phylloquinone given at the previous meal [5]. Use of stable isotopes indicate that labeled phylloquinone is cleared from circulation within 24 hours of intake [6]. These metabolic studies demonstrated that plasma phylloquinone concentrations are reflective of recent intake and decreases rapidly when a low vitamin K diet is consumed [5].

11.3.3   Undercarboxylated Vitamin K-Dependent Proteins

The degree to which a vitamin K-dependent protein is undercarboxylated has been exploited for the assessment of vitamin K nutritional status. As the vitamin K-dependent γ-carboxylation is a post-translational event, these measures are used as functional indicators of vitamin K status, whereas total concentrations of the proteins are influenced by other factors independent of vitamin K. The two proteins for which there are commercially available assays for undercarboxylated measures, although not currently available for clinical use in the United States, include prothrombin and osteocalcin. Undercarboxylated prothrombin, or PIVKA-II (proteins induced by vitamin K absence or antagonism-factor II), is sensitive to vitamin K deficiency, and has measurable, albeit modest, increases in response to dietary vitamin K restriction [7]. The assay is not appropriate for detecting differences in carboxylation of prothrombin to vitamin K supplementation because the dietary intakes required for maximal carboxylation of prothrombin are low compared with those of other extra-hepatic proteins such as osteocalcin.

Osteocalcin, a predominant non-collagenous protein in bone, is thought to be involved in the regulation of bone mineral maturation [8]. Synthesis of the protein is partially regulated by 1,25-dihydroxyvitamin D, but not by vitamin K. However, the mineral-binding capacity of osteocalcin is dependent on the vitamin K-dependent γ-carboxylation of its three glutamate residues, such that partially carboxylated osteocalcin may have reduced binding to the mineral in bone. Because total osteocalcin (tOC) concentrations respond to multiple factors, independent of available vitamin K, the undercarboxylated osteocalcin (ucOC) is expressed as the ratio of serum osteocalcin that is not carboxylated—i.e., as %ucOC or ucOC/tOC. The higher the ratio of undercarboxylated osteocalcin to total osteocalcin, the poorer the vitamin K status.

The multiple roles of vitamin K-dependent proteins are still an area of active investigation. The majority of the extra-hepatic proteins do not have commercially available assays for measurement of total protein concentrations, or, more importantly, for the discussion of vitamin K nutrition, the degree to which the individual proteins are carboxylated.

11.3.4   Urinary Measures

Whereas blood measures of vitamin K status can reflect recent dietary intake and availability of vitamin K in liver and bone, urinary measures have the capacity to reflect overall vitamin K metabolism. Urinary metabolites of vitamin K can be now be measured by high-performance liquid chromatography and reflect changes in dietary intake of vitamin K [9]. Advantages to measurement of urinary metabolites are that it is noninvasive and they directly reflect storage and transport of serum phylloquinone, in addition to the contribution of other forms of vitamin K, such as menaquinone-4 and endogenously produced longer chain menaquinones.

There is more collective experience with urinary Gla as a urinary measure of vitamin K status, primarily due to its availability as an assay for several decades. As Gla is not capable of being recycled, it is excreted in the urine following the turnover of the vitamin K-dependent proteins. Because this amino acid is common to all vitamin K-dependent proteins, it is therefore an overall measure of vitamin K-dependent proteins. Its use as a single measure of vitamin K status is not appropriate because absolute concentrations of urinary Gla are dependent on multiple factors independent of vitamin K intake, including, but not limited to, body composition. In contrast, the relative change of urinary Gla in response to manipulation of dietary vitamin K has been an effective measure of vitamin K status in metabolic studies [7].

11.4   DETERMINANTS OF VITAMIN K STATUS

11.4.1   DIETARY DETERMINANTS

11.4.1.1   Dietary Sources

Green vegetables contain the highest content of phylloquinone, and contribute up to 60% of total phylloquinone intake [4,10]. Plant oils and margarine found in spreads and salad dressings are also an important dietary source of phylloquinone in the U.S. diet [11,12]. Poultry products are the primary dietary sources of MK-4 in the U.S. diet because poultry feed is a rich source of menadione, which is subsequently converted to MK-4 in certain tissues [13,14]. Menaquinone-7 (MK-7) is primarily found in *natto*, a fermented soybean product. Certain cheeses contain some menaquinones [15]. It has been proposed that about 50% of the daily requirement for vitamin K is supplied by the production of endogenous menaquinones by gut flora. However, there is insufficient evidence to support this finding. [16].

11.4.1.2   Current Dietary Recommendations

There is no current recommended dietary allowance (RDA) for vitamin K. The adequate intake (AI) of a nutrient is the median level that is assumed to be adequate based on observation of groups of apparently healthy people. The AI in the United States for vitamin K is based on representative dietary intake data from healthy individuals from the Third Nutrition and Health Examination Survey (NHANES III), and is currently set at 120 and 90 µg/day, for men and women, respectively [17]. The adequacy of these intakes for promotion of health has not been determined because there are currently no physiological outcomes available that can be reliably used to assess nutritional adequacy.

There is considerable variability with respect to dietary vitamin K intake in nutritional surveys performed across different geographic regions and among different ages. Dietary surveys from the United Kingdom and Ireland have indicated that the elderly, in particular elderly women, consume amounts of phylloquinone below the AI set in the United States [18,19]. Nursing home residents have been reported to consume lower amounts of phylloquinone than free-living elderly [20]. In contrast, free-living elderly persons in areas of China and Hong Kong have significantly higher phylloquinone intakes than their counterparts in the United Kingdom [21]. This has been attributed to a greater intake of green vegetables in these populations. Phylloquinone intake in the United Kingdom has been decreasing over the last two decades, and has been associated with the decline in leafy green vegetable consumption [22]. In the United States, adults 70 years of age do not, on average, meet the AI [17]. These dietary surveys are all influenced by the type of dietary assessment and variability in nutrient databases used, which may result in measurement errors and thus wide reported ranges of vitamin K intakes within and between subgroups [23].

11.4.1.3   Safety of Supplementation

As new physiological roles for vitamin K are elucidated and there is growing enthusiasm for dietary supplements among the general public, supplemental vitamin K is now becoming more widely available in the forms of topical cream, capsules, tablets, and softgels. Many multivitamin formulations contain vitamin K in the form of phytonadione, ranging from 40 to 100 µg, which is well within normal dietary intakes in the U.S. adult population. Supplements containing vitamin K alone are also available in the forms of phytonadione or either MK-4 or MK-7, in daily doses of up to 4050 µg.

Vitamin K is considered safe at the recommended AI dosages discussed. There is no tolerable upper intake limit (UL) set because there are no known cases of toxicity with vitamin K. A common misconception is that excessive vitamin K will result in overcoagulation. However, the vitamin K-dependent proteins have a limited number of Glu residues capable of γ-carboxylation per molecule, beyond which there can be no further γ-carboxylation or excessive coagulation. However, for individuals on oral anticoagulants, such as warfarin, dietary vitamin K supplementation can influence stability of INR and needs to be monitored by health professionals. There is little collective experience on the potential toxicity or adverse events in sustained vitamin K supplementation in individuals with normal coagulation. As other forms of vitamin K are introduced into the dietary supplement market, it will be prudent to closely monitor any potential adverse consequences.

11.4.2 Non-Dietary Determinants of Vitamin K Status

11.4.2.1 Role of Plasma Lipids

Vitamin K is a fat-soluble vitamin, so its absorption occurs in the proximal intestine, and is dependent on bile and pancreatic secretions [24]. In the intestine, vitamin K is incorporated into nascent chylomicron particles that are secreted directly into the lymph and ultimately into the peripheral circulation. Vitamin K remains associated with these particles during delipidation in circulation and subsequent uptake by the liver. Triglyceride-rich lipoproteins, primarily chlyomicron remnants, and very low-density lipoproteins are thought to be the main transporters of phylloquinone [25–27].

In older adults, interpretation of elevated plasma phylloquinone concentrations is difficult, as there are concomitant increases in triglycerides with age and there is some indication that older adults consume more vitamin K in the form of green vegetables. Various techniques have been described for improving quantification of plasma phylloquinone in view of elevated lipid concentrations among the elderly. One technique employing high performance liquid chromatography (HPLC) noted a significant correlation (between phylloquinone and triglyceride concentrations in fasting plasma samples [28]. This finding suggests that interpretation of plasma phylloquinone in older adults, who are more likely to have elevated lipid concentrations, requires use of a correction factor for plasma triglycerides. However, if phylloquinone concentrations are adjusted for triglycerides, the adjusted plasma phylloquinone concentrations are lower in the elderly compared with younger adults [29]. Younger adults consistently have low phylloquinone intakes so it would be expected that their phylloquinone concentrations would be lower. Therefore, controversy currently exists as to whether adjustment of plasma phylloquinone for total plasma lipids will improve the predictive value of fasting plasma phylloquinone on health outcomes [30,31].

11.4.2.2 Hormonal Influences

In the rat model, estrogen stimulates the formation of prothrombin and reduces the requirement of vitamin K for the maximal γ-carboxylation of prothrombin by an unknown mechanism [32]. Among castrated male and female rats fed a vitamin K-deficient diet, prothrombin dropped in response to testosterone, but increased or was maintained in response to estradiol [32].

Vitamin K deficiency has been shown to reduce testosterone production in a rat model [33]. Levels of Cyp11a mRNA, a rate-limiting enzyme in testosterone synthesis, were found to be positively correlated with MK-4 concentrations in the testes. Comparing the control and vitamin K-supplemented rats with the vitamin K-deficient rats, there were decreased testosterone concentrations in plasma and testis in the deficient group, suggesting that vitamin K is involved in steroid production in the testes via regulation of Cyp11a.

There is a paucity of human studies examining the influence of sex hormones on vitamin K status. A small number of studies exist in postmenopausal women looking at estrogen effect, vitamin K, and bone metabolism; however, there are none at the time of this writing that have studied the effect of testosterone on vitamin K metabolism in men.

One study compared biochemical markers of bone metabolism, vitamin K status, and bone mineral density (BMD) measured by dual energy X-ray absorptiometry (DXA) in perimenopausal older women, cycling younger women, and early postmenopausal women receiving no estrogen supplementation [34]. Cycling older women were found to have similar estradiol and vitamin K status as cycling younger women, but lower total osteocalcin and BMD at the total hip. Comparing the cycling older women to the early postmenopausal women receiving no estrogen supplementation, BMD was similar at all sites, but total osteocalcin was elevated in the early postmenopausal group. In addition, circulating phylloquinone concentrations were highest in the early postmenopausal women, with %ucOC being higher when compared with all cycling women. The conclusions drawn were that premenopausal women showed reduced BMD despite normal estrogen profiles, and that %ucOC may be a specific bone marker of early postmenopause in healthy women.

11.4.2.3 Genetic Polymorphisms

As phylloquinone concentrations in circulation may be affected by lipid status, studies have examined the relationship of apolipoprotein E genotype to vitamin K status in older adults [19,35]. A study comparing vitamin K status in healthy older adults from China and the United Kingdom analyzed fasting plasma for phylloquinone, triacylglycerols, total osteocalcin, undercarboxylated osteocalcin, and apoE genotype, as well as hip bone mineral content (BMC) by DXA. Subjects were grouped according to apoE genotype as E2/3, E3/3 and [E3/4 + E4/4]. The mean plasma phylloquinone concentrations of the three genotype groups was significantly higher, and the %ucOC was lower in the Chinese than in the British subjects. Higher phylloquinone concentrations were found in subjects with [E3/4 + E4/4]. than those with either E2/3 or E3/3 in the United Kingdom. Ethnic differences in apoE genotype may also have an influence on osteocalcin γ-carboxylation status [35].

11.5 VITAMIN K AND BONE HEALTH

Osteoporosis, characterized by a loss of bone mass and micro-architectural deterioration of bone tissue, leads to an increase in the risk of skeletal fracture. Osteoporosis and osteopenia are major public health issues with our aging population. In the U.S., 10 million men and women have osteoporosis, and 34 million have low bone mass placing them at risk for the disease [36]. One out of every two women, and one in four men over 50 will have an osteoporosis-related fracture in their lifetime [36].

The micronutrients most highly studied and found to have the greatest importance in bone health to date are calcium and vitamin D. New research is emerging that suggest roles for other micronutrients, and in particular vitamin K, in bone metabolism. As discussed earlier, vitamin K may be involved in bone metabolism through the γ-carboxylation of proteins, such as osteocalcin.

Epidemiologic studies have described associations between biochemical markers of vitamin K status, specifically %ucOC, and risk of low bone mineral density and hip fracture. A recent review of observational studies summarized several reports of associations between low dietary phylloquinone intakes and hip fracture risk, especially among women [37]. Limitations of these studies include the potential confounding effect of overall poor diet and unhealthy lifestyle because vitamin K is primary found in foods associated with a healthy diet.

A recent systematic review and meta-analysis of randomized controlled trials concluded that supplementation with vitamin K, primarily in the form of MK-4, is associated with an increase in bone mineral density and reduced risk for fracture [38]. However, as acknowledged by the authors of this meta-analysis, the studies included were primarily limited to a small number of investigators from Japan, many of the studies were unblinded to investigators and participants, there was a wide range in co-supplementation with calcium or vitamin D, and supplementation was with 45 mg/day of MK-4. This dose, which is 450-fold higher than current U.S. dietary requirements for vitamin K, is currently in use as an anti-osteoporotic medication in Japan. Some authors have suggested that MK-4 effectiveness is due to the chemical structure of its side chain, which resembles the geranylgeraniol structure of the class of osteoporotic medications, bisphosphonates [39,40]. The magnitude of the reported protective effect of MK-4 in the meta-analysis was considerably greater than those effects associated with bisphosphonate use, which emphasizes the need for caution in the interpretation of this meta-analysis. More recently, an editorial suggested that unpublished industry data that was not included in the meta-analysis does not support conclusions that there is a protective effect of MK-4 on reduction in hip fracture risk in elderly women [41].

In comparison with the number of studies that report on the effect of MK-4 on BMD and fracture risk, reports of the effect of phylloquinone on these outcomes are few. Supplementation with a high dose of phylloquinone (1000 μg/day) was shown to reduce 3-year bone loss at the femoral neck, but not the lumbar spine, in postmenopausal women [42]. A recent 2-year randomized controlled trial that used a supplemental dose of 200 μg/day phylloquinone (an amount deemed attainable in the diet) reported a modest increase in BMC and BMD at the ultra distal radius in postmenopausal women who received phylloquinone with vitamin D_3 and calcium, compared with the women taking the same doses of phylloquinone and vitamin D_3 alone or a placebo. However, there were no differences in BMD or BMC at the femoral neck or trochanter among the treatment groups [43]. At the time of this writing, more clinical trials evaluating the effect of vitamin K supplementation on bone loss are nearing completion, which, when published, will provide a strong basis for making recommendations regarding the efficacy of vitamin K supplementation on reducing bone loss in the elderly.

11.6   VITAMIN K AND OSTEOARTHRITIS

It has been estimated that by the year 2020, 59.4 million Americans (18.2% of the population) will have some form of arthritis [44]. The proposed mechanism by which vitamin K may be involved in protection against osteoarthritis is by regulating bone and cartilage mineralization and growth plate cartilage calcification through the γ-carboxylation of the vitamin K-dependent matrix Gla protein (MGP). *In vivo* studies with MGP knockout mice models have demonstrated inappropriate calcification of various cartilages, including the growth plate, which leads to short stature, osteopenia, and fractures [45]. Osteoarthritis occurs due to abnormal cartilage repair and development of osteophytes. Low vitamin K leads to undercarboxylation of MGP, thus reducing protein function and affecting chondrocyte differentiation and endochondral bone formation.

An observational cohort study using the participants of the Framingham Offspring Study reported an association between low plasma vitamin K concentrations and increased prevalence of osteoarthritis manifestations in the hand and knee [46]. While promising, more research is required before vitamin K can be recommended as a preventive agent in progression of osteoarthritis.

11.7   VITAMIN K AND CARDIOVASCULAR HEALTH

Coronary artery calcification occurring in atherosclerosis is associated with increased risk for coronary heart disease. MGP is a vitamin K-dependent protein that inhibits calcification *in vivo*, as discussed in Section 11.6, and is expressed in smooth vascular muscle cells involved with the calcification process in coronary arteries [47,48]. In addition to abnormalities in cartilage formation, mouse models with targeted deletion of the MGP gene develop rapid calcification of the elastic lamellae of the arterial media, which is fatal within 2 months of age [45].

The association between serum MGP concentrations and prevalence of cardiovascular disease was examined in two cohorts of men and women [49]. One cohort was composed of men and women free of clinically apparent coronary heart disease from the Framingham Offspring Study, a longitudinal community-based study of men and women that identified risk factors for heart disease. The second cohort included healthy elderly men and women participating in a vitamin K supplementation trial prior to their randomization to treatment. Serum MGP concentrations were associated with risk factors for atherosclerosis in both groups, but no consistent associations were seen between MGP and coronary artery calcification after adjustment for coronary heart disease risk score. The commercially available assays for serum MGP only measure total MGP, which does not reflect the amount of the protein that is γ-carboxylated. This limits the interpretation on the role of vitamin K in vascular calcification based on serum MGP concentrations. Furthermore, it has been suggested that the effect of MGP on regulation of calcification is localized to the tissue of synthesis, such that circulating MGP cannot rescue the calcification effects of null MGP production in vascular smooth muscle cells of genetically manipulated mouse models, regardless of the degree to which the circulating MGP is carboxylated [50].

The association between dietary phylloquinone intake and cardiovascular disease has been examined in numerous cohorts, including the Health Professionals Follow-up Study, the Nurses' Health Study and the Framingham Heart Study [51–53]. These studies have consistently concluded that high phylloquinone intake is not an independent risk factor for cardiovascular disease, but rather, that higher phylloquinone intakes could be used as a marker of an overall heart-healthy dietary and lifestyle pattern because they track green vegetable consumption. In contrast, cross-sectional studies examining the potential role for vitamin K intake in the protection against vascular calcification report an inverse association between MK-4 intake and arterial calcification among cohorts in the Netherlands. Because intakes of menaquinones are primarily of limited animal sources, such as dairy products, it is not known if this is a protective effect specific to menaquinone intake or is simply tracking intake of factors present in these foods rich in menaquinones. In these latter studies, phylloquinone intake was not associated with arterial calcification, similar to the findings of the U.S. cohorts [54,55].

A single randomized controlled trial has been completed assessing the effect of supplemental phylloquinone on vascular health in postmenopausal women. Those who took a daily mineral supplement containing 1000 µg phylloquinone and 8 µg vitamin D had improved elasticity and compliance in the common carotid artery over 3 years of follow-up, compared with women taking the supplement without phylloquinone [56]. While the authors attribute this improvement to an increase in the vitamin K-dependent carboxylation of MGP, leading to a decrease in vascular calcium deposition, neither MGP nor vascular calcification was measured directly [56]. Additional studies are warranted to gain a better understanding of the role of vitamin K, at a dose obtainable in the diet, on the progression of vascular calcification.

11.8 DRUG AND NUTRIENT INTERACTIONS WITH VITAMIN K

11.8.1 Nutrient–Nutrient Interactions

An area that warrants further study is how vitamin K status is affected by interaction with other nutrients, in particular the other fat-soluble vitamins. Although vitamin K circulates in concentrations magnitudes lower than the other fat-soluble vitamins, there are common pathways of absorption and transport that could be a source of interaction. Furthermore, as new biochemical roles for vitamin K are being discovered, interactions through common pathways at the cellular level are also plausible. A study examining nutritional survey data of British adults reported that 10% of the variation in plasma phylloquinone concentrations was explained by intake of other fat-soluble vitamin concentrations [10].

Vitamin D promotes mineralization of bone, among other physiological roles currently emerging for this vitamin. Vitamin D is also involved in regulation of synthesis of the vitamin K-dependent bone proteins, osteocalcin, and matrix Gla protein [57]. Questions have arisen regarding whether there would be benefit to treatment and prophylaxis of osteoporosis with a combination of vitamin D and vitamin K. As described in Section 11.5, a two-year, double-blind, randomized, placebo control trial of supplementation with phylloquinone (200 µg/day), vitamin D3 (400 IU/day) plus calcium (1000 mg/day) or a combination (phylloquinone, vitamin D3, and calcium) examined the effect on bone health in older women [43]. Women who took combined vitamin K and vitamin D plus calcium showed a significant and sustained increase in both BMD and BMC at the site of the ultradistal radius. Similar changes were not seen in the vitamin K group alone or in the calcium plus vitamin D group, which suggests a possible synergistic role of the combination of these two fat-soluble vitamins. The amount of supplemental phylloquinone used in this trial was equivalent to that contained in ~50 g portion of leafy green vegetables, such as collards and spinach, and thus could be attained by dietary modification rather than from supplementation [43].

Vitamin E is one of the most frequently purchased single nutrient dietary supplements in the U.S., particularly among older adults [58]. Animal studies examining the relationship between vitamin E and vitamin K status indicate a potential nutrient–nutrient interaction. In chicks fed a diet high in vitamin E (4000 mg all rac-α-tocopheryl acetate/kg) but adequate in vitamin K (0.14 mg phylloquinone/kg), there was a threefold increase in prothrombin time and an increase in mortality rate (five out of 12 animals died from increased bleeding tendency) was observed. The inhibiting effect of high dietary vitamin E on procoagulant factors may be prevented by increasing dietary phylloquinone supplementation [59].

In adults with a normal coagulation status, supplemental doses of vitamin E at the tolerable upper limit of 1,000 IU RRR-α-tocopherol resulted in an increase of PIVKA-II, indicative of poor vitamin K status; however, other measures of vitamin K status (plasma phylloquinone concentration and percentage ucOC) did not change [60]. The mechanisms for this vitamin E-vitamin K interaction are currently unknown.

Although there has been some *in vitro* data to suggest an adverse effect of vitamin A on vitamin K status, there is currently no published literature available to support this nutrient–nutrient interaction in humans [61].

11.8.2 Drug–Nutrient Interaction

Warfarin is a commonly used oral anticoagulant in the elderly for prophylaxis against clot formation in states of arrhythmia, or in patients at risk for thromboembolic stroke. The mechanism of action of warfarin on prolongation of clotting times is through its inhibitory effect on the recycling of vitamin K, resulting in the incomplete γ-carboxylation of the Glu residues in vitamin K-dependent proteins due to inadequate substrate (Figure 11.2). As discussed in Section 11.3.1, clotting times are measured by INR in the clinical setting. In the general population with normal coagulation, the INR is between 1.0 to 1.2. In general, the goal for anticoagulation in the clinical setting of prophylaxis is for an INR between 2.0 to 3.0.

A recent review examining the potential interaction of dietary vitamin K and coagulation stability, particularly among the elderly patients, concluded that vitamin K intake of more than 250 µg/day decreased warfarin sensitivity in anticoagulated patients consuming regular diets [62]. In a randomized crossover study, patients who were allocated to an 80% decrease of phylloquinone intake increased their INR by almost 30% within 1 week of the intervention. Based on dietary records, it was estimated that for each increase in 100 µg of vitamin K intake, the INR would be reduced by 0.2 units [62]. Because vitamin K content of individual foods varies widely due to climate, soil conditions and other growing conditions, it is probable that INR would vary more widely with daily fluctuations in dietary intake than from daily intake of dietary supplements. However, initial intake and/or withdrawal of vitamin K through the use of dietary supplements would have impact on INR. This suggests that there is a clinically relevant interaction between dietary and/or supplemental vitamin K and warfarin, and that it has a major role in INR fluctuations in chronically anticoagulated patients.

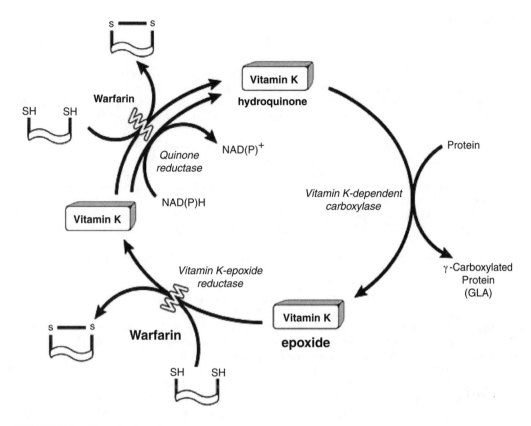

FIGURE 11.2 Vitamin K cycle.

11.9   SUMMARY

Poor vitamin K nutrition has been linked to several chronic diseases associated with abnormal calcification, which affect many elderly. On the whole, elderly persons consume more vitamin K than young adults, although there are subgroups of the elderly population who do not meet the current recommended dietary intakes for this nutrient.

However, the comparison of vitamin K status among different ages is hampered by our limited understanding of the influence of circulating lipids on the interpretation of measures of vitamin K status. Because the emphasis on vitamin K nutrition in the elderly has focused on its putative role on bone health, there are a disproportional number of studies conducted exclusively in postmenopausal women, with little known about vitamin K status in elderly men. More research is needed to determine what forms and amounts of vitamin K should be consumed to optimize health.

Development of novel techniques to measure vitamin K status have aided in improving the body of research in the field of vitamin K nutrition, but more research is required to identify non-dietary determinants of vitamin K status and their impact on the elderly. Areas of promising research include genetic and hormonal influences on vitamin K metabolism.

REFERENCES

1. Davidson, R.T., A.L. Foley, J.A. Engelke, and J.W. Suttie. 1998. Conversion of dietary phylloquinone to tissue menaquinone-4 in rats is not dependent on gut bacteria. *J Nutr*, 128(2): p. 220–3.
2. Ferland, G. 1998. The vitamin K-dependent proteins: An update. *Nutr Rev*, 56(8): p. 223–30.
3. Suttie, J.W. 1992. Vitamin K and human nutrition. *J Am Diet Assoc*, 92(5): p. 585–90.
4. McKeown, N.M., P.F. Jacques, C.M. Gundberg, J.W. Peterson, K.L. Tucker, D.P. Kiel, et al. 2002. Dietary and nondietary determinants of vitamin K biochemical measures in men and women. *J Nutr*, 132(6): p. 1329–34.
5. Booth, S.L., L. Martini, J.W. Peterson, E. Saltzman, G.E. Dallal, and R.J. Wood. 2003. Dietary phylloquinone depletion and repletion in older women. *J Nutr*, 133(8): p. 2565–9.
6. Erkkila, A.T., A.H. Lichtenstein, G.G. Dolnikowski, M.A. Grusak, S.M. Jalbert, K.A. Aquino, J.W. Peterson, and S.L. Booth. 2004. Plasma transport of vitamin K in men using deuterium-labeled collard greens. *Metabolism*, 53(2): p. 215–21.
7. Booth, S.L., M.E. O'Brien-Morse, G.E. Dallal, K.W. Davidson, and C.M. Gundberg. 1999. Response of vitamin K status to different intakes and sources of phylloquinone-rich foods: comparison of younger and older adults. *Am J Clin Nutr*, 70(3): p. 368–77.
8. Gundberg, C.M. 1998. Biology, physiology, and clinical chemistry of osteocalcin. *J Clin Ligand Assay*, 21: p. 128–138.
9. Harrington, D.J., S.L. Booth, D.J. Card, and M.J. Shearer. 2007. Excretion of the urinary 5C- and 7C-aglycone metabolites of vitamin K by young adults responds to changes in dietary phylloquinone and dihydrophylloquinone intakes. *J Nutr*, 137(7): p. 1763–8.
10. Thane, C.W., A.A. Paul, C.J. Bates, C. Bolton-Smith, A. Prentice, and M.J. Shearer. 2002. Intake and sources of phylloquinone (vitamin K1): Variation with socio-demographic and lifestyle factors in a national sample of British elderly people. *Br J Nutr*, 87(6): p. 605–13.
11. Peterson, J.W., Muzzey, K.L., Haytowitz, D., Exler, J., Lemar, L., and Booth, S.L. 2002. Phylloquinone (vitamin K–1) and dihydrophylloquinone content of fats and oils. *JAOCS*, 79: p. 641–646.
12. Piironen, V., Koivu T., Tammisalo, O., and Mattila, P. 1997. Determination of phylloquinone in oils, margarines and butter by high-performance liquid chromatography with electrochemical detection. *Food Chem*, 59: p. 473–480.
13. Elder, S.J., D.B. Haytowitz, J. Howe, J.W. Peterson, and S.L. Booth. 2006. Vitamin K contents of meat, dairy, and fast food in the U.S. Diet. *J Agric Food Chem*, 54(2): p. 463–7.
14. Ferreira, D.W., Haytowitz, D.B., Tassinari, M.S., Peterson, J.W., and Booth S.L. 2006. Vitamin K contents of grains, cereals, fast-food breakfasts, and baked goods. *J Food Sci*, 71: p. S66–S70.
15. Schurgers, L.J. and C. Vermeer. 2000. Determination of phylloquinone and menaquinones in food. Effect of food matrix on circulating vitamin K concentrations. *Haemostasis*, 30(6): p. 298–307.
16. Suttie, J.W. 1995. The importance of menaquinones in human nutrition. *Annu Rev Nutr*, 15: p. 399–417.
17. Institute of Medicine. 2001. U.S. Panel on Micronutrients, *Dietary reference intakes for vitamin A, vitamin K, arsenic, boron, chromium, copper, iodine, iron, manganese, molybdenum, nickel, silicon, vanadium, and zinc*, Washington, D.C.: National Academy Press.
18. Duggan, P., K.D. Cashman, A. Flynn, C. Bolton-Smith, and M. Kiely. 2004. Phylloquinone (vitamin K1) intakes and food sources in 18–64-year-old Irish adults. *Br J Nutr*, 92(1): p. 151–8.
19. Yan, L., B. Zhou, S. Nigdikar, X. Wang, J. Bennett, and A. Prentice. 2005. Effect of apolipoprotein E genotype on vitamin K status in healthy older adults from China and the UK. *Br J Nutr*, 94(6): p. 956–61.
20. Tse, S.L., T.Y. Chan, D.M. Wu, A.Y. Cheung, and T.C. Kwok. 2002. Deficient dietary vitamin K intake among elderly nursing home residents in Hong Kong. *Asia Pac J Clin Nutr*, 11(1): p. 62–5.
21. Yan, L., B. Zhou, D. Greenberg, L. Wang, S. Nigdikar, C. Prynne, and A. Prentice. 2004. Vitamin K status of older individuals in northern China is superior to that of older individuals in the UK. *Br J Nutr*, 92(6): p. 939–45.
22. Thane, C.W., L.Y. Wang, and W.A. Coward. 2006. Plasma phylloquinone (vitamin K1) concentration and its relationship to intake in British adults aged 19–64 years. *Br J Nutr*, 96(6): p. 1116–24.
23. Booth, S.L. and J.W. Suttie. 1998. Dietary intake and adequacy of vitamin K. *J Nutr*, 128(5): p. 785–8.
24. Shearer, M.J., A. McBurney, and P. Barkhan. 1974. Studies on the absorption and metabolism of phylloquinone (vitamin K1) in man. *Vitam Horm*, 32: p. 513–42.

25. Kohlmeier, M., A. Salomon, J. Saupe, and M.J. Shearer. 1996. Transport of vitamin K to bone in humans. *J Nutr*, 126(4 Suppl): p. 1192S–6S.
26. Lamon–Fava, S., J.A. Sadowski, K.W. Davidson, M.E. O'Brien, J.R. McNamara, and E.J. Schaefer. 1998. Plasma lipoproteins as carriers of phylloquinone (vitamin K1) in humans. *Am J Clin Nutr*, 67(6): p. 1226–31.
27. Schurgers, L.J. and C. Vermeer. 2002. Differential lipoprotein transport pathways of K-vitamins in healthy subjects. *Biochim Biophys Acta*, 1570(1): p. 27–32.
28. Azharuddin, M.K., D.S. O'Reilly, A. Gray, and D. Talwar. 2007. HPLC method for plasma vitamin K1: Effect of plasma triglyceride and acute-phase response on circulating concentrations. *Clin Chem*, 53(9): p. 1706–13.
29. Sadowski, J.A., S.J. Hood, G.E. Dallal, and P.J. Garry. 1989. Phylloquinone in plasma from elderly and young adults: Factors influencing its concentration. *Am J Clin Nutr*, 50(1): p. 100–8.
30. Cham, B.E., J.L. Smith, and D.M. Colquhoun. 1999. Interdependence of serum concentrations of vitamin K1, vitamin E, lipids, apolipoprotein A1, and apolipoprotein B: Importance in assessing vitamin status. *Clin Chim Acta*, 287(1–2): p. 45–57.
31. Traber, M.G. and I. Jialal. 2000. Measurement of lipid-soluble vitamins—further adjustment needed? *Lancet*, 355(9220): p. 2013–4.
32. Matschiner, J.T. and R.G. Bell. 1973. Effect of sex and sex hormones on plasma prothrombin and vitamin K deficiency. *Proc Soc Exp Biol Med*, 144(1): p. 316–20.
33. Shirakawa, H., Y. Ohsaki, Y. Minegishi, N. Takumi, K. Ohinata, Y. Furukawa, et al. 2006. Vitamin K deficiency reduces testosterone production in the testis through down-regulation of the Cyp11a a cholesterol side chain cleavage enzyme in rats. *Biochim Biophys Acta*, 1760(10): p. 1482–8.
34. Lukacs, J.L., S. Booth, M. Kleerekoper, R. Ansbacher, C.L. Rock, and N.E. Reame. 2006. Differential associations for menopause and age in measures of vitamin K, osteocalcin, and bone density: A cross-sectional exploratory study in healthy volunteers. *Menopause*, 13(5): p. 799–808.
35. Beavan, S.R., A. Prentice, D.M. Stirling, B. Dibba, L. Yan, D.J. Harrington, and M.J. Shearer. 2005. Ethnic differences in osteocalcin gamma-carboxylation, plasma phylloquinone (vitamin K1) and apolipoprotein E genotype. *Eur J Clin Nutr*, 59(1): p. 72–81.
36. National Institutes of Health. Osteoporosis. 2006 November 2006 [cited 2007 November 13, 2007].
37. Shea, M.K., and Booth, S.L. 2007. Role of vitamin K in the regulation of calcification. *Int Congr Ser*, 1297: p. 165–178.
38. Cockayne, S., J. Adamson, S. Lanham-New, M.J. Shearer, S. Gilbody, and D.J. Torgerson. 2006. Vitamin K and the prevention of fractures: Systematic review and meta-analysis of randomized controlled trials. *Arch Intern Med*, 166(12): p. 1256–61.
39. Binkley, N., D. Krueger, J. Engelke, T. Crenshaw, and J. Suttie. 2002. Vitamin K supplementation does not affect ovariectomy-induced bone loss in rats. *Bone*, 30(6): p. 897–900.
40. Hara, K., Y. Akiyama, T. Nakamura, S. Murota, and I. Morita. 1995. The inhibitory effect of vitamin K2 (menatetrenone) on bone resorption may be related to its side chain. *Bone*, 16(2): p. 179–84.
41. Tamura, T., S.L. Morgan, and H. Takimoto. 2007. Vitamin K and the prevention of fractures. *Arch Intern Med*, 167(1): p. 94; author reply 94–5.
42. Braam, L.A., M.H. Knapen, P. Geusens, F. Brouns, K. Hamulyak, M.J. Gerichhausen, and C. Vermeer. 2003. Vitamin K1 supplementation retards bone loss in postmenopausal women between 50 and 60 years of age. *Calcif Tissue Int*, 73(1): p. 21–6.
43. Bolton-Smith, C., M.E. McMurdo, C.R. Paterson, P.A. Mole, J.M. Harvey, S.T. Fenton, et al. 2007. Two-year randomized controlled trial of vitamin K1 (phylloquinone) and vitamin D3 plus calcium on the bone health of older women. *J Bone Miner Res*, 22(4): p. 509–19.
44. National Institutes of Health. *Arthritis prevalence rising as baby boomers grow older osteoarthritis second only to chronic heart disease in worksite disability.* 1998 [cited November 30, 2007]. http://www.nih.gov/news/pr/may98/niams-05.htm.
45. Luo, G., P. Ducy, M.D. McKee, G.J. Pinero, E. Loyer, R.R. Behringer, and G. Karsenty. 1997. Spontaneous calcification of arteries and cartilage in mice lacking matrix GLA protein. *Nature*, 386(6620): p. 78–81.
46. Neogi, T., Booth, S. L., Zhang, Y. Q., Jacques, P. F., Terkeltaub, R., Aliabadi, P., Felson, D. T. 2006. Low vitamin K status is associated with osteoarthritis in the hand and knee. *Arthritis Rheum*, 54(4): p. 1255–61.

47. Proudfoot, D., Skepper, J. N., Shanahan, C. M., Weissberg, P. L. 1998. Calcification of human vascular cells in vitro is correlated with high levels of matrix Gla protein and low levels of osteopontin expression. *Arterioscler Thromb Vasc Biol*, 18(3): p. 379–88.

48. Shanahan, C.M., Cary, N. R., Metcalfe, J. C., Weissberg, P. L. 1994. High expression of genes for calcification-regulating proteins in human atherosclerotic plaques. *J Clin Invest*, 93(6): p. 2393–402.

49. O'Donnell, C.J., M.K. Shea, P.A. Price, D.R. Gagnon, P.W. Wilson, M.G. Larson. 2006. Matrix Gla protein is associated with risk factors for atherosclerosis but not with coronary artery calcification. *Arterioscler Thromb Vasc Biol*, 26(12): p. 2769–74.

50. Murshed, M., T. Schinke, M.D. McKee, and G. Karsenty. 2004. Extracellular matrix mineralization is regulated locally; different roles of two gla-containing proteins. *J Cell Biol*, 165.5): p. 625–30.

51. Erkkila, A.T., S.L. Booth, F.B. Hu, P.F. Jacques, and A.H. Lichtenstein. 2007. Phylloquinone intake and risk of cardiovascular diseases in men. *Nutr Metab Cardiovasc Dis*, 17(1): p. 58–62.

52. Erkkila, A.T., S.L. Booth, F.B. Hu, P.F. Jacques, J.E. Manson, K.M. Rexrode. 2005. Phylloquinone intake as a marker for coronary heart disease risk but not stroke in women. *Eur J Clin Nutr*, 59(2): p. 196–204.

53. Braam, L., N. McKeown, P. Jacques, A. Lichtenstein, C. Vermeer, P. Wilson, and S. Booth. 2004. Dietary phylloquinone intake as a potential marker for a heart-healthy dietary pattern in the Framingham Offspring cohort. *J Am Diet Assoc*, 104(9): p. 1410–4.

54. Geleijnse, J.M., C. Vermeer, D.E. Grobbee, L.J. Schurgers, M.H. Knapen, I.M. van der Meer, A. Hofman, and J.C. Witteman. 2004. Dietary intake of menaquinone is associated with a reduced risk of coronary heart disease: The Rotterdam Study. *J Nutr*, 134(11): p. 3100–5.

55. Villines, T.C., C. Hatzigeorgiou, I.M. Feuerstein, P.G. O'Malley, and A.J. Taylor. 2005. Vitamin K1 intake and coronary calcification. *Coron Artery Dis*, 16(3): p. 199–203.

56. Braam, L.A., A.P. Hoeks, F. Brouns, K. Hamulyak, M.J. Gerichhausen, and C. Vermeer. 2004. Beneficial effects of vitamins D and K on the elastic properties of the vessel wall in postmenopausal women: A follow-up study. *Thromb Haemost*, 91(2): p. 373–80.

57. Shearer, M.J. 1997. The roles of vitamins D and K in bone health and osteoporosis prevention. *Proc Nutr Soc*, 56(3): p. 915–37.

58. Millen, A.E., K.W. Dodd, and A.F. Subar. 2004. Use of vitamin, mineral, nonvitamin, and nonmineral supplements in the United States: The 1987, 1992, and 2000 National Health Interview Survey results. *J Am Diet Assoc*, 104(6): p. 942–50.

59. Frank, J., H. Weiser, and H.K. Biesalski. 1997. Interaction of vitamins E and K: Effect of high dietary vitamin E on phylloquinone activity in chicks. *Int J Vitam Nutr Res*, 67(4): p. 242–7.

60. Booth, S.L., I. Golly, J.M. Sacheck, R. Roubenoff, G.E. Dallal, K. Hamada, and J.B. Blumberg. 2004. Effect of vitamin E supplementation on vitamin K status in adults with normal coagulation status. *Am J Clin Nutr*, 80(1): p. 143–8.

61. Matschiner, J.T. and Doisy, E.A. Jr. 1962. Role of vitamin A in induction of vitamin K deficiency in the rat. *Proc Soc Exp Biol Med*, 109: p. 139–142.

62. Rohde, L.E., M.C. de Assis, and E.R. Rabelo. 2007. Dietary vitamin K intake and anticoagulation in elderly patients. *Curr Opin Clin Nutr Metab Care*, 10(1): p. 1–5.

12 The Role of Diet in Slowing or Accelerating Aging

Saeed Hosseini and Reza Ghiasvand

CONTENTS

12.1 INTRODUCTION

Aging, which represents a great deal for both society and scientists, is usually defined as the progressive loss of function accompanied by decreasing fertility and increasing mortality with advancing age [1].

The literature provides evidence that proper nutrition is a powerful, modifiable lifestyle factor that may delay or prevent chronic diseases in later life and, more importantly, will potentially lead to additional years of health, productivity, and high functioning [2]. However, older adults may be at risk for inadequate nutrition because of physiological changes related to organ function declines, which can affect digestion, metabolism, and absorption of nutrients [3]. Additionally, older adults' nutritional intake may be compromised because of development of poor eating habits related to chewing or swallowing difficulties as well as diminished interest in food resulting from sensory loss (e.g., taste and smell) [4]. Physically active seniors' diets are relatively higher in dairy products and fruits than are the diets of sedentary older adults [5]. Proper nutrition, with an emphasis on consuming fruits and vegetables, has long-term health benefits, and contributes to physical, cognitive, and social functioning, overall health, and engagement with life [5,6].

Although there is evidence for the benefits of adequate nutrition, researchers have noted that many older adults are deficient in particular vitamins and minerals, including vitamins B6, B12, D, K, folic acid, and the antioxidant vitamins A, C, E, and beta carotene, as well as the minerals selenium, calcium, and iron, which are essential for overall health [2,7–10] Cognitive function has been found to be affected by nutrition in that malnutrition can cause long-term cognitive impairment [7]. Research findings also indicate that elders with various vitamin deficiencies, especially of B12, may be at risk for cognitive disorders (including dementia) that were previously considered to be due to "normal cognitive aging," while other nutrients such as antioxidants and vitamin C may be protective against cognitive decline [7,8].

Most leading causes of adult deaths in the United States, including coronary heart disease (CHD), cancer, and stroke, are influenced by diet [2]. Vitamin A has an association with vision and a healthy immune system; beta carotene has been associated with reduced risk for cancer and cataracts; and vitamins C, beta carotene, and folic acid may prevent heart disease [2,8–10]. In fact, there is strong evidence that a folic acid deficiency can increase risk for coronary artery disease (CAD) and stroke [8]. Other dietary factors associated with health in advancing age, particularly for women, may be the consumption of a significantly lower percentages of calories from fat and a higher percentage of calories from complex carbohydrates [11]. In relation to dietary fats, future health in both men and women was predicted by higher baseline high-density lipoprotein cholesterol levels, as well as lower low-density lipoprotein cholesterol levels for women. Eating a healthy diet, which has been found to assist with weight reduction and decrease serum cholesterol, is one of the most easily altered risk factors for chronic disease prevention and has been associated with decreasing CAD and osteoporosis, although these require early dietary intervention [5]. Additional findings suggested that optimal calcium intake is critically related to reducing the risk of bone loss and osteoporosis in both men and women and decreasing the incidence of fractures [2]. A diet with high soy protein combined with regular weight-bearing physical activity may protect against osteoporosis [5]. Osteoporosis can prevent optimal physical activity and, in turn, participation in social and community recreational activities, thus denying the benefits of such participation.

The studies cited previously noted the importance of maintaining consistent optimal nutrition. In addition, clinical and epidemiological studies in humans have found that dietary restriction, reduction in food intake, and consumption of a low-calorie diet (1600–2000 cal per day) may maximize life spans and positively affect antiaging and disease prevention [8]. Furthermore, caloric restriction has been found to decrease the risk of the most prominent age-related diseases in humans, including cardiovascular disease, diabetes, and cancers; may delay age-related functional deficits in the brain; reduce the risk of major neurodegenerative disorders including Alzheimer's and Parkinson's; and may promote successful brain aging in humans [8]. Dietary fiber intake is also an important health consideration since it has been found to be associated with lowering blood fat and glucose levels, which may be important in preventing heart disease and diabetes and in promoting colon health [2,11,12].

Degenerative changes of aging are believed to result, in part, from the oxidative destruction of cells and tissues [13]. A group of common food items referred to as "functional foods" (FF) has recently emerged as an active area of research [14,15]. Functional foods are usually defined as healthful foods or food ingredients that have a potential health benefit beyond their nutrient content when consumed regularly in typical quantities as part of a varied diet [14,16]. Their physiologically active components generally include antioxidants. Recent data from the Survey in Europe on Nutrition and the Elderly study show that antioxidant status is positively related to the number of vegetable servings consumed [17]. For example, whole grains, garlic (allyl compound) and soybeans are considered to decrease the risk of both heart disease and cancer [18,19]. Carrots (carotenoids) contain antioxidants that act as modulators of cell growth regulation, regulators of gene expression and immunoregulators [20,21]. Epidemiological evidence has linked tomatoes (lycopene) to protection against cardiovascular disease [22,23] and cancer [24]. Tea (polyphenols) may prevent cancer and CHD [25,26]. Fiber, both soluble and insoluble, may reduce the risk of heart disease and some types of cancer [14]. Finally, vegetables and fruit are associated with lower risk of cancer [27,28].

There are a number of observations consistent with the suggestion that the dipeptide carnosine (beta-alanyl-L-histidine) may exert important roles in aging. Carnosine is found in many long-lived, non-mitotic, mammalian tissues, sometimes at relatively high concentrations (up to 20 mM in human muscle) [29,30]. Evidence suggests that muscle levels of carnosine correlate with species maximum life-span [31,32), while in humans and rats at least, these values appear to decline with age [33]. A most striking observation is that carnosine can delay senescence in cultured human fibroblasts and temporarily reverse the senescence phenotype [34], thus generating a more juvenile appearance. Carnosine can also modify the senescent phenotype of cultured rodent fibroblasts [35]. More recently, Gallant et al. have shown that carnosine can influence age-associated changes and average life-span in senescence-accelerated (SAMP) mice, while lesser beneficial effects were observed in control (SAMR) mice [36].

The mechanism by which carnosine exerts its apparent antiaging effects is uncertain. Many proposals have been made for carnosine's *in vivo* role, which includes physiological buffer, metal ion chelator, antioxidant, and free-radical scavenger [29,30]. Oxygen free radicals are considered to play a primary role in the onset and progression of aging and related phenomena. Hence, it might be anticipated that carnosine's proposed antioxidant activities [37,38,39) could explain its beneficial effects to cultured fibroblasts.

Calorie restriction (dietary restriction), fiber intake, ω-3 fatty acid supplementation, and vitamin E supplementation have been extensively studied for their beneficial effects in delaying disease processes in experimental models. A key characteristic of each of these dietary regimens is their ability to delay or reduce the severity of a multitude of diseases such as autoimmune disease, certain types of cancer, heart disease, and aging. Aging and disease processes are often hard to separate, since thry tend to develop almost simultaneously.

Calorie restriction of 30–40% reduction in food intake is the only known dietary regimen to increase lifespan in all experimental models tested, including yeast, nematodes, flies, and rodents [40].

Aging in humans is manifest not only by the stereotypical changes in phenotype but also by a large increase in the onset of many diseases [41], such as hypertension, CHD, osteoporotic fractures, chronic obstructive pulmonary disease (COPD), malignancy, dementia, and Parkinson's disease.

12.2   HYPERTENSION

There is extensive evidence from both cross-sectional observations and intervention studies showing a positive association between salt intake and blood pressure. Hypertension is a risk factor for congestive heart failure, stroke and myocardial infarction. High salt intake per se may also directly cause heart failure. The Intersalt study showed that the rise in systolic blood pressure with age was only observed in populations with intakes greater than 100 mmol/day of salt [42], while a meta-analysis of 78 trials of salt reduction showed that blood pressure reductions were achieved by sufficiently reducing salt intake [43]. A reduction of 83 mmol of salt per day in elderly people aged 60–78 years was associated with a reduction of 7.2 mmHg in systolic and 3.2 mmHg in diastolic blood pressure in both normo- and hypertensive subjects [44]. Many countries recommend values of not more than 100 mmol of sodium per day. Since stroke is a cause of dementia, reduction in the prevalence of hypertension will also indirectly reduce the burden of dementia as a result of cerebrovascular disease. Apart from reducing salt intakes, diets rich in fruits and vegetables, low-fat dairy products and reduced saturated and total fat have been found to be effective in lowering blood pressure [45), as has oral potassium supplementation [46]. A diet high in potassium has been found to be inversely associated with the risk of developing stroke [47].

12.3   CORONARY HEART DISEASE

The relationship between serum cholesterol and CHD is well established. Widely accepted recommendations for cardiovascular health include a cholesterol intake of <300 mg per day, fat intake of < 30% of total energy, and percentage energy from saturated fats <10% [48].

Recently, the emphasis has been on increasing the intake of vegetable oils and fish, rather than just on lowering cholesterol intake [49]. The ratio of polyunsaturated to saturated fatty acids should be raised to 1.0 or more by increasing the intake of vegetable oils, particularly olive oil, and fish. A modest intake of oily fish (or fish oil capsules) resulted in a 29% reduction in total mortality during the first 2 year after a myocardial infarction (without any change in total plasma cholesterol concentration) [50], while no benefit was observed from conventional high-fiber and low saturated fat diets. The Mediterranean diet, high in antioxidants, vitamins, oleic acid, and ω-3 fatty acids, resulted in a 73% reduction in major cardiac events in patients recovering from a myocardial infarction [51].

In practice, it is likely that advice to adopt this type of diet might be more acceptable than the promotion of low-fat and low-cholesterol diets [52]. Other dietary components have been described to have protective effects: plant sterols [53], flavonoids [54], folate (acting by reducing blood levels of homocystein) [55], alcohol [56], and nuts [57].

12.4   OSTEOPOROTIC FRACTURES

Nutrients important in the prevention of osteoporotic fractures act by increasing bone strength, through increasing bone mineral density or increasing the strength of the bone matrix in other ways. Calcium, vitamin D, protein, and salt intake all play a role. Dietary habit throughout life will affect bone strength, particularly during the period for accretion of peak bone mass. In general, a high calcium intake is recommended in the elderly, because the efficiency of absorption is reduced with age. However, trials to determine the effectiveness of calcium supplementation in preventing fractures have shown conflicting results, some showing a reduction in risk [58, 59], some an increase [60]. Vitamin D and calcium have also been shown to prevent bone loss [61] and fractures [62]. High protein intake predisposes the body to bone loss by mobilizing calcium from the skeleton as a result of endogenous acid production, as well as increasing urinary calcium excretion. The incidence of hip fracture was related to per capita protein consumption [63]. However, very low protein intakes as observed in some elderly vegetarian communities is also associated with low bone mineral density [64], as well as decreased muscle mass, predisposing to falls and fractures. A high sodium intake, by increasing urinary calcium excretion, may also promote bone loss, although convincing evidence is lacking, and the effect may be ameliorated by increasing calcium intake [65].

12.5   CHRONIC OBSTRUCTIVE PULMONARY DISEASE

In patients with COPD, various factors, such as drugs inducing anorexia or shortness of breath, predispose to reduced dietary intake, and at the same time energy cost may be increased by the effort of breathing. Such patients are also prone to repeated episodes of infection, which may further compromise nutritional status. Elderly patients with COPD, similar to those with infection, heart failure, or malignancy, have poorer protein, energy, and vitamin status than healthier elderly people living in the community and long-term care institutions [66]. Energy balance studies in these patients show that there is a negative balance, which may compromise rehabilitation, as well as recovery from or susceptibility to infections. Nutritional supplementation resulted in an improvement of anthropometric indices, vitamin nutritional status, and some measures of well-being [67].

12.6   MALIGNANCY

An estimated 32% of cancers may be avoidable by changes in diet, with 20–42% of cancer deaths possibly avoidable by dietary change [68]. Dietary habits or food choices having an impact include type of food (plant vs. animal source), food preparation (fat and salt content, smoked or pickled foods, etc.), caloric intake, and amount of alcohol consumed. It has been observed that excess energy intake relative to requirements manifests as overweight has negative consequences with regard to several major cancers [69]. Increasing fruit and vegetable consumption possibly reduces cancer risk [70], while moderate wine drinking (two glasses per day) might reduce the risk of death from cancer by 22% [71]. The relationship between cancer and alcohol appears to be U-shape, but there is no clear evidence linking specific beverages to specific cancers [72]. The latest report of the committee on Medical Aspects of Food and Nutrition Policy (COMA) recommends an intake of five or more servings of fruits and vegetables per day, increasing dietary fiber and maintaining a BMI of 20–25 kg/m2. The consumption of red meat should be limited to 90 g daily [73]. Nutritional support should not be neglected in patients with cancer, particularly during therapy.

12.7 DEMENTIA

Deficiency of vitamin B12 can give rise to cognitive impairment ranging from memory defects to a potentially reversible dementia, even in the absence of hematological changes [74]. Antioxidants, such as vitamin E and selegiline [75] have been shown to play a role in retarding the progression of Alzheimer's disease. Estrogen has a beneficial effect on cognitive function, by acting directly on choline acetyl transferase, by stimulating neuronal regeneration, by promoting the breakdown of amyloid precursor protein, or by its antioxidant properties. In this regard, plant phytoestrogens may have a protective role. The Asian diet contains higher quantities of soy products that have a high phyto-estrogen content. This may partly explain the lower prevalence of Alzheimer's disease among Asians compared with Caucasians. It would be desirable to see if the incidence of Alzheimer's disease is lower among vegetarians in various parts of southern Asia.

12.8 PARKINSON'S DISEASE

Dietary factors have been implicated in the etiology of Parkinson's disease. An epidemiological study of environmental and genetic factors carried out in 215 Chinese patients and 313 controls showed that drinking tea regularly was a protective factor, while smoking, family history, and duration of pesticide (farming exposure) were risk factors [76], thus emphasizing the role of environmental toxins in disease causation.

REFERENCES

1. Kirwood, T.B.L., Austad, S.N., 2000. Why do we age? *Nature* 408, 233–238.
2. Shikany, J.M., White, G.L. Jr., 2000. Dietary guidelines for chronic disease prevention. *South Med J.* 93(12):1138–1151.
3. Lueckenotte, A.G., 2000. *Gerontologic Nursing.* 2nd ed. New York: Mosby.
4. Swartzberg, J.E., Margen, S., and the Editors of UC Berkley Wellness Letter, 2001. *The Complete Home Wellness Handbook: Home Remedies, Prevention, Self-Care.* New York: Rebus.
5. Lange-Collette, J., 2002. Promoting health among perimenopausal women through diet and exercise. *J Am Acad Nurs Pract* 14(4):172–177.
6. Pullen, C., Walker, S.N., 2002. Midlife and older rural women's adherence to U.S. dietary guidelines, across stages of change in healthy eating. *Pub Hlth Nurs* 19(3): 170–178.
7. Fillit, H.M., Butler, R.N., O'Connell, A.W., et al., 2002. Achieving and maintaining cognitive vitality with Aging. *Mayo Clin Proc* 77:681–696.
8. Mattson, M.P., Chan, S.L., Duan, W., 2002. Modification of brain aging and neurodegenerative disorders by genes, diet, and behavior. *Physiol Rev* 82(3):637–672.
9. Coutts, A., 2001. Nutrition and the life cycle 4: The healthy diet for the adult. *Br J Nurs* 10(6):362, 365–369.
10. Gonzalez-Gross, M., Marcos, A., Pietrzik, K., 2001. Nutrition and cognitive impairment in the elderly: Review. *Br J Nutr* 86:313–321.
11. Panel issues new guidelines for healthy eating. 2002. *Harvard Women's Health Watch* 10(3):1–3.
12. Fehrenbach, E., Northoff, H., 2001. Free radicals, exercise, apoptosis, and heat shock proteins. *Exerc Immunol Rev* 7:66–89.
13. Martin, A., Prior, R., Shukitt-Hale, B., Cao, G. and Joseph, J.A., 2000. Effects of fruits, vegetables or vitamin E rich diet on vitamins E and C distribution in peripheral and brain tissues: Implications for brain function. *J. Gerontol. Biol. Sci.* 55: B144–B151.
14. Hasler, C.M., 2000. The changing face of functional foods. *J. Am. Coll. Nutr.* 19: 499S–506S.
15. Functional Foods for Health (FFH). University of Illinois at Chicago and University of Illinois at Urbana–Champaign. www.ag.uiuc.edu/ffh (accessed January 2001).
16. American Dietetic Association (ADA). 1999. Position of The American Dietetic Association: functional foods. *J Am Diet Assoc* 99: 1278–1285.
17. Schlettwein-Gsell, D., Brubacher, D., Schroll Bjornsbo, K., Inelmen, E.M., Haller, J. and Van Staveren, W., 2002. Fruit and vegetable servings in ten SENECA towns and the impact of the midday meal. *Age Nutr* 5: 17–22.

18. Craig, W.J., 1997. Phytochemicals: Guardians of our health. *J Am Diet Assoc* 97(suppl.): 199S–204S.
19. Milner, J.A., 1996. Garlic: Its anticarcinogenic and antitumorigenic properties. *Nutr Rev* 54(suppl.): 82S–86S.
20. Rock, C.L., 1997. Carotenoids: Biology and treatment. *Pharmacol Ther* 75: 185–197.
21. Street, D.A., Comstock, G.W., Salkeld, R.M., Schuep, W. and Klag, M.J., 1994. Serum antioxidants and myocardial infarction: Are low levels of carotenoids and alpha-tocopherol risk factors for myocardial infarction? *Circulation* 90: 1154–1161.
22. Clinton, S.K., 1998. Lycopene: Chemistry, biology, and implications for human health and disease. *Nutr Rev* 56: 35–51.
23. Kohlmeier, L., Kark, J.D., Gomez-Gracia, E., Martin, B.C., Steck, S.E., Kardinaal, et al., 1997. Lycopene and myocardial infarction risk in the EURAMIC study. *Am J Epidemiol* 146: 618–626.
24. Tzonou, A., Signorello, L.B., Lagiou, P., Wuu, J., Trichopoulos, D. and Trichopoulou, A., 1999. Diet and cancer of the prostate: a case-control study in Greece. *Int J Cancer* 80: 704–708.
25. Yang, C.S., Chung, J.Y., Yang, G.-Y., Chhabra, S.K. and Lee, M.J., 2000. Tea and tea polyphenols in cancer prevention. *J Nutr* 130: 472S–478S.
26. Stensvold, I., Tverdal, A., Solvoll, K. and Foss, O.P., 1992. Tea consumption: Relationship to cholesterol, blood pressure, and coronary and total mortality. *Prev Med* 21: 546–553.
27. Block, G., Patterson, B. and Subar, A., 1992. Fruit, vegetables, and cancer prevention: A review of the epidemiological evidence. *Nutr Cancer* 18: 1–29.
28. American Cancer Society. Advisory Committee on Diet, Nutrition, and Cancer Prevention. 1996. Guidelines on diet, nutrition and cancer prevention: Reducing the risk of cancer with healthy food choices and physical activity. *CA Cancer J Clin* 46:325–341.
29. Quinn, P.R., Boldyrev, A.A., Formazuyk, V.E., 1992. Carnosine: Its properties, functions and potential therapeutic applications. *Mol Aspects Med* 13, 379–444.
30. Boldyrev, A.A., Formazyuk, V.E., Sergienko, V.I., 1994. Biological significance of histidine-containing dipeptides with special reference to carnosine: Chemistry, distribution, metabolism and medical applications. *Sov Sci Rev D Physicochem Biol* 13, 1–60.
31. Hipkiss, A.R., 2006. Would carnosine or a carnivorous diet help suppress Aging and associated pathologies? *Ann N Y Acad Sci* 1067, 369-74.
32. Munch, G., Thome, J., Foley, P., Schinzel, R., Riederer, P., 1997b. Advanced glycation end products in aging and Alzheimer's disease. *Brain Res Revs* 23, 134–143.
33. Stuerenburg, H.J., Kunze, K., 1999. Concentrations of free carnosine (a putative membrane-protective antioxidant) in human muscle biopsies and rat muscle. *Arch Geront Geriat* 29, 107–113.
34. McFarland, G.A., Holliday, R., 1999. Further evidence for the rejuvenating effects of the dipeptide L-carnosine on cultured human diploid fibroblasts. *Exptl Geront* 34, 35–45.
35. Kantha, S.S., Wada, S., Tanaka, H., Takeuchi, M., Watabe, S., Ochi, H., 1996. Carnosine sustains the retention of cell morphology in continuous fibroblast culture subjected to nutritional insult. *Biochem Biophys Res Commun* 223, 278–282.
36. Galant, S., Semyonova, M., Yuneva, M., 2000. Carnosine as a potential anti-senescence drug. *Biochemistry (Mosc).* 65(7), 866-8.
37. Kohen, R., Yamamoto, Y., Cundy, K.C., Ames, B.N., 1988. Antioxidant activity of carnosine, homocarnosine and anserine present in muscle and brain. *Proc Natl Acad Sci USA* 95, 2175– 2179.
38. Aruoma, O.I., Laughton, M.J., Halliwell, B., 1989. Carnosine, homocarnosine and anserine: Could they act as antioxidants in vivo? *Biochem J* 264, 863–869.
39. Kansci, G., Genot, C., Gandamer, G., 1994. Evaluation of antioxidant effect of carnosine on phospholipids by oxygen uptake and TBA test. *Sci des Aliments* 14, 663–671.
40. Jolly, C.A., 2004. Dietary restriction and immune function. *J Nutr* 134:1853– 1856.
41. Guarente, L., Kenyon, C., 2000. Genetic pathways that regulate aging in model organisms. *Nature* 408, 255–262.
42. Stamler, J., 1993. Dietary salt and blood pressure. In: The Third International Conference on Nutrition in Cardiovascular Diseases, eds. K.T. Lee, Y. Oike, T. Kanazawa. *Ann NY Acad Sci* 676, 122–156.
43. Law, M.R., Frost, C.D. and Wald, J., 1991. IV–Analysis of data from trials of salt reduction. *Br Med J* 302, 819 - 824.
44. Cappuccio, F.P., Markandu, N.D., Camey, C., Sagnella, G.A. and MacGregor, G.A., 1997. Double-blind randomised trial of modest salt restriction in older people. *Lancet* 350, 850–854.
45. Appel, L.J., Moore, T.J., Obarzanek, E., et al., 1997. A clinical trial of the effects of dietary patterns on blood pressure. *N Engl J Med* 277, 1624–1632.

46. Whelton, P.K., He, J., Cutler, J.A., et al., 1997. Effects of oral potassium on blood pressure. *JAMA* 277, 1624–1632.
47. Khaw, K.T. and Barret-Connor, E., 1987. Dietary potassium and stroke-associated mortality: A 12 y prospective population study. *N Engl J Med* 316, 235–240.
48. International Lipid Information Bureau. 1995. *The ILIB Lipid Handbook: Clinical Guide*. Houston, TX: International Lipid Information Bureau.
49. Oliver, M.F., 1998. Cholesterol lowering diets and coronary heart disease. *Br Med J* 317, 1253–1254.
50. Burr, M.L., Fehily, A.M., Gilbert, J.F. et al., 1989. Effects of changes in fat, fish, and fibre intakes on death and myocardial re-infarction: Diet and reinfarction trial (DART). *Lancet II*, 757–761.
51. De Lorgeril, M., Salen, P., Caillat-Vallet, E., Hanauer, M.T., Barthelemy, J.C., and Mamelle, N., 1997. Control of bias in dietary trial to prevent coronary recurrences: The Lyon diet heart study. *Eur J Clin Nutr* 51, 116–122.
52. Conway, S., 1998. Dietary advice should focus on promoting antioxidants and the right sort of fats. *Br Med J* 317, 1254–1255.
53. Miettinen, T.A., Puska, P., Gylling, H., Vanhanen, H., and Vartiainen, E., 1995. Reduction of serum cholesterol with sitostanol-ester margarine in a mildly hypercholesterolemic population. *N Engl J Med* 333, 1308–1312.
54. Kerry, N.L. and Abbey, M., 1997. Red wine and fractionated phenolic compounds prepared from red wine inhibit low density lipoprotein oxidation in vitro. *Atherosclerosis* 135, 93–102.
55. Omenn, G.S., Beresford S.A., and Motulsky A.G., 1998. Preventing coronary heart disease: B vitamins and homocysteine. *Circulation* 97, 421–424.
56. Woodward, M. and Tunstall, P.H., 1995. Alcohol consumption, diet, coronary risk factors, and prevalent coronary heart disease in men and women in the Scottish heart health study. *J Epidemiol Commun Hlth* 49, 354–362.
57. Hu, F.B., Stampfer, M.J., Manson, T.E. et al., 1998. Frequent nut consumption and risk of coronary heart disease in women: Prospective cohort study. *Br Med J* 317, 1341–1345.
58. Reid, I.R., Ames, R.W., Evans, M.C., Gamble, G.D., and Sharpe, S.J., 1995. Longterm effects of calcium supplementation on bone loss and fractures in postmenopausal women: A randomized controlled trial. *Am J Med* 98, 331–935.
59. Recker, R.R., Kimmel, D.B., Hinders, S., and Davies, K.M., 1994. Anti-fracture efficacy of calcium in elderly women. [abstract]. *J Bone Miner Res* 9 (Suppl 1), 135.
60. Cumming, R.G., Cummings, S.R., Nevitt, M.C. et al., 1997. Calcium intake and fracture risk: results from the study of osteoporotic fractures. *Am J Epidemiol* 145, 926–934.
61. Dawson-Hughes, B., Harris, S.S., Knoll, E.A., Gerard, E.D., 1997. Effect of calcium and vitamin D supplementation on bone density in men and women 65 y of age or older. *N Engl J Med* 337, 670–676.
62. Chapuy, M.C., Ariot, M.E., Delmas, P.D., and Meunier, P.J., 1994. Effect of calcium and cholecalciferol treatment for three years on hip fractures in elderly women. *Br Med J* 308, 1081–1082.
63. Abelow, B.J., Holford, T.R., and Insogna, K.L., 1992. Cross-cultural association between dietary animal protein and hip fracture: A hypothesis. *Calcif Tiss Int* 50, 14–18.
64. Lau, E.M.C., Kwok, T., Woo, J., and Ho, S.C., 1998. Bone mineral density in Chinese elderly female vegetarians, vegans, lacto-vegetarians and omnivores. *Eur J Clin Nutr* 52, 60–64.
65. Massey, L.K. and Whiting, S.J. (1996. Dietary salt, urinary calcium and bone loss. *J Bone Miner Res* 11, 731–736.
66. Woo, J., Swaminathan, R., and Mak, Y.T., 1991. Nutritional Status of general medical patients–influence of age and disease. *J Nutr Biochem* 2, 274–280.
67. Woo, J., Ho, S.C., Mak, Y.T., Law, L.K., and Cheung, A., 1994. Nutritional status of elderly patients during recovery from chest infection and the role of nutritional supplementation assessed by a prospective randomized single-blind trial. *Age Ageing* 23, 40–48.
68. Willett, W.C., 1995. Diet, nutrition, and avoidable cancer. *Enviro Hlth Perspect* 103(Suppl 8), 165–170.
69. Albanese, D., 1998. Height, early energy intake, and cancer. *Br Med J* 317, 1331–1332.
70. Ziegler, R.G., 1989. A review of epidemiological evidence that carotenoids reduce the risk of cancer. *J Nutr* 119, 116–122.
71. Dorozynski, A., 1998. Moderate wine drinking reduces all cause mortality. *Br Med J* 316, 645.
72. Sabroe, S., 1998. Alcohol and cancer. *Br Med J* 317, 827–830.
73. White, C., 1998. Report fuels confusion over red meat and cancer. *Br Med J* 316, 797–798.
74. Chiu, H., 1996. Vitamin B12 deficiency and dementia. *Int J Geriatr Psychiat* 11, 851–885.

75. Sano, M., Ernesto, C., Thomas, R.G., et al., 1997. A controlled trial of selegiline, alpha-tocopherol, or both as treatment for Alzheimer's disease. *N Engl J Med* 336, 1216–1222.

76. Chan, D.K.Y., Woo, J., Ho, S.C., et al., 1998. Genetic and environmental risk factors for Parkinson's disease in a Chinese population. *J Neurol Neurosurg Psychiat* 65, 781–784.

13 Nutrition and Cancer Prevention:
An Overview

Elaine B. Trujillo and John A. Milner

CONTENTS

13.1   INTRODUCTION

Cancer is no longer recognized as a consequence of genetic predisposition or an inevitable result of aging. In fact, a plethora of evidence points to environmental factors, including dietary habits, as the primary contributor to about 90% of all cancers. Overall, dietary habits are thought to account for approximately 30% of cancers—a percentage close to that associated with tobacco usage. The actual percentage related to diet is highly dependent on the composition of the diet, the genetics of the consumer, and the type of cancer [1]. Humans are likely exposed to thousands of bioactive food components daily. A host of these compounds, including both essential, and nonessential nutrients, arising from plants (phytochemicals), along with zoochemicals coming from animal products, fungochemicals from mushrooms, and bacterochemicals arising from bacteria in the gastrointestinal tract, may be physiologically relevant modifiers of cancer risk. While literature inconsistencies exist, the basic premise that dietary factors influence cancer risk is undeniable [2].

During the past 30 years epidemiological, and preclinical studies have helped define the linkages between diet, and cancer prevention, and have served as the basis for clinical intervention trials. Evidence–based dietary guidance for reducing cancer risk has surfaced from organizations worldwide. In 2007, The World Cancer Research Fund/American Institute for Cancer Research (WCRF/AICR) global report recommended that individuals be as lean as possible, limit energy-dense foods, avoid sugary drinks, consume "fast foods" sparingly, eat mostly foods of plant origin, limit intake of red meat, avoid processed meat, and limit alcoholic intake [2]. While these

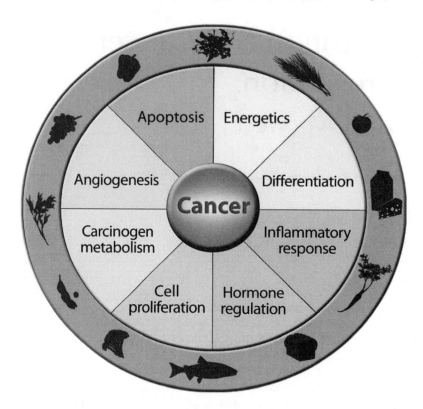

FIGURE 13.1 Foods and their bioactive components can influence multiple processes associated with cancer. Understanding which ones account for a change in cancer risk and tumor behavior is fundamental to understanding the role of diet in cancer prevention. (Davis, C.D. and Milner, J.A. 2007. Molecular targets for nutritional preemption of cancer. *Curr Cancer Drug Targets* 7. With permission.

population-based recommendations are founded on the totality of existing evidence there remains a dearth of information about which specific dietary bioactive food constituents are responsible for a change in cancer risk, the mechanism(s) by which these food components exert their biological effects, and how dietary patterns or composition may affect the response, and how interindividual genetic variations influence the carcinogenic or anticarcinogenic effects of foods or their components [3].

Nevertheless, a host of foods, and their components are reported to modify numerous cancer-related cellular processes including carcinogen metabolism, hormonal balance, cell signaling, cell cycle control, differentiation, apoptosis, and angiogenesis (Figure 13.1) [4]. Identifying which of these processes are being modified singly or in combination, and the dietary exposure needed to bring about a desired outcome in humans, is fundamental to developing effective intervention programs.

The genetic revolution, and the associated "omics" technologies are undeniably providing new insights into the role of nutrition in cancer prevention, particularly through the development of nutritional preemption strategies that builds on an individual's personal profile for providing the best prevention, and therapeutic advice. This approach is based on a personalized understanding of nutrigenomics, proteomics, and metabolomics, sometimes referred to as the "omics" of nutrition, and is fundamental for identifying those who will benefit or be placed at risk because of dietary modification [4].

This review is centered on a select few foods, and beverages (soy, spinach, fish, garlic, tea, wine, tomato, broccoli, oats, and nuts) as a proof-of-principle about how dietary habits can influence cancer risk, and tumor behavior. While the information is not meant to be all-inclusive, the foods were

TABLE 13.1

Selected Foods and their Bioactive Components with Potential Protective Effects Against Cancer

Dietary Sources	Bioactive Component
Berries, grapes	Anthocyanadins
Citrus fruit, carrots, squash, pumpkin	β–Carotene, terpenes
Cruciferous vegetables	Isothiocyanates, Indoles
Fatty Fish	n–3 fatty acids
Grains	Polysaccharides, Lunacin
Meat	Conjugated linoleic acid, selenium
Strawberries, raspberries, walnuts	Ellagic acid
Grapes skin., red wine	Resveratrol
Onions, garlic, leeks	Allyl sulfur compounds, Quercetin
Soybeans, and other legumes	Isoflavones, Bowman-Birk inhibitor
Tea, berries	Catechins
Tomatoes, and related tomato products, guava, watermelon	Lycopene
Dark green leafy vegetables	Carotenoids, Folate
Nuts	Flavonoids, Proanthocyanidins

selected based on their potential for promoting overall health, and in particular cancer prevention. Table 13.1 provides selected foods, and their respective bioactive food components.

13.2 SOY

Soy, a member of the legume family, has been a staple food for Asians for thousands of years. Its beans are used to make a variety of foods such as tofu, as well as flours, and sauces. Pure soy protein, also known as soy isolate, has been used in a variety of meat substitutes, such as burgers, and chicken. In addition, soy protein isolates, and genistein (1000 mg tablets) are available as dietary supplements.

Historically, the chances of breast and prostate cancer was considerably lower in Asians compared with individuals residing in the United States; suggesting that lifestyle factors might be contributing to risk [5,6]. Evidence for this hypothesis was supported by migration studies involving Asian immigrants to the U.S. who acquired a greater prostate cancer incidence within two generations of relocating [7]. Likewise, breast cancer risk tended to increase, especially when Western-style dietary habits were rapidly adopted [8]. Since that era, epidemiological studies have generally linked higher soy intake with a lower cancer risk; however, considerable variability is noted. At least part of this variation likely relates to the quantity, and duration of exposure to soy, the type of soy preparation examined, and interactions between dietary constituents or genes. It should be noted that monitoring soy intake or exposure to its active components is hampered by assessment methodologies, which unfortunately is also true for estimating the intake of most foods, and their constituents. Unquestionably assessing the quantity, and type of soy-related product consumed is fundamental to evaluating its nutritional or pharmacological effects [9].

A meta-analysis of 18 soy studies (12 case-control studies, and 6 cohort studies) provided evidence that a high intake was modestly associated with reduced breast cancer risk (odds ratio = 0.86, 95% CI 0.75–0.99) [10]. When exposure was analyzed in terms of grams per day, a statistically significant association was observed only among premenopausal women [10]. These findings are similar to a meta-analysis of four studies (three cohort, and 11 case-control studies) reported in

2004 that indicated soy food consumption was associated with a lower risk of breast cancer (odds ratio = 0.78, 95% CI 0.68–0.91). In this case, a significant association between high soy intake, and lower risk of breast cancer was also observed in postmenopausal women (odds ratio = 0.64, 95% CI 0.47–0.88) [11]. Although these studies are suggestive of a protection, considerable variability across the studies is evident. At least some of this variability in response to increasing soy may relate to the genetics of the individual. Polymorphisms in enzymes associated with estrogen regulation or metabolism of genistein or other soy active components may influence the overall response [12]. Recent studies suggest that specific polymorphisms in estrogen receptor (ER)–μ can potentially influence the response to soy in men [13].

One of the mechanisms by which soy may function is by modifying estrogen exposure [14,15]. It is generally recognized that a greater lifetime exposure to estrogen is associated with an increase in breast cancer risk. The similarities in structure between the isoflavones in soy, and natural estrogen have fostered numerous studies in animal models to determine if they promote or antagonize this hormone. Generally, phytoestrogens in soy have been shown in animal models to have anti-estrogenic properties, thus supporting the belief that soy dampens estrogen's effects [14,15]. The few human intervention trials published to date have been inconclusive about soy's being a significant modifier of estrogen homeostasis; at least as reflected by changes in the menstrual cycle [16–20]. Overall, a wide range of soy interventions have been used, yet most have not identified a significant change in menstrual cycle duration [20]. A double-blind, randomized trial with 30 healthy premenopausal women evaluated the role of isoflavones on mammographic breast density [19], and could not detect a significant change in mammographic density when 100 mg of isoflavones were consumed daily for 12 months, suggesting that isoflavones do not exert an estrogenic effect—at least at this exposure.

However, some studies do suggest that soy can exert estrogenic effects. For example, the influence of a 60 g soy supplement (45 mg isoflavones) taken twice daily for 14 days on cell proliferation was examined in 48 premenopausal women who were about to undergo breast biopsy for benign or malignant breast disease [17]. Proliferation rates of breast lobular epithelium increased in those who received soy supplementation, suggesting that soy supplements might increase the proliferation of breast neoplasm [17]. Findings from another intervention study were also suggestive of detrimental effects on breast secretion in both pre- and postmenopausal women [21]. In a 12-month study in women (n = 24) who received 38 g of soy protein isolate (38 mg of genistein), there was a two- to sixfold increase in nipple aspirate fluid volume in premenopausal women, although there was no consistent response in postmenopausal women. During the months of soy consumption, plasma estradiol levels were found to increase, which was related to epithelial hyperplasia in at least 29% of the women [21]. This study suggests isoflavones offered an estrogenic boost when provided as a soy protein isolate. Unquestionably, more research is needed to determine whether soy brings about a different response in normal vs. neoplastic cells.

Timing of soy consumption may also be an important variable. Preclinical evidence in animal models, and epidemiological studies in children suggest that exposure to soy or genistein early in life may reduce subsequent breast cancer risk more than if exposure occurs during later life [22]. The response to soy when introduced later in life remains controversial, since few studies have reported a reduction in estrogen or a decrease in menopausal symptoms, as mentioned previously [14]. Part of this response during earlier life may relate to increased sensitivity to changes in hormonal status or to differentiation changes within terminal end buds in the mammary gland.

The anticancer properties of soy are not limited to women, since its intake may also modify prostate cancer risk, possibly by influencing hormonal status [20], although the evidence is relatively weak [2]. In an evidence-based report involving four studies, a nonsignificant decrease in testosterone levels was associated with soy intake, and thus the response may relate to other metabolic changes. However, the small total number of subjects, and multiple confounding factors make firm conclusions difficult [20]. In a study of over 18,000 Japanese men who were followed for incident prostate cancer, there was a nonsignificant decreased risk for those consuming the highest soy intake when compared with the lowest (relative risk of 0.79, 95% CI 0.53–1.18) [23]. One study involving over 12,000 men reported a statistically significant decreased risk with frequent consumption (more than once/day) of soy milk (relative risk of 0.3, 95% CI 0.1–1.0) [24]. Yet another study reported no relationship between soy bean paste soup intake, and prostate cancer [25]. Finally, a study among men of Japanese ancestry in Hawaii reported a nonsignificant beneficial effect for tofu (relative risk of 0.35, 95% CI 0.08–1.43) [26]. Overall, cohort studies have reported a range of biological responses, and thus firm conclusions about benefits remain elusive [23–26]. Four case-control studies did point to a nonsignificant decreased prostate cancer risk with increased intake [27–32].

Preclinical studies provide evidence that genistein can slow the development of stomach cancers by increasing apoptosis, and lowering cell proliferation, and blood vessel growth [33]. Such findings are consistent with rodent studies showing that miso inhibits N-nitrosamine-induced stomach tumors [34]. Several case-control studies suggest a decreased stomach cancer risk in those consuming the highest intake of soy compared with those consuming the lowest amounts [35–43], however, only five of the studies had statistical significance [35, 37–39, 43]. In a cohort study in Korea, there was a nonsignificant decreased risk of stomach cancer with high intakes of soy foods (relative risk 0.60, 95% CI 0.40–1.10) [44]. In Japan, a cohort study provided evidence for a significant inverse association with death from stomach cancer in both men (relative risk of 0.50, 95% CI 0.26–0.93), and women (relative risk of 0.49, 95% CI 0.22–1.13) [45], and in a dose-dependent response.

Soy foods contain a variety of compounds that may contribute to their anticancer effects, including protease inhibitors, saponins, phenolic acids, and isoflavones [5]. These compounds also have been shown to have antioxidant potential, inhibit angiogenesis, and, depending on the exposure, increase apoptosis, and depress cell proliferation [6,47]. Soy-induced changes in estrogen metabolism, as mentioned above, may lead to epigenetic changes by influencing gene promoter regions or by inducing histone modifications that affect chromatin transcription [46].

Soy is known to contain the Bowman-Birk inhibitor (BBI), a small water-soluble protein. BBI is stable within the pH range encountered in most foods, can withstand boiling water temperature for 10 minutes, is resistant to the pH range, and proteolytic enzymes of the gastrointestinal tract, is bioavailable, and is not allergenic. BBI has been reported to reduce the proteolytic activities of trypsin, chymotrypsin, elastase, cathepsin G, chymase, serine protease-dependent matrix metalloproteinases, urokinase protein activator, mitogen-activated protein kinase, and PI3 kinase, and upregulates connexin 43 (Cx43) expression [48]. Several studies have demonstrated the efficacy of BBI against tumor cells *in vitro*, animal models, and human phase IIa clinical trials [48].

13.3 SPINACH

Spinach, *Spinacia oleracea*, is a flowering plant in the family of Amaranthaceae. It contains many essential, and nonessential nutrients. It is a rich source of folate, a B-vitamin that is essential for health. Folate is involved in critical metabolic pathways, including the synthesis of purines, and pyrimidines, which are important for DNA synthesis, and cell replication. Folate is found in dietary supplements, and fortified foods as folic acid. There is evidence that folate is associated with decreased risk of certain cancers, such as colorectal, pancreatic, and esophageal; however, the evidence is primarily derived from epidemiological studies, and randomized intervention trials of folate for cancer prevention are few in number.

Evidence exists that foods containing folate offer protection against colorectal cancer [2]. While there is considerable epidemiological evidence to suggest a dose–response relationship, there are multiple unexplained inconsistencies coupled with potential confounding factors such as dietary fiber [2]. A protective effect of folate intake (0.84, 95% CI 0.76–0.93) per 100 µg/day, with low heterogeneity was found in a meta-analysis of four cohort studies [49–52]. Another meta-analysis of seven cohort studies, and nine case-control studies found a decreased risk of colorectal cancer for those consuming the highest dietary folate intake when compared with the lowest (0.75, 95% CI 0.64–0.89) [53]. In these cohort studies, the association between folate consumption, and colorectal cancer risk was stronger for dietary folate from foods alone (relative risk for high vs. low intake of 0.75, 95% CI 0.64–0.89) than for folate from foods, and supplements (relative risk 0.95, 95% CI 0.81–1.11). The results of these meta-analyses point to a small protective effect of folate against colorectal cancer, especially when marginal intakes are consumed.

The use of blood folate as a predictor of cancer risk, especially with colorectal cancer, has been mixed. In a nested case-control study including 105 cases, and 523 matched controls from the New York University Women's Health Study cohort, there was a statistically significant inverse association between serum folate, and colorectal cancer incidence. The risk of colorectal cancer in individuals in the highest quartile of serum folate was half that of those in the lowest quartile (odds ratio of 0.52, 95% CI 0.27–0.97) [54]. In another case-control study, nested within the Alpha-Tocopherol Beta-Carotene study (ATBC) cohort of male smokers, there was no statistically significant association between serum values, and colorectal cancer [55]. Two case-control studies found red cell or plasma folate were significantly lower in cases than controls [56–58].

Results from a randomized double-blind intervention trial in more than 1,000 participants with a history of colorectal adenomas received either 1 mg of folic acid or placebo or aspirin have been published. Folic acid was associated with higher risks of having three or more adenomas [59]. As adenomas are a risk factor for colon cancer, this study suggests a potentially harmful effect of supplemental folate intake.

It has been hypothesized that diets having lower methyl-group availability, such as a low folate diet, may have increased pancreatic cancer risk, although the evidence is limited [2]. In a nested case-control study within the ATBC study cohort of male Finnish smokers, pancreatic cancer was inversely related to serum folate concentrations, with the highest serum tertiles having approximately half the risk of the lowest (OR of 0.45, 95% CI 0.24–0.82) [60]. Thus, the response to folate may vary depending on the tissue examined.

In another study within the ATBC study cohort, dietary folate intake (not from supplements) was significantly inversely associated with the risk of pancreatic cancer with those in the highest quintile (> 373 µg folate/day) having approximately half the risk compared with those in the lowest quintile (adjusted hazards ratio of 0.52, 95% CI 0.31–0.87) [61]. However, the results of two large U.S. cohorts (Nurses' Health Study, and Health Professionals Follow-up Study) found no association between folate intake (from food, and supplements), and the risk of pancreatic cancer [62]. There was a nonsignificant suggestion of an inverse relation of folate from food (not from supplements) with pancreatic cancer in both cohorts [62]. A meta-analysis of these three cohort studies revealed a summary effect estimate of 0.94 (95% CI 0.80–1.11) per 100 µg/day, with high heterogeneity [61,62] not indicative of a strong association of folate on pancreatic cancer risk.

A large cohort study in Swedish men and women provided evidence that increased intake of folate from food sources, but not from supplements, may reduce pancreatic cancer [63]. Dietary, and total folate intakes were inversely associated with risk of pancreatic cancer. The multivariable rate ratios of pancreatic cancer for those in the highest category of folate intake (≥350 µg/day) compared with the lowest category of intake (< 200 µg/day) were 0.25 (95% CI, 0.11–0.59), and 0.33 (95% CI, 0.15–0.72) for total folate (dietary, and supplemental sources). No association was observed with only folate supplements [63]. This differential effect between folate from foods, and from supplements may be explained by folate's serving as a marker for fruit, and vegetable intake, by a different metabolic response to folic acid in supplements, or as a result of confounders associated with foods vs. supplement usage.

There is also limited evidence that folate protects against esophageal cancer. Eight case-control studies [64–71] all showed a decreased risk for the highest folate intake compared with the lowest, although there was statistical significance in only two of the studies [69,71].

Preclinical evidence suggests that an inadequate intake of folate increases the risk of colorectal cancer possibly by leading to global DNA hypomethylation, which interferes with gene expression, and impairs DNA repair, or by causing uracil misincorporation leading to DNA breaks, and instability [53,72]. Cellular changes, which are linked to an increased risk, appear to occur during inadequacy, and oversupplementation. The ability of folate to increase risk during inadequacy, and excess may actually be reflecting cellular events that are being modified by folate status in normal, and neoplastic cells respectively.

13.4 FISH

Fish, especially saltwater fish, are a source of omega-3 fatty acids, which have been implicated in the prevention of cardiovascular disease, arthritis, asthma, and some cancers. Fish can also be a significant source of selenium, and vitamin D, both of which may have implications in cancer prevention. Epidemiological studies have found total, and saturated fat intake correlates with breast cancer risk. Preclinical studies suggest that saturated fats promote colon carcinogenesis, and that polyunsaturated fat (PUFA) promotes cancers at various sites, including the mammary gland [73]. The PUFA that has been most often linked with tumor promotion in animals is linoleic acid, a member of the omega-6 fatty acids. Linoleic acid is found primarily in vegetable oils such as sunflower, corn, and soybean. Omega-3 fatty acids have been demonstrated to suppress mammary tumor formation, and proliferation in animal models. Likewise, epidemiological studies provide evidence that individuals consuming diets high in omega-3 fatty acids experience a lower prevalence of some cancers. In addition, small trials have assessed the effects of omega-3 fatty acids on immunocompetence by adding omega-3 fatty acids to diets, either through foods rich in this fatty acid or through supplements [74].

Results of omega-3 fatty acid intervention studies to reduce the risk of cancer have been mixed. A systematic review of 38 articles published from 1966 to 2005 concluded that there is insufficient evidence to suggest a significant association between omega-3 fatty acids, and cancer incidence, and that supplementation with omega-3 fatty acids is unlikely to prevent cancer [74]. However, this conclusion is based on an inadequate appreciation of the interactions of omega-3 fatty acids with the total fat content of the diet, the ratio of omega-3 to omega-6 fatty acids provided, and the genetic makeup of the consumer. Regardless, among 65 estimates of associations calculated from 20 different cohorts for 11 different types of cancer, and six different ways to assess omega-3 fatty acids consumption, 10 associations were statistically significant—cancers of the breast, lung, and prostate, and associations were significant for both increased risk, and decreased risk. It should be noted that there was a significant positive association between skin cancer, and the intake of omega-3 fatty acids [74].

Although numerous cohort, and case-control studies [75–96] have investigated fish, and colorectal cancer, only limited evidence suggests that it is protective [2]. A decreased risk for those consuming the highest amounts of fish when compared with the lowest was found in nine cohort studies [75,79–81,83,85,86,89,92,93,95], and was statistically significant in only two [79,80]. A meta-analysis of seven cohort studies [2] gave a summary effect estimate of 0.96 (95% CI 0.92–1.00) per serving/week, with low heterogeneity [75,76,78,82,83,93,95]. The variability in these studies may be partially explained by differing definitions of fish in the studies that included fresh, salted, or dried fish. It also is possible that high fish intake is associated with low meat intake, a potential confounder [2].

Fish oils can inhibit the formation of lymphoid, and hemopoietic cancers in animals. Although most human trials (cohort, and case-control studies) have found nonsignificant relationships with reduced incidence of lymphoid, and hemopoietic cancers [2], two case-control studies found a statistically significant association for nonHodgkins lymphoma [97,98].

Fish is known to be an important natural source of iodine in the diets of different populations, and therefore an association between fish intake, and thyroid cancer risk may be mediated by iodine [2]. In a pooled analysis of 13 case-control studies that investigated fish consumption, there was a significantly reduced incidence of thyroid cancer with increased fish consumption in areas of endemic iodine deficiency, but none in areas where iodine intake were high [99].

Cantonese-style salted fish is probably associated with increased risk of nasopharyngeal cancer [2]. Salted fish contains nitrates, and nitrosamines, which are known mutagens, and animal carcinogens that induce gene mutation. Many case-control studies have investigated the association between Cantonese–style salted fish, and nasopharyngeal cancer risk. A meta-analysis of nine studies suggest an effect estimate of 1.28 (95% CI 1.13–1.44) per serving/week [2]

Adding fish oils to animal diets is typically associated with reduced tumors [73]. Possible mechanisms are thought to revolve around a reduction in omega-6 PUFA-derived eicosanoid biosynthesis (eicosanoids promote inflammation), and direct inhibition of cyclooxygenase-2 (COX-2), an enzyme involved in the production of prostaglandins [74].

13.5 GARLIC

Garlic (*Allium sativum*) is a vegetable that belongs to the Allium class of bulb-shaped plants that also includes onions, chives, and leeks. It has been valued for its medicinal properties for centuries. Garlic has been reported to possess a variety of health benefits, notably antimicrobial, anticarcinogenic, and protective against cardiovascular disease [100]. Garlic has a characteristic flavor, and odor. It is unique because of its high sulfur content, which is most likely involved in its anticancer properties. Garlic also contains other substances that may be beneficial to health, including arginine, selenium, potassium, calcium, magnesium, phosphorus, vitamin C, and folate. Garlic is used for flavoring in cooking, and for its health benefits as garlic supplements, which are available as essential oil, garlic oil macerate, garlic powder, and garlic extract.

Preclinical studies provide some of the strongest evidence that garlic, and its associated sulfur components can suppress tumor incidence in breast, colon, skin, uterine, esophagus, and lung cancers. The mechanisms for this protection may include blockage of nitrosamine formation, suppression in the bioactivation of several carcinogens, enhanced DNA repair, reduced cell proliferation, or induction of apoptosis [101]. It has been postulated that several of these cellular events are occurring simultaneously, and account for the protection observed experimentally by garlic supplementation [101]. Considerable preclinical evidence with model carcinogens, and transplantable tumors supports an anticancer effect of garlic, and some of its allyl sulfur that effectively inhibits colon tumor formation, and also can inhibit cell growth in the laboratory [102–105].

Epidemiological studies suggest that garlic intake may reduce the risk of developing several types of cancer, particularly those related to the gastrointestinal tract, such as cancer of the stomach, esophagus, and colon, as well as breast, and prostate cancer. Many of the studies on garlic, and cancer prevention use different types of garlic preparations, and in varying amounts, which makes it difficult to draw conclusions about the results.

The evidence from epidemiological studies is consistent with a dose–response relationship for garlic, and colorectal cancer prevention [2]. An analysis of data from seven epidemiological studies (three case-control studies, three cohort studies, and one case-control study on colorectal polyps) suggest a protective effect of high intake of raw or cooked garlic on colorectal cancer [106]. Two of the three case-control studies showed a significant inverse association for the uppermost level of raw or cooked garlic consumption, and colorectal cancer [107,108], and the third case-control study found a nonsignificant dose–response trend [109]. One case-control study examining the relationship with colorectal polyps, and garlic intake suggested a significant protective effect [110]. Both cohort studies reported nonsignificant decreased risk when comparing the highest with the lowest garlic intake groups, and a significant inverse association for cancer of the distal colon [77,111]. The only study to examine garlic supplements did not find an association with colorectal cancer incidence [112].

Only a few clinical trials have examined the anticancer effects of garlic. A double-blind randomized study in Japan examined the effect of aged garlic extract (2.4 mL vs. 0.16 mL garlic extract daily) on individuals with colorectal adenomas. At the end of 12 months, those receiving the higher dose of garlic extract had reduced the risk of new colorectal adenomas compared with those receiving the lower dose [113].

Allium vegetables probably protect against stomach cancer [2]. A review of three case-control studies, and one cohort study found a protective effect of raw or cooked garlic, but not for garlic supplement use, for gastric cancer [106,114–117]. Seven case-control studies pointed to a significant decreased risk of stomach cancer when comparing highest with lowest garlic intakes [35,115,118–122]. A meta-analysis of five case-control studies indicated protection with a summary effect estimate of 0.41 (95% CI 0.23–0.73) per serving/day [2,35,41,114,118,119].

In a double–blind randomized trial, more than 5,000 Chinese men, and women with a high risk for stomach cancer received 200 mg of synthetic allitridium (an extract of garlic) daily, and 100 micrograms of selenium every other day or placebo [123,124]. The 5-year follow-up suggested that the intervention was effective in reducing stomach cancer incidence in men (0.36, 95% CI 0.14–0.92) but not in women (1.14, 95% CI 0.22–5.76) [123]. The statistically significant protective effect for men had dissipated at the 10-year follow-up [124]. Another randomized trial in China involving individuals with stomach lesions found that garlic supplementation of 800 mg garlic extract plus 4 mg steam-distilled garlic oil daily for 7 years did not reduce the incidence of stomach cancer [125].

The mechanism(s) by which garlic may influence cancer risk, and tumor behavior remain an area of active investigation. It is known that garlic has antibiotic properties that may act directly against *H. pylori*, and thereby reduce stomach cancer by influencing nitrosamine formation. Other cancer related processes influenced by garlic are depressed carcinogen bioactivation, decreased cellular proliferation, and increased neoplastic apoptosis [105].

13.6 TEA

Tea is one of the most ancient, and popular beverages consumed worldwide. Derived from the leaf of the plant *Camillia sinensis,* it is consumed as black tea, green tea, oolong tea, and white tea. Tea contains polyphenolic compounds—the amount varies depending on the type of tea, and the processing. Most of the research in the area of tea, and cancer prevention has used green tea, and to a lesser extent black tea. Green tea is the result of fresh tea leaves being immediately steamed, and dried, and results in higher amounts of the polyphenol catechin. The most active, and abundant catechin is epigallocatechin-3-gallate (EGCG). Other active polyphenols in green tea include epigallocatechin (EGC), epicatechin-3-gallate (ECG), and epicatechin (EC). Black tea is produced by extended oxidation of tea leaves, and results in more of the complex polyphenols, such as thearubigins, and theaflavins. Oolong tea is partially oxidized, and contains a mixture of the simple, and complex polyphenols. White tea is processed the least, and has an EGCG content similar to that of green tea but differs in the amounts of other polyphenols, and caffeine. Canned, and bottled tea drinks are popular worldwide but they do not retain the polyphenol content that is contained in the traditionally brewed teas [126].

Dietary supplements containing green tea extracts are available, and generally contain varying polyphenol contents. Polyphenon E is a standardized decaffeinated green tea mixture that has been used in animal, and human studies as a preventive agent [127,128]. It contains 200 mg EGCG, 37 mg EGC, 31 mg EC, and other green tea polyphenols per capsule. In comparison, a cup of green tea may contain 100 mg to 200 mg of EGCG, and 120 to 205 mg polyphenols [129]. Preclinical studies have demonstrated the inhibitory action of tea against tumorigenesis in skin, lung, oral cavity, esophagus, stomach, small intestine, colon, liver, pancreas, and mammary gland [130]. Epidemiological studies have linked tea intake to a reduced risk of cancer, including cancer of the colon, stomach, breast, ovary, and prostate. However, results of these trials have been inconsistent; some studies have shown reduced cancer incidence, and recurrence associated with tea consumption, others have failed to show an effect [131]. A case-control study nested within the Shanghai Cohort Study of the 18,244 men compared with 772 cohort controls used a urinary tea polyphenol marker to determine the association between urinary polyphenol concentration, and stomach, and esophageal cancer risk [132]. Urinary EGC positivity showed a statistically significant inverse association with stomach cancer (OR 0.52, 95% CI 0.28–0.97). Although this biomarker study suggests a preventive effect of tea on stomach cancer, several others studies yield conflicting results. A wealth of evidence does not support that green tea possibly protects against stomach cancer [2], and nine epidemiological trials of green tea consumption on gastrointestinal cancers in Japan, and China had conflicting results [133–141].

Epidemiological studies have investigated the role of tea on breast cancer risk. In a prospective study of 1,160 Japanese women with invasive breast cancer, there was a significantly decreased risk with a consumption of three or more cups of green tea daily (HR 0.69, 95% CI 0.47–1.0). The reduction was particularly noteworthy in women with stage I breast cancer (HR 0.43, 95% CI 0.22–0.84) [142]. A case-control study of Asian American women in the United States also reported a significant decreased risk with increasing amounts of green tea intake in association with none, 0–85.7 mL (approximately 3 ounces), and > 85.7 mL of green tea per day. Interestingly, there was no association between black tea consumption, and breast cancer risk [143]. It should be noted, however, that in a pooled analysis of two prospective studies involving 35,004 women that drinking up to five or more cups of green tea daily was not associated with a lower breast cancer risk, and, likewise, no association was found for black tea [144]. Epidemiological studies of other cancers, including cancers of the pancreas, kidney, bladder, lung, prostate, and ovary also have been inconsistent.

Few clinical trials have investigated the role of tea in cancer prevention, and again the results are inconclusive. The role of tea on serum pepsinogen levels has been examined as this is considered a marker for stomach atrophy, and stomach cancer. In a study of 163 individuals who consumed 100 mg capsules of tea polyphenols for 1 year, there was no significant decrease in serum pepsinogen levels [145].

The role of green tea supplements (5 mg of decaffeinated green tea extract) was investigated in 200 Chinese with esophageal precancerous lesions. After 12 months, there was no difference in those receiving the green tea extract, and the controls in terms of precancerous lesions [146].

There is some evidence for a protective effect of tea on oral cancer as evidenced in a double–blind intervention study of 59 oral mucosa leukoplakia patients who received 3 g of mixed tea orally, and topically or a placebo (orally, and topically). After 6 months, the size of the oral lesions was significantly decreased in 38% of those in the tea group compared with 10% in the placebo group. In addition, pathological examination revealed significantly decreased cell proliferation in the tea group, indicating a protective effect of tea on oral cancer [147].

Several studies have examined tea consumption, and the risk of prostate cancer. In a double-blind study of 60 men with high-grade intra-epithelial neoplasia who received 200 mg of green tea catechin or a placebo three times daily for 1 year, significantly fewer prostate cancers were detected in the tea group (3% compared with the placebo group (30%) [148].

The association of tea consumption, and cancer risk has been investigated using a marker for DNA oxidative damage, 8-hydroxydeoxyguanosine (8-OHdG). Although direct evidence that links 8-OHdG with cancer risk is lacking, urinary 8-OhdG has been found to be higher in individuals with lung cancer. In addition, human cancer cells from the breast, lung, liver, kidney, brain, stomach, and ovary have higher contents for 8-OHdG than tissues without tumors [149]. Two randomized controlled studies found associations of tea consumption, and decreased 8-OHdG levels [149,150]. In a study of 133 heavy smokers who were randomized to receive either four cups/day of decaffeinated green tea, decaffeinated black tea, or water for 4 months, there were significantly decreased urinary 8-OHdG levels in the green tea group, and no change in the black tea group [149]. In a double–blind study of 124 individuals at risk for hepatic cancer who received either placebo, 500 mg green tea polyphenol supplement, or 1,000 mg green tea polyphenol supplement, those in the green tea supplement groups showed a significant decrease in urinary 8-OHdG levels compared with the placebo group [150]. These studies suggest that green tea polyphenols reduce DNA damage, and potentially may reduce the risk for cancer.

Many mechanisms have been proposed for the inhibition of carcinogenesis by tea, including the modulation of signal transduction pathways that leads to the inhibition of cell proliferation, and transformation, induction of apoptosis of preneoplastic, and neoplastic cells, and the inhibition of tumor invasion, and angiogenesis [130]. Not only have a host of studies provided evidence that EGCG can block carcinogenesis in a variety of tissues, it can inhibit mitogen-activated protein kinases (MAPK), activation of activator protein 1 (AP-1), and nuclear factor-B (NF-kappaB), topoisomerase I, matrix metalloproteinases, and potentially several other specific targets (151).

Not all the anticancer effects linked to tea can be associated with polyphenols. L-theanine is another compound found in tea with potential anticancer properties (152). Clinical studies provide evidence that the oral consumption of this tea component enhances γδ T-cell proliferation, and interferon–⊠ secretion suggesting a role in immunocompetence. The significance of these studies awaits additional examination of the influence of exposures, and duration on these, and other food components. (152)

13.7 WINE

Wine is an alcoholic beverage made from the fermentation of grape juice. Its history dates back to 6000 to 5000 B.C. A popular beverage, it is used to accompany, and enhance various cuisines, and has been used for many years in religious ceremonies in many cultures, and regions. Moderate consumption of no more than two drinks per day is associated with lower overall mortality, primarily due to lower cardiovascular deaths. However, heavy drinking has deleterious effects, both physically, and socially, and it has been estimated that 3% of all cancer deaths in the United States can be attributed to alcohol consumption [1]. Large quantities of alcohol are associated with increased risk of cancer of the gastrointestinal tract [153–155]. Alcoholic drinks have been implicated as a factor for premenopausal, and postmenopausal breast cancer. Rather convincing evidence exists that cancers of the mouth, pharynx, larynx, and esophagus are linked to alcoholic drinks. The same case is likely for liver cancer [2]. Potential beneficial effects of moderate alcohol consumption are suggested by a J-shaped association between low consumption of wine with cancer, although such data are difficult to interpret [156].

Unlike other alcoholic beverages, wine, particularly red wine, contains substantial amounts of polyphenolic substances such as flavonoids (flavones, flavanones, anthocyanins, catechins), and nonflavonoid phenols. Proposed preventive/therapeutic properties of polyphenols include increased levels of HDL cholesterol, decreased platelet aggregation, and endothelial adhesion, antioxidant activity, free radical scavenging, inhibition of cell proliferation, and angiogenesis [156]. One particular nonflavonoid polyphenolic compound, resveratrol, has received more attention for its potential preventive properties [153]. Resveratrol is synthesized in the skin of grapes, and, as the skins are removed much earlier for the preparation of white wine, red wine contains much higher amounts of resveratrol [156]. A few studies have evaluated the effects of specific alcoholic beverages, including beer, wine, and spirits, on cancer mortality. In a large prospective study of middle-aged men in France, mortality from cancer was observed for those consuming two to five drinks per day (RR of 0.81), and approximately 82% of alcohol intake was attributed to wine consumption [157]. Studies from a pooled cohort from Denmark showed different effects of moderate drinking, and wine intake. There was no change in cancer risk for light drinkers (eight to 21 drinks per week) [158] overall, but some differences in types of alcohol consumed. Light consumption of beer and spirits slightly increased the risk of cancer, and similar consumption of wine decreased mortality from all causes, and from cancer. Wine drinkers had a lower risk of death from cancer at all levels of alcohol intake than nonwine drinkers. However, the relative risk for wine drinkers became higher than one for cancer when the daily consumption was more than three drinks per day [158]. In this same cohort, the risk of lung cancer in men was significantly decreased by consumption of more than 13 drinks of wine per week (RR of 0.44, 95% CI 0.22–0.86) while consumption of corresponding amounts of beer, and spirits increased the risk [159]. Similarly, in the same cohort, consumption of seven or more drinks of beer or spirits per week significantly increased the risk of cancer of the upper digestive tract, while the same consumption of wine gave a relative risk of 0.4 (0.2–0.8) [160]. When the proportion of wine in total alcohol intake was over 30%, consumption of seven to

21 drinks per week was associated with a relative risk of 0.5 (0.2–1.4) while subjects who drank the same amount of alcohol but no wine had a relative risk of three [160].

There is substantial evidence that alcohol intake is an important factor in determining esophageal cancer risk [2]. Ten case-control studies [161–169], one cross-sectional study [170], and five ecological studies provide a wealth of evidence linking drinking habits with esophageal cancer [171–175]. All but one of the case-control studies identified wine intake with an increased risk of esophageal cancer [162], which was statistically significant in seven [163–165,167,169].

Alcohol is a cause of cirrhosis, which predisposes to liver cancer, but the factors that determine why some people are susceptible to cirrhosis are not known. According to the WCRF/AICR report, alcoholic drinks are a probable cause of liver cancer [2]. One cohort study identified a nonsignificant increased risk with increased wine intake [176], two studies showed that there was no significant effect on liver cancer risk [177,178], and a case-control study indicated a nonsignificant increased risk [179].

The evidence that alcoholic drinks are a cause of mouth, pharynx, and larynx cancers is rather compelling [2]. Several case-control studies that specifically evaluated cancers of the mouth, pharynx, and larynx showed increased risk with increased wine intake [180–195], which was statistically significant in some [181–184,186,187,189,196,197]. Five studies provided evidence for a depression in risk [196–200], which was statistically different in one [199,200]. A meta–analysis of 11 case-control studies provided a summary effect estimate of 1.02 (95% CI, 1.01–1.03), with rather high heterogeneity [2,181,182,184,186–189,191,192,195,198]. Evidence that alcohol consumption is associated with increased breast cancer risk in both premenopausal, and postmenopausal women is convincing, and is based on ample data from cohort, and case-control studies [2]. There is less evidence for a role of wine consumption on breast cancer risk.

A prospective study in Canada reported the risk of death from breast cancer increased with intakes of total alcohol of 10–20 g per day, and greater than 20 g per day, and this increase was contributed largely by the intake of wine, a 15% increase in risk at intakes higher than 10 g per day of alcohol from wine [201]. Other studies failed to show that wine was associated with an increase in breast cancer risk. In the Framingham Study, the risk of breast cancer was not significantly associated to consumption of wine, beer, or spirits [202]. The pooling Project of Prospective Cohort Studies in the United States reported approximately a 10% increase of breast cancer risk by each daily increase of 10 g of alcohol (approximately 0.75 to one drink per day); the effect of wine was not significant (RR of 1.05, CI 0.98–1.12), and was similar to the effect of beer, and spirits [203].

Resveratrol has been proposed to affect initiation or promotion, and progression of the cancer process [204,205], and it has been postulated to affect inhibition of cytochrome P450 enzymes [206], antioxidant properties [207], anti-inflammatory activities [206], and effects on cell cycle, cell proliferation, and apoptosis [208]. Thus, it is possible that the overall response is pleitrophic. The effective concentrations of resveratrol needed to bring about these changes *in vivo* remains unclear.

13.8 TOMATO

Tomato, *Lycopersicon esculentum*, is a member of the Solanaceae family, and, although it is generally consumed as a vegetable, the tomato is a fruit. Tomatoes are consumed worldwide in the form of processed foods such as juices, purees, paste, sauces, and soups. Several beneficial nutrients are contained in tomatoes, and have received attention for their potential preventive effects. Tomatoes contain carbohydrates, fiber, minerals, proteins, vitamins, and a variety of antioxidants, including ascorbic acid, β-carotene, chlorogenic acid, rutin, tocopherol, copper, iron, and chromium. Rightly or wrongly, the beneficial effects of tomatoes have largely been attributed to the carotenoids they contain. Lycopene, the most abundant carotenoid in tomatoes, is what makes the tomato red. Green tomatoes do not contain lycopene—they contain high amounts of chlorophyll. Other carotenoids in tomatoes include phytoene, phytofluene, α-carotene, β-carotene, and γ-carotene [209].

The bioavailability of lycopene is influenced by food processing, cooking, and other components in the meal, including lipids, and fiber. Lycopene is absorbed more efficiently from heat-processed foods than from unprocessed sources, and from lipid-rich diets. The Mediterranean style of consuming tomatoes cooked in olive oil facilitates release of lycopene from tomatoes, and favors its maximal absorption. The *cis* isomer has been shown to be more bioavailable than the *trans* isomer [209].

Several clinical studies have reported an inverse association between tomato or lycopene intake, and the risk of some types of cancer. A systematic review of 72 epidemiological studies reported a consistent inverse relationship between intakes of tomatoes, and plasma lycopene levels, and prostate, lung, and stomach cancer [210]. There is a substantial amount of consistent evidence that foods containing lycopene probably protect against prostate cancer [2]. In a cohort of the Health Professionals Follow-up study, lycopene intake was significantly related to lower risk of prostate cancer. The combined intake of tomatoes, tomato sauce, tomato juice, and pizza, which accounted for 82% of lycopene intake, was inversely associated with the risk of prostate cancer (relative risk of 0.65, 95% CI 0.44–0.95) for consumption frequency greater than 10 vs. fewer than 1.5 servings per week [211]. Additional data from this same cohort confirmed that frequent tomato or lycopene intake was associated with a reduced risk of prostate cancer. The relative risk for high vs. low quintiles of intake were 0.84 (95% CI 0.73–0.96), and the intake of tomato sauce, the primary source of bioavailable lycopene, was associated with an even greater reduction in prostate cancer risk with a relative risk for ≥ 2 servings/week vs. < 1 serving/month of 0.77 (95% CI 0.66–0.90) [212]. In a cohort study involving approximately 14,000 Seventh-day Adventist men, increasing consumption of tomatoes conferred significant protection against prostate cancer [213]. However, other cohort studies have found no significant association [214] or a nonsignificant increased risk of prostate cancer with tomato intake [215]. A meta-analysis on four cohort studies found a summary effect estimate of 0.69 (95% CI 0.43–1.08) per serving/day, with moderate heterogeneity [2], suggesting a protective effect of tomatoes on prostate cancer risk.

The evidence that tomato intake is associated with stomach cancer is less compelling. In two large cohort studies, the Netherlands Cohort, and the Japan Collaborative Cohort, there was no significant association of tomato intake, and stomach cancer risk [216,217]. Most case-control studies that have examined the relationship of tomato intake, and stomach cancer risk have shown decreased risk with increased intake [41,115,116,119,120,218–223].

Cellular, and molecular studies have shown lycopene to be one of the most potent antioxidants. It has been suggested to prevent oxidations of critical biomolecules including DNA, proteins, and lipids [209,224]. Lycopene exhibits radical quenching activity twice that of β-carotene, and 10 times that of β-tocopherol [227]. Lycopene has been demonstrated to induce phase II detoxification enzymes that are regulated by the antioxidant response element, and the transcription nuclear factor E2-related factor 2 [209,226]. Lycopene is hypothesized to suppress carcinogen-induced phosphorylation of regulatory proteins such as p53, and retinoblastoma, and stop cell division at the G_0–G_1 cell cycle phase [209].

13.9 BROCCOLI

Broccoli, *Brassica oleracea*, a plant of the cabbage family (Brassicaceae), is considered a cruciferous vegetable, along with cauliflower, cabbage, and Brussels sprouts. These contain multiple nutrients, and phytochemicals including folate, fiber, carotenoids, and chlorophyll, with potential cancer preventive properties. Cruciferous vegetables are rich sources of glucosinolates, sulfur-containing compounds that are responsible for the pungent aroma, and bitter taste of the vegetables. The hydrolysis of glucosinolates by plant enzymes results in the formation of biologically active compounds, including indoles, and isothiocyanates. Broccoli, and broccoli sprouts are a good source of glucoraphanin, the glucosinolate precursor of sulforaphane, and glucobrassicin, the precursor of indole-3-carbinol [227]. Sulforaphane has been shown to be an effective preventive agent in cell culture, and in carcinogen-induced, and genetic animal models [228–229].

Intriguing evidence linking broccoli intake with reduced cancer risk has surfaced in studies in China. Broccoli consumption was linked to a reduced liver cancer risk in a randomized, placebo-controlled trial in Qidong, People's Republic of China. The individuals living in Qidong are at high risk for the development of hepatocellular carcinoma, in part because of the consumption of aflatoxin-contaminated foods and exposure to high levels of phenanthrene, a sentinel of hydrocarbon air toxics. Two hundred residents were given hot drinking water infused with 3-day-old broccoli sprouts (containing either 400 or < 3 μmol glucoraphanin nightly for 2 weeks). There was an inverse association for the excretion of dithiocarbamates, and urinary aflatoxin–DNA adducts, and *trans*, anti-phenanthrene tetraol, a metabolite of the combustion product phenanthrene in the intervention arm. An inverse correlation between sulforaphane treatment, and excretion of carcinogens was detected, suggesting induction of one or more phase II enzymes [228].

Sulforaphane metabolites arising from broccoli have also been observed in human breast tissue epithelial cells following an oral dose of a broccoli sprout preparation (200 mμmol of sulforaphane), suggesting that bioactive compounds within this food can reach multiple target sites [229]. A clinical trial involving 20 men determined that the consumption of 250 g/day (9 oz/day) of broccoli, and 250 g/day of Brussels sprouts significantly increased the urinary excretion of a potential carcinogen found in well–done meat, namely the heterocyclic amine, 2-amino-1-methyl-6-phenylimidazo[4,5-*b*]pyridine (PhIP) [230]. Thus, these data provide evidence that a high cruciferous vegetable intake may decrease colorectal cancer risk by enhancing the conjugation, and elimination of some carcinogens.

Cohort studies in the United States, Europe, Shanghai, and Singapore provide evidence that enhanced cruciferous vegetable intake is associated with a reduction in cancer risk at several sites, including the lung, breast, colon, rectum, and prostate [231]. A population-based case-control study of prostate cancer evaluated the induction of phase II enzymes, including glutathione S-transferases (GSTs). In this study of 428 men with incident prostate cancer, and 537 community controls, intakes of cruciferous vegetables, and of broccoli, the greatest source of sulforaphane, were associated with decreased prostate cancer risk at all levels above the lowest consumers (adjusted fourth quartile odds ratio of 0.58, 95% CI 0.38, 0.89, and 0.72, 95% CI 0.49, 1.06), respectively. In relation to genotypes, there was a nonsignificant increase in risk with the GSTT1 null genotype (OR of 1.51, 95% CI 0.98, 2.31) but no effects of GSTM1 genotype. However, men with GSTM1-present genotype, and high broccoli intake had the greatest reduction in risk (odds ratio 0.49, 95% CI 0.27, 0.89) [232]. These findings suggest that two or more servings per month of cruciferous vegetables may reduce risk of prostate cancer, especially among men with GSTM1-present alleles.

In vitro, and *in vivo* studies have shown that sulforaphane affects many steps of cancer development, including modulating the early stages of the carcinogenetic process (initiation) or affecting events, such as apoptosis, cell proliferation, and angiogenesis [233]. Pathways that block metabolic activation of carcinogens can effectively hamper initiating events in the carcinogenetic process. Evidence suggests that sulforaphane attenuates the effects of carcinogens via inhibition of phase I enzymes, and induction of phase II enzymes [233–235]. Sulforaphane protects DNA from chemical insult, and is a potent inhibitor of genotoxicity induced by compounds acting through different mechanisms [233,236]. Several studies demonstrated the ability of sulforaphane to modulate events involved in the clonal expansion of transformed cells, and in the formation of a premalignant lesion, such as cell-cycle progression, apoptosis, and autophagy [233,237,238]. Sulforaphane has been identified as a novel histone deacetylase (HDAC) inhibitor, which has been shown to induce apoptosis via de-repression of genes such as p21, and bax [233,239]. Finally, sulforaphane can interfere with essential steps that characterize the progression phase of the carcinogenetic process, such as the progression of benign to malignant tumors, angiogenesis, and metastasis formation [233, 240–242].

A small human study found a single dose of 68 g broccoli sprouts markedly inhibited histone deacetylase activity in peripheral blood mononuclear cells within a few hours following consumption. These findings provided evidence of one genetic mechanism through which sulforaphane may bring about multiple cellular changes simultaneously [239].

13.10   OATS

The common oat plant, *Avena sativa*, is a species of cereal grain grown for its seed. Oats have numerous uses in food, most commonly they are rolled or crushed into oatmeal or ground into fine oat flour. Oats are widely known for their cholesterol-lowering properties, and potential to reduce the risk of heart diseases. In 1988, the Food, and Drug Administration allowed a health claim on food labels containing soluble fiber from whole oats (oat bran, oat flour, and rolled oats)—three grams of soluble fiber daily from these foods, in conjunction with a diet low in saturated fat, cholesterol, and fat, may reduce the risk of heart disease.

Dietary fiber, composed of plant cell walls, and components obtained from those walls, also includes nonstarch polysaccharides from sources other than plant cells walls [243]. Dietary fiber is frequently classified as soluble, and insoluble. Generally, soluble dietary fibers are quickly, and extensively degraded, and fermented in the colon; examples include psyllium, and pectin. Insoluble fibers are degraded much more slowly, and with a much slower production of short chain fatty acids, and include fruits, vegetables, and wheat [243].

Oats contain a soluble fiber known as β-glucan, which is widely found in grains, barley, yeast, bacteria, algae, and mushrooms. β-glucan has been evaluated with regard to its various effects, including its anticarcinogenic effects. *In vitro*, complement activation causes soluble yeast β-glucan to prime neutrophils or natural killer cells for cytotoxicity against specific tumors [244]. Thus, β-glucan-mediated tumor immunotherapy utilizes a novel mechanism by which innate immune effector cells are primed to kill tumor cells [244]. There have been numerous randomized controlled studies on the use of β-glucan in cancer treatment, primarily from Japan, and using the yeast form of β-glucan [245]. Although yeast glucan administered to cancer patients has been shown to enhance the effect of chemotherapy or radiation therapy, and had a positive effect on survival, and quality of life, most of the studies were carried out in one area of the world, and largely by one research team, thus raising questions about the applicability to other circumstances [245].

A plethora of data suggests that foods containing dietary fiber protect against colorectal cancer. This hypothesis evolved from the observation that rural Africans whose diets contained large amounts of unprocessed food plants, especially cereals, had a low incidence of colorectal cancer [246]. Since then, there have been numerous epidemiological studies. A review of the literature by the American Gastroenterological Association concluded that correlation studies showed a strong inverse relationship between dietary fiber intake, and risk of colorectal cancer [247]. The recent WCRF/AICR report suggests that dietary fiber probably protects against colorectal cancer, although the evidence for cereals, and grains was too limited to make a conclusion [2].

Several studies have examined specific types of dietary fiber as modifiers of cancer risk. In a meta–analysis, nine out of 10 case-control studies reported an inverse association between whole grain consumption, and risk of colorectal cancer or adenoma with an odds ratio for the highest compared with the lowest consumption of 0.79 [248]. Two cohort studies reported no association between overall whole grain consumption, and risk of colorectal cancer [81,249]. In the Swedish Mammography Cohort of over 61,000 women, high consumption of whole grains was associated with a lower risk of colon cancer with a rate ratio of 0.67 (95% CI, 0.47–0.96) for the higher whole grain consumers (≥ 4.5 servings/day) compared with the lower consumers (< 1.5 servings/day) [250]. Additionally, in the National Institutes of Health–AARP Diet and Health Study of over 225,000 men, and women, dietary fiber intake was not associated with colorectal cancer but fiber from grains was significantly associated with a lower risk of colorectal cancer (relative risk of 0.86, 95% CI 0.76–0.98) [251].

There have been several proposed mechanisms for how dietary fiber protects against colorectal cancer. It has been suggested that the consumption of increased amounts of dietary fiber leads to an increase in fecal weight, and a decrease in transit time, and thereby decreases the probability of carcinogen interaction with the colonic mucosa [243]. This mechanism also could lead to enhanced removal of secondary bile acids, thought to be tumor promoters, and increased excretion of estrogens, thereby protecting against breast cancer [243,252]. Another possible mechanism is thought to be related to the production of short chain fatty acids (SCFA) in the colon. The production of SCFA can change the colonic microflora, leading to functional changes that include the production of microbial enzymes, which are considered important in carcinogen activation. SCFAs provide the primary energy source for the growth of the normal mucosa. The SCFA butyrate has been studied for its ability to induce differentiation, and apoptosis of colonic tumor cells in tissue culture [253], and affect the expression of several key genes in carcinogenesis [254]. Other hypotheses include dietary fiber modulating glycemia, and insulemia, and the production of antioxidant properties from bacterial growth in the colon [243].

13.11   NUTS

Nuts are the oily kernels found within a shell, and used in food. They are used in cooking, eaten raw, roasted, or pressed for oil used in cookery, and cosmetics, and are considered an important component of a healthy diet. Nuts are nutrient-dense, and provide protein, fat, dietary fiber, and many bioactive food components such as folic acid, niacin, vitamin E, vitamin B6, copper, magnesium, potassium, zinc, carotenoids, flavonoids, proanthocyanidins, and phytoestrogens [255].

Nuts are touted to promote heart health, primarily due to their fatty acid composition. They are high in unsaturated fats, especially monounsaturated fatty acids, and some nuts. Walnuts, in particular, contain high amounts of the omega-3 fatty acid alpha-linolenic acid. Although there is evidence to suggest that omega-3 fatty acids from eicosapetnanoic acid, and docosahexanoic acid (primarily from fish) may be protective of some types of cancer, the role of alpha-linolenic acid in cancer prevention is less clear. A meta-analysis of nine cohort, and case-control studies that reported on the association between alpha-linolenic acid, and the incidence of prevalence of prostate cancer showed an increased risk of prostate cancer in men with a high intake or elevated blood level of alpha-linolenic acid (relative risk of 1.7) [256].

Cohort, and case-control studies suggest a reduction in colon cancer risk with increased nut intake. In a prospective observational cohort study, the Adventist Health Study, the protection (relative risk) from nuts on colon cancer risk for intakes of one to four times per week compared with less than once per week were 67 (95% CI 0.45–0.98), but not for higher intakes [257]. However, three human case-control studies have provided mixed results. There was either no protective effect of combined higher intake of nuts and legumes [258,259], or a significant linear dose–response protective effect with higher combined intake of pulses, nuts, and seeds in women, but not in men [260]. Unfortunately, these studies did not separate the effects of nuts, and seeds from legumes, which could potentially be related to the observed variation in results.

An animal study assessed the effect of almonds on colon cancer, specifically by examining aberrant crypt foci (ACF), possible precursors of colon cancer. Rats fed an isocaloric, macronutrient-matched high-fat, low-fiber diet formulated using whole almonds, almond meal, or almond oil had a large, and statistically significant dietary treatment-related decline in ACF [261]. These results suggest that almond consumption may be an effective preventive agent, but further studies in multiple models are needed.

Other bioactive food components in nuts are preventive properties, including selenium, and vitamin E. Few epidemiologic studies have investigated the association of cancer risk with diets providing large amounts of vitamin E. The WCRF/AICR report concluded that there is limited evidence suggesting that foods containing vitamin E protect against esophageal, and prostate cancer [2]. International evidence suggests an inverse association between selenium status, and cancer mortality [262]. There is limited evidence that foods containing selenium protect against lung, colorectal, or stomach cancer; however, evidence from cohort, and case-control studies is consistent for a dose–response relationship that foods containing selenium probably protect against prostate cancer [2]. The ongoing Selenium, and Vitamin E Cancer Prevention Trial, which is investigating the role of vitamin E, and selenium in prostate cancer prevention, may provide insights into the abilities, and possible mechanisms by which vitamin E, and selenium might function as preventive agents.

13.12 FUTURE DIRECTIONS

Evidence continues to mount that foods eaten can profoundly influence cancer risk, and tumor behavior. However, the response is likely dependent on the interactions of thousands of bioactive components that occur in the foods consumed, and the genetics of the consumer. These effects, which may be inhibitory or stimulatory, depending on the specific bioactive food component, are surely mediated through multiple, and diverse biological mechanisms. The identification, and elucidation of the specific molecular sites for food components is critical for identifying those individuals who will benefit maximally or be placed at risk from dietary change. Until this information is available it remains prudent to eat a variety of foods, and to maintain a healthy weight through controlling caloric intake, and exercise.

It is becoming increasing apparent that not all individuals respond identically to foods or their isolated components. Additional research aimed at determining the physiological consequences of nutrigenomics—which includes nutrigenetic (genetic profiles that modulate the response to food components), nutritional transcriptomics (influence of food components on gene expression profiles), and nutritional epigenomics (influence of food components on DNA methylation, and other epigenetic events, and vice versa)—should help with preemptive strategies for reducing cancer risk or suppressing the aggressiveness of neoplasms [263]. New reports are constantly surfacing that population studies are underestimating the significance of diet in overall cancer prevention, and therapy, and that subpopulations may be particularly sensitive to subtle changes in eating behaviors. Advances in the understanding of the diet, and cancer prevention interrelationship will require a greater understanding of (1) exposures needed to bring about a desired response, (2) which change in a biological process can be used to predict a change in cancer risk, and (3) what gene–nutrient, and nutrient–nutrient interactions are critical for determining a positive or negative response. As the science of nutrition unfolds, a clearer understanding will surely emerge about how foods, and their components can be effectively used to reduce cancer burdens, and how agronomic or biological technologies can be used to modify the food supply. While the challenges to unraveling the relationships between diet, and cancer prevention are enormous, so are the societal, and health benefits.

REFERENCES

1. Doll, R. and Peto, R. 1981. The causes of cancer: Quantitative estimates of avoidable risks of cancer in the United States today. *J Natl Cancer Inst* 66, 1191–1308.
2. World Cancer Research Fund/American Institute for Cancer Research. 2007. Food, nutrition, physical activity, and the prevention of cancer: A global perspective. Report. AICR, Washington DC.
3. Greenwald, P., Clifford, C. K., and Milner, J. A. 2001. Diet and cancer prevention. *Eur J Cancer* 37, 948–965.
4. Davis, C.D. and Milner, J.A. 2007. Molecular targets for nutritional preemption of cancer. *Curr Cancer Drug Targets* 7, 410–5 .
5. Parker, S. L., Tong, T., Bolden, S., and Wingo, P. A. 1997. Cancer statistics, 1997. *CA Cancer J Clin* 47, 5–27.
6. Parkin, D. M. and Muir, C. S. 1992. Cancer incidence in five continents. Comparability and quality of data. *IARC Sci Publ*, 45–173.
7. Muir, C. S., Nectoux, J., and Staszewski, J. 1991. The epidemiology of prostatic cancer: Geographical distribution and time-trends. *Acta Oncol* 30, 133–140
8. Ziegler, R. G., Hoover, R. N., Pike, M. C., Hildesheim, A., Nomura, A. M., West, D. W., et al. 1993. Migration patterns and breast cancer risk in Asian-American women. *J Natl Cancer Inst* 85, 1819–1827.
9. Allred, C. D., Allred, K. F., Ju, Y. H., Goeppinger, T. S., Doerge, D. R., and Helferich, W. G. 2004. Soy processing influences growth of estrogen-dependent breast cancer tumors. *Carcinogenesis* 25, 1649–1657.

10. Trock, B. J., Hilakivi-Clarke, L., and Clarke, R. 2006. Meta-analysis of soy intake and breast cancer risk. *J Natl Cancer Inst* 98, 459–471.
11. Yan, L. and Spitznagel, E. 2004. A meta-analysis of soyfoods and risk of breast cancer in women. *Int J Cancer Prev* 1, 281–29312.
12. Xu, W.H., Dai, Q., Xiang, Y.B., Long, J.R., Ruan, Z.X., Cheng, J.R., et al. 2007. Interaction of soy food and tea consumption with CYP19A1 genetic polymorphisms in the development of endometrial cancer. *Am J Epidemiol* 166, 1420–30.
13. Hedelin, M., Bälter, K.A., Chang, E.T., Bellocco, R., Klint, A., Johansson, J.E., et al. 2006. Dietary intake of phytoestrogens, estrogen receptor-beta polymorphisms and the risk of prostate cancer. *Prostate* 66, 1512–20.
14. Duffy, C., Perez, K., and Partridge, A. 2007. Implications of phytoestrogen intake for breast cancer. *CA Cancer J Clin* 57, 260–277.
15. de Lemos, M. L. 2001. Effects of soy phytoestrogens genistein and daidzein on breast cancer growth. *Ann Pharmacother* 35, 1118–1121.
16. Xu, X., Duncan, A. M., Wangen, K. E., and Kurzer, M. S. 2000. Soy consumption alters endogenous estrogen metabolism in postmenopausal women. *Cancer Epidemiol Biomarkers Prev* 9, 781–786.
17. McMichael-Phillips, D. F., Harding, C., Morton, M., Roberts, S. A., Howell, A., Potten, C. S., and Bundred, N. J. 1998. Effects of soy-protein supplementation on epithelial proliferation in the histologically normal human breast. *Am J Clin Nutr* 68, 1431S–1435S.
18. Kumar, N. B., Cantor, A., Allen, K., Riccardi, D., and Cox, C. E. 2002. The specific role of isoflavones on estrogen metabolism in premenopausal women. *Cancer* 94, 1166–1174.
19. Maskarinec, G., Williams, A. E., and Carlin, L. 2003. Mammographic densities in a one-year isoflavone intervention. *Eur J Cancer Prev* 12, 165–169.
20. Balk, E., Chung, M., Chew, P., Ip, S., Raman, G., Kupelnick, B., et al. 2005. Effects of soy on health outcomes. *Evid Rep Technol Assess Summ.*, 1–8.
21. Petrakis, N. L., Barnes, S., King, E. B., Lowenstein, J., Wiencke, J., Lee, M. M., et al. 1996. Stimulatory influence of soy protein isolate on breast secretion in pre- and postmenopausal women. *Cancer Epidemiol Biomarkers Prev* 5, 785–794.
22. Wu, A. H., Wan, P., Hankin, J., Tseng, C. C., Yu, M. C., and Pike, M. C. 2002. Adolescent, and adult soy intake and risk of breast cancer in Asian-Americans. *Carcinogenesis* 23, 1491–1496.
23. Allen, N. E., Sauvaget, C., Roddam, A. W., Appleby, P., Nagano, J., Suzuki, G., et al. 2004. A prospective study of diet and prostate cancer in Japanese men. *Cancer Causes Control* 15, 911–920.
24. Jacobsen, B. K., Knutsen, S. F., and Fraser, G. E. 1998. Does high soy milk intake reduce prostate cancer incidence? The Adventist Health Study United States. *Cancer Causes Control* 9, 553–557.
25. Hirayama, T. 1979. Epidemiology of prostate cancer with special reference to the role of diet. *Natl Cancer Inst Monogr*, 149–155.
26. Severson, R. K., Nomura, A. M., Grove, J. S., and Stemmermann, G. N. 1989. A prospective study of demographics, diet, and prostate cancer among men of Japanese ancestry in Hawaii. *Cancer Res* 49, 1857–1860.
27. Jian, L., Zhang, D. H., Lee, A. H., and Binns, C. W. 2004. Do preserved foods increase prostate cancer risk? *Br J Cancer* 90, 1792–1795.
28. Lee, M. M., Gomez, S. L., Chang, J. S., Wey, M., Wang, R. T., and Hsing, A. W. 2003. Soy, and isoflavone consumption in relation to prostate cancer risk in China. *Cancer Epidemiol Biomarkers Prev* 12, 665–668.
29. Sung, J. F., Lin, R. S., Pu, Y. S., Chen, Y. C., Chang, H. C., and Lai, M. K. 1999. Risk factors for prostate carcinoma in Taiwan: A case-control study in a Chinese population. *Cancer* 86, 484–491.
30. Lee, M. M., Wang, R. T., Hsing, A. W., Gu, F. L., Wang, T., and Spitz, M. 1998. Case-control study of diet and prostate cancer in China. *Cancer Causes Control* 9, 545–552.
31. Sonoda, T., Nagata, Y., Mori, M., Miyanaga, N., Takashima, N., Okumura, K., et al. 2004. A case-control study of diet and prostate cancer in Japan: Possible protective effect of traditional Japanese diet. *Cancer Sci* 95, 238–242.
32. Kolonel, L. N., Hankin, J. H., Whittemore, A. S., Wu, A. H., Gallagher, R. P., Wilkens, et al. 2000. Vegetables, fruits, legumes, and prostate cancer: A multiethnic case-control study. *Cancer Epidemiol Biomarkers Prev* 9, 795–804.
33. Tatsuta, M., Iishi, H., Baba, M., Yano, H., Uehara, H., and Nakaizumi, A. 1999. Attenuation by genistein of sodium-chloride-enhanced gastric carcinogenesis induced by N-methyl-N'-nitro-N-nitrosoguanidine in Wistar rats. *Int J Cancer* 80, 396–399.

34. Watanabe, H., Uesaka, T., Kido, S., Ishimura, Y., Shiraki, K., Kuramoto, K., et al. 1999. Influence of concomitant miso or NaCl treatment on induction of gastric tumors by N-methyl-N'-nitro-N-nitroso-guanidine in rats. *Oncol Rep* 6, 989–993.

35. Gao, C. M., Takezaki, T., Ding, J. H., Li, M. S., and Tajima, K. 1999. Protective effect of allium vegetables against both esophageal and stomach cancer: A simultaneous case-referent study of a high-epidemic area in Jiangsu Province, China. *Jpn J Cancer Res* 90, 614–621.

36. Hamada, G. S., Kowalski, L. P., Nishimoto, I. N., Rodrigues, J. J., Iriya, K., Sasazuki, S., et al. 2002. Risk factors for stomach cancer in Brazil. II: A case-control study among Japanese Brazilians in Sao Paulo. *Jpn J Clin Oncol* 32, 284–290.

37. Hoshiyama, Y. and Sasaba, T. 1992. A case-control study of stomach cancer and its relation to diet, cigarettes, and alcohol consumption in Saitama Prefecture, Japan. *Cancer Causes Control* 3, 441–448.

38. Ji, B. T., Chow, W. H., Yang, G., McLaughlin, J. K., Zheng, W., Shu, X. O., et al. 1998. Dietary habits and stomach cancer in Shanghai, China. *Int J Cancer* 76, 659–664.

39. Kim, H. J., Chang, W. K., Kim, M. K., Lee, S. S., and Choi, B. Y. 2002. Dietary factors and gastric cancer in Korea: A case-control study. *Int J Cancer* 97, 531–535.

40. Nan, H. M., Park, J. W., Song, Y. J., Yun, H. Y., Park, J. S., Hyun, T., et al. 2005. Kimchi and soybean pastes are risk factors of gastric cancer. *World J Gastroenterol* 11, 3175–3181.

41. Takezaki, T., Gao, C. M., Wu, J. Z., Ding, J. H., Liu, Y. T., Zhang, Y., et al. 2001. Dietary protective and risk factors for esophageal and stomach cancers in a low-epidemic area for stomach cancer in Jiangsu Province, China: Comparison with those in a high-epidemic area. *Jpn J Cancer Res* 92, 1157–1165.

42. Takezaki, T., Gao, C. M., Wu, J. Z., Li, Z. Y., Wang, J. D., Ding, J. H., et al. 2002. hOGG1 Ser326.Cys polymorphism and modification by environmental factors of stomach cancer risk in Chinese. *Int J Cancer* 99, 624–627.

43. You, W. C., Blot, W. J., Chang, Y. S., Ershow, A. G., Yang, Z. T., An, Q., et al. 1988. Diet and high risk of stomach cancer in Shandong, China. *Cancer Res* 48, 3518–3523.

44. Ahn, Y. O. 1997. Diet and stomach cancer in Korea. *Int J Cancer Suppl* 10, 7–9.

45. Nagata, C., Takatsuka, N., Kawakami, N., and Shimizu, H. 2002. A prospective cohort study of soy product intake and stomach cancer death. *Br J Cancer* 87, 31–36.

46. Hilakivi-Clarke, L. 2007. Nutritional modulation of terminal end buds: Its relevance to breast cancer prevention. *Curr Cancer Drug Targets* 7, 465–474.

47. Whitsett, T. G., Jr. and Lamartiniere, C. A. 2006. Genistein and resveratrol: Mammary cancer chemoprevention and mechanisms of action in the rat. *Expert Rev Anticancer Ther* 6, 1699–1706.

48. Losso, J. N. 2008. The biochemical and functional food properties of the bowman-birk inhibitor. *Crit Rev Food Sci Nutr* 48, 94–118.

49. Konings, E. J., Goldbohm, R. A., Brants, H. A., Saris, W. H., and van den Brandt, P. A. 2002. Intake of dietary folate vitamers and risk of colorectal carcinoma: Results from The Netherlands Cohort Study. *Cancer* 95, 1421–143353.

50. Larsson, S. C., Giovannucci, E., and Wolk, A. 2005. A prospective study of dietary folate intake and risk of colorectal cancer: Modification by caffeine intake and cigarette smoking. *Cancer Epidemiol Biomarkers Prev* 14, 740–743.

51. Su, L. J., and Arab, L. 2001. Nutritional status of folate and colon cancer risk: Evidence from NHANES I epidemiologic follow-up study. *Ann Epidemiol* 11, 65–72.

52. Giovannucci, E., Stampfer, M. J., Colditz, G. A., Hunter, D. J., Fuchs, C., Rosner, B. A., et al. 1998. Multivitamin use, folate, and colon cancer in women in the Nurses' Health Study. *Ann Intern Med* 129, 517–524.

53. Sanjoaquin, M. A., Allen, N., Couto, E., Roddam, A. W., and Key, T. J. 2005. Folate intake and colorectal cancer risk: A meta-analytical approach. *Int J Cancer* 113, 825–828.

54. Kato, I., Dnistrian, A. M., Schwartz, M., Toniolo, P., Koenig, K., Shore, R. E., et al. 1999. Serum folate, homocysteine, and colorectal cancer risk in women: A nested case-control study. *Br J Cancer* 79, 1917–1922.

55. Glynn, S. A., Albanes, D., Pietinen, P., Brown, C. C., Rautalahti, M., Tangrea, J. A., et al. 1996. Colorectal cancer and folate status: A nested case-control study among male smokers. *Cancer Epidemiol Biomarkers Prev* 5, 487–494.

56. Jaskiewicz, K. 1989. Oesophageal carcinoma: Cytopathology and nutritional aspects in aetiology. *Anticancer Res* 9, 1847–1852.

57. Jaskiewicz, K., Marasas, W. F., Lazarus, C., Beyers, A. D., and Van Helden, P. D. 1988. Association of esophageal cytological abnormalities with vitamin and lipotrope deficiencies in populations at risk for esophageal cancer. *Anticancer Res* 8, 711–715.

58. Tan, W., Miao, X., Wang, L., Yu, C., Xiong, P., Liang, G., et al. 2005. Significant increase in risk of gastroesophageal cancer is associated with interaction between promoter polymorphisms in thymidylate synthase and serum folate status. *Carcinogenesis* 26, 1430–1435.

59. Cole, B. F., Baron, J. A., Sandler, R. S., Haile, R. W., Ahnen, D. J., Bresalier, R. S., et al. 2007. Folic acid for the prevention of colorectal adenomas: A randomized clinical trial. *JAMA* 297, 2351–2359.

60. Stolzenberg-Solomon, R. Z., Albanes, D., Nieto, F. J., Hartman, T. J., Tangrea, J. A., Rautalahti, M., et al. 1999. Pancreatic cancer risk and nutrition-related methyl-group availability indicators in male smokers. *J Natl Cancer Inst* 91, 535–541.

61. Stolzenberg-Solomon, R. Z., Pietinen, P., Barrett, M. J., Taylor, P. R., Virtamo, J., and Albanes, D. 2001. Dietary, and other methyl-group availability factors and pancreatic cancer risk in a cohort of male smokers. *Am J Epidemiol* 153, 680–687.

62. Skinner, H. G., Michaud, D. S., Giovannucci, E. L., Rimm, E. B., Stampfer, M. J., Willett, W. C., et al. 2004. A prospective study of folate intake and the risk of pancreatic cancer in men and women. *Am J Epidemiol* 160, 248–258.

63. Larsson, S. C., Hakansson, N., Giovannucci, E., and Wolk, A. 2006. Folate intake and pancreatic cancer incidence: A prospective study of Swedish women and men. *J Natl Cancer Inst* 98, 407–413.

64. Brown, L. M., Blot, W. J., Schuman, S. H., Smith, V. M., Ershow, A. G., Marks, R. D., and Fraumeni, J. F., Jr. 1988. Environmental factors and high risk of esophageal cancer among men in coastal South Carolina. *J Natl Cancer Inst* 80, 1620–1625.

65. Brown, L. M., Swanson, C. A., Gridley, G., Swanson, G. M., Schoenberg, J. B., Greenberg, R. S., et al. 1995. Adenocarcinoma of the esophagus: Role of obesity and diet. *J Natl Cancer Inst* 87, 104–109.

66. Zhang, Z. F., Kurtz, R. C., Yu, G. P., Sun, M., Gargon, N., Karpeh, M., Jr., et al. 1997. Adenocarcinomas of the esophagus and gastric cardia: The role of diet. *Nutr Cancer* 27, 298–309.

67. Tavani, A., Negri, E., Franceschi, S., and La Vecchia, C. 1993. Risk factors for esophageal cancer in women in northern Italy. *Cancer* 72, 2531–2536.

68. De Stefani, E., Ronco, A., Mendilaharsu, M., and Deneo-Pellegrini, H. 1999. Diet and risk of cancer of the upper aerodigestive tract. II. Nutrients. *Oral Oncol* 35, 22–26.

69. Mayne, S. T., Risch, H. A., Dubrow, R., Chow, W. H., Gammon, M. D., Vaughan, T. L., et al. 2001. Nutrient intake and risk of subtypes of esophageal and gastric cancer. *Cancer Epidemiol Biomarkers Prev* 10, 1055–1062.

70. Franceschi, S., Bidoli, E., Negri, E., Zambon, P., Talamini, R., Ruol, A., et al. 2000. Role of macronutrients, vitamins, and minerals in the aetiology of squamous-cell carcinoma of the oesophagus. *Int J Cancer* 86, 626–631.

71. Chen, H., Tucker, K. L., Graubard, B. I., Heineman, E. F., Markin, R. S., Potischman, N. A., et al. 2002. Nutrient intakes and adenocarcinoma of the esophagus and distal stomach. *Nutr Cancer* 42, 33–40.

72. Ross, S. A. 2003. Diet, and DNA methylation interactions in cancer prevention. *Ann N Y Acad Sci* 983, 197–20751.

73. Rao, C. V., Hirose, Y., Indranie, C., and Reddy, B. S. 2001. Modulation of experimental colon tumorigenesis by types and amounts of dietary fatty acids. *Cancer Res* 61, 1927–1933.

74. MacLean, C. H., Newberry, S. J., Mojica, W. A., Khanna, P., Issa, A. M., Suttorp, M. J., et al. 2006. Effects of omega-3 fatty acids on cancer risk: A systematic review. *JAMA* 295, 403–415.

75. Bostick, R. M., Potter, J. D., Kushi, L. H., Sellers, T. A., Steinmetz, K. A., McKenzie, D. R., et al. 1994. Sugar, meat, and fat intake, and non-dietary risk factors for colon cancer incidence in Iowa women United States. *Cancer Causes Control* 5, 38–52.

76. Willett, W. C., Stampfer, M. J., Colditz, G. A., Rosner, B. A., and Speizer, F. E. 1990. Relation of meat, fat, and fiber intake to the risk of colon cancer in a prospective study among women. *N Engl J Med* 323, 1664–1672.

77. Giovannucci, E., Rimm, E. B., Stampfer, M. J., Colditz, G. A., Ascherio, A., and Willett, W. C. 1994. Intake of fat, meat, and fiber in relation to risk of colon cancer in men. *Cancer Res* 54, 2390–2397.

78. English, D. R., MacInnis, R. J., Hodge, A. M., Hopper, J. L., Haydon, A. M., and Giles, G. G. 2004. Red meat, chicken, and fish consumption and risk of colorectal cancer. *Cancer Epidemiol Biomarkers Prev* 13, 1509–1514.

79. Norat, T., Bingham, S., Ferrari, P., Slimani, N., Jenab, M., Mazuir, M., et al. 2005. Meat, fish, and colorectal cancer risk: The European Prospective Investigation into cancer and nutrition. *J Natl Cancer Inst* 97, 906–916.

80. Kato, I., Akhmedkhanov, A., Koenig, K., Toniolo, P. G., Shore, R. E., and Riboli, E. 1997. Prospective study of diet, and female colorectal cancer: The New York University Women's Health Study. *Nutr Cancer* 28, 276–281.

81. Pietinen, P., Malila, N., Virtanen, M., Hartman, T. J., Tangrea, J. A., Albanes, D., and Virtamo, J. 1999. Diet and risk of colorectal cancer in a cohort of Finnish men. *Cancer Causes Control* 10, 387–396

82. Larsson, S. C., Rafter, J., Holmberg, L., Bergkvist, L., and Wolk, A. 2005. Red meat consumption and risk of cancers of the proximal colon, distal colon, and rectum: The Swedish Mammography Cohort. *Int J Cancer* 113, 829–834.

83. Tiemersma, E. W., Kampman, E., Bueno de Mesquita, H. B., Bunschoten, A., van Schothorst, E. M., Kok, F. J., and Kromhout, D. 2002. Meat consumption, cigarette smoking, and genetic susceptibility in the etiology of colorectal cancer: Results from a Dutch prospective study. *Cancer Causes Control* 13, 383–393.

84. Phillips, R. L. 1975. Role of life-style, and dietary habits in risk of cancer among Seventh-Day Adventists. *Cancer Res* 35, 3513–3522.

85. Khan, M. M., Goto, R., Kobayashi, K., Suzumura, S., Nagata, Y., Sonoda, T., et al. 2004. Dietary habits and cancer mortality among middle aged and older Japanese living in Hokkaido, Japan by cancer site and sex. *Asian Pac J Cancer Prev* 5, 58–65.

86. Goldbohm, R. A., van den Brandt, P. A., van 't Veer, P., Brants, H. A., Dorant, E., Sturmans, F., and Hermus, R. J. 1994. A prospective cohort study on the relation between meat consumption and the risk of colon cancer. *Cancer Res* 54, 718–723.

87. Hsing, A. W., McLaughlin, J. K., Chow, W. H., Schuman, L. M., Co Chien, H. T., Gridley, G.,et al. 1998. Risk factors for colorectal cancer in a prospective study among U.S. white men. *Int J Cancer* 77, 549–553.

88. Hirayama, T. 1989. Association between alcohol consumption and cancer of the sigmoid colon: Observations from a Japanese cohort study. *Lancet* 2, 725–727

89. Kearney, J., Giovannucci, E., Rimm, E. B., Ascherio, A., Stampfer, M. J., Colditz, G. A., et al. 1996. Calcium, vitamin D, and dairy foods and the occurrence of colon cancer in men. *Am J Epidemiol* 143, 907–917.

90. Knekt, P., Jarvinen, R., Dich, J., and Hakulinen, T. 1999. Risk of colorectal and other gastro-intestinal cancers after exposure to nitrate, nitrite, and N-nitroso compounds: A follow-up study. *Int J Cancer* 80, 852–856.

91. Sanjoaquin, M. A., Appleby, P. N., Thorogood, M., Mann, J. I., and Key, T. J. 2004. Nutrition, lifestyle, and colorectal cancer incidence: A prospective investigation of 10998 vegetarians and non-vegetarians in the United Kingdom. *Br J Cancer* 90, 118–121.

92. Kojima, M., Wakai, K., Tamakoshi, K., Tokudome, S., Toyoshima, H., Watanabe, Y., et al. 2004. Diet, and colorectal cancer mortality: Results from the Japan Collaborative Cohort Study. *Nutr Cancer* 50, 23–32.

93. Ma, J., Giovannucci, E., Pollak, M., Chan, J. M., Gaziano, J. M., Willett, W., and Stampfer, M. J. 2001. Milk intake, circulating levels of insulin-like growth factor-I, and risk of colorectal cancer in men. *J Natl Cancer Inst* 93, 1330–1336.

94. Luchtenborg, M., Weijenberg, M. P., de Goeij, A. F., Wark, P. A., Brink, M., Roemen, G. M., et al. 2005. Meat and fish consumption, APC gene mutations, and hMLH1 expression in colon and rectal cancer: A prospective cohort study The Netherlands. *Cancer Causes Control* 16, 1041–1054.

95. Gaard, M., Tretli, S., and Loken, E. B. 1996. Dietary factors and risk of colon cancer: a prospective study of 50,535 young Norwegian men and women. *Eur J Cancer Prev* 5, 445–454.

96. Phillips, R. L., and Snowdon, D. A. 1985. Dietary relationships with fatal colorectal cancer among Seventh-Day Adventists. *J Natl Cancer Inst* 74, 307–317.

97. Zheng, T., Holford, T. R., Leaderer, B., Zhang, Y., Zahm, S. H., Flynn, S., et al. 2004. Diet and nutrient intakes and risk of non-Hodgkin's lymphoma in Connecticut women. *Am J Epidemiol* 159, 454–466.

98. Fritschi, L., Ambrosini, G. L., Kliewer, E. V., and Johnson, K. C. 2004. Dietary fish intake and risk of leukaemia, multiple myeloma, and non-Hodgkin lymphoma. *Cancer Epidemiol Biomarkers Prev* 13, 532–537.

99. Bosetti, C., Kolonel, L., Negri, E., Ron, E., Franceschi, S., Dal Maso, L., et al. 2001. A pooled analysis of case-control studies of thyroid cancer. VI. Fish and shellfish consumption. *Cancer Causes Control* 12, 375–382.

100. Ross, S. A. and Milner, J. 2007. Garlic: The mystical food in health promotion. In *Handbook of Nutraceuticals and Functional Foods*, Wildman, R. E. C., (Ed.), pp. 73–99, CRC Press, Boca Raton.

101. Milner, J. A. 2001. A historical perspective on garlic and cancer. *J Nutr* 131, 1027S–1031S.

102. Xiao, D., Lew, K. L., Kim, Y. A., Zeng, Y., Hahm, E. R., Dhir, R., and Singh, S. V. 2006. Diallyl trisulfide suppresses growth of PC-3 human prostate cancer xenograft in vivo in association with Bax and Bak induction. *Clin Cancer Res* 12, 6836–6843.

103. Chu, Q., Lee, D. T., Tsao, S. W., Wang, X., and Wong, Y. C. 2007. S-allylcysteine, a water-soluble garlic derivative, suppresses the growth of a human, androgen-independent prostate cancer xenograft, CWR22R, under in vivo conditions. *BJU Int* 99, 925–932.

104. Shukla, Y. and Kalra, N. 2007. Cancer chemoprevention with garlic and its constituents. *Cancer Lett* 247, 167–181.

105. Milner, J. A. 2006. Preclinical perspectives on garlic and cancer. *J Nutr* 136, 827S–831S.

106. Fleischauer, A. T., and Arab, L. 2001. Garlic, and cancer: A critical review of the epidemiologic literature. *J Nutr* 131, 1032S–1040S.

107. Iscovich, J. M., L'Abbe, K. A., Castelleto, R., Calzona, A., Bernedo, A., Chopita, N. A., et al. 1992. Colon cancer in Argentina. I: Risk from intake of dietary items. *Int J Cancer* 51, 851–857.

108. Hu, J. F., Liu, Y. Y., Yu, Y. K., Zhao, T. Z., Liu, S. D., and Wang, Q. Q. 1991. Diet and cancer of the colon and rectum: A case-control study in China. *Int J Epidemiol* 20, 362–367.

109. Le Marchand, L., Hankin, J. H., Wilkens, L. R., Kolonel, L. N., Englyst, H. N., and Lyu, L. C. 1997. Dietary fiber and colorectal cancer risk. *Epidemiology* 8, 658–665.

110. Witte, J. S., Longnecker, M. P., Bird, C. L., Lee, E. R., Frankl, H. D., and Haile, R. W. 1996. Relation of vegetable, fruit, and grain consumption to colorectal adenomatous polyps. *Am J Epidemiol* 144, 1015–1025.

111. Steinmetz, K. A., Kushi, L. H., Bostick, R. M., Folsom, A. R., and Potter, J. D. 1994. Vegetables, fruit, and colon cancer in the Iowa Women's Health Study. *Am J Epidemiol* 139, 1–15.

112. Dorant, E., van den Brandt, P. A., and Goldbohm, R. A. 1996. A prospective cohort study on the relationship between onion and leek consumption, garlic supplement use, and the risk of colorectal carcinoma in The Netherlands. *Carcinogenesis* 17, 477–484.

113. Tanaka, S., Haruma, K., Kunihiro, M., Nagata, S., Kitadai, Y., Manabe, N., et al. 2004. Effects of aged garlic extract (AGE) on colorectal adenomas: A double-blinded study. *Hiroshima J Med Sci* 53, 39–45.

114. You, W. C., Blot, W. J., Chang, Y. S., Ershow, A., Yang, Z. T., An, Q., et al. 1989. Allium vegetables, and reduced risk of stomach cancer. *J Natl Cancer Inst* 81, 162–164.

115. Buiatti, E., Palli, D., Decarli, A., Amadori, D., Avellini, C., Bianchi, S., et al. 1989. A case-control study of gastric cancer and diet in Italy. *Int J Cancer* 44, 611–616.

116. Hansson, L. E., Nyren, O., Bergstrom, R., Wolk, A., Lindgren, A., Baron, J., and Adami, H. O. 1993. Diet and risk of gastric cancer. A population-based case-control study in Sweden. *Int J Cancer* 55, 181–189.

117. Dorant, E., van den Brandt, P. A., Goldbohm, R. A., and Sturmans, F. 1996. Consumption of onions and a reduced risk of stomach carcinoma. *Gastroenterology* 110, 12–20.

118. Munoz, N., Plummer, M., Vivas, J., Moreno, V., De Sanjose, S., Lopez, G., and Oliver, W. 2001. A case-control study of gastric cancer in Venezuela. *Int J Cancer* 93, 417–423.

119. Zickute, J., Strumylaite, L., Dregval, L., Petrauskiene, J., Dudzevicius, J., and Stratilatovas, E. 2005. [Vegetables and fruits and risk of stomach cancer.] *Medicina Kaunas.* 41, 733–740.

120. Li, X. X. 1986. [Case-control study of gastric cancer in high-incidence areas.] *Zhonghua Liu Xing Bing Xue Za Zhi* 7, 340–342.

121. Xu, H. X. 1985. [Relation between the diet of the residents and the incidence of gastric cancer in Yantai District]. *Zhonghua Liu Xing Bing Xue Za Zhi* 6, 245–247.

122. Li, H., Chen, X. L., and Li, H. Q. 2005. Polymorphism of CYPIA1, and GSTM1 genes associated with susceptibility of gastric cancer in Shandong Province of China. *World J Gastroenterol* 11, 5757–5762.

123. Li, H., Li, H. Q., Wang, Y., Xu, H. X., Fan, W. T., Wang, M. L., et al. 2004. An intervention study to prevent gastric cancer by micro-selenium and large dose of allitridum. *Chin Med J Engl.* 117, 1155–1160.

124. Zheng, G. H., Li, H., Fan, W. T., and Li, H. Q. 2005. [Study on the long-time effect on allitridum and selenium in prevention of digestive system cancers]. *Zhonghua Liu Xing Bing Xue Za Zhi* 26, 110–112.

125. You, W. C., Brown, L. M., Zhang, L., Li, J. Y., Jin, M. L., Chang, Y. S., et al. 2006. Randomized double-blind factorial trial of three treatments to reduce the prevalence of precancerous gastric lesions. *J Natl Cancer Inst* 98, 974–983.

126. Chen, Z., Zhu, Q. Y., Tsang, D., and Huang, Y. 2001. Degradation of green tea catechins in tea drinks. *J Agric Food Chem* 49, 477–482.

127. Yan, Y., Cook, J., McQuillan, J., Zhang, G., Hitzman, C. J., Wang, Y., et al. 2007. Chemopreventive effect of aerosolized polyphenon E on lung tumorigenesis in A/J mice. *Neoplasia* 9, 401–405.

128. Hede, K. 2007. Imprinting may provide cancer prevention tools. *J Natl Cancer Inst* 99, 424–426.

129. Henning, S. M., Fajardo-Lira, C., Lee, H. W., Youssefian, A. A., Go, V. L., and Heber, D. 2003. Catechin content of 18 teas and a green tea extract supplement correlates with the antioxidant capacity. *Nutr Cancer* 45, 226–235.

130. Yang, C. S., Maliakal, P., and Meng, X. 2002. Inhibition of carcinogenesis by tea. *Annu Rev Pharmacol Toxicol* 42, 25–54.

131. Cabrera, C., Artacho, R., and Gimenez, R. 2006. Beneficial effects of green tea—a review. *J Am Coll Nutr* 25, 79–99.

132. Sun, C. L., Yuan, J. M., Lee, M. J., Yang, C. S., Gao, Y. T., Ross, R. K., and Yu, M. C. 2002. Urinary tea polyphenols in relation to gastric and esophageal cancers: A prospective study of men in Shanghai, China. *Carcinogenesis* 23, 1497–1503.

133. Shibata, K., Moriyama, M., Fukushima, T., Kaetsu, A., Miyazaki, M., and Une, H. 2000. Green tea consumption and chronic atrophic gastritis: A cross-sectional study in a green tea production village. *J Epidemiol* 10, 310–316.

134. Kuwahara, Y., Kono, S., Eguchi, H., Hamada, H., Shinchi, K., and Imanishi, K. 2000. Relationship between serologically diagnosed chronic atrophic gastritis, Helicobacter pylori, and environmental factors in Japanese men. *Scand J Gastroenterol* 35, 476–481.

135. Nakachi, K., Matsuyama, S., Miyake, S., Suganuma, M., and Imai, K. 2000. Preventive effects of drinking green tea on cancer and cardiovascular disease: Epidemiological evidence for multiple targeting prevention. *Biofactors* 13, 49–54.

136. Nagano, J., Kono, S., Preston, D. L., and Mabuchi, K. 2001. A prospective study of green tea consumption and cancer incidence, Hiroshima, and Nagasaki Japan. *Cancer Causes Control* 12, 501–508.

137. Setiawan, V. W., Zhang, Z. F., Yu, G. P., Lu, Q. Y., Li, Y. L., et al. 2001. Protective effect of green tea on the risks of chronic gastritis and stomach cancer. *Int J Cancer* 92, 600–604.

138. Tsubono, Y., Nishino, Y., Komatsu, S., Hsieh, C. C., Kanemura, S., Tsuji, I., et al. 2001. Green tea and the risk of gastric cancer in Japan. *N Engl J Med* 344, 632–636.

139. Hoshiyama, Y., Kawaguchi, T., Miura, Y., Mizoue, T., Tokui, N., Yatsuya, H., et al. 2002. A prospective study of stomach cancer death in relation to green tea consumption in Japan. *Br J Cancer* 87, 309–313.

140. Fujino, Y., Tamakoshi, A., Ohno, Y., Mizoue, T., Tokui, N., and Yoshimura, T. 2002. Prospective study of educational background and stomach cancer in Japan. *Prev Med* 35, 121–127.

141. Hoshiyama, Y., Kawaguchi, T., Miura, Y., Mizoue, T., Tokui, N., Yatsuya, H., et al. 2004. A nested case-control study of stomach cancer in relation to green tea consumption in Japan. *Br J Cancer* 90, 135–138.

142. Inoue, M., Tajima, K., Mizutani, M., Iwata, H., Iwase, T., Miura, S., et al. 2001. Regular consumption of green tea and the risk of breast cancer recurrence: Follow-up study from the Hospital-Based Epidemiologic Research Program at Aichi Cancer Center HERPACC, Japan. *Cancer Lett* 167, 175–182.

143. Wu, A. H., Yu, M. C., Tseng, C. C., Hankin, J., and Pike, M. C. 2003. Green tea and risk of breast cancer in Asian Americans. *Int J Cancer* 106, 574–579.

144. Suzuki, Y., Tsubono, Y., Nakaya, N., Suzuki, Y., Koizumi, Y., and Tsuji, I. 2004. Green tea and the risk of breast cancer: Pooled analysis of two prospective studies in Japan. *Br J Cancer* 90, 1361–1363.

145. Hamajima, N., Tajima, K., Tominaga, S., Matsuura, A., Kuwabara, M., and Okuma, K. 1999. Tea polyphenol intake and changes in serum pepsinogen levels. *Jpn J Cancer Res* 90, 136–143.

146. Wang, L. D., Zhou, Q., Feng, C. W., Liu, B., Qi, Y. J., Zhang, Y. R., et al. 2002. Intervention and follow-up on human esophageal precancerous lesions in Henan, northern China, a high-incidence area for esophageal cancer. *Gan To Kagaku Ryoho* 29 Suppl 1, 159–172.

147. Li, N., Sun, Z., Han, C., and Chen, J. 1999. The chemopreventive effects of tea on human oral precancerous mucosa lesions. *Proc Soc Exp Biol Med* 220, 218–224.

148. Bettuzzi, S., Brausi, M., Rizzi, F., Castagnetti, G., Peracchia, G., and Corti, A. 2006. Chemoprevention of human prostate cancer by oral administration of green tea catechins in volunteers with high-grade prostate intraepithelial neoplasia: A preliminary report from a one-year proof-of-principle study. *Cancer Res* 66, 1234–1240.

149. Hakim, I. A., Harris, R. B., Brown, S., Chow, H. H., Wiseman, S., Agarwal, S., and Talbot, W. 2003. Effect of increased tea consumption on oxidative DNA damage among smokers: A randomized controlled study. *J Nutr* 133, 3303S–3309S.

150. Luo, H., Tang, L., Tang, M., Billam, M., Huang, T., Yu, J., et al. 2006. Phase IIa chemoprevention trial of green tea polyphenols in high-risk individuals of liver cancer: Modulation of urinary excretion of green tea polyphenols and 8-hydroxydeoxyguanosine. *Carcinogenesis* 27, 262–268.

151. Chen L, Zhang HY.2007. Cancer preventive mechanisms of the green tea polyphenol (-) epigallocatechin-3-gallate. *Molecules* 125, 946–57.

152. Percival SS, Bukowski JF, Milner J. 2008. Bioactive food components that enhance gammadelta T cell function may play a role in cancer prevention. *J Nutr* 1381, 1–4.

153. Visioli, F., Grande, S., Bogani, P., and Galli, C. 2004. The role of antioxidants in the mediterranean diets: Focus on cancer. *Eur J Cancer Prev* 13, 337–343.

154. Longnecker, M. P., and Enger, S. M. 1996. Epidemiologic data on alcoholic beverage consumption and risk of cancer. *Clin Chim Acta* 246, 121–141.

155. Burns, J., Crozier, A., and Lean, M. E. 2001. Alcohol consumption and mortality: Is wine different from other alcoholic beverages? *Nutr Metab Cardiovasc Dis* 11, 249–258.

156. Bianchini, F. and Vainio, H. 2003. Wine and resveratrol: Mechanisms of cancer prevention? *Eur J Cancer Prev* 12, 417–425

157. Renaud, S. C., Gueguen, R., Schenker, J., and d'Houtaud, A. 1998. Alcohol and mortality in middle-aged men from eastern France. *Epidemiology* 9, 184–188.

158. Gronbaek, M., Becker, U., Johansen, D., Gottschau, A., Schnohr, P., Hein, H. O., et al. 2000. Type of alcohol consumed and mortality from all causes, coronary heart disease, and cancer. *Ann Intern Med* 133, 411–419.

159. Prescott, E., Gronbaek, M., Becker, U., and Sorensen, T. I. 1999. Alcohol intake and the risk of lung cancer: Influence of type of alcoholic beverage. *Am J Epidemiol* 149, 463–470.

160. Gronbaek, M., Becker, U., Johansen, D., Tonnesen, H., Jensen, G., and Sorensen, T. I. 1998. Population based cohort study of the association between alcohol intake and cancer of the upper digestive tract. *BMJ* 317, 844–847.

161. Zhang, Z. F., Kurtz, R. C., Sun, M., Karpeh, M., Jr., Yu, G. P., Gargon, N., et al. 1996. Adenocarcinomas of the esophagus and gastric cardia: Medical conditions, tobacco, alcohol, and socioeconomic factors. *Cancer Epidemiol Biomarkers Prev* 5, 761–768.

162. Gammon, M. D., Schoenberg, J. B., Ahsan, H., Risch, H. A., Vaughan, T. L., Chow, W. H., et al. 1997. Tobacco, alcohol, and socioeconomic status and adenocarcinomas of the esophagus and gastric cardia. *J Natl Cancer Inst* 89, 1277–1284.

163. Valsecchi, M. G. 1992. Modelling the relative risk of esophageal cancer in a case-control study. *J Clin Epidemiol* 45, 347–355.

164. Castelletto, R., Castellsague, X., Munoz, N., Iscovich, J., Chopita, N., and Jmelnitsky, A. 1994. Alcohol, tobacco, diet, mate drinking, and esophageal cancer in Argentina. *Cancer Epidemiol Biomarkers Prev* 3, 557–564.

165. Bosetti, C., La Vecchia, C., Negri, E., and Franceschi, S. 2000. Wine and other types of alcoholic beverages and the risk of esophageal cancer. *Eur J Clin Nutr* 54, 918–920.

166. Wu, M. M., Kuo, T. L., Hwang, Y. H., and Chen, C. J. 1989. Dose–response relation between arsenic concentration in well water and mortality from cancers and vascular diseases. *Am J Epidemiol* 130, 1123–1132.

167. De Jong, U. W., Breslow, N., Hong, J. G., Sridharan, M., and Shanmugaratnam, K. 1974. Aetiological factors in oesophageal cancer in Singapore Chinese. *Int J Cancer* 13, 291–303.

168. Victora, C. G., Munoz, N., Day, N. E., Barcelos, L. B., Peccin, D. A., and Braga, N. M. 1987. Hot beverages and oesophageal cancer in southern Brazil: A case-control study. *Int J Cancer* 39, 710–716.

169. Yu, M. C., Garabrant, D. H., Peters, J. M., and Mack, T. M. 1988. Tobacco, alcohol, diet, occupation, and carcinoma of the esophagus. *Cancer Res* 48, 3843–3848.

170. Hinds, M. W., Kolonel, L. N., Lee, J., and Hirohata, T. 1980. Associations between cancer incidence and alcohol/cigarette consumption among five ethnic groups in Hawaii. *Br J Cancer* 41, 929–940.

171. Razvodovsky, Y. 2003. Aggregate level time series association between alcohol consumption and cancer mortality rate. *Alcoholism* 39, 11–20.
172. Schrauzer, G. N. 1976. Cancer mortality correlation studies. II. Regional associations of mortalities with the consumptions of foods and other commodities. *Med Hypotheses* 2, 39–49.
173. Breslow, N. E., and Enstrom, J. E. 1974. Geographic correlations between cancer mortality rates and alcohol/tobacco consumption in the United States. *J Natl Cancer Inst* 53, 631–639.
174. Kono, S. and Ikeda, M. 1979. Correlation between cancer mortality and alcoholic beverage in Japan. *Br J Cancer* 40, 449–455.
175. Chilvers, C., Fraser, P., and Beral, V. 1979. Alcohol and oesophageal cancer: An assessment of the evidence from routinely collected data. *J Epidemiol Commun Hlth* 33, 127–133.
176. Goodman, M. T., Moriwaki, H., Vaeth, M., Akiba, S., Hayabuchi, H., and Mabuchi, K. 1995. Prospective cohort study of risk factors for primary liver cancer in Hiroshima and Nagasaki, Japan. *Epidemiology* 6, 36–41.
177. Prior, P. 1988. Long-term cancer risk in alcoholism. *Alcohol Alcohol* 23, 163–171.
178. Kato, I., Nomura, A. M., Stemmermann, G. N., and Chyou, P. H. 1992. Prospective study of the association of alcohol with cancer of the upper aerodigestive tract and other sites. *Cancer Causes Control* 3, 145–151.
179. Austin, H., Delzell, E., Grufferman, S., Levine, R., Morrison, A. S., Stolley, P. D., and Cole, P. 1986. A case-control study of hepatocellular carcinoma and the hepatitis B virus, cigarette smoking, and alcohol consumption. *Cancer Res* 46, 962–966.
180. Franco, E. L., Kowalski, L. P., Oliveira, B. V., Curado, M. P., Pereira, R. N., Silva, M. E., et al. 1989. Risk factors for oral cancer in Brazil: A case-control study. *Int J Cancer* 43, 992–1000.
181. Franceschi, S., Barra, S., La Vecchia, C., Bidoli, E., Negri, E., and Talamini, R. 1992. Risk factors for cancer of the tongue and the mouth. A case-control study from northern Italy. *Cancer* 70, 2227–2233.
182. Franceschi, S., Talamini, R., Barra, S., Baron, A. E., Negri, E., Bidoli, E., et al. 1990. Smoking and drinking in relation to cancers of the oral cavity, pharynx, larynx, and esophagus in northern Italy. *Cancer Res* 50, 6502–6507.
183. Fioretti, F., Bosetti, C., Tavani, A., Franceschi, S., and La Vecchia, C. 1999. Risk factors for oral and pharyngeal cancer in never smokers. *Oral Oncol* 35, 375–378.
184. Zavras, A. I., Douglass, C. W., Joshipura, K., Wu, T., Laskaris, G., Petridou, E., et al. 2001. Smoking and alcohol in the etiology of oral cancer: Gender-specific risk profiles in the south of Greece. *Oral Oncol* 37, 28–35.
185. Schlecht, N. F., Pintos, J., Kowalski, L. P., and Franco, E. L. 2001. Effect of type of alcoholic beverage on the risks of upper aerodigestive tract cancers in Brazil. *Cancer Causes Control* 12, 579–587.
186. Talamini, R., Bosetti, C., La Vecchia, C., Dal Maso, L., Levi, F., Bidoli, E., et al. 2002. Combined effect of tobacco and alcohol on laryngeal cancer risk: A case-control study. *Cancer Causes Control* 13, 957–964.
187. Lissowska, J., Pilarska, A., Pilarski, P., Samolczyk-Wanyura, D., Piekarczyk, J., Bardin-Mikollajczak, A., et al. 2003. Smoking, alcohol, diet, dentition, and sexual practices in the epidemiology of oral cancer in Poland. *Eur J Cancer Prev* 12, 25–33.
188. Day, G. L., Blot, W. J., Austin, D. F., Bernstein, L., Greenberg, R. S., Preston-Martin, S., et al. 1993. Racial differences in risk of oral and pharyngeal cancer: Alcohol, tobacco, and other determinants. *J Natl Cancer Inst* 85, 465–473.
189. Altieri, A., Bosetti, C., Gallus, S., Franceschi, S., Dal Maso, L., Talamini, R., et al. 2004. Wine, beer, and spirits, and risk of oral, and pharyngeal cancer: A case-control study from Italy and Switzerland. *Oral Oncol* 40, 904–909.
190. Spitz, M. R., Fueger, J. J., Goepfert, H., Hong, W. K., and Newell, G. R. 1988. Squamous cell carcinoma of the upper aerodigestive tract. A case comparison analysis. *Cancer* 61, 203–208.
191. Kabat, G. C., Chang, C. J., and Wynder, E. L. 1994. The role of tobacco, alcohol use, and body mass index in oral and pharyngeal cancer. *Int J Epidemiol* 23, 1137–1144.
192. Huang, W. Y., Winn, D. M., Brown, L. M., Gridley, G., Bravo-Otero, E., Diehl, S. R., et al. 2003. Alcohol concentration and risk of oral cancer in Puerto Rico. *Am J Epidemiol* 157, 881–887.
193. De Stefani, E., Deneo-Pellegrini, H., Mendilaharsu, M., and Ronco, A. 1999. Diet and risk of cancer of the upper aerodigestive tract. I. Foods. *Oral Oncol* 35, 17–21.
194. De Stefani, E., Correa, P., Oreggia, F., Deneo-Pellegrini, H., Fernandez, G., Zavala, D., et al. 1988. Black tobacco, wine, and mate in oropharyngeal cancer. A case-control study from Uruguay. *Rev Epidemiol Sante Publique* 36, 389–394.

195. Oreggia, F., De Stefani, E., Correa, P., and Fierro, L. 1991. Risk factors for cancer of the tongue in Uruguay. *Cancer* 67, 180–183.

196. Merletti, F., Boffetta, P., Ciccone, G., Mashberg, A., and Terracini, B. 1989. Role of tobacco, and alcoholic beverages in the etiology of cancer of the oral cavity/oropharynx in Torino, Italy. *Cancer Res* 49, 4919–4924.

197. Garrote, L. F., Herrero, R., Reyes, R. M., Vaccarella, S., Anta, J. L., Ferbeye, L., et al. 2001. Risk factors for cancer of the oral cavity, and oro-pharynx in Cuba. *Br J Cancer* 85, 46–54.

198. Blot, W. J., McLaughlin, J. K., Winn, D. M., Austin, D. F., Greenberg, R. S., Preston-Martin, S., et al. 1988. Smoking and drinking in relation to oral and pharyngeal cancer. *Cancer Res* 48, 3282–3287.

199. Burch, J. D., Howe, G. R., Miller, A. B., and Semenciw, R. 1981. Tobacco, alcohol, asbestos, and nickel in the etiology of cancer of the larynx: A case-control study. *J Natl Cancer Inst* 67, 1219–1224.

200. Olsen, J., Sabreo, S., and Fasting, U. 1985. Interaction of alcohol and tobacco as risk factors in cancer of the laryngeal region. *J Epidemiol Commun Hlth* 39, 165–168.

201. Jain, M. G., Ferrenc, R. G., Rehm, J. T., Bondy, S. J., Rohan, T. E., Ashley, M. J. et al. 2000. Alcohol and breast cancer mortality in a cohort study. *Breast Cancer Res Treat* 64, 201–209.

202. Zhang, Y., Kreger, B. E., Dorgan, J. F., Splansky, G. L., Cupples, L. A., and Ellison, R. C. 1999. Alcohol consumption and risk of breast cancer: The Framingham Study revisited. *Am J Epidemiol* 149, 93–101.

203. Smith-Warner, S. A., Spiegelman, D., Yaun, S. S., van den Brandt, P. A., Folsom, A. R., Goldbohm, R. A., et al. 1998. Alcohol and breast cancer in women: A pooled analysis of cohort studies. *JAMA* 279, 535–540.

204. de la Lastra C. A. and Villegas I. 2007. Resveratrol as an antioxidant and prooxidant agent: Mechanisms, and clinical implications. *Biochem Soc Trans.* 35Pt 5, 1156–60.

205. Jang, M., Cai, L., Udeani, G. O., Slowing, K. V., Thomas, C. F., Beecher, C. W., et al. 1997. Cancer chemopreventive activity of resveratrol, a natural product derived from grapes. *Science* 275, 218–220.

206. Ciolino, H. P. and Yeh, G. C. 1999. Inhibition of aryl hydrocarbon-induced cytochrome P-450 1A1 enzyme activity, and CYP1A1 expression by resveratrol. *Mol Pharmacol* 56, 760–767.

207. Sgambato, A., Ardito, R., Faraglia, B., Boninsegna, A., Wolf, F. I., and Cittadini, A. 2001. Resveratrol, a natural phenolic compound, inhibits cell proliferation and prevents oxidative DNA damage. *Mutat Res* 496, 171–180.

208. Gusman, J., Malonne, H., and Atassi, G. 2001. A reappraisal of the potential chemopreventive and chemotherapeutic properties of resveratrol. *Carcinogenesis* 22, 1111–1117.

209. Bhuvaneswari, V. and Nagini, S. 2005. Lycopene: A review of its potential as an anticancer agent. *Curr Med Chem Anticancer Agents* 5, 627–635.

210. Giovannucci, E. 1999. Tomatoes, tomato-based products, lycopene, and cancer: Review of the epidemiologic literature. *J Natl Cancer Inst* 91, 317–331.

211. Giovannucci, E., Ascherio, A., Rimm, E. B., Stampfer, M. J., Colditz, G. A., and Willett, W. C. 1995. Intake of carotenoids and retinol in relation to risk of prostate cancer. *J Natl Cancer Inst* 87, 1767–1776.

212. Giovannucci, E., Rimm, E. B., Liu, Y., Stampfer, M. J., and Willett, W. C. 2002. A prospective study of tomato products, lycopene, and prostate cancer risk. *J Natl Cancer Inst* 94, 391–398.

213. Mills, P. K., Beeson, W. L., Phillips, R. L., and Fraser, G. E. 1989. Cohort study of diet, lifestyle, and prostate cancer in Adventist men. *Cancer* 64, 598–604.

214. Hsing, A. W., McLaughlin, J. K., Schuman, L. M., Bjelke, E., Gridley, G., Wacholder, S., et al. 1990. Diet, tobacco use, and fatal prostate cancer: results from the Lutheran Brotherhood Cohort Study. *Cancer Res* 50, 6836–6840.

215. Schuurman, A. G., Goldbohm, R. A., Dorant, E., and van den Brandt, P. A. 1998. Vegetable, and fruit consumption, and prostate cancer risk: A cohort study in The Netherlands. *Cancer Epidemiol Biomarkers Prev* 7, 673–680.

216. Platz, E. A., De Marzo, A. M., Erlinger, T. P., Rifai, N., Visvanathan, K., Hoffman, S. C., and Helzlsouer, K. J. 2004. No association between pre-diagnostic plasma C-reactive protein concentration and subsequent prostate cancer. *Prostate* 59, 393–400

217. Botterweck, A. A., van den Brandt, P. A., and Goldbohm, R. A. 1998. A prospective cohort study on vegetable and fruit consumption and stomach cancer risk in The Netherlands. *Am J Epidemiol* 148, 842–853

218. Tokui, N., Yoshimura, T., Fujino, Y., Mizoue, T., Hoshiyama, Y., Yatsuya, H., et al. 2005. Dietary habits and stomach cancer risk in the JACC Study. *J Epidemiol* 15 Suppl 2, S98–108.

219. Franceschi, S., Bidoli, E., La Vecchia, C., Talamini, R., D'Avanzo, B., and Negri, E. 1994. Tomatoes and risk of digestive-tract cancers. *Int J Cancer* 59, 181–184.
220. Haenszel, W., Kurihara, M., Segi, M., and Lee, R. K. 1972. Stomach cancer among Japanese in Hawaii. *J Natl Cancer Inst* 49, 969–988.
221. Correa, P., Fontham, E., Pickle, L. W., Chen, V., Lin, Y. P., and Haenszel, W. 1985. Dietary determinants of gastric cancer in south Louisiana inhabitants. *J Natl Cancer Inst* 75, 645–654.
222. Boeing, H., Jedrychowski, W., Wahrendorf, J., Popiela, T., Tobiasz–Adamczyk, B., and Kulig, A. 1991. Dietary risk factors in intestinal and diffuse types of stomach cancer: A multicenter case-control study in Poland. *Cancer Causes Control* 2, 227–233.
223. Graham, S., Haughey, B., Marshall, J., Brasure, J., Zielezny, M., Freudenheim, J., et al. 1990. Diet in the epidemiology of gastric cancer. *Nutr Cancer* 13, 19–34.
224. Basu, A. and Imrhan, V. 2007. Tomatoes vs. lycopene in oxidative stress and carcinogenesis: Conclusions from clinical trials. *Eur J Clin Nutr* 61, 295–303.
225. Di Mascio, P., Kaiser, S., and Sies, H. 1989. Lycopene as the most efficient biological carotenoid singlet oxygen quencher. *Arch Biochem Biophys* 274, 532–538.
226. Ben-Dor, A., Steiner, M., Gheber, L., Danilenko, M., Dubi, N., Linnewiel, K., et al. 2005. Carotenoids activate the antioxidant response element transcription system. *Mol Cancer Ther* 4, 177–186.
227. Higdon, J. V., Delage, B., Williams, D. E., and Dashwood, R. H. 2007. Cruciferous vegetables and human cancer risk: Epidemiologic evidence and mechanistic basis. *Pharmacol Res* 55, 224–236.
228. Kensler, T. W., Chen, J. G., Egner, P. A., Fahey, J. W., Jacobson, L. P., Stephenson, K. K., et al. P. 2005. Effects of glucosinolate-rich broccoli sprouts on urinary levels of aflatoxin-DNA adducts, and phenanthrene tetraols in a randomized clinical trial in He Zuo township, Qidong, People's Republic of China. *Cancer Epidemiol Biomarkers Prev* 14, 2605–2613.
229. Cornblatt, B. S., Ye, L., Dinkova-Kostova, A. T., Erb, M., Fahey, J. W., Singh, N. K., et al. 2007. Preclinical and clinical evaluation of sulforaphane for chemoprevention in the breast. *Carcinogenesis* 28, 1485–1490.
230. Walters, D. G., Young, P. J., Agus, C., Knize, M. G., Boobis, A. R., Gooderham, N. J., and Lake, B. G. 2004. Cruciferous vegetable consumption alters the metabolism of the dietary carcinogen 2-amino-1-methyl-6-phenylimidazo[4,5-b]pyridine PhIP in humans. *Carcinogenesis* 25, 1659–1669.
231. Juge, N., Mithen, R. F., and Traka, M. 2007. Molecular basis for chemoprevention by sulforaphane: A comprehensive review. *Cell Mol Life Sci* 64, 1105–1127.
232. Joseph, M. A., Moysich, K. B., Freudenheim, J. L., Shields, P. G., Bowman, E. D., Zhang, Y., et al. 2004. Cruciferous vegetables, genetic polymorphisms in glutathione S-transferases M1 and T1 and prostate cancer risk. *Nutr Cancer* 50, 206–213.
233. Fimognari, C., and Hrelia, P. 2007. Sulforaphane as a promising molecule for fighting cancer. *Mutat Res* 635, 90–104.
234. Dashwood, R. H. 2002. Modulation of heterocyclic amine-induced mutagenicity, and carcinogenicity: An 'A-to-Z' guide to chemopreventive agents, promoters, and transgenic models. *Mutat Res* 511, 89–112.
235. Zhang, Y., Talalay, P., Cho, C. G., and Posner, G. H. 1992. A major inducer of anticarcinogenic protective enzymes from broccoli: Isolation, and elucidation of structure. *Proc Natl Acad Sci USA* 89, 2399–2403.
236. Barcelo, S., Gardiner, J. M., Gescher, A., and Chipman, J. K. 1996. CYP2E1-mediated mechanism of anti-genotoxicity of the broccoli constituent sulforaphane. *Carcinogenesis* 17, 277–282.
237. Pham, N. A., Jacobberger, J. W., Schimmer, A. D., Cao, P., Gronda, M., and Hedley, D. W. 2004. The dietary isothiocyanate sulforaphane targets pathways of apoptosis, cell cycle arrest, and oxidative stress in human pancreatic cancer cells and inhibits tumor growth in severe combined immunodeficient mice. *Mol Cancer Ther* 3, 1239–1248.
238. Herman-Antosiewicz, A., Johnson, D. E., and Singh, S. V. 2006. Sulforaphane causes autophagy to inhibit release of cytochrome C, and apoptosis in human prostate cancer cells. *Cancer Res* 66, 5828–5835.
239. Myzak, M. C., Tong, P., Dashwood, W. M., Dashwood, R. H., and Ho, E. 2007. Sulforaphane retards the growth of human PC-3 xenografts and inhibits HDAC activity in human subjects. *Exp Biol Med Maywood.* 232, 227–234.
240. Conaway, C. C., Wang, C. X., Pittman, B., Yang, Y. M., Schwartz, J. E., Tian, D., et al. 2005. Phenethyl isothiocyanate, and sulforaphane, and their N-acetylcysteine conjugates inhibit malignant progression of lung adenomas induced by tobacco carcinogens in A/J mice. *Cancer Res* 65, 8548–8557.

241. Bertl, E., Bartsch, H., and Gerhauser, C. 2006. Inhibition of angiogenesis and endothelial cell functions are novel sulforaphane-mediated mechanisms in chemoprevention. *Mol Cancer Ther* 5, 575–585.
242. Thejass, P. and Kuttan, G. 2006. Antimetastatic activity of Sulforaphane. *Life Sci* 78, 3043–3050.
243. Ferguson, L. R., Chavan, R. R., and Harris, P. J. 2001. Changing concepts of dietary fiber: Implications for carcinogenesis. *Nutr Cancer* 39, 155–169.
244. Yan, J., Allendorf, D. J., and Brandley, B. 2005. Yeast whole glucan particle (WGP) Beta-glucan in conjunction with antitumour monoclonal antibodies to treat cancer. *Expert Opin Biol Ther* 5, 691–702.
245. Kim, S. Y., Song, H. J., Lee, Y. Y., Cho, K. H., and Roh, Y. K. 2006. Biomedical issues of dietary fiber beta-glucan. *J Korean Med* Sci 21, 781–789.
246. Burkitt, D. P. 1969. Related disease—related cause? *Lancet* 2, 1229–1231.
247. Kim, Y. I. 2000. AGA technical review: Impact of dietary fiber on colon cancer occurrence. *Gastroenterology* 118, 1235–1257.
248. Jacobs, D. R., Jr., Marquart, L., Slavin, J., and Kushi, L. H. 1998. Whole-grain intake, and cancer: An expanded review and meta-analysis. *Nutr Cancer* 30, 85–96.
249. McCullough, M. L., Robertson, A. S., Chao, A., Jacobs, E. J., Stampfer, M. J., Jacobs, D. R., et al. 2003. A prospective study of whole grains, fruits, vegetables, and colon cancer risk. *Cancer Causes Control* 14, 959–970.
250. Larsson, S. C., Giovannucci, E., Bergkvist, L., and Wolk, A. 2005. Whole grain consumption and risk of colorectal cancer: A population-based cohort of 60,000 women. *Br J Cancer* 92, 1803–1807.
251. Schatzkin, A., Mouw, T., Park, Y., Subar, A. F., Kipnis, V., Hollenbeck, A., et al. 2007. Dietary fiber and whole-grain consumption in relation to colorectal cancer in the NIH-AARP Diet and Health Study. *Am J Clin Nutr* 85, 1353–1360.
252. Cohen, L. A., Zhao, Z., Zang, E. A., Wynn, T. T., Simi, B., and Rivenson, A. 1996. Wheat bran and psyllium diets: Effects on N-methylnitrosourea-induced mammary tumorigenesis in F344 rats. *J Natl Cancer Inst* 88, 899–907.
253. Hague, A. and Paraskeva, C. 1995. The short-chain fatty acid butyrate induces apoptosis in colorectal tumour cell lines. *Eur J Cancer Prev* 4, 359–364.
254. Smith, J. G., Yokoyama, W. H., and German, J. B. 1998. Butyric acid from the diet: Actions at the level of gene expression. *Crit Rev Food Sci Nutr* 38, 259–297.
255. Jenab, M., Ferrari, P., Slimani, N., Norat, T., Casagrande, C., Overad, K., et al. 2004. Association of nut, and seed intake with colorectal cancer risk in the European Prospective Investigation into Cancer, and Nutrition. *Cancer Epidemiol Biomarkers Prev* 13, 1595–1603.
256. Brouwer, I. A., Katan, M. B., and Zock, P. L. 2004. Dietary alpha-linolenic acid is associated with reduced risk of fatal coronary heart disease, but increased prostate cancer risk: A meta-analysis. *J Nutr* 134, 919–922.
257. Singh, P. N. and Fraser, G. E. 1998. Dietary risk factors for colon cancer in a low-risk population. *Am J Epidemiol* 148, 761–774.
258. Peters, R. K., Pike, M. C., Garabrant, D., and Mack, T. M. 1992. Diet and colon cancer in Los Angeles County, California. *Cancer Causes Control* 3, 457–473.
259. Pickle, L. W., Greene, M. H., Ziegler, R. G., Toledo, A., Hoover, R., Lynch, H. T., and Fraumeni, J. F., Jr. 1984. Colorectal cancer in rural Nebraska. *Cancer Res* 44, 363–369.
260. Kune, S., Kune, G. A., and Watson, L. F. 1987. Case-control study of dietary etiological factors: The Melbourne Colorectal Cancer Study. *Nutr Cancer* 9, 21–42.
261. Davis, P. A. and Iwahashi, C. K. 2001. Whole almonds, and almond fractions reduce aberrant crypt foci in a rat model of colon carcinogenesis. *Cancer Lett* 165, 27–33.
262. Zeng H. and Combs, G.F. Jr. 2008. Selenium as an anticancer nutrient: Roles in cell proliferation and tumor cell invasion. *J Nutr Biochem*. 191, 1–7
263. Trujillo, E., Davis, C., and Milner, J. 2006. Nutrigenomics, proteomics, metabolomics, and the practice of dietetics. *J Am Diet Assoc* 106, 403–13.

Section III

Bioactive Foods as Nutrients
in Health Promotion

14 Potential Role of Resveratrol in Preventing Inflammation and Diseases Associated with Obesity and Aging

Kathleen LaPoint and Michael K. McIntosh

CONTENTS

14.1 OBESITY, INFLAMMATION, AND CHRONIC DISEASE

14.1.1 OBESITY AND INSULIN RESISTANCE

Obesity and its associated pathologies are the most common metabolic diseases in the United States, affecting over 30% of the adult population, and is increasing at an alarming rate among all age groups in the country. Currently, in all but four states at least 20% of their population are classified as obese (body mass index [BMI] > 30.0) [1]. This rapid rise in obesity is accompanied by a similar increase in insulin resistance or type II diabetes [2]. In fact, approximately 80% of individuals with type II diabetes are overweight (BMI 25.0–29.9) or obesity (BMI > 30.0), suggesting a strong positive relationship between the two diseases [3,4]. Interestingly, decreasing body fat is one of the most effective ways to improve insulin sensitivity. Thus, overnutrition relative to inadequate energy expenditure leads to increased adiposity and insulin resistance, and vice versa.

14.1.2 OBESITY AND THE METABOLIC SYNDROME

Along with insulin resistance, obesity is also positively associated with atherosclerosis and hypertension [5]. This cluster of obesity-related diseases is referred to as the metabolic syndrome. The clinical criterion for diagnosis of the metabolic syndrome defined by the World Health Organization (WHO) is a diagnosis of diabetes together with two or more of the following: (1) hypertriglyceridemia or low high-density lipoprotein cholesterol (HDL), (2) microalbuminuria, (3) hypertension, or (4) obesity [6]. The metabolic syndrome is not only a major predictor of early mortality, but also of morbidity. For example, kidney disease and renal failure, both debilitating and life-shortening, are positively correlated with the incidence of metabolic syndrome [7]. Stroke, gall bladder disease, osteoarthritis, sleep apnea, and certain types of cancer (e.g., endometrial, breast, colon) are linked to obesity as well [4].

14.1.3 METABOLIC SYNDROME, LOW GRADE INFLAMMATION, AND WHITE ADIPOSE TISSUE

Interestingly, the metabolic syndrome has recently been associated with low grade inflammation [8]. One emerging feature of obesity is the linkage between obesity and chronic inflammation characterized by increased cytokine and chemokine production and acute-phase inflammatory signaling in white adipose tissue (WAT) [9]. WAT is no longer considered an inert depot of stored energy, but an active endocrine organ secreting a diverse array of proinflammatory "adipokines" such as leptin, interleukin (IL)-1β, IL-6, IL-8, tumor necrosis factor (TNF)-α, monocyte chemoattractant protein-1 (MCP-1), and macrophage migration inhibitory factor (MIF) [10], all of which have been linked to insulin resistance [11, 12]. Acute phase proteins such as plasminogen-activator inhibitor 1 (PAI-1) and C-reactive protein (CRP), which promote hypertension and atherogenesis, respectively, are also secreted from WAT [13]. However, the exact role of cells composing adipose tissue in mediating inflammation and causing insulin resistance is still unclear.

It has been suggested that, in adult WAT, nonadipocytes (i.e., stromal vascular cells or cells from the supporting matrix) are the major producers of IL-6 and TNF-α rather than adipocytes [14,15]. Similarly, preadipocytes have been reported to act as macrophage-like cells and secrete an array of cytokines [16]. Intriguingly, Charrière et al. [17] reported plasticity of preadipocytes showing evidence that 3T3-L1 cells have the ability to acquire phagocytic phenotypes and properties in the presence of macrophages. Consistent with this notion, our group demonstrated that human preadipocytes are more potent mediators of inflammation than human adipocytes [18].

Conversely, it has been proposed that macrophages residing in adipose tissue are responsible for most of the secreted cytokines [19]. Weisberg et al. [20] reported that adipose tissue recruits circulating monocytes/macrophages from bone. Thus, WAT consists of a variety of cells with the capacity to promote low-grade chronic inflammation via the release of adipokines, acute phase proteins, fatty acids, prostaglandins, and other compounds. This capacity of WAT to secrete inflammatory agents increases in proportion to its mass, thereby contributing to the pathologies of the metabolic syndrome.

14.1.4 LOCATION, LOCATION, LOCATION—THE INFLAMMATORY ROLE OF CENTRAL WAT

Upper-body or visceral obesity appears to be a better predictor of systemic insulin resistance and metabolic syndrome than subcutaneous or lower-body obesity. It has been proposed that this central location of WAT provides inflammatory mediators directly to nearby organs such as liver, pancreas, heart, and kidneys, thereby promoting insulin resistance, hyperlipidemia, hypertension, or kidney failure [21].

An alternative hypothesis is that visceral or central WAT secretes unique adipokines that promote disease, or it fails to secrete adipokines that prevent disease. For example, the inflammatory cytokines IL-6 and IL-8 have been reported to be more abundant in visceral WAT compared with subcutaneous WAT [21]. Interestingly, retinol binding protein 4 (RBP4), six-transmembrane protein of prostate 2 (STAMP2), visfatin, inhibitor of apoptosis 2 (cIAP2), and resistin have been proposed to be preferentially secreted from visceral WAT compared with subcutaneous WAT, and are positively linked to insulin resistance [9].

As an example, serum levels of RBP4 have been recently shown to be positively correlated with body fat levels [22]. RBP4 mRNA levels were higher in visceral WAT than in subcutaneous WAT of the study participants. RBP4 levels were twofold higher in participants with type II diabetes than in those without diabetes. Elevated RBP4 levels were negatively correlated with the levels of the insulin-responsive glucose transporter 4 (GLUT4), a protein that mediates insulin-stimulated glucose disposal. Thus, elevated levels of RBP4, which are associated with increased visceral WAT, contribute to insulin resistance, in part, by reducing the levels of GLUT4.

It has been proposed that obese individuals, particularly those with increased visceral WAT, lack certain adipokines that prevent disease. One such adipokine is adiponectin, an insulin-sensitizing protein secreted exclusively from WAT [23]. Adiponectin improves insulin sensitivity by decreasing hepatic glucose output and enhancing glucose and fatty acid oxidation, in part, by activating AMP kinase [24]. Indeed, the levels of adiponectin have been shown to be lower in obese subjects compared to lean subjects [25]. Intriguingly, overexpression of adiponectin in obese mice prevents them from developing of insulin resistance, demonstrating the important role of adiponectin in maintaining insulin sensitivity [26]. Thus, a lack of sufficient adiponectin may lead to insulin resistance and hyperlipidemia.

14.1.5 THERAPIES FOR PREVENTING INFLAMMATION FROM WAT

Consuming a prudent diet that provides calories that are proportional to energy expenditure theoretically impedes the development of overweight and obesity. However, successful weight loss and maintenance are difficult even when resources abound on how to eat healthfully and remain active. Weight control using pharmacological approaches has not proven to be an effective solution to the obesity epidemic or its comorbidities.

On the other hand, exciting data are emerging suggesting that consuming foods, beverages, or supplements rich in phenolic phytochemicals may attenuate inflammatory-related diseases, including those associated with metabolic syndrome [27]. Although these compounds may not initially promote weight or fat loss, they appear to effectively reduce certain morbidities associated with obesity. One of the proposed mechanisms by which they prevent the development of these morbidities is suppressing chronic low-grade inflammation. In the next section of this chapter we will discuss (1) the major classes of phenol phytochemicals and their structure-function relationships, (2) relative bioavailability, (3) proposed health benefits, and (4) proposed mechanisms by which they reduce inflammation. We have chosen to focus primarily on resveratrol (a stilbene found in grapes, berries, and peanuts), based on exciting data suggesting its potential role as an anti-inflammatory dietary ingredient.

14.2 POLYPHENOLS

14.2.1 CHEMISTRY

Polyphenols are a group of chemical compounds found in plants, generally produced as part of the plant's chemical defense against UV radiation, predators, or pests [28]. They are classified according to their carbon skeletons into the following groups:

- Phenolic acids
- Flavonoids
- Tannins
- Stilbenes
- Coumarins
- Lignans

Phenolic acids and flavonoids are plentiful in the foods we eat; stilbenes and lignans are less common [29].

Polyphenols are abundant in fruits, chocolate, coffee, tea, wine, and beer; vegetables, legumes, and grains are also good sources of certain polyphenols [30]. Quantifying the types and amounts of polyphenols in the diet is difficult for a number of reasons, but total intake of polyphenols has been estimated at roughly 1 g per day [30]. The polyphenol content of a plant is variable, influenced by factors such as the plant cultivar, growing conditions, and stage of maturation [28,29]. These compounds are more concentrated in the peels of fruits and vegetables and in the outer layer of grains, so processing of foods for consumption can result in substantial decrease in polyphenol content [30]. Additionally, these compounds are highly reactive and good substrates for enzymes such as polyphenoloxidases, peroxidases, glycosidases, and esterases [29]. Enzymatic reactions occurring during storage and processing of food can produce compounds that may have properties different from their precursors. For example, oxidation of polyphenols can reduce the quality of some foods, but it is essential in the processing of chocolate, tea, and coffee [29]. In another example, only half the polyphenols found in a 2-year-old red wine were grape polyphenols. The other half were unknown polyphenol species produced during fermentation and aging [29].

All plant phenols are derived from shikimic acid and share least one aromatic ring structure with one or more hydroxyl groups [31]. Polyphenols range from simple molecules to highly polymerized compounds that exhibit a wide range of properties that depend on their structures. They contribute to the colors and flavors of foods, are scavengers of reactive oxygen species, and have the ability to complex with proteins. Their chemical properties are a largely a function of the number and accessibility of phenol groups. [29].

14.2.2 BENEFICIAL EFFECTS

Most of the evidence for the beneficial effects of polyphenols comes from studies in animal models and human cell lines. Polyphenols trap and scavenge free radicals, directly interact with receptors and enzymes, and modulate signal transduction pathways [31]. As the most abundant antioxidants in diet, they may protect the body against cancers, cardiovascular diseases (CVD), and inflammatory diseases by preventing oxidative stress [30,32]. The polyphenol curcumin, for example, has been the subject of many studies demonstrating its anti-inflammatory, antibacterial, antiviral, antifungal, antitumor, antispasmodic, and hepatoprotective effects [27]. Additionally, some polyphenols appear to have estrogenic-like properties, and may be able to prevent breast cancer and osteoporosis [33,34].

Epidemiologic studies have been inconsistent, but there appears to be a correlation between a diet rich in polyphenols and reduced risk of CVD, asthma, and osteoporosis, as well as lung, endometrial, ovarian, thyroid, breast, and colorectal cancers [30,32]. However, results from *in vitro* or animal experiments were obtained using much higher doses of unmetabolized polyphenols than what is possible through diet [31]. Polyphenols are metabolized by the phase II conjugation pathways producing methylated, glucuronidated, and sulfated compounds [30]. Studies in humans demonstrate variation in the extent of metabolism according to the specific polyphenol and by subject [30]. More studies are required to help clarify whether proposed health benefits are due to the polyphenols or other dietary factors.

14.2.3 POLYPHENOL SUPPLEMENTATION

Polyphenol supplements are becoming popular and some supplement manufacturers recommend intakes of 100 times higher than what is achievable through diet [35]. Supplementation could provide doses similar to those that produced such dramatic results in *in vitro* and animal experiments, but may result in undesirable outcomes. Polyphenols can interfere with thyroid hormone biosynthesis and iron absorption, and can be carcinogenic or genotoxic at high doses [35,36]. High doses of phytoestrogen isoflavones are associated with antiluteinizing hormone effects in premenopausal women and there are concerns about sexual maturation of infants fed soy formula [35]. Polyphenols may affect an administered drug's efficacy or increase its toxicity through competition for the same metabolic pathway [37]. Furthermore, because polyphenols are highly unstable, the method of extraction may alter the polyphenols, raising concerns about the safety supplements [35].

14.3 RESVERATROL

Epidemiologic studies have demonstrated an inverse correlation between red wine consumption and coronary heart disease in France. Known as the French paradox, this apparent protective effect of red wine was seen despite a diet high in saturated fat [38]. Although alcohol itself appears to have cardioprotective effects, resveratrol appeared to add to those effects [39].

14.3.1 CHEMISTRY

Resveratrol (3,5,4'-trihydroxystilbene) is a stilbene phytoalexin that exists as *cis*-resveratrol or *trans*-resveratrol [40]. *Trans*-resveratrol is the more stable, abundant, and bioactive isomer [41]. In addition to red wine, grapes, berries, soy, peanuts, and peanut butter are important sources of resveratrol in the Western diet; it is also present in relatively high concentrations in the plant *Polygonum cuspidatum*, an herbal remedy used in Japanese and Chinese medicine [42]. Resveratrol glucoside or piceid is the primary form of resveratrol found in grapes, but because free resveratrol is more abundant in wines, the sugar group appears to be cleaved during fermentation and aging [43,44]. Because resveratrol is synthesized in the skin rather than the flesh of the grape, red wines fermented with the skin have higher resveratrol concentrations than white wines [42]. The average resveratrol content in red wine is 1.9 ± 1.7 mg/L, ranging from undetectable to 14 mg/L [44].

14.3.2 BENEFICIAL EFFECTS

Cardiovascular disease, cancers, diabetes, and neurodegenerative diseases are associated with aging; oxidative stress and inflammation appear to be common contributing factors. Obesity, characterized by inflammation, appears to accelerate aging and increase the risk of age-related diseases [42,45,46]. *In vivo* evidence for resveratrol as a potential therapy for obesity and age-related diseases is accumulating. Resveratrol's cancer chemopreventive and chemotherapeutic properties have been demonstrated in multiple rodent models [43]. Isolated rodent hearts showed improved recovery in function and were protected from ischemia/reperfusion injury when resveratrol was administered before the ischemic injury [8]. Mice fed a high-calorie diet supplemented with resveratrol showed improved insulin sensitivity compared with mice fed the high-calorie diet without resveratrol [47], and resveratrol appears to protect rodents from brain damage after cerebral ischemia [8]. Additional anti-aging effects observed are enhanced aerobic capacity, improved motor function, resistance to obesity in mice [48], increased survival in obese mice [49], and increased lifespan in *Saccharomyces cerevisae, Caenorhabditis elegans, Drosophila melanogaster,* and the fish species *Nothobranchius furzeri* [49].

14.3.3 MECHANISMS

Mechanisms by which resveratrol might potentially exert antiaging, anticancer, cardioprotective, and neuroprotective effects are numerous. Resveratrol's antioxidant properties may account for many of its beneficial effects. Reactive oxygen species cause oxidative injury to cellular proteins, nucleic acids, and lipids; oxidative stress occurs when the body cannot repair or remove the damage from reactive oxygen species at the rate at which the damage is induced. Like other polyphenols, resveratrol is a free radical scavenger; drinking red wine has been shown to increase serum antioxidant capacity in humans [40]. Resveratrol appears to inhibit the oxidation of low-density lipoproteins, a key event in atherosclerosis, by chelating copper [50]. Resveratrol also inhibits lipid peroxidation in cellular membranes [33]. Induction of glutathione and antioxidant enzymes in rat aortic smooth muscle cells and induction of neuroprotective heme oxidase 1 in primary neuronal cultures and aortic smooth muscle cells demonstrated that the modulation of antioxidant pathways is another mechanism by which resveratrol may protect against oxidative stress [43].

Resveratrol appears to offer additional protection against age-related pathologies by downregulating uncontrolled inflammatory response. Both direct interaction with enzymes and inhibition of signal transduction pathways have been demonstrated *in vitro*. Resveratrol suppresses prostaglandin and thrombroxane production by inhibiting activity and transcription of cyclooxygenase-2 [27,51]. Proinflammatory metabolites of arachidonic acid are also reduced by resveratrol's inhibition of the lipooxygenase pathway [52]. Nitric oxide and cytokines involved in inflammatory processes are also suppressed by resveratrol [27,53]. Downregulation of these proinflammatory targets appear to be mediated through the inhibition of transcription factors nuclear factor ☒ B and activator protein-1 [53,54].

Calorie restriction has been shown to slow aging and delay the onset of age-related diseases in organisms from yeast to rodents and perhaps primates [55]. Sirtuins appear to mediate this anti-aging response by deacetylating histones and transcription factors regulating stress, metabolism, and survival pathways [46]. The ability of resveratrol to improve survival, aerobic capacity, motor function, and insulin sensitivity may be mediated, in part, by induction of the sirtuin SIRT1 [49,56]. The effect of resveratrol on health and longevity through SIRT1 is proposed to be due to induction of adaptive stress responses [48].

14.3.4 PHARMACOKINETICS

In vitro experiments identifying these molecular targets have typically required high concentrations of resveratrol. The relevance of these studies *in vivo* depends upon absorption, metabolism, and distribution of resveratrol in the body. Pharmacokinetic studies show that resveratrol is absorbed by intestinal epithelial cells through rapid passive diffusion, and absorbance in human subjects is estimated to be at least 70% after supplementation of 25 mg [57]. However, resveratrol is extensively metabolized to sulfate and glucuronide conjugates in both the duodenum and the liver [58,59,60]. About 99% of the resveratrol transferred across the intestine was determined to be resveratrol glucuronide [61]. Resveratrol glucoside requires the sodium-dependent glucose co-transporter for uptake, and is deglycosylated to resveratrol before glucuronide conjugation [62]. Metabolism of resveratrol in the intestine appears to be inhibited at high resveratrol concentrations achievable by supplementation [63]. Only trace amounts of circulating free resveratrol were detected in healthy human subjects after drinking wine, although resveratrol glucuronide was found in higher concentrations in some subjects [60]. After administration of 25 mg resveratrol per 70 kg body weight, peak unconjugated resveratrol concentrations were only 10-40 nmol/L [59]. However, after single dose supplementation of 0.5 to 5 g resveratrol in human subjects, concentrations of free resveratrol peaked at 0.3 µM–2.4 µM, reaching the concentrations found to have beneficial effect in *in vitro* systems [64]. Serum concentrations of resveratrol glucuronide and resveratrol sulfate were 3 to 8 times the concentration of free resveratrol in those subjects.

Large variations in circulating resveratrol and its metabolites were found in subjects after administration, but absorption and bioavailability do not appear to be influenced by amount or type of food consumed with wine or by the matrix in which supplementation is given [59,60]. Resveratrol in its various forms reaches peak concentration in the serum after about 30–60 minutes [57,59,60]. Most of the resveratrol is excreted as a glucuronide in the urine [65].

The extensive glucuronidation and sulfation of resveratrol are presumed to lead to rapid clearance and low bioavailability of resveratrol, preventing its accumulation in target tissues. Nevertheless, free resveratrol was detected in the liver, heart, lungs, and brain of rats 18 hours after administration, despite the very low concentrations of unconjugated resveratrol in circulation [66]. The low concentrations of free serum resveratrol *in vivo* may be due, in part, to low aqueous solubility. Resveratrol has been shown to bind to albumin, which may be an important carrier in the serum

[67,68]. Alternatively, the accumulation of free resveratrol in tissues could be the result of ⊠-glucuronidase activity. The enzyme is widely expressed and may release free resveratrol in target tissues by cleaving the glucuronide conjugate [69]. It is also important to note that wine contains abundant polyphenols in addition to resveratrol. Flavonoids such as quercetin have been shown to inhibit sulfation and glucuronidation of resveratrol, which may increase its bioavailability *in vivo* [66,70].

14.4 SUMMARY AND CONCLUSION

The rapid rise in obesity in the United States is accompanied by an increased risk for developing age-related diseases. Excess WAT, in particular intra-abdominal visceral WAT, promotes low-grade chronic inflammation through the release of adipokines, acute phase proteins, fatty acids, prostaglandins, and other compounds. Inflammation appears to be an important contributing factor for insulin resistance, hypertension, cardiovascular disease, kidney failure, and certain types of cancer, metabolic disorders, and neurodegenerative diseases.

Accumulating data has demonstrated that resveratrol may prevent or slow the progression of these diseases, as well as increase lifespan and resistance to stress. However, results obtained with high doses of resveratrol used for *in vitro* experiments may not be physiologically relevant. Rapid and extensive metabolism of resveratrol results in circulating concentrations of free resveratrol much lower than concentrations typically required to achieve *in vitro* effects. More experiments are required to determine whether resveratrol can accumulate in tissues and whether metabolites can activate targets.

A significant increase in the consumption of resveratrol, as for many other polyphenols, may not be without risk. Like other polyphenols, resveratrol undergoes the same biotransformation processes that also mediate the bioavailability of pharmaceutical agents. And like other polyphenols, resveratrol is unstable, raising concerns about the safety of supplements. There is currently not enough evidence to recommend supplementation, but resveratrol is already being tested in human subjects to assess oral bioavailability, pharmacokinetics, and toxicity

REFERENCES

1. Department of Health and Human Services Centers for Disease Control and Prevention. 2007. U.S. Obesity trends 1985–2006. http://www.cdc.gov/nccdphp/dnpa/obesity/trend/maps/index.htm (accessed November 27, 2007).
2. Department of Health and Human Services Centers for Disease Control and Prevention. 2007. Diabetes Data and Trends. http://www.cdc.gov/diabetes/statistics/prev/national/figpersons.htm (accessed November 27, 2007).
3. Department of Health and Human Services Centers for Disease Control and Prevention. 2007. Overweight and obesity health consequences. http://www.cdc.gov/nccdphp/dnpa/obesity/consequences.htm (accessed November 27, 2007).
4. Centers for Disease Control and Prevention. 2007. BMI–0 Body Mass Index. http://www.cdc.gov/nccdphp/dnpa/bmi/adult_BMI/about_adult_BMI.htm (accessed November 28, 2007).
5. Ford, E., Giles, W., and Mokdad, A. 2004. Increasing prevalence of the metabolic syndrome among U.S. adults. *Diabetes Care* 27, 2444–2449.
6. Reynolds, K. and He, J. 2005. Epidemiology of the metabolic syndrome. *Am. J. Med. Sci.* 330, 273–279.
7. National Kidney and Urologic Diseases Information Clearinghouse. 2007. Kidney and urologic diseases statistics for the United States. http://kidney.niddk.nih.gov/kudiseases/pubs/kustats/index.htm#kp accessed November 28, 2007.
8. Wellen, K. and Hotamisligil, G. 2005. Inflammation, stress, and diabetes. *J. Clin. Invest.* 115, 1111–1119.
9. Hotamisligil G. 2006. Inflammation and metabolic disorders. *Nature* 444, 860–867.
10. Trayhurn, P. 2005. Endocrine and signaling role of adipose tissue: New perspective on fat. *Acta Physiol. Scand.* 184, 285–293.

11. Hutley, L. and Prins, J. 2005. Fat as an Endocrine Organ: Relationship to the metabolic syndrome. *Am. J. Med. Sci.* 330, 280–289.

12. Qatanani, M. and Lazar, M. 2007. Mechanisms of obesity-associated insulin resistance: Many choices on the menu. *Genes Dev.* 21, 1443–1455.

13. Ford, E. 2003. The metabolic syndrome and C-reactive protein, fibrinogen, and leukocyte count: Findings from the Third National Health and Nutrition Examination Survey. *Atherosclerosis* 168, 351–358.

14. Fain, J., Madan, A., Hiler, M., Cheema, P., and Bahouth, S. 2004. Comparison of the release of cytokines by adipose tissue, adipose tissue matrix, and adipocytes from visceral and subcutaneous abdominal adipose tissues of obese humans. *Endocrinology* 145, 2273–2282.

15. Fain, J., Bahouth, S., and Madan, A. 2004. TNF-α release by the nonfat cells of human adipose tissue. *Int. J. Obesity* 28, 616–623.

16. Cousin, B., Munoz, O., and Andre, M. 1999. A role for preadipocytes as macrophage-like cells. *FASEB J* 13, 305–312.

17. Charrière, G., Cousin, B., Arnaud, E., André, M., Bacou, F., Pénicaud, L., and Casteilla, L. 2003. Preadipocyte conversion to macrophage. *J. Biol. Chem.* 278, 9850–9855.

18. Chung, S., LaPoint, K., Kennedy A., Martinez, K., Boysen-Sandberg, M., and McIntosh M. 2006. Preadipocytes mediated LPS-induced inflammation and insulin resistance in primary cultures of newly differentiated human adipocytes. *Endocrinology* 147, 5340–51.

19. Xu, H., Barnes, G., Yang, Q., Tan, G., Yang, D., Chou, C., et al. 2003. Chronic inflammation in fat plays a crucial role in the development of obesity-related insulin resistance. *J. Clin. Invest.* 112, 1821–1830.

20. Weisberg, S., McCann, D., Desai, M., Rosenbaum, M., Leibel, R., and Ferrante A. 2003. Obesity is associated with macrophage accumulation in adipose tissue. *J. Clin. Invest.* 112, 1796–1808.

21. Bruun, J., Lihn A., Madan, A., Pedersen, S., Schiott, K., Fain, J., and Richelsen, B. 2003. Higher production of IL-8 in visceral vs. subcutaneous adipose tissue. Implication of nonadipose cells in adipose tissue. *Am. J. Physiol. Endocrinol. Metab.* 286, 8–13.

22. Kloting, N., Graham, T., Berndt, J., Kralisch, S., Kovacs, P., Wason C., et al. 2007. Serum retinol-binding protein is more highly expressed in visceral than in subcutaneous adipose tissue and is a marker of intra-abdominal fat mass. *Cell Metab.* 6, 79–87.

23. Trujillo, M. and Scherer, P. 2005. Adiponectin—journey from an adipocyte secretory protein to biomarker of the metabolic syndrome. *J. Int Med.* 257, 167–175.

24. Yamauchi, T., Kamon, J., Minokoshi, Y., Ito, Y. Waki, H., Uchida, S., et al. 2002. Adiponectin stimulates glucose utilization and fatty acid oxidation by activating AMP-activated protein kinase. *Nature Med.* 8, 1288–1295.

25. Pajvani, U., Hawkins, M., Combs, T., Rajala, M., Doebber, T., Berger, J., et al. 2004. Complex distribution, not absolute amount of adiponectin, correlates with thiazolidinedione-mediated improvements in insulin sensitivity. *J. Biol. Chem.* 279, 12152–12162.

26. Kim, J.-Y., van de Wall, E., Laplante, M., Azzara, A., Trujillo, M., Hofmann, S., et al. 2007. Obesity-associated improvements in metabolic syndrome profile through expansion of adipose tissue. *J. Clin. Invest.* 117, 2621–2636.

27. Rahman, I., Biswas, S., and Kirkham, P. 2006. Regulation of inflammation and redox signaling by dietary polyphenols. *Biochem. Pharmacol.* 72, 1439–52.

28. Manach, C., Scalbert, A., Morand, C., Rémésy, C., Jiménez, L. 2004. Polyphenols: Food sources and bioavailability. *Am. J. Clin. Nutr.* 79, 727–747.

29. Cheynier, V. 2005. Polyphenols in foods are more complex than often thought. *Am. J. Clin. Nutr.* 81, 223S–229S.

30. Scalbert, A., Williamson, G. 2000. Dietary intake and bioavailability of polyphenols. *J. Nutr.* 130, 2073S–2085S.

31. Scalbert, A., Johnson, I., and Saltmarsh, M. 2005 Polyphenols: Antioxidants and beyond. *Am. J. Clin. Nutr.* 81, 215S–217S.

32. Arts, I. and Hollman, P. 2005. Polyphenols and disease risk in epidemiologic studies. *Am. J. Clin. Nutr.* 81, 317S–325S.

33. Yamaguchi, M. 2002. Isoflavone and bone metabolism: Its cellular mechanism and preventive role in bone loss. *J. Health Sci.* 48, 209–222.

34. Duncan, A., Phipps, W., and Kurzer, M. 2003. Phyto-oestrogens. *Best Pract. Res. Clin. Endocrinol. Metab.* 17, 253–271.

35. Mennen, L., Walker, R., Bennetau-Pelissero, C., and Scalbert, A. 2005. Risk and safety of polyphenol consumption. *Am. J. Clin.* 81, 326S–329S.

36. Verster, A. and van der Pols, J. 1995. Anaemia in the Eastern Mediterranean region. *E. Med. Health J.* 1, 64–79.
37. Lambert, J., Sang, S., Lu, A., and Yang, C. 2007. Metabolism of dietary polyphenols and possible interactions with drugs. *Curr. Drug Metab.* 8, 499–507.
38. Renaud, S. and de Lorgeril, M. 1992. Wine, alcohol, platelets, and the French paradox for coronary heart disease. *Lancet* 339, 1523–1526.
39. Siemann, E. and Creasy, L. 1992. Concentration of the phytoalexin resveratrol in wine. *Am. J. Eno. Vitic.* 43, 49–52.
40. Whitehead, T., Robinson, D., Allaway, S., Syms, J., and Hale, A. 1995. Effect of red wine ingestion on the antioxidant capacity of serum. *Clin. Chem.* 41, 32–35.
41. King, R., Bomser, J., and Min, D. 2006 Bioactivity of resveratrol. *Comp. Rev. Food Sci. Food Safety* 5, 65–70.
42. Burns, J., Yokota, T., Ashihara, H., Lean, M., and Crozier, A. 2002. Plant foods and herbal sources of resveratrol. *J. Agric. Food Chem.* 50, 3337–3340.
43. Szende, B., Tyihák, E., and Király–Véghely, Z. 2000. Dose-dependent effect of resveratrol on proliferation and apoptosis in endothelial and tumor cell cultures. *Exp. Mol. Med.* 32, 88–92.
44. Stervbo, U., Vang, O., and Bonnensen, C. 2007. A review of the content of the putative chemopreventive phytoalexin resveratrol in wine. *Food Chem.* 101, 449–457.
45. Valdes, A., Andrew, T., Gardner, J., Kimura, M., Oelsner, E., Cherkas, L., et al. 2005. Obesity, cigarette smoking, and telomere length in women. *Lancet* 366, 662–4.
46. Fontana, L. and Klein, S. 2007. Aging, adiposity, and calorie restriction. *JAMA* 297, 986–994.
47. Baur, J. and Sinclair, D. 2006. Therapeutic potential of resveratrol: The in vivo evidence. *Nat. Rev. Drug Discov.* 5, 493–506.
48. Mattson, M. 2007 Dietary factors, hormesis and health. *Ageing Res. Rev.* Sept 1; [Epub ahead of print].
49. Baur, J., Pearson, K., Price, N., Jamieson, H., Lerin, C., Kalra, A., et al. 2006. Resveratrol improves health and survival of mice on a high-calorie diet. *Nature* 444, 337–342.
50. Saiko, P., Szakmary, A., Jaeger, W., and Szekeres, T. 2007. Resveratrol and its analogs: Defense against cancer, coronary disease and neurodegenerative maladies or just a fad? *Mutat. Res.* Aug 17; [Epub ahead of print].
51. Subbaramaiah, K., Chung, W., Michaluart, P., Telang, N., Tanabe, T., Inoue, H., et al. 1998. Resveratrol inhibits cyclooxygenase-2 transcription and activity in phorbol ester-treated human mammary epithelial cells. *J. Biol. Chem.* 273, 21875–21882.
52. Pace-Asciak, C., Hahn, S., Diamandis, E., Soleas, G., and Goldberg, D. 1995. The red wine phenolics trans-resveratrol and quercetin block human platelet aggregation and eicosanoid synthesis: Implications for protection against coronary heart disease. *Clin. Chim. Acta* 235, 207–219.
53. Tsai, S.-H., Lin-Siau, S.-Y., and Lin, J.-K. 1999. Suppression of nitric oxide synthase and the down-regulation of the activation of NFκB in macrophages by resveratrol. *Br. J. Pharmacol.* 126, 784–790.
54. Kundu, J. and Surh, Y. 2004. Molecular basis of chemoprevention by resveratrol: NF-kappaB and AP-1 as potential targets. *Mutat. Res.* 555, 65–80.
55. Guarente, L. 2006. Sirtuins as potential targets for metabolic syndrome. *Nature* 444, 868–875.
56. Lagouge, M., Argmann, C., Gerhart-Hines, Z., Meziane, H., Lerin, C., Daussin, F., et al. 2006. Resveratrol improves mitochondrial function and protects against metabolic disease by activating SIRT1 and PGC-1α. *Cell* 127, 1109–1122.
57. Walle, T., Hsieh, F., DeLegge, M., Oatis, J., and Walle, U. 2004. High Absorption but very low bioavailability of oral resveratrol in humans. *Drug Metab. Disp.* 32, 1377–1382.
58. Kaldas, M., Walle, U., and Walle, T. 2003. Resveratrol transport and metabolism by human intestinal CaCo-2 cells. *J. Pharm. Pharmacol.* 55, 307–312.
59. Goldberg, D., Yan, J., and Soleas, G. 2003. Absorption of three wine-related polyphenols in three different matrices by healthy subjects. *Clin. Biochem.* 36, 79–87.
60. Vitaglione, P., Sforza, S., Galaverna, G., Ghidine, C., Caporaso, N., Vescovi, P., et al. 2005. Bioavailability of *trans*-resveratrol from red wine in humans. *Mol. Nutr. Food Res.* 49, 495–504.
61. Kuhnle, G., Spencer, J., Chowrimootoo, G., Schroeter, H., Debnam, E., et al. 2001 Resveratrol is absorbed in the small intestine as resveratrol glucuronide. *Biochem. Biophys. Res. Commun.* 272 212–217.
62. Henry-Vitrac, C., Desmoulière, A., Girard, D., Mérillon, J.-M., and Krisa, S. 2006. Transport, deglycosylation, and metabolism of trans-piceid by small intestinal epithelial cells. *Eur. J. Nutr.* 45, 376–382.

63. Maier-Salamon, A., Hagenauer, B., Wirth, M., Gabor, F., Szekeres, T., and Jager, W. 2006. Increased transport of resveratrol across monolayers of the human intestinal Caco-2 cells is mediated by inhibition and saturation of metabolites. *Pharm. Res.* 23, 2107–2115.

64. Boocock, D., Faust, G., Patel, K., Schinas, A., Brown, V., Ducharme, M., et al. 2007. Phase I dose escalation pharmacokinetic study in healthy volunteers of resveratrol, a potential cancer chemopreventive agent. *Cancer Epidemiol. Biomarkers Prev.* 16, 1246–1252.

65. Wenzel. E. and Somoza, V. 2005. Metabolism and bioavailability of trans-resveratrol. *Mol. Nutr. Food Res.* 49, 472–481.

66. Abd El-Mohsen, M., Bayele, H., Kuhnle, G., Gibson, G., Debnam, E., Srai, S., et al. 2006. Distribution of [³H]*trans*-resveratrol in rat tissues following oral administration. *Br. J. Nutr.* 96, 62–70.

67. Jannin, B., Menzel, M., Berlot, J., Delmas, D., Lancon, A., and Latruffe, N. 2004. Transport of resveratrol, a cancer chemopreventive agent, to cellular targets: Plasmatic protein binding and cell uptake. *Biochem. Pharmacol.* 68, 1113–1118.

68. Lu, Z., Zhang, Y., Liu, H., Yuan, J., Zheng, Z., and Zou, G. 2007. Transport of a cancer chemopreventive polyphenol, resveratrol: Interaction with serum albumin and hemoglobin. *J. Fluoresc.* 17, 580–587.

69. Wang, LX., Heredia, A., Song, H., Zhang, Z., Yu, B., Davis, C., and Redfield, R. 2004. Resveratrol glucuronides as the metabolites of resveratrol in humans: Characterization, synthesis, and anti-HIV activity. *J. Pharm. Sci.* 93, 2448–2457.

70. de Santi, C., Pietrabissa, A., Spisni, R., Mosca, F., and Pacifici, G. 2000. Sulphation of resveratrol, a natural compound present in wine, and its inhibition by natural flavonoids. *Xenobiotica* 30, 857–866.

15 Health Benefits of Phytochemicals for Older Adults

Giuliana Noratto, Rosemary Walzem,
Lisbeth Pacheco, and Susanne U. Mertens-Talcott

CONTENTS

15.1 SPECIAL NEEDS AND CONDITIONS OF THE ELDERLY

Aging is the progressive accumulation of changes over time that are associated with or responsible for the increasing susceptibility to disease and death. Although several theories try to explain the aging process, the free radical theory offer significant insight into the process [1]. Epidemiological evidence demonstrates that diets rich in fruit and vegetables promote health, and attenuate, or delay, the onset of various diseases, including cardiovascular disease, certain cancers, and several other age-related degenerative disorders [2–4]. Relating to plant components, polyphenols are a group of phytochemicals that are gaining acceptance as responsible for the health benefits attributed to fruit and vegetables. These chemical components, the molecular mechanisms exerted by them, and the reduced risk of age-related disorders are matters of intense research.

Plant polyphenols are the most abundant antioxidants in the human diet. Because of their chemical structure, they are able to scavenge free radicals and inactivate other pro-oxidants. Flavonoids, a chemically defined family of polyphenols, have a basic structure (Figure 15.1A), and several subclasses of flavonoids are characterized by a substitution pattern in the B- and C-rings. The main subclasses include flavan-3-ols, flavanones, flavones, isoflavones, flavonols, and anthocyanidins [5]. Their chemical structure (several hydroxyl groups directly associated with a cyclic benzene ring) favors antioxidant actions, i.e., scavenging radicals and chelating redox-active metals (Figure 15.1B). These characteristics are due to the hydrogen of the phenoxyl groups, which is prone to be donated to a radical. After the reaction, they retain key features of their structure, which is chemically stabilized by resonance [6]. They may also offer indirect protection by activating endogenous defense systems and by modulating cellular signaling processes [7]. The alternative molecular mechanisms, not directly related to their free radical scavenging or metal chelating properties, are the subject of extensive study aimed to provide scientific support for relating the consumption of plant polyphenols to human health.

Although significant progress has been made, some critical areas still need to be elucidated in order to define mechanisms linking plant polyphenol consumption and health. This chapter reviews aspects of the biological actions of polyphenols in the prevention and treatment of the most common age-related diseases.

15.2 CHRONIC DISEASES RELEVANT TO THE ELDERLY

15.2.1 CARDIOVASCULAR DISEASE

Epidemiological evidence suggests that high consumption of polyphenol-rich foods (fruits, vegetables, cocoa, etc.) or beverages (wine, tea, grape juice, etc.) is inversely correlated with the risk of cardiovascular disease (CVD) and all causes of mortality in the general U.S. population [4,6–9]. Several studies have reported the antioxidant properties of dietary polyphenols and their ability to inhibit the oxidation of low-density lipoprotein (LDL), which results in a marked decrease in the susceptibility of the lipoprotein to aggregation, a hallmark in early atherosclerosis [9]. However, it has also been shown that beneficial effects of polyphenols can be brought about by other mechanisms. For example, flavonoids can inhibit platelet aggregation and adhesion, inhibit enzymes involved in lipid metabolism, and induce endothelium-dependent vasodilation [10].

Vascular endothelium cells form a layer that separates blood from the vessel wall. These control many important functions including maintenance of blood circulation and fluidity, as well as regulation of vascular tone, coagulation, and inflammatory responses [11,12]. The control of endothelium function is mediated by the phosphorylation of endothelial nitric oxide synthase (eNOS), which produces nitric oxide (NO) and thus leads to vasodilation. Proinflammatory or pro-oxidant stimuli may directly stimulate or sensitize vascular cells to generate reactive oxygen species (ROS) where the formation may exceed the capacity of the antioxidant defense system. ROS may oxidize LDL cholesterol and initiate a series of events that begin with cell activation, endothelial dysfunction, local inflammation, and a procoagulant vascular surface [11–13]. The endothelial dysfunction is associated to loss of nitric oxide (NO) bioactivity in the vessel wall that may result in a cascade of events activating angiogenic growth factors, such as vascular endothelial growth factor (VEGF).

15.2.1.1 Role of Polyphenols in CVD

Several studies have established the concept of the "French paradox," in which epidemiological studies have demonstrated relatively low incidence of coronary heart disease in the French population, despite high saturated fat consumption, a well-known risk for coronary disease [14,15]. The

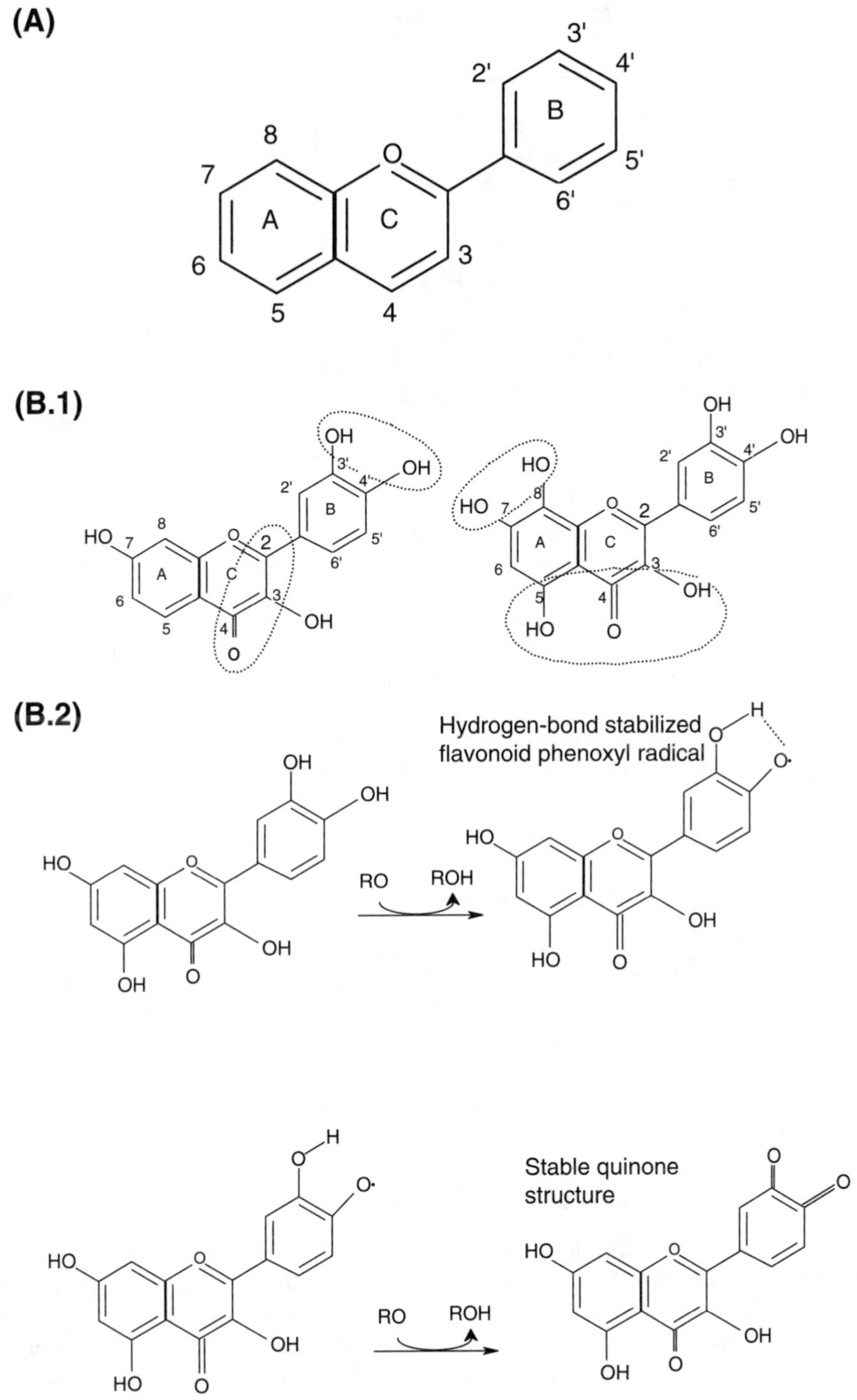

FIGURE 15.1. (A) Chemical structure of flavonoids: Rings (A, C, and B) and substitution numbers. (B.1) Chemical structure of polyphenols and features that confer multiple functional activities to them. (B.2) Mechanism of antioxidant action of 3′, 4′-diOH polyphenols [125].

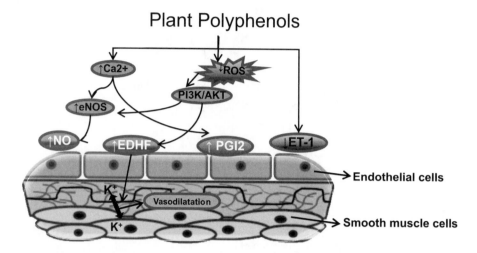

FIGURE 15.2 Effects of polyphenols in CVD through the improvement of endothelium function. Plant polyphenols induce NO synthesis mediated by an increase in (a) Ca2+ and (b) phosphorylation of eNOS by the PI3-kinase/Akt pathway; in addition, plant polyphenols cause endothelium-derived hyperpolarizing factor (EDHF)-mediated relaxations by opening K+ channels through controlling the formation of superoxide anions leading to the activation of the PI3-kinase/Akt pathway. Polyphenols also increase endothelial prostacyclin by influx of Ca2+ and inhibit the synthesis and the effects of endothelin-1. All these mechanisms might help to explain the vasodilatory, vasoprotective, and antihypertensive effects of polyphenols *in vivo* [24].

elevated consumption of wine may be involved in the French paradox [16] since its content of polyphenols is high compared with other foods. The effective protection of polyphenols against CVD has been attributed to (a) their antioxidant and radical scavenger properties, (b) their capacity to enhance endothelium function, and (c) their anti-angiogenic activity (Figure 15.2).

15.2.1.2   Antioxidant Properties of Polyphenols

The antioxidant properties of polyphenols may protect blood vessels against the oxidative stress associated with many cardiovascular risk factors. It has been reported that procyanidins (oligomers of flavan-3-ol and flavan 3,4-diol) can protect endothelial cells from membrane lipid oxidation and cytotoxicity by scavenging peroxynitrite free radicals [17]. Furthermore, the antioxidant properties of polyphenols might protect vascular endothelial function against deleterious consequences of oxidation of LDLs. Cholesterol derivatives in oxidized LDL can reduce maximal arterial relaxation through a specific effect on vascular endothelial cells [18].

15.2.1.3   Improvement of Endothelium Function

The relaxing factors contributing to the improvement of endothelium function are the increase of endothelial production of NO, prostacyclin (PGI2), endothelium-derived hyperpolarizing factor (EDHF), and the decrease of the contracting factor endothelin-1. The endothelial production of NO has a number of important functions in the vessel wall, such as inhibition of platelet aggregation and adhesion, molecule expression, prevention of smooth muscle proliferation, and modulation of vascular growth. Synthesis of NO exerted by red wine polyphenols (RWP) has been linked to phosphorylation of endothelium nitric oxide synthetase (eNOS).

PGI2 is a prostanoid required for cardiovascular homeostasis that prevents platelet aggregation, induces vasodilation, and downregulates expression of endothelial cell adhesion molecules [19]. Some plant polyphenols, especially from the 3-flavanol subclass, such as procyanidins found in grapes and cocoa, have shown to favorably alter eicosanoid synthesis and inhibit platelet activation and inflammatory processes that contribute to CVD [17]. The EDHF causes hyperpolarization and relaxation by opening K+ channels [20]. Plant polyphenols that include RWPs, resveratrol [21], and other traditional Chinese medicinal herbs containing polyphenols [22] have been shown to induce endothelium-dependent vasorelaxations as well as hyperpolarization of smooth muscle cells through both NO and EDHF. The signaling pathways leading to polyphenol-induced NO and EDHF formation share the activation of the PI3K/AKT pathway as a common step (Figure 15.2). The inhibition of endothelin-1 synthesis, which is pro-inflammatory and promotes fibrosis, arterial remodeling, and vascular injury, may be mediated by plant polyphenols, indeed reducing the development of atherosclerosis. Resveratrol, a phytoalexin found in wine and grapes, has been reported to inhibit endothelin-1 gene expression, partially by interfering with the ERK1/2 pathway through attenuation of reactive oxygen species formation [23].

15.2.1.4 Anti-Angiogenic Activity of Polyphenols

Angiogenesis in CVD is characterized by migration and proliferation of endothelial cells and the maturation of new blood vessels in response to local pro-angiogenic factors and activation of matrix metalloproteinases that degrade the extracellular matrix [24]. The anti-angiogenic activity of polyphenols in blood vessels has been associated with inhibition of matrix metalloproteinases (MMP) activation, inhibition of vascular endothelial growth factor (VEGF) expression, and prevention of migration and proliferation of vascular cells. The inhibition of matrix metalloproteinases (MMP) activation has been reported for epicagallocatechin 3-gallate (EGCG), the major catechin in tea and wine [25,26]. The inhibition of vascular endothelial growth factor (VEGF) expression, a major pro-angiogenic factor that stimulates endothelial cell migration and proliferation and also the formation of new blood vessels *in vitro* and *in vivo* [27], has been prevented by RWP and the anthocyanins delphinidin and cyanidin through the p38 MAPK pathway [28]. Finally, RWP [29] and tea polyphenols, especially epigallocatechin-3-gallate (EGCG) and epicatechin-3-gallate (ECG) [30], have shown activity in prevention of migration and proliferation of vascular cells. Overall, polyphenols participate in vascular protection and exert antiangiogenic effects that are also involved in their anticancer activity.

15.2.2 CANCER

Cancer is a multistep process that takes place over a period of time due to the accumulation of mutations in a single cell, resulting in gradual phenotypic changes from a normal to a preneoplastic cell that progresses to neoplastic. The different stages in carcinogenesis are: Initiation (days), promotion (5–10 years), and progression (1–5 years) [31,32]. Initiation is irreversible and includes an initial chemical or physical carcinogenic stimulus directly targeting DNA. Promotion is usually a relatively slow and reversible process leading to an accumulation of premalignant cells abnormally dividing. Progression is generally irreversible and leads to the final stage of carcinogenesis with tumor growth and acquisition of invasiveness and metastatic potential [33]. The six essential alterations in cell physiology that lead to malignant growth are [33]:

1. Self-sufficiency in growth signals
2. Insensitivity to growth-inhibitory (antigrowth) signals
3. Evasion of programmed cell death (apoptosis)
4. Unlimited replicative potential
5. Sustained angiogenesis
6. Tissue invasion and metastasis

The passage from pre-malignant to malignant cell involves activation of proto-oncogenes or inactivation of tumor suppressor genes, resulting in the generation of consequently mutant cells with selective advantages. One of the well-known factors of these systems is the p53 tumor suppressor

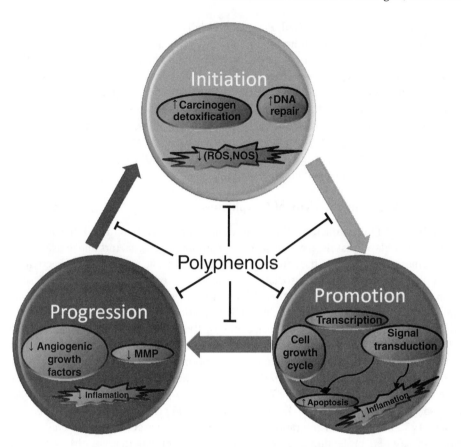

FIGURE 15.3 Plant polyphenols act at different stages in the carcinogenesis process. During initiation, they act as cancer-blocking agents by scavenging free radicals,, regulating detoxifying enzymes, and enhancing DNA repair. During promotion and progression, they play a role as cancer-suppressing agents by regulating the cell growth cycle, signal transduction pathways, transcriptional regulation (expression of pro-apoptotic genes, i.e., p53 or downregulation of oncogenic genes, i.e., RAS), inflamation (i.e., by blocking the activation or transcriptional activity of NF-kB) and induction of apoptosis. Additionally, during progression, they downregulate the expression and activation of angiogenic growth factors and decrease matrix metalloproteinases (MMPs) and cell adhesion molecules, which play an important role in the angiogenesis process for tumor progression and metastasis [42].

protein, which, in response to DNA damage, elicits either cell cycle arrest to allow DNA repair to take place or apoptosis if the damage is excessive [34].

15.2.2.1   Role of Polyphenols in Cancer

Dietary increase of antioxidant defense capacity has been considered a reasonable way to prevent ROS-mediated carcinogenicity [35]. Epidemiological and human studies indicate that a low risk of cancer is related to antioxidant-rich diets [2,36]. Plant polyphenols have shown potential as natural anticarcinogenic compounds that, according to their mechanisms of action, may have potential as cancer-blocking or cancer-suppressing agents (Figure 15.3).

Cancer-blocking agents act during the initiation stage of protecting cellular targets by scavenging ROS and other oxidative species, enhancing carcinogen detoxification, modifying the carcinogen uptake and metabolism, and enhancing DNA repair. Cancer-suppressing agents inhibit the promotion and progression stages after the formation of preneoplastic cells by interfering with cell cycle regulation (cyclin dependent proteins), regulation of signal transduction pathways (MAP kinase,

TGF-β serine-threonine kinase signaling and β-catenin pathways) [37], transcription (NF-kB activation), and apoptosis (activation of pro-apoptotic genes and pro-apoptotic proteins) [38,37].

Plant polyphenols may target one or more of the molecular pathways in cancer cells with only low toxicity in normal cells. Curcumin, resveratrol, and caffeic acid phenylester have been shown to regulate the expression of genes involved in inflammatory processes through blocking the activation or transcriptional activity of NF-kB, and modulation of signal-transduction pathways such as tyrosine kinase inhibitors [37,39]. The anti-inflamatory activity is mediated through inhibition of expression of COX-2 and inducible nitric oxide synthase (iNOS) by blocking improper NF-kB activation [40,41]. Therefore, the anti-inflammatory activity of antioxidants may be mediated by several mechanisms, some of which may be unrelated to its intrinsic antioxidant activity.

Finally, during progression, tumor angiogenesis is critically important for the growth of solid tumors and is mediated by the initiation of blood vessel formation. The angiogenesis process has been shown to be an important target to suppress tumor growth and metastasis, since it is mediated by endothelial cells in which it is easy to achieve active concentrations of antiangiogenic agents [42]. Dietary polyphenols have shown anti-angiogenic activity by acting via different mechanisms: (1) regulation of angiogenic growth factors (VEGF, bFGF and IGF-1), (2) decrease of inflammatory angiogenic molecules (IL-8, COX-2 and iNOS), and (3) decreasing matrix metalloproteinases (MMPs) and cell adhesion molecules. These factors play an important role in the angiogenesis process for tumor progression and metastasis [42].

The combined effects of different phytochemicals, as they are found naturally in foods, may be greater in cancer chemoprevention than the effects of single compounds, a phenomenon known as "combination chemoprevention." This effect explains why low doses of chemopreventive agents differing in their mode of action may act together at high efficiency due to synergistic mechanisms [32]. Effective chemopreventive agents can extend the latency period for onset of cancer, with an immense impact on raising the quality of life for millions of people [39].

15.2.3 DEGENERATIVE COGNITIVE BRAIN FUNCTION

Brain cells, mainly neurons, are highly vulnerable to the detrimental effects of ROS. This vulnerability is due to many factors: High metabolic activity, rich composition of polyunsaturated fatty acids, high intracellular concentration of transition metals that may catalyze the formation of reactive hydroxyl radicals, low levels of antioxidants, and low capability to regenerate [43].

Glial cells (microglia and astrocytes) provide support and protection for neurons; they surround and hold them in place, supply nutrients and oxygen, insulate one neuron from another, and destroy pathogens and remove dead neurons. However, during neuroinflammatory processes, they produce free radicals that are the key pathogenic elements in neurodegenerative diseases such Alzheimer's disease (AD) and Parkinson's disease (PD) [43]. Free radicals have the capacity to attack proteins, polysaccharides, lipids bilayers, and DNA, causing oxidative cellular damage in neurons. These events lead to neuronal injury, the pathogenic feature of AD and PD.

Even though microglia cells have the function of protecting the nervous system, they also participate in inflammatory process when they are activated by neurotoxic factors. When pro-oxidants exceed the endogenous antioxidant defenses, the oxidative stress causes protein misfolding and aggregation, which exert the microglial activation [43]. Genetic mutations also associated to AD and PD cause the irregular processing of misfolded proteins, which results in deposition of protein aggregates in the cytosol, extracellular spaces, or nucleus, leading to central nervous system (CNS) amyloidosis [44]. The primary protein deposits found in tissues of patients with AD are amyloid-β (Aβ) and, in patients with PD, α-synuclein is found [43]. Microglial activation results from interactions with aggregated proteins; this process augments the inflammatory process through the production of neurotoxic factors such as quinolinic acid, superoxide anions, matrix metalloproteinases, NO, arachidonic acid and its metabolites, proinflamatory cytokines and excitotoxins that can kill or injure neurons [43]. All these factors maintain the neuroinflammatory cascade.

15.2.3.1   Role of Polyphenols in Neurodegenerative Disorders

Given that neurodegenerative disorders are strongly associated with inflammation and oxidative stress, the rationale for studying the effects of dietary antioxidants is based on the hypothesis that neurodegenerative disorders may be slowed and possibly even reversed by appropriately increasing levels of antioxidants or decreasing overproduction of free radicals in the body. The effectiveness of polyphenols for protection against neurodegenerative disorders is based on their ability to modulate different molecular mechanisms in brain cells (Figure 15.4). The rate-limiting step for the effective protection of polyphenols will depend on their ability to cross the blood–brain barrier according to their properties, such as charged state, lipophilicity, and interactions with efflux transporters, with possible relative specificity of polyphenols for different brain areas [45].

Several reports indicate the efficacy of polyphenols on neuronal function and behavior by using *in vitro* and *in vivo* models [46–49]. It has been shown that polyphenols found in blueberries can reverse age-related declines in neuronal signal transduction as well as cognitive performance via combined mechanisms that include neurogenesis, insulin-like growth factor 1 (IGF-1) and its receptor (IGF-1R), and MAPK signal transduction cascades [50]. The hippocampus is one of the brain regions with the capacity to generate neurons (neurogenesis), but this ability is diminished during aging and accompanied by cognitive decline. There is an agreement between *in vitro* and *in vivo* studies showing that EGCG attenuates Aβ-induced toxicity in hippocampal neurons [51]. Grape seed extract (GSE), enriched in proanthocyanidins, oligomers of the catechins, has shown neuroprotective activity *in vivo* as well. The effective protection was related to synthesis of proteins that are involved in energy generation, protein folding (heat shock protein), cytoskeletal proteins, and glial fibrillary acidic protein; all these proteins were affected in a direction opposite to that detected for the same protein in AD [52]. Pomegranate juice has influenced both behavior and neuropathology in an animal model of AD. The beneficial effects were associated to a decrease in accumulation of soluble Aβ and amyloid deposition in the hippocampus [53].

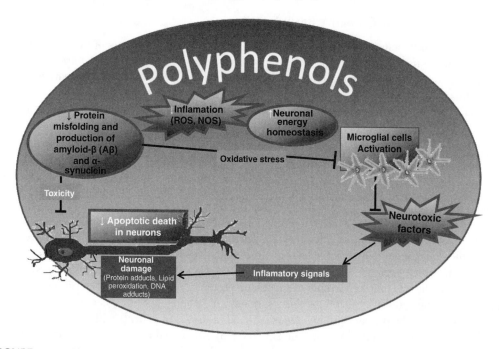

FIGURE15. 4   Plant polyphenols target markers of inflammation and oxidative stress that cause neurodegenerative disorders. Polyphenols can additionally deactivate activated microglia, protect neurons against Amyloi-β(Aβ), α-synuclein-induced toxicity, and inflammatory signals, thus protecting neuronal cell from death [43].

Additionally, reservatrol from red wine, the green tea catechins, and the turmeric extract curcumin have received special attention for potential disease prevention or treatment of AD. Resveratrol has shown to exert neuronal protection in AD by targeting multiple molecular pathways [54]:

- Repression of p53 activity promoted by Aβ in neurons
- Protection of neurons against Aβ-induced toxicity
- Modulation of the ubiquitin proteasome system to promote Aβ degradation
- Preventing reactive oxygen species-induced Aβ production
- Blocking inflammatory cascades and preventing apoptosis of neurons

Additionally, resveratrol has been shown to stimulate neuronal energy homeostasis, similar to that achieved in caloric restriction and associated with increased life span and delay in the onset of diseases associated with aging. This is based on the hypothesis that diets high in carbohydrates may alter metabolism of cellular membrane proteins and trigger excessive cell signaling cascades, leading to neuronal damage [55]. Curcumin has the potential to suppress the AD pathogenic cascade at multiple sites: inhibition of expression of inflammatory cytokines, COX-2, and NOS mediated by regulation of gene transcription [56], and inhibition of the activity and expression of β-secretase enzyme that makes the initial step in amyloid production [57]. Tea catechins may protect against neuronal diseases through their radical scavenging and iron chelating activity or regulation of antioxidant protective enzymes. Even more, EGCG (the most abundant catechin derivative in tea) appears to protect neuronal cells from death by inhibition of mitochondria mediated apoptosis [58].

15.2.4 OTHER AGE-RELATED AILMENTS

15.2.4.1 Macular Degeneration and Arthritis

Age-related macular degeneration (AMD) is the leading cause of blindness for the western world [59]. The retina is particularly susceptible to oxidative stress caused by reactive oxygen species due to its high consumption of oxygen, its high proportion of polyunsaturated fatty acids, and its exposure to visible light [60]. *In vitro* studies have shown that the retinal injury caused by oxidative stress photochemical may be prevented by antioxidants. Among plant phytochemicals (carotenoids, polyphenols, alkaloids, nitrogen-containing and organosulfur compounds) [61], the carotenoids (lutein and zeaxanthin) are the only xanthophylls detected in the human lens [62]. They may act to protect the eye from ultraviolet phototoxicity via quenching reactive oxygen species, and interact synergistically with other antioxidants such as α-tocopherol [63], which is an effective scavenger of free radicals and present in high quantities in human retina [64]. Though the pathophysiology of cataract and AMD is complex and contains both environmental and genetic components, research studies suggest that dietary factors including antioxidant vitamins and xanthophylls may contribute to a reduction in the risk of these degenerative eye diseases [65]. Observational studies have shown that high intake of lutein and zeaxanthin, particularly from certain xanthophyll-rich foods like spinach, broccoli, and eggs, significantly reduce the risk for cataract (up to 20%) and for AMD (up to 40%) [66]. This is supported by studies showing that lutein and zeaxanthin are significantly lower in the macula and whole retina of eyes with early AMD than in healthy eyes [67].

15.2.4.2 Arthritis

Arthritis is a chronic disease that results from an inflammation of the joints. It results from dysregulation of pro-inflammatory cytokines (e.g. tumor necrosis factor and interleukin-1b) and proinflammatory enzymes that mediate the production of prostaglandins (e.g., cyclooxygenase-2) and leukotrienes (e.g. lipooxygenase), together with the expression of adhesion molecules and matrix metalloproteinases, and hyperproliferation of synovial fibroblasts. These cell signals are regulated by the activation of the transcription factor NF-kB. Therefore, agents that suppress the activation of NF-kB and expression of pro-inflammatory cytokines and pro-inflammatory enzymes may have potential for the treatment of arthritis [68]. The fact that numerous plant polyphenols may have potential for arthritis treatment is supported by several preclinical and clinical studies showing their suppression effect of cell signaling networks, which mediates the inflammatory response during arthritis. Among these natural plant compounds, most research has been made on curcumin (from turmeric), resveratrol (red grapes, cranberries, and peanuts), tea polyphenols, genistein (soy), quercetin (onions), silymarin (artichoke), guggulsterone (guggul), boswellic acid (salai guggul), and withanolides (ashwagandha). The common characteristic among these natural plant compounds is their ability to inhibit NF-kB activation and downregulate the expression of inflammatory gene products, which are major players in the development of arthritis [68].

15.3   ANTIOXIDANT MECHANISMS OF PHYTOCHEMICALS

Several degenerative diseases, including cancers, CVD, and neurodegenerative diseases, are generally associated with aging. Oxidative damage to cell components, DNA, proteins, and lipids accumulates with age and contributes to cell degeneration and to the pathogenesis of these diseases [69]. Natural defense mechanisms against oxidative damage include antioxidant enzymes, such as glutathione peroxidase, catalase, and superoxide disumutase, which metabolize superoxide, hydrogen peroxide, and lipid peroxides, thus preventing the formation of toxic hydroxyl and peroxyl radicals [70]. An imbalance between the generation of reactive oxygen species and the antioxidant defense mechanisms results in a condition known as "oxidative stress," which is considered to be an important contributing factor to the development of degenerative diseases, particularly those mediated by chronic inflammation [71].

High intake of fruits and vegetables has been associated with a lowered incidence of several degenerative diseases, including cancer [24]. Protective effects from fruit and vegetable consumption have been attributed to the presence in these foods of naturally occurring phytochemicals, which have the ability to act as antioxidants and inhibit oxidative stress *in vivo* [72]. Mechanisms by which phytochemicals contribute to natural antioxidant defense systems include the inhibition of reactive oxygen species formation and interruption of radical chain reactions. Phytochemical antioxidants prevent the formation of reactive oxygen species by inhibiting enzymes or chelating trace elements involved in free radical production [70]. Such antioxidants interrupt radical chain reactions by scavenging reactive oxygen species and free radicals, which are considered to be the predominant antioxidant mechanism [73].

Free radical scavenging by antioxidants is conceptually a redox transition involving the donation of a single electron or hydrogen atom to a free radical, which transfers the radical character to the antioxidant and leads to a more stable compound [74]. Thus, a phytochemical antioxidant must delay or prevent autoxidation or free radical-mediated oxidation, and also result in a stable radical [75]. Chemical properties of phytochemicals, in terms of the availability of the phytochemical hydrogens as hydrogen-donating radical scavengers, may predict their antioxidant activity [76]. In addition to their antioxidant properties, many phytochemicals have been shown to be biologically active and protect against disease-related biological pathways, such as cell signaling, cell cycle regulation, oxidative stress, and inflammation [77].

15.4   FOODS HIGH IN PHYTOCHEMICALS

15.4.1   GREEN TEA

Tea, derived from the leaves of Camellia sinensis, is a rich source of catechins, the water-soluble polyphenolic constituents that account for 30–42% of its dry weight. The main catechins in green tea are epicatechin (EC), ECG, epigallocatechin (EGC) and EGCG. EGCG is the major catechin, accounting for up to 50% of the total polyphenols, and is also considered the most active polyphenolic ingredient in tea [78]. This catechin has several biological and pharmacological properties including free radical scavenging activity, antioxidant actions, iron-chelating capabilities and attenuation of lipid peroxidation due to various forms of radicals [79].

Tea has been a matter of intense research and the subject of the "Asian paradox," a paradox that has been postulated as result of epidemiological data that indicate that even though consumption of tobacco is high, Asia, and Japan in particular, have among the lowest incidences of arteriosclerosis and lung cancer per capita [80]. On the basis of numerous *in vitro, in vivo*, and epidemiological studies, green tea is now accepted as a cancer preventive as well as a potential agent in reduction of CVD. A cohort study of a Japanese population with 13-year follow-up data found an evident delay of cancer onset and death [81,82] and protection against cardiovascular disease [3], and this was associated with increased consumption of green tea. Green tea has been shown to protect against all stages of carcinogenesis in several animal tumor bioassay systems [83]. The multiple mechanisms involved in the anticancer activity of tea polyphenols include, but are not limited to, induction of apoptosis, cell cycle arrest, induction of p53, and modulation of cell signaling pathways. In summary, studies of green tea show a promising effect on delaying the aging process, protecting against most diseases that older people would suffer, thus avoiding premature death.

14.4.2 Wine

Wine is a complex beverage made from the juice of *Vitis vinifera*. The color, alcohol content, and phytochemical composition of wine vary widely and depend upon the variety of grapes used, the environment in which the grapes were grown, and the vintification techniques employed [84].

Epidemiological studies consistently find that traditional dietary patterns that feature regular moderate wine consumption are associated with reduced total and cardiovascular mortality [85–87]. Much research has focused on determining the separate health effects of alcohol and polyphenolic components of wine as well as whether consumption within a particular dietary or lifestyle context is needed to gain benefit. A number of reviews detail possible mechanisms by which these compounds could confer cardioprotective benefit [16] as well as more general anti-inflammatory, insulin sensitizing, and vasomotor actions [16,88].

Red wine contains more polyphenols than white wine does, and white wine does not contain anthocyanins. The complex mixture present in wines includes flavonoids primarily as anthocyanins and flavan-3-ols, and non-flavonoids such as stilbenes (e.g., resveratrol) and gallic acid. Flavan-3-ols predominate in wine, with oligomeric and polymeric procyanidins (condensed tannins) typically making up 25–50% of total phenolic constituents [84,89]. Recent studies in traditionally wine-consuming regions of France and Italy identified oligomeric procyanidins (<5 monomers) as the most important red wine component to be associated with longevity [90]. The Italian Longitudinal Study on Aging (ILSA) found that vascular risk factors influenced incident mild cognitive impairment and the rate of progression to dementia [91,92]. The link between vascular and long-term cognitive health suggests that dietary components that reduce vascular risk may also reduce risk of cognitive decline or Alzheimer's disease development. Indeed, Orgogozo et al., 1997 [93] found that moderate wine drinking was associated with reduced risk of incident dementia (odds ratio = 0.19) and Alzheimer's (OR = 0.28), following adjustment for confounders. These authors concluded there was no reason to advise regular wine consumers over the age of 65 to stop drinking. To add to this, a very recent outcome from the ILSA study found that consumption of up to one drink per day of wine or alcohol by patients with mild cognitive impairment may decrease the rate of progression to dementia [94].

Ramassamy (2006) [95], recently reviewed possible intracellular targets of a number of polyphenolic compounds found in wine, albeit the review did not focus on wine per se, with the potential for intervention in a number of neurodegenerative diseases including Alzheimer's and Parkinson's disease. In this regard, of interest is the recent observation by de la Torre et al. (2006) [96] that red wine also contains hydroxytyrosol, a dopamine metabolite and a key biologically active phenol in olive oil. This group further reported that ethanol-containing wine, as opposed to nonalcoholic grape juice, increased urinary hydroxytyrosol excretion well above the amount that could be explained by the test wine's hydroxytyrosol content. This type of metabolic effect could be specific to wine, which combines alcohol and polyphenolic compounds, although diets rich in fruits and vegetables and a nonwine source of ethanol would also need to be evaluated.

Initiation of wine drinking by the elderly should not be taken lightly due to the higher rates of hypertension and prescription medication intake among those over 65 years of age [97,98]. A recent well-designed crossover study showed that red wine elevated blood pressure in a predicable ethanol-dependent manner [99]. In addition, other studies have found that individuals from traditionally nonwine-drinking ethnic groups may not gain as much benefit as individuals derived from traditional wine-drinking ethnic groups [100]. Drug interactions are ascribable to both the ethanol and polyphenolic components of wine.

15.4.3 SOY

Soybeans and their products are consumed in many Asian countries, and many epidemiological reports describe the health benefits of soy consumption related to the prevention of cancer, CVD, decrease of climacteric symptoms, and prevention of osteoporosis [101–103]. Soybeans are a rich source of phytoestrogen isoflavones, such as daidzein and genistein; they exhibit similar chemical structure to the mammalian steroid hormone 17β-oestradiol and so have been linked to the low incidence of hormone-related cancers [104,105]. Although epidemiological studies have related the low breast cancer incidence in Asian nations and the high consumption of foods rich in phytoestrogens, some human intervention trials failed to show the precise effect of dietary phytoestrogens on the proliferation of mammary tissue [106]. One factor causing these discrepancies may be the time of intake. Higher protection may be achieved by exposure to a dietary factor that decreases the breast cancer risk early in life.

This hypothesis has been supported by epidemiological and rodent studies showing that breast cancer chemoprevention, exerted by dietary phytoestrogens, is dependent on ingestion before puberty, when the mammary gland is relatively immature. On the other hand, it has also been shown that low doses of phytoestrogens may promote cancer cell growth of estrogen-dependent breast cancer cells, consequentially increasing the risk of development of preexisting breast tumors [106]. According to these results, consumption of phytoestrogens may be a double-edged sword, because many phytoestrogen supplements are marketed for use of postmenopausal women as natural and safe alternatives to hormone replacement.

An alternative protection exerted by phytoestrogens may be through inhibition of enzymes involved in estrogen synthesis such sulfotransferases and aromatases [107,108]. Finally, soy phytoestrogens may be acting in synergy with other soy phytochemicals that may enhance their health benefits. In summary, soy has many health benefits; however, older people should consume soy products with caution, especially if soy has not been a regular part of their diet.

15.4.4 BRASSICA

Brassica vegetables, including cabbage, kale, broccoli, cauliflower, Brussels sprouts, kohlrabi, rapeseed, rutabaga, and turnip contain the sulfur-containing phytochemicals glucosinolates (previously known as thioglucosides). Epidemiological data suggest that high consumption of brassica vegetables is associated with a decreased risk of cancer; this has been coupled to the relatively high content of glucosinolates and related compounds [109]. This association appears to be most consistent for lung, stomach, colon, and rectal cancer, and least consistent for prostatic, endometrial, and ovarian cancer [110,111]. The degradation products of glucosinolates by myrosinase, an enzyme that is released from damaged plant cells, seems necessary for the anticarcinogenic effects of glucosinolates; the released isothiocyanates or indoles may be the active forms. The mechanisms for this protection have been found to be related to the ability to modify xenobiotic metabolizing enzymes and induce cell cycle arrest and apoptosis [112]. The influence of these compounds on the activity of phase 1 and phase 2 metabolizing enzymes may protect against chemical carcinogens through modulation of metabolism of carcinogenic/mutagenic compounds, thereby preventing the formation of electrophilic intermediates that may damage DNA.

Cytochrome P450 enzymes are responsible for phase 1 metabolism, which involves oxidation, reduction, and hydrolysis reactions. By this means, xenobiotics can be chemically more reactive and act as promutagens/procarcinogens. Glutathione S-transferases (GST) and UDP-glucuronyl transferases are responsible for phase 2 metabolism, which is a detoxifying mechanism; it comprises conjugation reactions making phase 1 metabolites more polar and readily excretable [113]. Alterations on the activity of these enzymes have implications on the level of toxicity of chemicals [114], and indoles and isothiocyanates have been shown to induce GST and inhibit of cytochrome-P450 enzyme [115].

Most evidence regarding the anticarcinogenic effects of glucosinolate hydrolysis products and brassica vegetables has come from studies in animals. However, because of interspecies differences and because the dose of both the anticarcinogenic and the carcinogenic compound used in animal studies often exceeds their estimated levels in a normal human diet, it is difficult to extrapolate results from animal studies to humans. Therefore, more studies are required to confirm the effective protection of these compounds in humans.

15.4.5 POMEGRANATE

Pomegranate (*Punica granatum, Punicaceae*), native to Persia, is an edible fruit cultivated in Mediterranean countries and some parts of the United States. Pomegranate has been extensively used as a folk medicine by many cultures [116]. This fruit is a rich source of two types of polyphenolic compounds: (1) anthocyanins (such as delphinidin, cyanidin, and pelargonidin), which give the fruit and juice its red color; and (2) hydrolyzable tannins (such as punicalagin and ellagic acid derivatives) [117]. Commercial pomegranate juices show an antioxidant activity three times higher than red wine and a green tea infusion; the hydrolyzable tannins, particularly punicalagin, are one of the most active ingredients responsible for ~87% of the juice's antioxidative potential [117].

Pomegranate juice has been reported to exert potent antioxidant capacity against lipid peroxidation, to inhibit serum angiotensin converting enzyme (ACE) activity (potent vasoconstrictor glycoprotein), and to reduce systolic blood pressure [118]. The possible mechanisms by which the ACE inhibitors may affect atherosclerosis are associated to lowering of blood pressure, antiproliferation of vascular cells, inhibition of platelet aggregation, and inhibition of lipid peroxidation effects [119,120]. Alternatively, it has been shown how different pomegranate fractions inhibit cancer cell proliferation and invasion and promote apoptosis of breast [121] and prostate cancer cells [122]. The active components of pomegranate fruit extract, anthocyanin and hydrolyzable tannin-rich fractions, may possess chemopreventive activity in a wide range of tumor models through the modulation of MAPK and NF-kB pathways [123]. In conclusion, there is evidence to support the wide range of protection that pomegranate juice consumption can offer against cardiovascular diseases and cancer.

15.5 SUMMARY

The effective protection of plant polyphenols against age-related diseases has been supported by epidemiological evidence and corroborated by several *in vitro* and *in vivo* studies. The biological activity of plant polyphenols on cardiovascular protection has been related to the antioxidant and radical scavenger properties, thus keeping cells from oxidative stress as well as the capacity to enhance the endothelium function and anti-angiogenic activity by inhibition of cell proliferation and modulation of different molecular pathways in the vascular system. The activity of polyphenols in cancer has also been related to dietary increase of the endogenous antioxidant defense as a reasonable way to prevent ROS-mediated carcinogenicity, thus acting as cancer-blocking agents. They may also offer protection as cancer-suppressing agents by modulating cellular signaling processes that are involved in cell physiology alterations that lead to malignant growth: self-sufficiency in growth signals, insensitivity to growth-inhibitory (antigrowth) signals, evasion of programmed cell death (apoptosis), unlimited replicative potential, sustained angiogenesis, tissue invasion, and metastasis. Likewise, the protection of polyphenols in brain function may be achieved through the modulation of neuronal pathogenic cascade at multiple sites: protection of neurons against neurotoxic factors (Aβ and α-synuclein, ROS, activated microglial cells), modulation of the neuronal energy homeostasis, the inhibition of expression of inflammatory proteins by regulation of gene transcription, and modulation of the ubiquitin proteasome system to promote Aβ degradation [54]. Therefore, the biological protection of polyphenols is related to their ability to cross brain membranes and target the pathogenic cascade of events that lead to the development of neurodegenerative diseases.

Overall, there is evidence that oxidative stress plays a significant role in the development of many diseases during the aging process. Therefore, it is likely that strategies intended to keep a balance between ROS production and antioxidant defenses will be significant in keeping a low rate at which cellular damage accumulates, thus effectively supporting optimal aging and retarding the onset of age-related diseases. Indeed, as demonstrated in several studies, the consumption of combinations of different plant phytochemicals, as they naturally occur in foods, may be a more effective strategy in retarding or preventing diseases associated with aging. However, these plant phytochemicals should be ingested with caution, because intake of dietary supplements in which the levels are higher than those obtained from a typical vegetable-rich diet may cause adverse effects that overcome the beneficial ones [124].

In summary, through awareness of the beneficial properties of plant foods, the practice of eating better could result in longer and better quality of life for the increasing aging population.

REFERENCES

1. Halliwell, B. 1991. Reactive oxygen species in living systems: Source, biochemistry, and role in human disease. *Am J Med* 91, 14S–22S.
2. Block, G., Patterson, B., and Subar, A. 1992. Fruit, vegetables, and cancer prevention: A review of the epidemiological evidence. *Nutr Cancer* 18, 1–29.
3. Nakachi, K., Matsuyama, S., Miyake, S., Suganuma, M., and Imai, K. 2000. Preventive effects of drinking green tea on cancer and cardiovascular disease: Epidemiological evidence for multiple targeting prevention. *Biofactors* 13, 49–54.
4. Bazzano, L. A., He, J., Ogden, L. G., Loria, C. M., Vupputuri, S., Myers, L., and Whelton, P. K. 2002. Fruit and vegetable intake and risk of cardiovascular disease in US adults: the first National Health and Nutrition Examination Survey Epidemiologic Follow-up Study. *Am J Clin Nutr* 76, 93–9.
5. Crozier, A., Jaganath, I. B., and Clifford, M. N., Eds. 2006. Phenols, polyphenols and tannins: An overview. In *Plant secondary metabolites*. Crozier, A., Clifford, M. N., and Ashihara, H. (Eds.). Oxford: Blackwell Publishing Ltd.
6. Fraga, C. G. 2007. Plant polyphenols: How to translate their in vitro antioxidant actions to in vivo conditions. *Iubmb Life* 59, 308–315.
7. Han, X. Z., Shen, T., and Lou, H. X. 2007. Dietary polyphenols and their biological significance. *Int J Molec Sci* 8, 950–988.
8. Joshipura, K. J., Hu, F. B., Manson, J. E., Stampfer, M. J., Rimm, E. B., Speizer, F. E., et al. 2001. The effect of fruit and vegetable intake on risk for coronary heart disease. *Ann Intern Med* 134, 1106–14.
9. Aviram, M. and Fuhrman, B. 1998. Polyphenolic flavonoids inhibit macrophage-mediated oxidation of LDL and attenuate atherogenesis. *Atherosclerosis* 137 Suppl, S45–50.
10. Reed, J. 2002. Cranberry flavonoids, atherosclerosis and cardiovascular health. *Crit Rev Food Sci Nutr* 42, 301–16.
11. Gonzalez, M. A. and Selwyn, A. P. 2003. Endothelial function, inflammation, and prognosis in cardiovascular disease. *Am J Med* 115 Suppl 8A, 99S–106S.

12. Behrendt, D. and Ganz, P. 2002. Endothelial function. From vascular biology to clinical applications. *Am J Cardiol* 90, 40L–48L.
13. Murohara, T., Kugiyama, K., Ohgushi, M., Sugiyama, S., Ohta, Y., and Yasue, H. 1994. LPC in oxidized LDL elicits vasocontraction and inhibits endothelium-dependent relaxation. *Am J Physiol* 267, H2441–9.
14. Artaud-Wild, S. M., Connor, S. L., Sexton, G., and Connor, W. E. 1993. Differences in coronary mortality can be explained by differences in cholesterol and saturated fat intakes in 40 countries but not in France and Finland. A paradox. *Circulation* 88, 2771–9.
15. Criqui, M. H. and Ringel, B. L. 1994. Does diet or alcohol explain the French paradox? *Lancet* 344, 1719–23.
16. German, J. B. and Walzem, R. L. 2000. The health benefits of wine. *Annu Rev Nutr* 20, 561–93.
17. Aldini, G., Carini, M., Piccoli, A., Rossoni, G., and Facino, R. M. 2003. Procyanidins from grape seeds protect endothelial cells from peroxynitrite damage and enhance endothelium-dependent relaxation in human artery: New evidences for cardio-protection. *Life Sci* 73, 2883–98.
18. Deckert, V., Persegol, L., Viens, L., Lizard, G., Athias, A., Lallemant, C., et al. 1997. Inhibitors of arterial relaxation among components of human oxidized low-density lipoproteins. Cholesterol derivatives oxidized in position 7 are potent inhibitors of endothelium-dependent relaxation. *Circulation* 95, 723–31.
19. Noguchi, K., Iwasaki, K., Endo, H., Kondo, H., Shitashige, M., and Ishikawa, I. 2000. Prostaglandins E2 and I2 downregulate tumor necrosis factor alpha-induced intercellular adhesion molecule-1 expression in human oral gingival epithelial cells. *Oral Microbiol Immunol* 15, 299–304.
20. Ndiaye, M., Chataigneau, T., Chataigneau, M., and Schini-Kerth, V. B. 2004. Red wine polyphenols induce EDHF-mediated relaxations in porcine coronary arteries through the redox-sensitive activation of the PI3-kinase/Akt pathway. *Br J Pharmacol* 142, 1131–6.
21. Li, H. F., Chen, S. A., and Wu, S. N. 2000. Evidence for the stimulatory effect of resveratrol on Ca2+–activated K+ current in vascular endothelial cells. *Cardiovasc Res* 45, 1035–45.
22. Kwan, C. Y., Zhang, W. B., Deyama, T., and Nishibe, S. 2004. Endothelium-dependent vascular relaxation induced by Eucommia ulmoides Oliv. bark extract is mediated by NO and EDHF in small vessels. Naunyn Schmiedebergs. *Arch Pharmacol* 369, 206–11.
23. Liu, J. C., Chen, J. J., Chan, P., Cheng, C. F., and Cheng, T. H. 2003. Inhibition of cyclic strain-induced endothelin-1 gene expression by resveratrol. *Hypertension* 42, 1198–205.
24. Stoclet, J. C., Chataigneau, T., Ndiaye, M., Oak, M. H., El Bedoui, J., et al. 2004. Vascular protection by dietary polyphenols. *Eur J Pharmacol* 500, 299–313.
25. Zhen, M. C., Huang, X. H., Wang, Q., Sun, K., Liu, Y. J., Li, W., et al. 2006. Green tea polyphenol epigallocatechin-3-gallate suppresses rat hepatic stellate cell invasion by inhibition of MMP-2 expression and its activation. *Acta Pharmacol Sin* 27, 1600–7.
26. Annabi, B., Lachambre, M. P., Bousquet–Gagnon, N., Page, M., Gingras, D., and Beliveau, R. 2002. Green tea polyphenol-epigallocatechin 3-gallate inhibits MMP-2 secretion and MT1-MMP-driven migration in glioblastoma cells. *Biochim Biophys Acta* 1542, 209–20.
27. Ferrara, N. and Davis-Smyth, T. 1997. The biology of vascular endothelial growth factor. *Endocr Rev* 18, 4–25.
28. Oak, M. H., Chataigneau, M., Keravis, T., Chataigneau, T., Beretz, A., Andriantsitohaina, R., Stoclet, J. C., et al. 2003. Red wine polyphenolic compounds inhibit vascular endothelial growth factor expression in vascular smooth muscle cells by preventing the activation of the p38 mitogen-activated protein kinase pathway. *Arterioscler Thromb Vasc Biol* 23, 1001–7.
29. Iijima, K., Yoshizumi, M., Hashimoto, M., Akishita, M., Kozaki, K., Ako, J., et al. 2002. Red wine polyphenols inhibit vascular smooth muscle cell migration through two distinct signaling pathways. *Circulation* 105, 2404–10.
30. Lo, H. M., Hung, C. F., Huang, Y. Y., and Wu, W. B. 2007. Tea polyphenols inhibit rat vascular smooth muscle cell adhesion and migration on collagen and laminin via interference with cell–ECM interaction. *J Biomed Sci* 14, 637–645.
31. Veronesi, U. and Bonanni, B. 2005. Chemoprevention: From research to clinical oncology. *Eur J Cancer* 41, 1833–41.
32. Russo, G. L. 2007. Ins and outs of dietary phytochemicals in cancer chemoprevention. *Biochem Pharmacol*, 74 533–544.
33. Hanahan, D. and Weinberg, R. A. 2000. The hallmarks of cancer. *Cell* 100, 57–70.
34. Levine, A. J. 1997. p53, the cellular gatekeeper for growth and division. *Cell* 88, 323–31.

35. Lee, K. W. and Lee, H. J. 2006. Biphasic effects of dietary antioxidants on oxidative stress-mediated carcinogenesis. *Mech Ageing Dev* 127, 424–31.
36. Steinmetz, K. A. and Potter, J. D. 1991. Vegetables, Fruit, and Cancer 2. Mechanisms. *Cancer Causes Control* 2, 427–442.
37. Surh, Y. J. 2003. Cancer chemoprevention with dietary phytochemicals. *Nat Rev Cancer* 3, 768–80.
38. Greenwald, P., Clifford, C. K., and Milner, J. A. 2001. Diet and cancer prevention. *Eur J Cancer* 37, 948–65.
39. Sporn, M. B. and Suh, N. 2002. Chemoprevention: An essential approach to controlling cancer. *Nat Rev Cancer* 2, 537–43.
40. Subbaramaiah, K. and Dannenberg, A. J. 2001. Resveratrol inhibits the expression of cyclooxygenase-2 in mammary epithelial cells. *Adv Exp Med Biol* 492, 147–57.
41. Surh, Y. J., Chun, K. S., Cha, H. H., Han, S. S., Keum, Y. S., Park, K. K., and Lee, S. S. 2001. Molecular mechanisms underlying chemopreventive activities of anti-inflammatory phytochemicals: Downregulation of COX-2 and iNOS through suppression of NF-kappa B activation. *Mutat Res* 480–481, 243–68.
42. Bhat, T. A. and Singh, R. P. 2007. Tumor angiogenesis: A potential target in cancer chemoprevention. *Food Chem Toxicol.*
43. Reynolds, A., Laurie, C., Mosley, R. L., and Gendelman, H. E. 2007. Oxidative stress and the pathogenesis of neurodegenerative disorders. *Int Rev Neurobiol* 82, 297–325.
44. Sipe, J. D. and Cohen, A. S. 2000. Review: History of the amyloid fibril. *J Struct Biol* 130, 88–98.
45. Youdim, K. A., Shukitt-Hale, B., and Joseph, J. A. 2004. Flavonoids and the brain: Interactions at the blood–brain barrier and their physiological effects on the central nervous system. *Free Radic Biol Med* 37, 1683–93.
46. Shukitt-Hale, B., Carey, A. N., Jenkins, D., Rabin, B. M., and Joseph, J. A. 2007. Beneficial effects of fruit extracts on neuronal function and behavior in a rodent model of accelerated aging. *Neurobiol Aging* 28, 1187–94.
47. Schaffer, S., Podstawa, M., Visioli, F., Bogani, P., Muller, W. E., and Eckert, G. P. 2007. Hydroxytyrosol-rich olive mill wastewater extract protects brain cells in vitro and ex vivo. *J Agric Food Chem* 55, 5043–9.
48. Dasgupta, B. and Milbrandt, J. 2007. Resveratrol stimulates AMP kinase activity in neurons. *Proc Natl Acad Sci USA* 104, 7217–22.
49. Frautschy, S. A., Hu, W., Kim, P., Miller, S. A., Chu, T., Harris-White, M. E., and Cole, G. M. 2001. Phenolic anti-inflammatory antioxidant reversal of Abeta-induced cognitive deficits and neuropathology. *Neurobiol Aging* 22, 993–1005.
50. Lau, F. C., Shukitt-Hale, B., and Joseph, J. A. 2005. The beneficial effects of fruit polyphenols on brain aging. *Neurobiol Aging* 26 Suppl 1, 128–32.
51. Brown, M. K., Evans, J. L., and Luo, Y. 2006. Beneficial effects of natural antioxidants EGCG and alpha-lipoic acid on life span and age-dependent behavioral declines in Caenorhabditis elegans. *Pharmacol Biochem Behav* 85, 620–8.
52. Kim, H., Deshane, J., Barnes, S., and Meleth, S. 2006. Proteomics analysis of the actions of grape seed extract in rat brain: Technological and biological implications for the study of the actions of psychoactive compounds. *Life Sci* 78, 2060–5.
53. Hartman, R. E., Shah, A., Fagan, A. M., Schwetye, K. E., Parsadanian, M., Schulman, R. N., et al. 2006. Pomegranate juice decreases amyloid load and improves behavior in a mouse model of Alzheimer's disease. *Neurobiol Dis* 24, 506–15.
54. Anekonda, T. S. 2006. Resveratrol––A boon for treating Alzheimer's disease? *Brain Res Rev* 52, 316–26.
55. Henderson, S. T. 2004. High carbohydrate diets and Alzheimer's disease. *Med Hypotheses* 62, 689–700.
56. Aggarwal, B. B., Kumar, A., and Bharti, A. C. 2003. Anticancer potential of curcumin: Preclinical and clinical studies. *Anticancer Res* 23, 363–98.
57. Cole, G. M., Lim, G. P., Yang, F., Teter, B., Begum, A., Ma, Q., et al. 2005. Prevention of Alzheimer's disease: Omega-3 fatty acid and phenolic antioxidant interventions. *Neurobiol Aging* 26 Suppl 1, 133–6.
58. Weinreb, O., Mandel, S., Amit, T., and Youdim, M. B. 2004. Neurological mechanisms of green tea polyphenols in Alzheimer's and Parkinson's diseases. *J Nutr Biochem* 15, 506–16.

59. Klein, R., Wang, Q., Klein, B. E., Moss, S. E., and Meuer, S. M. 1995. The relationship of age-related maculopathy, cataract, and glaucoma to visual acuity. *Invest Ophthal Vis Sci* 36, 182–91.

60. Beatty, S., Koh, H., Phil, M., Henson, D., and Boulton, M. 2000. The role of oxidative stress in the pathogenesis of age-related macular degeneration. *Surv Ophthalmol* 45, 115–34.

61. Liu, R. H. 2004. Potential synergy of phytochemicals in cancer prevention: Mechanism of action. *J Nutr* 134, 3479S–3485S.

62. Snodderly, D. M., Auran, J. D., and Delori, F. C. 1984. The macular pigment. II. Spatial distribution in primate retinas. *Invest Ophthalmol Vis Sci* 25, 674–85.

63. Palozza, P. and Krinsky, N. I. 1992. Beta-Carotene and alpha-tocopherol are synergistic antioxidants. *Arch Biochem Biophys* 297, 184–7.

64. Friedrichson, T., Kalbach, H. L., Buck, P., and van Kuijk, F. J. 1995. Vitamin E in macular and peripheral tissues of the human eye. *Curr Eye Res* 14, 693–701.

65. Yeum, K. J., Taylor, A., Tang, G., and Russell, R. M. 1995. Measurement of carotenoids, retinoids, and tocopherols in human lenses. *Invest Ophthalmol Vis Sci* 36, 2756–61.

66. Moeller, S. M., Jacques, P. F., and Blumberg, J. B. 2000. The potential role of dietary xanthophylls in cataract and age-related macular degeneration. *J Am Coll Nutr* 19, 522S–527S.

67. Landrum, J. T., Bone, R. A., and Kilburn, M. D. 1997. The macular pigment: A possible role in protection from age-related macular degeneration. *Adv Pharmacol* 38, 537–56.

68. Khanna, D., Sethi, G., Ahn, K. S., Pandey, M. K., Kunnumakkara, A. B., Sung, B., et al. 2007. Natural products as a gold mine for arthritis treatment. *Curr Opin Pharmacol* 7, 344–51.

69. Scalbert, A., Manach, C., Morand, C., Remesy, C., and Jimenez, L. 2005. Dietary polyphenols and the prevention of diseases. *Crit Rev Food Sci Nutr* 45, 287–306.

70. Pietta, P. G. 2000. Flavonoids as antioxidants. *J Nat Prod* 63, 1035–1042.

71. Liu, R. H. and Hotchkiss, J. H. 1995. Potential genotoxicity of chronically elevated nitric oxide: A review. *Mutat Res* 339, 73–89.

72. Chun, O. K., Kim, D. O., Smith, N., Schroeder, D., Han, J. T., and Lee, C. Y. 2005. Daily consumption of phenolics and total antioxidant capacity from fruit and vegetables in the American diet. *J Sci Food Agric* 85, 1715–1724.

73. Shahidi, F. and Wanasundara, P. K. 1992. Phenolic antioxidants. *Crit Rev Food Sci Nutr* 32, 67–103.

74. Cos, P., De Bruyne, T., Hermans, N., Apers, S., Berghe, D. V., and Vlietinck, A. J. 2004. Proanthocyanidins in health care: Current and new trends. *Curr Med Chem* 11, 1345–1359.

75. Rice–Evans, C. A., Miller, N. J., and Paganga, G. 1996. Structure–antioxidant activity relationships of flavonoids and phenolic acids. *Free Radic Biol Med* 20, 933–56.

76. Robbins, R. J. 2003. Phenolic acids in foods: An overview of analytical methodology. *J Agric Food Chem* 51, 2866–87.

77. Le Marchand, L. 2002. Cancer preventive effects of flavonoids—a review. *Biomed Pharmacother* 56, 296–301.

78. Yang, C. S. and Wang, Z. Y. 1993. Tea and cancer. *J Natl Cancer Inst* 85, 1038–49.

79. Guo, Q., Zhao, B., Li, M., Shen, S., and Xin, W. 1996. Studies on protective mechanisms of four components of green tea polyphenols against lipid peroxidation in synaptosomes. *Biochim Biophys Acta* 1304, 210–22.

80. Sumpio, B. E., Cordova, A. C., Berke–Schlessel, D. W., Qin, F., and Chen, Q. H. 2006. Green tea, the "Asian paradox," and cardiovascular disease. *J Am Coll Surg* 202, 813–25.

81. Imai, K., Suga, K., and Nakachi, K. 1997. Cancer-preventive effects of drinking green tea among a Japanese population. *Prev Med* 26, 769–75.

82. Nakachi, K., Eguchi, H., and Imai, K. 2003. Can teatime increase one's lifetime? *Ageing Res Rev* 2, 1–10.

83. Adhami, V. M. and Mukhtar, H. 2006. Polyphenols from green tea and pomegranate for prevention of prostate cancer. *Free Radic Res* 40, 1095–104.

84. Walzem, R. and German, J., Eds. 2004. The French Paradox: Mechanisms of action of non-alcoholic wine components on cardiovascular disease. In *Beverages in Nutrition and Health*. Wilson, N. J. T. (Ed.). Totowa, NJ: Humana Press.

85. DiCastlenuovo, A., Rotondo, S., Iacoviello, L., Donati, M. B., and de Gaeteno, G. 2002. Meta-analysis of wine and beer consumption in relation to vascular risk. *Circulation* 105, 2836–2844.

86. Renaud, S. C., Gueguen, R., Siest, G., and Salamon, R. 1999. Wine, beer, and mortality in middle-aged men from eastern France. *Arch Int Med* 159, 1865–1870.

87. St. Leger, A. S., Chochrane, A. L., and Moore, F. 1979. Factors associated with cardiac mortality in developed countries with particular reference to the consumption of wine. *Lancet* 12, 1017–1020.

88. Koppes, L. L. J., Dekker, J. M., Hendriks, H. F. J., Bouter, L. M., and Heine, R. J. 2006. Meta-analysis of the relationship beteen alcohol consumption and coronary heart disease and mortality in type 2 diabetic patients. *Diabetologica* 49, 648–652.

89. Waterhouse, A. L. 2002. Wine phenolics. *Ann NY Acad Sci* 957, 21–36.

90. Corder, R., Mullen, W., Khan, N. Q., Marks, S. C., Wood, E. G., Carrier, M. J., and Crozier, A. 2006. Oenology: Red wine procyanidins and vascular health. *Nature* 444, 566.

91. Panza, F., D'Introno, A., Colacicco, A. M., Capurso, C., Del Parigi, A., Caselli, R. J., et al. 2005. Current epidemiology of mild cognitive impairmant and other predementia syndromes. *Am J Geriat Psychiat* 13, 633–644.

92. Solfrizzi, V., Panza, F., Colacicco, A. M., D'Introno, A., Capurso, C., Torres, F., et al. 2004. Vascular risk factors, incidence of MCI, and rates of progression to dementia. *Neurology* 63, 1882–1891.

93. Orgogozo, J. M., Dartigues, J. F., Lafont, S., Letenneur, L., Commenges, D., Salamon, R., et al. 1997. Wine consumption and dementia in the elderly: A prospective community study in the Bordeaux area. *Rev Neurol Paris* 153, 185–92.

94. Solfrizzi, V., D'Introno, A., Colacicco, A. M., Capurso, C., Del Parigi, A., Baldassarre, G., et al. 2007. Alcohol consumption, mild cognitive impairment, and progression to dementia. *Neurology* 68, 1790–9.

95. Ramassamy, C. 2006. Emerging role of polyphenolic compounds in the treatment of neurodegenerative diseases: A review of their intracellular targets. *Eur J Pharmacol* 545, 51–64.

96. de la Torre, R., Covas, M. I., Pujadas, M. A., Fito, M., and Farre, M. 2006. Is dopamine behind the health benefits of red wine? *Eur J Nutr* 45, 307–10.

97. Beilin, L. J. and Puddey, I. B. 2006. Alcohol and hypertension: An update. *Hypertension* 47, 1035–8.

98. Fuchs, F. D. 2005. Vascular effects of alcoholic beverages: Is it only alcohol that matters? *Hypertension* 45, 851–2.

99. Zilkens, R. R., Burke, V., Hodgson, J. M., Barden, A., Beilin, L. J., and Puddey, I. B. 2005. Red wine and beer elevate blood pressure in normotensive men. *Hypertension* 45, 874–9.

100. Fuchs, F. D., Chambless, L. E., Folsom, A. R., Eigenbrodt, M. L., Duncan, B. B., Gilbert, A., and Szklo, M. 2004. Association between alcoholic beverage consumption and incidence of coronary heart disease in whites and blacks: The Atherosclerosis Risk in Communities Study. *Am J Epidemiol* 160, 455–472.

101. Adlercreutz, C. H. T., Goldin, B. R., Gorbach, S. L., Hockerstedt, K. A. V., Watanabe, S., Hamalainen, E. K., et al. 1995. Soybean phytoestrogen intake and cancer risk. *J Nutr* 125, S757–S770.

102. Finkel, E. 1998. Phyto-oestrogens: The way to postmenopausal health? *Lancet* 352, 1762.

103. Yamori, Y., Miura, A., and Taira, K. 2001. Implications from and for food cultures for cardiovascular diseases: Japanese food, particularly Okinawan diets. *Asia Pac J Clin Nutr* 10, 144–5.

104. Watanabe, S., Uesugi, S., and Kikuchi, Y. 2002. Isoflavones for prevention of cancer, cardiovascular diseases, gynecological problems and possible immune potentiation. *Biomed Pharmacother* 56, 302–12.

105. Barnes, S. 1998. Phytoestrogens and breast cancer. *Baillieres Clin Endocrinol Metab* 12, 559–79.

106. Limer, J. L. and Speirs, V. 2004. Phyto-oestrogens and breast cancer chemoprevention. *Breast Cancer Res* 6, 119–27.

107. Kirk, C. J., Harris, R. M., Wood, D. M., Waring, R. H., and Hughes, P. J. 2001. Do dietary phytoestrogens influence susceptibility to hormone–dependent cancer by disrupting the metabolism of endogenous oestrogens? *Biochem Soc Trans* 29, 209–16.

108. Grube, B. J., Eng, E. T., Kao, Y. C., Kwon, A., and Chen, S. 2001. White button mushroom phytochemicals inhibit aromatase activity and breast cancer cell proliferation. *J Nutr* 131, 3288–93.

109. Kristal, A. R. and Lampe, J. W. 2002. Brassica vegetables and prostate cancer risk: A review of the epidemiological evidence. *Nutr Cancer* 42, 1–9.

110. Verhoeven, D. T., Goldbohm, R. A., van Poppel, G., Verhagen, H., and van den Brandt, P. A. 1996. Epidemiological studies on brassica vegetables and cancer risk. *Cancer Epidemiol Biomarkers Prev* 5, 733–48.

111. van Poppel, G., Verhoeven, D. T., Verhagen, H., and Goldbohm, R. A. 1999. Brassica vegetables and cancer prevention: Epidemiology and mechanisms. *Adv Exp Med Biol* 472, 159–68.

112. Lund, E. 2003. Non-nutritive bioactive constituents of plants: Dietary sources and health benefits of glucosinolates. *Int J Vitam Nutr Res* 73, 135–43.

113. Verhoeven, D. T., Verhagen, H., Goldbohm, R. A., van den Brandt, P. A., and van Poppel, G. 1997. A review of mechanisms underlying anticarcinogenicity by brassica vegetables. *Chem Biol Interact* 103, 79–129.

114. Wilkinson, J. T. and Clapper, M. L. 1997. Detoxication enzymes and chemoprevention. *Proc Soc Exp Biol Med* 216, 192–200.

115. Steinkellner, H., Rabot, S., Freywald, C., Nobis, E., Scharf, G., Chabicovsky, M., et al. 2001. Effects of cruciferous vegetables and their constituents on drug metabolizing enzymes involved in the bioactivation of DNA-reactive dietary carcinogens. *Mutat Res* 480–481, 285–97.

116. Langley, P. 2000. Why a pomegranate? *BMJ* 321, 1153–4.

117. Gil, M. I., Tomas-Barberan, F. A., Hess-Pierce, B., Holcroft, D. M., and Kader, A. A. 2000. Antioxidant activity of pomegranate juice and its relationship with phenolic composition and processing. *J Agric Food Chem* 48, 4581–9.

118. Aviram, M. and Dornfeld, L. 2001. Pomegranate juice consumption inhibits serum angiotensin converting enzyme activity and reduces systolic blood pressure. *Atherosclerosis* 158, 195–8.

119. Griendling, K. K., Tsuda, T., Berk, B. C., and Alexander, R. W. 1989. Angiotensin II stimulation of vascular smooth muscle. *J Cardiovasc Pharmacol* 14 Suppl 6, S27–33.

120. Keidar, S., Kaplan, M., Shapira, C., Brook, J. G., and Aviram, M. 1994. Low density lipoprotein isolated from patients with essential hypertension exhibits increased propensity for oxidation and enhanced uptake by macrophages: A possible role for angiotensin II. *Atherosclerosis* 107, 71–84.

121. Kim, N. D., Mehta, R., Yu, W., Neeman, I., Livney, T., Amichay, A., et al. 2002. Chemopreventive and adjuvant therapeutic potential of pomegranate Punica granatum for human breast cancer. *Breast Cancer Res Treat* 71, 203–17.

122. Albrecht, M., Jiang, W., Kumi-Diaka, J., Lansky, E. P., Gommersall, L. M., Patel, A., et al. 2004. Pomegranate extracts potently suppress proliferation, xenograft growth, and invasion of human prostate cancer cells. *J Med Food* 7, 274–83.

123. Lansky, E. P. and Newman, R. A. 2007. Punica granatum pomegranate and its potential for prevention and treatment of inflammation and cancer. *J Ethnopharmacol* 109, 177–206.

124. Skibola, C. F. and Smith, M. T. 2000. Potential health impacts of excessive flavonoid intake. *Free Radic Biol Med* 29, 375–83.

125. Trinajstic, N. 2007. Structure-Property/Activity Modeling of Polyphenols. *Int. J. Mol. Sci.*

16 Management of Insulin Resistance with Chinese Herbs

Jianping Ye and Jun Yin

CONTENTS

16.1 INSULIN RESISTANCE

Insulin is a hormone whose major function is to reduce blood glucose. Insulin resistance is a state wherein the body loses its response to insulin. It has a high prevalence in obese subjects and aging people. The main damage from insulin resistance is development of type 2 diabetes and cardiovascular diseases (CVD). Often associated with metabolic syndrome, insulin resistance was discovered 70 years ago by Himsworth [1]. The clinical evidence of insulin resistance was that diabetic patients lost response to regular dose of insulin. A higher dose of insulin was required to control the blood glucose in these patients.

16.1.1 Physiology of Insulin

16.1.1.1 Control of Blood Glucose

Blood glucose is determined by a balance of glucose absorption in the intestine and glucose disposal in peripheral tissues in a fed condition. After a meal, the blood glucose is increased by absorbed glucose from the food. In the fasting condition, the blood glucose comes mainly from the liver through gluconeogenesis, and is controlled by a balance between glucose production in the liver and glucose disposal in the peripheral tissues.

As a source of energy, blood glucose is consumed by every tissue in the body, such as skeletal muscle, brain, heart, and liver. However, the consumption can be promoted by insulin in certain tissue or organs. These tissue/organs include skeletal muscle, heart, and adipose tissue. The response of these organs leads to a reduction in blood glucose. The reason for this tissue-specific effect of insulin is determined by the expression of glucose transporter 4 (GLUT4), which is expressed only in skeletal myotubes, cardiomyocytes, and adipocytes. In response to insulin, GLUT4 in the cell surface will be increased, leading to enhancement in glucose uptake. By increasing glucose disposal in these peripheral tissues, insulin reduces blood glucose. With insulin resistance, the response of these peripheral tissues to insulin is attenuated, and they are not able to take glucose as efficiently as they should. Therefore, blood glucose may increase in the presence of normal levels of insulin.

In the fasting condition, a major source of blood glucose is the liver, which produces glucose from amino acids or lactic acids. In response to insulin, the liver will reduce glucose production. With insulin resistance, insulin will not be able to efficiently reduce glucose production by the liver. This will lead to hyperglycemia in the fasting condition. In the fed condition, the liver insulin resistance may contribute to postprandial hyperglycemia in type 2 diabetes. This is because, even with a high level of insulin after a meal, the liver is still not able to shut down its glucose production. Therefore, insulin reduces blood glucose through two major activities: (a) stimulation of glucose disposal in muscle and fat and (b) inhibition of hepatic glucose production.

16.1.1.2 Improvement of Microcirculation

In addition to these effects, insulin also improves microcirculation through induction of nitric oxide (NO) production in endothelial cells. This activity induces vascular dilation, which promotes glucose uptake by muscle as more muscle cells are exposed to the blood glucose when vascular dilation occurs. Insulin also stimulates growth of the small blood vessels. These activities of insulin may constitute the mechanism of beneficial effects of insulin in the treatment of patients in the intensive care unit (ICU).

16.1.2 Physiological Insulin Resistance

In the physiological condition, insulin resistance is a part of the stress response, which protects the body from hypoglycemic shock. In the fasting condition, insulin resistance in the skeletal muscle is able to reduce glucose consumption by muscle, and save the limited glucose for the brain, which can only use glucose for energy. The insulin resistance in muscle may be a result of a high level of free fatty acids in the blood. Free fatty acids (FFA) are a major source of energy in the fasting condition. Blood FFA usually reaches to the highest level in the fasting condition, where it is used as an alternative fuel in skeletal muscle and heart in the absence of sufficient glucose. At the same time, FFA also reduces insulin sensitivity in the muscle and heart to reduce glucose utilization, a mechanism that is important for the protection of the body from hypoglycemic shock. In the fasting condition, if muscle continues to consume a large amount of glucose, the brain will not be able to overcome muscle consumption, as skeletal muscle accounts for 40% of body weight, and the brain accounts for only about 5–10% of body weight. When the brain cannot get sufficient energy, the body will suffer a shock. Therefore, FFA-induced insulin resistance in the muscle provides protection of the body from hypoglycemic shock.

During mental stress, insulin resistance may contribute to the increased blood glucose when glucocorticoid secretion is increased. Blood glucose is higher under many mental stress conditions, such as fighting, defense, or anger. Glucocorticoid is able to induce insulin resistance and elevate blood glucose. Under mental stress, secretion of the hormone glucocorticoid is increased in the body. Glucocorticoid has many activities in the regulation of glucose metabolism. In the liver, it increases glucose production. This activity is against insulin function and is responsible for liver insulin resistance. Glucocorticoid also induces insulin resistance in muscle. This activity of glucocorticoid leads to reduced glucose uptake by muscle. Additionally, the glucocorticoid may cause muscle to release large amounts of amino acids through hydrolysis of the muscle proteins. Insulin stimulates protein synthesis and inhibits protein degradation. This activity of insulin is reduced by glucocorticoid.

16.1.3 CELLULAR MECHANISM OF INSULIN SENSITIVITY

Systemic insulin resistance is determined by insulin sensitivity in the insulin target tissues, such as muscle (skeletal muscle and cardiomyocytes), liver, and fat. Muscle insulin resistance accounts for a major part of systemic insulin resistance.

The skeletal muscle has been considered to be the major site of insulin-stimulated glucose disposal *in vivo*. In response to insulin, muscle takes at least 10 times more glucose than white adipose tissue (WAT) does on the basis of per milligram of tissue in the resting condition [2]. Because muscle mass is considerably greater than WAT mass in lean subjects, this observation has indicated the prominent role of muscle in glucose disposal. Although a muscle-specific knockout of insulin receptor failed to result in systemic insulin resistance or disorder in glucose metabolism, the role of skeletal muscle in determination of systemic insulin sensitivity is well accepted. In the muscle insulin receptor knockout mice, muscle insulin resistance led to an increase in fat mass and disorder of lipid metabolism, such as an increase in serum triglycerides and FFA, but no disorder in glucose metabolism or type 2 diabetes. The blood glucose, insulin, and glucose tolerance were normal in the muscle-specific insulin receptor knockout mice in the conscious and unrestricted condition [3]. This is because the glucose uptake in skeletal muscle can be induced by muscle contraction. Skeletal muscle contraction may replace insulin signal in the induction of glucose uptake. Muscle contraction may induce glucose uptake by muscle cells through calcium mobilization and hypoxia. The contraction-induced glucose uptake in muscle contributes to the beneficial effect of physical exercise in the regulation of blood glucose.

The liver has two major functions in the regulation of systemic insulin sensitivity. The first is synthesis of glucose and the second is clearance of blood insulin. Production of glucose is a major function of the liver in the maintenance of homeostasis of blood glucose in the fasting condition. Removal of insulin from blood by the liver is important in the control of insulin levels. Most (75%) insulin in the blood is degraded in the liver. When this function of the liver is reduced, insulin levels will be increased in the blood and lead to insulin resistance. This is demonstrated in the liver-specific knockout mice for insulin receptor.

Adipose tissue regulates insulin sensitivity through at least two functions. The first is regulation of blood FFAs. Adipocyte is able to remove FFAs from blood and convert them into fat triglycerides (TG). If this function is reduced in adipose tissue, blood FFAs will have no place to go and will induce insulin resistance. This often happens in the presence of obesity. The second function of adipose tissue in the control of insulin sensitivity is the endocrine function. Adipose tissue is able to produce many cytokines including adiponectin, leptin, IL-6 (interleukin 6), TNF-α (Tumor Necrosis Factor α) and RBP4 (Rentinol Binding Protein 4). These cytokines can be divided into two groups on the basis of their functions. The first group, such as adiponectin, is able to enhance insulin sensitivity. In obesity, reduction of adiponectin is often associated with insulin resistance. The second group, such as TNF-a, can reduce insulin sensitivity. In obesity or chronic inflammation, the TNF-α level is often elevated and involved in development of insulin resistance. TNF-α is able to inhibit insulin signaling activity by targeting insulin receptor substrate 1 (IRS-1) and peroxisome proliferator-activated receptor g (PPARg).

16.1.4 PATHOLOGICAL INSULIN RESISTANCE AND ITS CHARACTERISTICS

In the physiological condition, insulin resistance is transient under stress. When the stress disappears, insulin sensitivity will be restored automatically. Therefore, a change in insulin sensitivity is a physiological phenomenon in the body. It constitutes a part of physiological response of the body to stress. However, when insulin resistance persists in the body, it will lead to development of type 2 diabetes.

Insulin resistance has the following characteristics:

- Hyperinsulinemia
- Postprandial hyperglycemia
- Decreased glucose infusion rate
- Increased hepatic glucose production
- Impaired glucose tolerance
- Hyperglycemia
- Increased HbA1c
- Hyperlipidemia
- Impaired insulin tolerance
- Loss of first phase secretion of insulin
- Hypoadiponectinemia
- Increased inflammatory markers
- Hypertension

16.1.5 RISK FACTORS FOR INSULIN RESISTANCE

Several factors are known to induce insulin resistance. These include:

- Obesity
- Aging
- Genetic background
- Inflammation
- FFA
- Oxidative stress
- Hyperinsulinemia
- Endoplasmic reticulum (ER) stress
- Mitochondrial dysfunction
- Fatty liver
- Adipose tissue hypoxia
- Hyperlipidemia;
- Lipodystrophy [10]
- Pregnancy

16.1.5.1 Obesity

Obesity is a status where body mass index (BMI) (weight in kg/height in m^2) is above 27. Obesity can be divided into peripheral obesity and central (or abdominal) obesity. In peripheral obesity, waist circumference and a waist-to-hip ratio are close to the normal range, the fat is evenly distributed in the body, and the subjects have less risk of insulin resistance. In central obesity, the subjects exhibit extra accumulation of fat in the abdomen area and have a large ratio of waist circumference and waist-to-hip (> 0.95). The best indicator of central obesity is an increase in waist circumference. It is mainly due to an increase in fat deposit in the abdominal cavity, not in the abdominal subcutaneous fat. The increase is often observed in the omentum, the mesenteric, and retroperitoneal regions in the abdominal cavity. The fat tissues in these regions are usually called visceral fat, which is positively and independently associated with insulin resistance [11]. Therefore, central obese subjects suffer a high risk of insulin resistance. Accumulation of the visceral fat is often a result of imbalance of sex hormones, overintake of sucrose, and lack of physical exercise. Lack of androgen in aging subjects and in men contributes to the development of central obesity. An increase in cortisol or glucocorticoid also increases visceral fat for central obesity. Therefore, central obesity is a risk factor of insulin resistance.

16.1.5.2 Aging

Insulin resistance occurs frequently in the aging population. This is related to an increased prevalence of central obesity. Imbalance of sex hormone and lack of physical exercise contribute to this central obesity in aging people. Removal of visceral fat is able to prevent insulin resistance in aging [12]. Other factors include free radicals, which lead to oxidative stress in aging, and mitochondrial dysfunction [13–15]. Oxidative stress and mitochondrial dysfunction are known to increase the risk of insulin resistance [13,14,16].

16.1.5.3 Genetic Background

Although insulin resistance is determined by multiple factors, genetic background is key. This is supported by several lines of evidence. The first is that insulin-resistant patients and high-risk populations are often associated with a family history of type 2 diabetes. The second is a high risk of insulin resistance in certain ethnic groups, as indicated by epidemiology studies. In the United States, black Americans and Pima Indians have a higher risk of insulin resistance than Caucasians. East Indians and Chinese are also at high risk of insulin resistance. Within each ethnic group, the genetic background is similar among different individuals. This genetic nature determines their susceptibility to certain diseases. Central obesity, mitochondrial dysfunction, hypoadiponectinemia, and increase in inflammatory mediators are possible links to the gene background [17–19].

16.1.6 Treatment of Insulin Resistance

In most cases, insulin resistance is a result of lipid accumulation that is most commonly observed in obese patients and aging subjects. It may be a consequence of chronic inflammation or infection. The treatment strategy is to remove the cause. In the treatment of insulin resistance in obese subjects, the first choice is to reduce obesity or body weight. This can be accomplished by increasing physical exercise and adopting caloric restriction. The second choice is medicine. This is recommended after failure of exercise and caloric restriction in the control of blood glucose. Medications include insulin, metformin, thiazolidinedione (TZD), α-glucosidase inhibitors, glucagon-like peptide derivatives, and lipid reducing medicine. The third choice is surgery, such as bariatric surgery.

16.2 CHINESE HERBS IN THE MANAGEMENT OF INSULIN SENSITIVITY

16.2.1 Traditional Chinese Medicine

Traditional Chinese Medicine (TCM) is a medical system developed on the basis of Taoist philosophy. The theory of TCM was first documented in *Huangdi Neijing* (*Yellow Thearch's Inner Classic*), an ancient Chinese book that was composed 2000 years ago in China [14]. The book provides the foundation for diagnostic methods and therapeutic strategies, including acupuncture. It proposes that the human body contains *Yin, Yang,* and Five Elements (agents). The Five Elements are metal, wood, water, fire, and earth. A perfect balance among these elements is required for the maintenance of health in the body. A disease is a consequence of imbalance of Yin and Yang or the Five Elements from cold, heat, emotions, or other influences. *Qi* (air) and blood serve as mediators in communication between Yin and Yang, and among the Five Elements. The primary aim in the treatment of illness is to restore the balance, and replenish Qi or blood. Herbal medicines, acupuncture, and massage are often used to restore the balance in the clinical practice in TCM [15].

Obesity and type 2 diabetes are two major diseases in the metabolic syndrome. According to *Huangdi Neijing,* obesity is a result of overeating, and diabetes is referred as *Xiaoke* disease, which is a consequence of obesity. The complications of Xiaoke disease include stroke, carbuncle, and foot gangrene [16,17]. In Chinese, *Xiao* means losing body weight and *Ke* means thirsty, which are similar to the symptoms of diabetes, which exhibits loss of body weight in the presence of increased drinking, eating, and urination. In the TCM theory, Xiaoke is considered to be a result of Yin deficiency with dryness-heat. The treatment of diabetes should be focused on replenishing Yin (fluid) and evacuating fire (heat) from the body [18].

TCM prefers herbology, a Chinese art of combining different medical herbs into one therapy through prescription [19]. According to TCM, a disease may have a set of identical symptoms among different patients, but the background (*Qi*, blood, *Yin, Yang,* and Five Elements) for development of the same disease is quite different in different patients. Each patient should receive personalized herbology because of the difference in his or her background. In the personalized treatment, multiple herbs are often prescribed to form a special formula and a single herb is not often used individually.

The bioactivities of many Chinese herbs have been identified with modern technologies in chemistry and pharmacology. With pharmacological concepts in medicine, many scientists try to isolate and purify bioactive components in herbs with the hope of enriching the therapeutic activities. This strategy is used widely to study Chinese herbs in China and many other countries. Hundreds of traditional Chinese herbs and active components have been tested for treatment of diabetes, dyslipidemia, and obesity. In this chapter, 22 of the herbs were selected from the literature to represent the current understanding of Chinese herbs in the treatment of metabolic syndrome (Table 16.1). Among these, the most commonly recognized herbs are ginseng, coptis, bitter melon, and tea.

In TCM, the major function of Asian ginseng is to replenish Qi, and American ginseng is used to restore Yin. Coptis and bitter melon are both bitter herbs that may serve to evacuate fire from the human body. In the theory of TCM, these herbs are beneficial to patients with obesity and diabetes.

16.2.2 Treatment of Insulin Resistance with Chinese Herbs

16.2.2.1 Ginseng

Ginseng is one of the most popular Chinese herbal medicines. In TCM, ginseng is referred as the root of *Panax ginseng* C. A. Mey only. However, the root of *Panax quinquefolium* L. (American ginseng) is also called ginseng sometimes. Since the major effects of ginseng include adaptogen, aphrodisiac, and nourishing stimulant, which are required for treatment of aging, ginseng has been historically used in the treatment of most ageing-associated diseases [20]. Ginseng has been widely studied for treatment of diabetes, dyslipidemia, and obesity. Interestingly, in addition to ginseng root, ginseng berry and leaf were also shown to reduce blood glucose in diabetic models [21,22].

Ginseng contains many bioactive compounds. The representative compounds are ginseng-specific saponins (ginsenosides), which have clear bioactivities in the reduction of blood glucose and blood pressure. Ginseng inhibits body weight gain, decreases blood glucose, TG, and FFA levels, and improves insulin sensitivity [23]. Efficacy and safety of ginseng on glucose metabolism have been confirmed in patients with type 2 diabetes in double-blinded placebo-controlled studies [24,25].

In addition to glucose metabolism, ginseng is also shown to regulate lipid metabolism [26]. American ginseng and Chinese red ginseng reduce cholesterol and TG levels in liver and serum of

TABLE 16.1

Effects of Traditional Chinese Herbs on Metabolism

Name	Botanical Name	Action	Reference
Aloe vera leaves	*Aloevera L. var. chinensis Haw. Berger*	FBG, TC, TG, FFA, hepatic transaminases ↓ Insulin ↑	68–70
Cortex Cinnamomi (cassia bark)	*Cinnamomum zeylanicum*	FBG, insulin, TC, TG ↓ HDL ↑	71–75
Crataegus (hawthorn)	*Crataegus cuneats Sieb. et Zucc.*	TC, TG, LDL, VLDL, lipid deposits in liver and aorta, FBG ↓	76,77
Fructus Corni (dogwood)	*Cornus officinalis Sieb. et Zucc.*	Lipid accumulation in liver, TG, body weight, FBG ↓Insulin, C-peptide ↑	78,79
Fructus Ligustri Lucidi (glossy privet fruit)	*Ligustrum lucidum Ait.*	FBG ↓	81
Fructus Lycii (wolfberry)	*Lycium barbarum L.*	Anti-oxidative, FBG, TC, TG ↓ HDL, SOD activity ↑	82–84
Ganoderma Lucidum (medicinal mushroom)	*Ganoderma lucidum (Leyss. ex Fr.) Karst.*	TC, TG, LDL, LPO, FBG ↓Insulin, HDL↑	85–90
Rhizoma Zingiberis (dried ginger)	*Zingiber officinale Roscoe*	FBG, TC, TG, blood pressure, body weight, LDL oxidation, atherosclerosis, LPO, lipoproteins ↓ Insulin, HDL ↑	91–98
Radix Glycyrrhizae (licorice)	*Glycyrriza uralensis Fisch.G.Glabra L.*	FBG, visceral adipose tissues, body weight ↓	99–101
Radix Notoginseng (Chinese ginseng)	*Panax notoginseng (Burk.) F.H. Chen*	TC, TG, LDL, FBG ↓	102–105
Radix Platycodi (platycodon root)	*Platycodon grandiflorum*	TG, LDL, TG, liver surface fat pads, calorie intake, body weight ↓	106–108
Pumpkin	*Cucurbita moschata (Duch. ex Lam.) Duch. ex Poiret*	Fatty liver, TC, TG, FBG ↓ Glucose tolerance, insulin ↑	109,110
Radix Astragali seu Hedysari (astragalus root)	*Astragalus membranaceus (Fisch.) Bunge var. mongholicus (Bunge) Hsiao and Astragalus membranaceus (Fisch.) Bunge*	FBG ↓Insulin sensitivity, glucose-insulin tolerance, ACTH, insulin ↑	111–113
Radix et Rhizom Rhei (rhubarb)	*Rheum palmatum L.*	FBG, LPO ↓ Oral glucose tolerance ↑	105,114, 115
Radix Puerariae (kudzuvine root)	*Pueraria lobata (Willd.) Ohwi.*	FBG, glycation products, insulin, abdominal fat, TC, TG, body mass ↓	116–122
Radix Rehmanniae (rehmannia root)	*Rehmannia glutinosa Libosch.*	FBG ↓	123
Radix Salviae Miltiorrhizae (danshen root)	*Salvia miltiorrhiza Bge.*	TG ↓	105,124,125
Rhizoma Polygonati (Solomonseal root)	*Polygonatum sibiricum Red.*	FBG ↓	126–129
Rhizoma Polygonati Odorati (coastal glehnia root)	*Polygonatum odoratum (Mill.) Druce*	FBG, TG, glycosylated hemoglobin ↓	130,131

TABLE 16.1 (CONTINUED)
Effects of Traditional Chinese Herbs on Metabolism

Name	Botanical Name	Action	Reference
Salix matsudana leaves	*Salix matsudana Koidz.*	Body weight, parametrial adipose tissue weights, TC ↓	132,133
Semen Cassiae (flatstem milkvetch seed)	*Cassia obtusifolia L.*	TC, TG, LDL, apoB, body weight, insulin ↓	134,135
Tea	*Camellia sinensis*	FBG, body weight, TC, TG, FFA, LDL, systolic blood pressure, LPO ↓ Vitamin, glucose tolerance, adiponectin, LDL particle size, insulin, HDL ↑	136–142

FBG–fasting blood glucose; FFA–free fatty acids; HDL–high-density lipoprotein; LDL–low-density lipoprotein; LPO–lipid peroxidation; SOD–superoxidase dismutase; TC–total cholesterol; TG–triglycerides; VLDL–very low-density lipoprotein.

animal. The decrease of cholesterol and low-density lipoprotein-cholesterol (LDL-C) was related to the suppression of β-hydroxy-β-methylglutaryl-CoA (HMG-CoA) reductase and cholesterol 7 α-hydroxylase activities [26]. In rats and patients fed on high-cholesterol diets for hyperlipidemia, red ginseng powder reduced plasma total cholesterol, TG, FFAs, and platelet adhesiveness, and increased HDL-C significantly [27]. In a clinical trial, administration of ginseng extract led to reduction of total cholesterol, TG and LDL-C, and induction of HDL [28].

Ginsenosides are considered to be the active components in the regulation of lipid and glucose metabolism. Some studies suggest that ginseng is able to increase insulin secretion [29–31]. Impaired insulin response to glucose in the mice was restored after ginseng administration, and insulin release, especially glucose-induced insulin release from isolated rat pancreases, was stimulated by the ginseng extracts [29].

In summary, ginseng has antihyperglycemia and antiobesity effects (Figure 16.1). The mechanism of action is related to insulin sensitization, insulin secretion, β-cell protection, thermogenesis, and antioxidation. It's a promising herbal remedy in the treatment of metabolic syndrome. However, the cellular and molecular mechanisms of the metabolic activities of ginseng remain largely unknown. More research is required to establish the signaling pathway for ginseng.

16.2.2.2 Berberine

Berberine, a botanical alkaloid in the root and bark of several plants, is the major active component of rhizoma coptidis, a popular traditional Chinese medication in the treatment of diabetes and infections. In about A.D. 500, the anti-diabetes activity of Rhizoma Coptidis was recorded for the first time in *Note of Elite Physicians* by Hongjing Tao. Berberine is the bioactive compound in Rhizoma Coptidis for anti-diabetes and anti-infection. Berberine has a well-established antimicrobial activity in the control of infection by bacteria, viruses, fungi, protozoans, and helminthes [8,14]. In China, berberine is an over-the-counter drug for the treatment of gastrointestinal infections such as bacterial diarrhea. In 1988, the hypoglycemic effect of berberine was found when it was used to treat diarrhea in diabetic patients in China [13]. Since then, berberine has been used as an antihyperglycemic agent by many physicians in China. There are substantial numbers of clinical reports about the hypoglycemic action of berberine in Chinese literature.

Berberine was reported to have a comparable activity to sulphonureas or metformin in reducing blood glucose in diabetic patients in the Chinese literature. Our study confirmed that administration of berberine (0.5 g t.i.d.) at the beginning of each major meal was able to reduce fasting blood glucose (FBG) as well as post prandial blood glucose (PBG), increase insulin sensitivity in adult

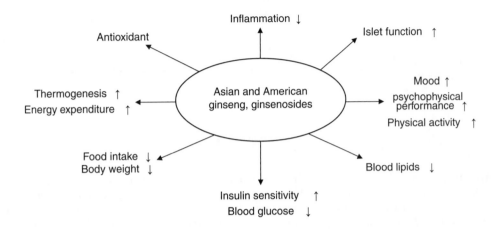

FIGURE 16.1 Ginseng is able to improve glucose metabolism through multiple pathways: (1) Glucose disposal is increased partially due to activation of insulin signaling pathway and GLUT4 translocation by ginseng; (2) food intake is suppressed through inhibition of NPY expression in hypothalamus; (3) Physical activity is increased through improvement of mood and psychophysical performance; 4) Fat composition and body weight are reduced partially related to upregulation of thermogenesis and energy expenditure; (5) Antioxidant and anti-inflammation properties may be involved in the mechanisms of insulin sensitization. (6) islet function is protected through antioxidant activity and inhibition of β cell apoptosis.

patients with newly diagnosed type 2 diabetes or poorly controlled diabetes [32]. Besides the hypoglycemic action, a beneficial effect of berberine on lipid metabolism was also observed [32,33]. However, up to now, there is no multicenter, well controlled, long-term clinical trial to evaluate the efficacy of berberine in the treatment of diabetes.

Effects of berberine on lipid metabolism were evaluated in animals and human subjects. Two clinical trials demonstrated that berberine was able to decrease TG, serum cholesterol, and LDL-C in subjects with dyslipidemia [33,34]. In animals, TG deposition in liver and muscle was reduced significantly, and liver steatosis was prevented by berberine administration [35,36]. In *in vitro* study, berberine was shown to suppress adipocyte differentiation and reduce lipid accumulation in 3T3-L1 adipocytes. In the cells treated by berberine, expression of lipogenic genes was inhibited significantly [37–41].

In summary, berberine, a single compound identified from a Chinese herb, has a promising activity in the control of blood glucose and lipid in patients (Figure 16.2). The metabolic activity has been confirmed in various animal models, and the action mechanism may include induction of glycolysis, α-glucosidase inhibition, and elevation of hepatic LDL receptor level.

16.2.2.3 Bitter Melon

Bitter melon (bitter gourd, karolla, or cerasee) is a popular vegetable as well as an herb in China. The species name of bitter melon is *Momordica charantia*. Bitter melon has been used as an herb for at least 600 years in South China [42].

Bitter melon is known for its "plant insulin," a polypeptide with 166 residues, which exerts a potent hypoglycemic effect after subcutaneous injection [43]. Oral administration of "plant insulin" is not effective in the regulation of glucose metabolism as the peptide is inactivated in the gut. Requirement for injection limited its clinical application. In addition to the "plant insulin," bitter melon may also contain unknown bioactive components, as a substantial number of reports indicate that bitter melon is able to exert a hypoglycemic effect in a variety of animal models through oral administration.

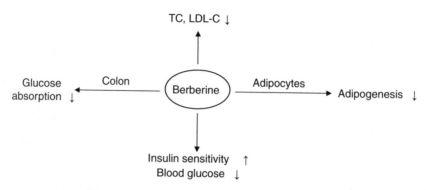

FIGURE 16.2 Mechanism of berberine in regulation of metabolism: (1) Enhances glucose uptake through induction of glycolysis, which is due to inhibition of aerobic respiratory; (2) adipogenesis suppressed through inhibition of peroxisome proliferator-activated receptor (PPAR) γ and CCAAT-enhancer-binding protein (C/EBP) α function; (3) intestinal glucose absorption decreased by inhibition of α-glucosidase; (4) low-density lipoprotein receptor (LDLR) expression upregulated through increasing LDLR mRNA, which is related to inactivation of extracellular signal-regulated kinase (ERK) and activation of c-Jun NH(2)-terminal kinase (JNK) pathway.

In diabetic mice or rats, oral administration of bitter melon extracts decreased blood glucose and increased insulin sensitivity [44–46]. Furthermore, administration of bitter melon extracts decreased serum cholesterol, triglycerides, LDL-C, urea, creatinine, alanine transaminase (ALT), and aspartate transaminase (AST), and increased serum HDL-C, suggesting that bitter melon may correct hyperlipidemia and protect hepatic-renal functions [47–49]. Ten weeks' administration of bitter melon fruit extract nearly restored the increased TG, total cholesterol (TC), and lipid peroxide together with decreased HDL-C [50]. Once the bitter melon extract was withdrawn, the hyperglycemia and dyslipidemia appeared again [51].

The hypoglycemic effect of bitter melon extract was also tested in more than 100 patients with type 2 diabetes. Administration of the fruit juice or homogenized suspension of bitter melon led to significant reduction of both FBG and PBG [52,53]. Nearly 75% of the patients had good response to bitter melon. Bitter melon administrated together with a 50% dose of metformin or glibenclamide led to a greater reduction in blood glucose than that by full doses of the drugs, which indicated that bitter melon had a synergistic effect with other oral hypoglycemic agents [54]. However, these results are not supported by a recent randomized, double-blind, placebo-controlled clinical trial with 40 patients [55]. In that study, HbA1c was decreased by 0.22% in favor of bitter melon, a difference that is not significant. No significant effects were observed in FBG, total cholesterol and body weight under treatment with bitter melon. Thus, the clinical application of bitter melon needs more evidence from clinical trials.

In summary, bitter melon has some activities in the regulation of glucose and lipid metabolism (Figure 16.3), which were tested in animals and patients. Antioxidant and protection of β-cells are considered the major mechanisms of bitter melon in the treatment of diabetes. Additionally, bitter melon may also act through inhibition of glucose absorption and enhancement of glucose disposal. However, the clinical outcomes of bitter melon on diabetes are controversial. The therapeutic efficacy of bitter melon needs to be evaluated in clinical trials with larger sample size.

16.2.2.4   Tea

Tea is one of the most popular beverages in the world. The earliest legend about tea originates from Shennong, the mythical emperor of China who invented agriculture and Chinese medicine. Tea, including green, black, and oolong tea, is prepared from the leaves of *Camelia sinensis,* which is native to the area that includes the northern part of Burma and southwest China; it now has been cultivated in half the world. The major bioactive component of tea is catechins, which are

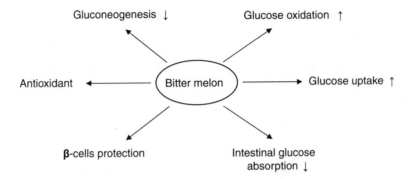

FIGURE 16.3 Mechanism of bitter melon in reduction of blood glucose. Antioxidant and β-cells protection are considered the major mechanisms of bitter melon action in the treatment of diabetes. Additionally, bitter melon is able to inhibit glucose absorption in intestine, reduce hepatic gluconeogenesis, and increase glucose uptake, glucose oxidation, and hepatic glycogen content.

polyphenolic antioxidant plant metabolites. Green and white teas have much more catechins (30%) than black tea has (10%) because fermentation reduces the polyphenols in black or oolong tea. Among the catechins, epigallocatechin gallate (EGCG) is the most abundant in tea and represents the bioactive component of tea in many studies.

Tea has been reported to have anti-aging, anticancer, antidiabetic, anti-obesity, anti-inflammatory, and anticardiovascular disease effects [56–60]. In a randomized controlled clinical trial with 60 patients of glucose abnormalities, 544 mg polyphenols (456 mg catechins) administration daily for 2 months reduced HbA1c and diastolic blood pressure significantly [61]. In the rat model of insulin resistance induced by fructose, green tea restored metabolic disorders such as hyperglycemia, hyperinsulinemia, and hypertension [62].

Tea polyphenols were reported to have beneficial effects on obesity and dyslipidemia. In a randomized triple-crossover clinical trial, nine male subjects with mild or borderline hypertriglycerolaemia were chosen to test the effects of tea catechins. The results demonstrated that tea catechins attenuated the postprandial increase in plasma triglycerol levels following a fat load [63]. In a randomized double blind, placebo-controlled, cross-over pilot study with six overweight men, EGCG showed the potential effect on increasing fat oxidation [64]. In another study using metabolic chamber, green tea extract was shown to have thermogenic properties and promote fat oxidation beyond the effect by its caffeine content alone. The study indicated that the sympathetic nerve system is involved in stimulation of thermogenesis and this activity is increased by a synergistic interaction between catechins and caffeine [65,66]. In animal experiments, EGCG injection reduced body weight, food intake, lipid absorption, plasma triglycerides, cholesterol, leptin and insulin levels [67].

In summary, tea and its bioactive component catechins or EGCG have potential effects on reduction of blood glucose and lipids. It may increase insulin sensitivity and attenuate diet-induced obesity through inhibition of energy intake and increase in fat oxidation. Tea is a healthy beverage with beneficial effects on metabolism.

16.3 CONCLUSION

Traditional Chinese Medicine is an excellent system in complementary and alternative medicine. It holds great and unique potential in the management of insulin resistance and metabolic syndrome, especially in the control of glucose and lipid metabolism. It also holds potential in the treatment of diabetic complications. The metabolic activities of many Chinese herbal medicines have been proven in well-designed animal experiments. The mechanisms of action remain to be investigated for these herbs, as large-scale clinical trials have not been conducted for these herbal medicines.

REFERENCES.

1. Himsworth H: Diabetes Mellitus: Its differentiation into insulin-sensitive and insulin-insensitive types *Lancet* 1:127–130, 1936.
2. Kraegen EW, James DE, Jenkins AB, Chisholm DJ: Dose–response curves for in vivo insulin sensitivity in individual tissues in rats. *Am J Physiol* 248:E353–362, 1985.
3. Bruning JC, Michael MD, Winnay JN, Hayashi T, Horsch D, Accili D, Goodyear LJ, Kahn CR: A muscle-specific insulin receptor knockout exhibits features of the metabolic syndrome of NIDDM without altering glucose tolerance. *Mol Cell* 2:559–569, 1998.
4. Shimomura I, Hammer RE, Ikemoto S, Brown MS, Goldstein JL: Leptin reverses insulin resistance and diabetes mellitus in mice with congenital lipodystrophy. *Nature* 401:73–76, 1999.
5. Ross R, Aru J, Freeman J, Hudson R, Janssen I: Abdominal adiposity and insulin resistance in obese men. *Am J Physiol Endocrinol Metab* 282:E657–663, 2002.
6. Gabriely I, Ma XH, Yang XM, Atzmon G, Rajala MW, Berg AH, et al.: Removal of visceral fat prevents insulin resistance and glucose intolerance of aging: an adipokine-mediated process? *Diabetes* 51:2951–2958, 2002.
7. Petersen KF, Befroy D, Dufour S, Dziura J, Ariyan C, Rothman DL, et al.: Mitochondrial dysfunction in the elderly: possible role in insulin resistance. *Science* 300:1140–1142, 2003.
8. Lowell BB, Shulman GI: Mitochondrial Dysfunction and Type 2 Diabetes. *Science* 307:384–387, 2005.
9. Reznick RM, Zong H, Li J, Morino K, Moore IK, Yu HJ, Liu ZX, et al.: Aging-associated reductions in AMP-activated protein kinase activity and mitochondrial biogenesis. *Cell Metab* 5:151–156, 2007.
10. Houstis N, Rosen ED, Lander ES: Reactive oxygen species have a causal role in multiple forms of insulin resistance. *Nature* 440:944–948, 2006.
11. Petersen KF, Dufour S, Befroy D, Garcia R, Shulman GI: Impaired mitochondrial activity in the insulin-resistant offspring of patients with type 2 diabetes. *N Engl J Med* 350:664–671, 2004.
12. Weyer C, Funahashi T, Tanaka S, Hotta K, Matsuzawa Y, Pratley RE, Tataranni PA: Hypoadiponectinemia in Obesity and Type 2 Diabetes: Close association with insulin resistance and hyperinsulinemia. *J Clin Endocrinol Metab* 86:1930–1935, 2001.
13. Vozarova B, Stefan N, Hanson R, Lindsay RS, Bogardus C, Tataranni PA, et al.: Plasma concentrations of macrophage migration inhibitory factor are elevated in Pima Indians compared to Caucasians and are associated with insulin resistance. *Diabetologia* 45:1739–1741, 2002.
14. Wang B: *Huangdi Neijing*. 1 ed. Beijing, Ancient Books of Traditional Chinese Medicine Press, 2003.
15. Tang X: Basic theories of traditional Chinese medicine. 1 ed. Shanghai, Shanghai University of Traditional Chinese Medicine Press, 2006.
16. Wang QQ: Experience in clinical practice of doctrines in Huangdi Neijing: Part 1. *Zhong Xi Yi Jie He Xue Bao* 3:486–488, 2005.
17. Yao S, Liu A: Analyze the content of Xiaoke and its complications in *Neijing J Beijing U TCM* 23, 2000.
18. Li WL, Zheng HC, Bukuru J, De Kimpe N: Natural medicines used in the traditional Chinese medical system for therapy of diabetes mellitus. *J Ethnopharmacol* 92:1–21, 2004.
19. Qu R: *Herbology*. 1 ed. Shanghai, Shanghai University of Traditional Chinese Medicine Press, 2006.
20. Ren shen: In *Chinese Materia Medica dictionary*, 1 ed. School JNM, Ed. Shanghai, Shanghai Scientific & Technical Publishers, 1986, p. 29–36.
21. Vuksan V, Sievenpiper JL: Herbal remedies in the management of diabetes: Lessons learned from the study of ginseng. *Nutr Metab Cardiovasc Dis* 15:149–160, 2005.
22. Xie JT, McHendale S, Yuan CS: Ginseng and diabetes. *Am J Chin Med* 33:397–404, 2005.
23. Yun SN, Moon SJ, Ko SK, Im BO, Chung SH: Wild ginseng prevents the onset of high-fat diet induced hyperglycemia and obesity in ICR mice. *Arch Pharm Res* 27:790–796, 2004.
24. Sotaniemi EA, Haapakoski E, Rautio A: Ginseng therapy in non-insulin-dependent diabetic patients. *Diabetes Care* 18:1373–1375, 1995.
25. Vuksan V, Sung MK, Sievenpiper JL, Stavro PM, Jenkins AL, Di Buono M, et al.: Korean red ginseng (Panax ginseng) improves glucose and insulin regulation in well-controlled, type 2 diabetes: Results of a randomized, double-blind, placebo-controlled study of efficacy and safety. *Nutr Metab Cardiovasc Dis*, 2006.

26. Qureshi AA, Abuirmeileh N, Din ZZ, Ahmad Y, Burger WC, Elson CE: Suppression of cholesterogenesis and reduction of LDL cholesterol by dietary ginseng and its fractions in chicken liver. *Atherosclerosis* 48:81–94, 1983.

27. Yamamoto M, Uemura T, Nakama S, Uemiya M, Kumagai A: Serum HDL-cholesterol-increasing and fatty liver-improving actions of Panax ginseng in high cholesterol diet-fed rats with clinical effect on hyperlipidemia in man. *Am J Chin Med* 11:96–101, 1983.

28. Kim SH, Park KS: Effects of Panax ginseng extract on lipid metabolism in humans. *Pharmacol Res* 48:511–513, 2003.

29. Kimura M, Waki I, Chujo T, Kikuchi T, Hiyama C, Yamazaki K, Tanaka O: Effects of hypoglycemic components in ginseng radix on blood insulin level in alloxan diabetic mice and on insulin release from perfused rat pancreas. *J Pharmacobiodyn* 4:410–417, 1981.

30. Lee WK, Kao ST, Liu IM, Cheng JT: Increase of insulin secretion by ginsenoside Rh2 to lower plasma glucose in Wistar rats. *Exp Pharmacol Physiol* 33:27–32, 2006.

31. Waki I, Kyo H, Yasuda M, Kimura M: Effects of a hypoglycemic component of ginseng radix on insulin biosynthesis in normal and diabetic animals. *J Pharmacobiodyn* 5:547–554, 1982.

32. Yin J, Xing H, Ye J: Efficacy of berberine in patients with type 2 diabetes. *Metabolism* 57:712–717, 2008.

33. Kong W, Wei J, Abidi P, Lin M, Inaba S, Li C, et al.: Berberine is a novel cholesterol-lowering drug working through a unique mechanism distinct from statins. *Nat Med* 10:1344–1351, 2004.

34. Cicero AF, Rovati LC, Setnikar I: Eulipidemic effects of berberine administered alone or in combination with other natural cholesterol-lowering agents. A single-blind clinical investigation. *Arzneimittelforschung* 57:26–30, 2007.

35. Yin J, Chen M, Tang J, Li F, Zhou L, Yang Y, Chen J: Effects of berberine on glucose and lipid metabolism in animal experiment. *Chin J Diabetes* 12:215–218, 2004.

36. Yin J, Chen M, Yang Y, Tang J, Li F: Effects of berberine on lipid metabolism in rats. *Acta Universitatis Medicinalis Secondae Shanghai* 23:28–30, 2003.

37. Lee YS, Kim WS, Kim KH, Yoon MJ, Cho HJ, Shen Y, et al.: Berberine, a natural plant product, activates AMP-activated protein kinase with beneficial metabolic effects in diabetic and insulin-resistant states. *Diabetes* 55:2256–2264, 2006.

38. Huang C, Zhang Y, Gong Z, Sheng X, Li Z, Zhang W, Qin Y: Berberine inhibits 3T3-L1 adipocyte differentiation through the PPARgamma pathway. *Biochem Biophys Res Commun* 348:571–578, 2006.

39. Choi BH, Ahn IS, Kim YH, Park JW, Lee SY, Hyun CK, Do MS: Berberine reduces the expression of adipogenic enzymes and inflammatory molecules of 3T3-L1 adipocyte. *Exp Mol Med* 38:599–605, 2006.

40. Wang SH, Wang WJ, Wang XF, Chen W: Effect of Astragalus polysaccharides and berberine on carbohydrate metabolism and cell differentiation in 3T3-L1 adipocytes. *Zhongguo Zhong Xi Yi Jie He Za Zhi* 24:926–928, 2004.

41. Zhou LB, Chen MD, Wang X, Song HD, Yang Y, Tang JF, et al.: Effect of berberine on the differentiation of adipocyte. *Zhonghua Yi Xue Za Zhi* 83:338–340, 2003.

42. Ku gua: In *Chinese Materia Medica Dictionary*, 1 ed. School JNM, Ed. Shanghai, Shanghai Scientific & Technical Publishers, 1986, p. 1281.

43. Khanna P, Jain SC, Panagariya A, Dixit VP: Hypoglycemic activity of polypeptide-p from a plant source. *J Nat Prod* 44:648–655, 1981.

44. Miura T, Itoh C, Iwamoto N, Kato M, Kawai M, Park SR, Suzuki I: Hypoglycemic activity of the fruit of the *Momordica charantia* in type 2 diabetic mice. *J Nutr Sci Vitaminol (Tokyo)* 47:340–344, 2001.

45. Miura T, Itoh Y, Iwamoto N, Kato M, Ishida T: Suppressive activity of the fruit of *Momordica charantia* with exercise on blood glucose in type 2 diabetic mice. *Biol Pharm Bull* 27:248–250, 2004.

46. Srivastava Y, Venkatakrishna-Bhatt H, Verma Y: Effect of *Momordica charantia Linn.* pomous aqueous extract on cataractogenesis in murrin alloxan diabetics. *Pharmacol Res Commun* 20:201–209, 1988.

47. Chaturvedi P, George S, Milinganyo M, Tripathi YB: Effect of *Momordica charantia* on lipid profile and oral glucose tolerance in diabetic rats. *Phytother Res* 18:954–956, 2004.

48. Fernandes NP, Lagishetty CV, Panda VS, Naik SR: An experimental evaluation of the antidiabetic and antilipidemic properties of a standardized *Momordica charantia* fruit extract. *BMC Complement Altern Med* 7:29, 2007.

49. Abd El Sattar El Batran S, El–Gengaihi SE, El Shabrawy OA: Some toxicological studies of *Momordica charantia* L. on albino rats in normal and alloxan diabetic rats. *J Ethnopharmacol* 108:236–242, 2006.

50. Ahmed I, Lakhani MS, Gillett M, John A, Raza H: Hypotriglyceridemic and hypocholesterolemic effects of anti-diabetic *Momordica charantia* (karela) fruit extract in streptozotocin-induced diabetic rats. *Diabetes Res Clin Pract* 51:155–161, 2001.

51. Chaturvedi P: Role of *Momordica charantia* in maintaining the normal levels of lipids and glucose in diabetic rats fed a high-fat and low-carbohydrate diet. *Br J Biomed Sci* 62:124–126, 2005.

52. Ahmad N, Hassan MR, Halder H, Bennoor KS: Effect of *Momordica charantia* (Karolla) extracts on fasting and postprandial serum glucose levels in NIDDM patients. *Bangladesh Med Res Counc Bull* 25:11–13, 1999.

53. Welihinda J, Karunanayake EH, Sheriff MH, Jayasinghe KS: Effect of *Momordica charantia* on the glucose tolerance in maturity onset diabetes. *J Ethnopharmacol* 17:277–282, 1986.

54. Tongia A, Tongia SK, Dave M: Phytochemical determination and extraction of *Momordica charantia* fruit and its hypoglycemic potentiation of oral hypoglycemic drugs in diabetes mellitus (NIDDM). *Indian J Physiol Pharmacol* 48:241–244, 2004.

55. Dans AM, Villarruz MV, Jimeno CA, Javelosa MA, Chua J, Bautista R, Velez GG: The effect of *Momordica charantia* capsule preparation on glycemic control in type 2 diabetes mellitus needs further studies. *J Clin Epidemiol* 60:554–559, 2007.

56. Wolfram S: Effects of green tea and EGCG on cardiovascular and metabolic health. *J Am Coll Nutr* 26:373S–388S, 2007.

57. Chen L, Zhang HY: Cancer preventive mechanisms of the green tea polyphenol (–)-epigallocatechin-3-gallate. *Molecules* 12:946–957, 2007.

58. Basu A, Lucas EA: Mechanisms and effects of green tea on cardiovascular health. *Nutr Rev* 65:361–375, 2007.

59. Ross SM: Green tea chings: on health, longevity, and a cup of humanity. *Holist Nurs Pract* 21:280–282, 2007.

60. Tipoe GL, Leung TM, Hung MW, Fung ML: Green tea polyphenols as an anti-oxidant and anti-inflammatory agent for cardiovascular protection. *Cardiovasc Hematol Disord Drug Targets* 7:135–144, 2007.

61. Fukino Y, Ikeda A, Maruyama K, Aoki N, Okubo T, Iso H: Randomized controlled trial for an effect of green tea-extract powder supplementation on glucose abnormalities. *Eur J Clin Nutr*, 2007.

62. Wu LY, Juan CC, Hwang LS, Hsu YP, Ho PH, Ho LT: Green tea supplementation ameliorates insulin resistance and increases glucose transporter IV content in a fructose-fed rat model. *Eur J Nutr* 43:116–124, 2004.

63. Unno T, Tago M, Suzuki Y, Nozawa A, Sagesaka YM, Kakuda T, et al: Effect of tea catechins on postprandial plasma lipid responses in human subjects. *Br J Nutr* 93:543–547, 2005.

64. Boschmann M, Thielecke F: The effects of epigallocatechin-3-gallate on thermogenesis and fat oxidation in obese men: a pilot study. *J Am Coll Nutr* 26:389S–395S, 2007.

65. Dulloo AG, Seydoux J, Girardier L, Chantre P, Vandermander J: Green tea and thermogenesis: Interactions between catechin-polyphenols, caffeine and sympathetic activity. *Int J Obes Relat Metab Disord* 24:252–258, 2000.

66. Dulloo AG, Duret C, Rohrer D, Girardier L, Mensi N, Fathi M, et al.: Efficacy of a green tea extract rich in catechin polyphenols and caffeine in increasing 24-h energy expenditure and fat oxidation in humans. *Am J Clin Nutr* 70:1040–1045, 1999.

67. Kao YH, Hiipakka RA, Liao S: Modulation of endocrine systems and food intake by green tea epigallocatechin gallate. *Endocrinology* 141:980–987, 2000.

68. Okyar A, Can A, Akev N, Baktir G, Sutlupinar N: Effect of aloe vera leaves on blood glucose level in type I and type II diabetic rat models. *Phytother Res* 15:157–161, 2001.

69. Rajasekaran S, Sivagnanam K, Subramanian S: Modulatory effects of Aloe vera leaf gel extract on oxidative stress in rats treated with streptozotocin. *J Pharm Pharmacol* 57:241–246, 2005.

70. Rajasekaran S, Ravi K, Sivagnanam K, Subramanian S: Beneficial effects of aloe vera leaf gel extract on lipid profile status in rats with streptozotocin diabetes. *Clin Exp Pharmacol Physiol* 33:232–237, 2006.

71. Kannappan S, Jayaraman T, Rajasekar P, Ravichandran MK, Anuradha CV: Cinnamon bark extract improves glucose metabolism and lipid profile in the fructose-fed rat. *Singapore Med J* 47:858–863, 2006.

72. Mang B, Wolters M, Schmitt B, Kelb K, Lichtinghagen R, Stichtenoth DO, Hahn A: Effects of a cinnamon extract on plasma glucose, HbA, and serum lipids in diabetes mellitus type 2. *Eur J Clin Invest* 36:340–344, 2006.

73. Kim SH, Hyun SH, Choung SY: Anti-diabetic effect of cinnamon extract on blood glucose in db/db mice. *J Ethnopharmacol* 104:119–123, 2006.
74. Qin B, Nagasaki M, Ren M, Bajotto G, Oshida Y, Sato Y: Cinnamon extract prevents the insulin resistance induced by a high-fructose diet. *Horm Metab Res* 36:119–125, 2004.
75. Qin B, Nagasaki M, Ren M, Bajotto G, Oshida Y, Sato Y: Cinnamon extract (traditional herb) potentiates in vivo insulin-regulated glucose utilization via enhancing insulin signaling in rats. *Diabetes Res Clin Pract* 62:139–148, 2003.
76. Shanthi S, Parasakthy K, Deepalakshmi PD, Devaraj SN: Hypolipidemic activity of tincture of Crataegus in rats. *Indian J Biochem Biophys* 31:143–146, 1994.
77. Jouad H, Lemhadri A, Maghrani M, Burcelin R, Eddouks M: Hawthorn evokes a potent anti-hyperglycemic capacity in streptozotocin-induced diabetic rats. *J Herb Pharmacother* 3:19–29, 2003.
78. Jayaprakasam B, Olson LK, Schutzki RE, Tai MH, Nair MG: Amelioration of obesity and glucose intolerance in high-fat-fed C57BL/6 mice by anthocyanins and ursolic acid in Cornelian cherry (*Cornus mas*). *J Agric Food Chem* 54:243–248, 2006.
79. Qian DS, Zhu YF, Zhu Q: Effect of alcohol extract of *Cornus officinalis Sieb*. et Zucc on GLUT4 expression in skeletal muscle in type 2 (non-insulin-dependent) diabetic mellitus rats. *Zhongguo Zhong Yao Za Zhi* 26:859–862, 2001.
80. Hsu JH, Wu YC, Liu IM, Cheng JT: Release of acetylcholine to raise insulin secretion in Wistar rats by oleanolic acid, one of the active principles contained in *Cornus officinalis*. *Neurosci Lett* 404:112–116, 2006.
81. Hao Z, Hang B, Wang Y: Hypoglycemic effect of *fructus Ligustri Lucidi*. *Zhongguo Zhong Yao Za Zhi* 17:429–431, 447, 1992.
82. Li XM: Protective effect of Lycium barbarum polysaccharides on streptozotocin-induced oxidative stress in rats. *Int J Biol Macromol* 40:461–465, 2007.
83. Luo Q, Cai Y, Yan J, Sun M, Corke H: Hypoglycemic and hypolipidemic effects and antioxidant activity of fruit extracts from *Lycium barbarum*. *Life Sci* 76:137–149, 2004.
84. Xu M, Zhang H, Wang Y: The protective effects of Lycium barbarum polysaccharide on alloxan–induced isolated islet cells damage in rats. *Zhong Yao Cai* 25:649–651, 2002.
85. Chen WQ, Luo SH, Ll HZ, Yang H: Effects of ganoderma lucidum polysaccharides on serum lipids and lipoperoxidation in experimental hyperlipidemic rats. *Zhongguo Zhong Yao Za Zhi* 30:1358–1360, 2005.
86. Berger A, Rein D, Kratky E, Monnard I, Hajjaj H, Meirim I, et al.: Cholesterol-lowering properties of *Ganoderma lucidum* in vitro, ex vivo, and in hamsters and minipigs. *Lipids Health Dis* 3:2, 2004.
87. Zhang HN, He JH, Yuan L, Lin ZB: In vitro and in vivo protective effect of *Ganoderma lucidum* polysaccharides on alloxan-induced pancreatic islets damage. *Life Sci* 73:2307–2319, 2003.
88. He CY, Li WD, Guo SX, Lin SQ, Lin ZB: Effect of polysaccharides from *Ganoderma lucidum* on streptozotocin-induced diabetic nephropathy in mice. *J Asian Nat Prod Res* 8:705–711, 2006.
89. Zhang HN, Lin ZB: Hypoglycemic effect of *Ganoderma lucidum* polysaccharides. *Acta Pharmacol Sin* 25:191–195, 2004.
90. Hikino H, Ishiyama M, Suzuki Y, Konno C: Mechanisms of hypoglycemic activity of ganoderan B: a glycan of *Ganoderma lucidum* fruit bodies. *Planta Med* 55:423–428, 1989.
91. Al-Amin ZM, Thomson M, Al-Qattan KK, PeltonenShalaby R, Ali M: Anti-diabetic and hypolipidaemic properties of ginger (*Zingiber officinale*) in streptozotocin-induced diabetic rats. *Br J Nutr* 96:660–666, 2006.
92. Akhani SP, Vishwakarma SL, Goyal RK: Anti-diabetic activity of *Zingiber officinale* in streptozotocin-induced type I diabetic rats. *J Pharm Pharmacol* 56:101–105, 2004.
93. Ojewole JA: Analgesic, antiinflammatory and hypoglycaemic effects of ethanol extract of *Zingiber officinale* (Roscoe) rhizomes (Zingiberaceae) in mice and rats. *Phytother Res* 20:764–772, 2006.
94. Bhandari U, Kanojia R, Pillai KK: Effect of ethanolic extract of *Zingiber officinale* on dyslipidaemia in diabetic rats. *J Ethnopharmacol* 97:227–230, 2005.
95. Kadnur SV, Goyal RK: Beneficial effects of *Zingiber officinale Roscoe* on fructose induced hyperlipidemia and hyperinsulinemia in rats. *Indian J Exp Biol* 43:1161–1164, 2005.
96. Fuhrman B, Rosenblat M, Hayek T, Coleman R, Aviram M: Ginger extract consumption reduces plasma cholesterol, inhibits LDL oxidation and attenuates development of atherosclerosis in atherosclerotic, apolipoprotein E–deficient mice. *J Nutr* 130:1124–1131, 2000.
97. Liu N, Huo G, Zhang L, Zhang X: Effect of *Zingiber Officinale Roscoe* on lipid peroxidation in hyperlipidemia rats. *Wei Sheng Yan Jiu* 32:22–23, 2003.

98. Bhandari U, Sharma JN, Zafar R: The protective action of ethanolic ginger (*Zingiber officinale*) extract in cholesterol fed rabbits. *J Ethnopharmacol* 61:167–171, 1998.
99. Mae T, Kishida H, Nishiyama T, Tsukagawa M, Konishi E, Kuroda M, et al.: A licorice ethanolic extract with peroxisome proliferator-activated receptor-gamma ligand-binding activity affects diabetes in KK-Ay mice, abdominal obesity in diet-induced obese C57BL mice and hypertension in spontaneously hypertensive rats. *J Nutr* 133:3369–3377, 2003.
100. Aoki F, Honda S, Kishida H, Kitano M, Arai N, Tanaka H, et al.: Suppression by licorice flavonoids of abdominal fat accumulation and body weight gain in high-fat diet-induced obese C57BL/6J mice. *Biosci Biotechnol Biochem* 71:206–214, 2007.
101. Nakagawa K, Kishida H, Arai N, Nishiyama T, Mae T: Licorice flavonoids suppress abdominal fat accumulation and increase in blood glucose level in obese diabetic KK-A(y) mice. *Biol Pharm Bull* 27:1775–1778, 2004.
102. Ji W, Gong BQ: Hypolipidemic effects and mechanisms of *Panax notoginseng* on lipid profile in hyperlipidemic rats. *J Ethnopharmacol* 113:318–324, 2007.
103. Cicero AF, Vitale G, Savino G, Arletti R: *Panax notoginseng* (*Burk.*) effects on fibrinogen and lipid plasma level in rats fed on a high-fat diet. *Phytother Res* 17:174–178, 2003.
104. Gong YH, Jiang JX, Li Z, Zhu LH, Zhang ZZ: Hypoglycemic effect of sanchinoside C1 in alloxan-diabetic mice. *Yao Xue Xue Bao* 26:81–85, 1991.
105. Wen C, Xu H, Huang QF: Effect of drugs for promoting blood circulation on blood lipids and inflammatory reaction of atherosclerotic plaques in ApoE gene deficiency mice. *Zhongguo Zhong Xi Yi Jie He Za Zhi* 25:345–349, 2005.
106. Han LK, Zheng YN, Xu BJ, Okuda H, Kimura Y: Saponins from platycodi radix ameliorate high fat diet-induced obesity in mice. *J Nutr* 132:2241–2245, 2002.
107. Han LK, Xu BJ, Kimura Y, Zheng Y, Okuda H: Platycodi radix affects lipid metabolism in mice with high fat diet-induced obesity. *J Nutr* 130:2760–2764, 2000.
108. Zhao HL, Sim JS, Shim SH, Ha YW, Kang SS, Kim YS: Antiobese and hypolipidemic effects of platycodin saponins in diet-induced obese rats: Evidences for lipase inhibition and calorie intake restriction. *Int J Obes (Lond)* 29:983–990, 2005.
109. Choi H, Eo H, Park K, Jin M, Park EJ, Kim SH, et al.: A water-soluble extract from *Cucurbita moschata* shows anti-obesity effects by controlling lipid metabolism in a high fat diet–induced obesity mouse model. *Biochem Biophys Res Commun* 359:419–425, 2007.
110. Quanhong L, Caili F, Yukui R, Guanghui H, Tongyi C: Effects of protein-bound polysaccharide isolated from pumpkin on insulin in diabetic rats. *Plant Foods Hum Nutr* 60:13–16, 2005.
111. Xie JT, Wang CZ, Wang AB, Wu J, Basila D, Yuan CS: Antihyperglycemic effects of total ginsenosides from leaves and stem of *Panax ginseng*. *Acta Pharmacol Sin* 26:1104–1110, 2005.
112. Lu J, Zou D, Zhang J: Preventive effect of radix Astragali on insulin resistance caused by tumor necrosis factor-alpha. *Zhongguo Zhong Xi Yi Jie He Za Zhi* 19:420–422, 1999.
113. Li RJ, Qiu SD, Chen HX, Tian H, Wang HX: The immunotherapeutic effects of *Astragalus* polysaccharide in type 1 diabetic mice. *Biol Pharm Bull* 30:470–476, 2007.
114. Wu Y, Cao Y, Shi X, Shi Y: Inhibitory effect of radix et rhizoma Rhei on the production of lipid peroxides (LPO) in mice liver. *Zhongguo Zhong Yao Za Zhi* 21:240–242 inside backcover, 1996.
115. Choi SB, Ko BS, Park SK, Jang JS, Park S: Insulin sensitizing and alpha-glucoamylase inhibitory action of sennosides, rheins and rhaponticin in Rhei Rhizoma. *Life Sci* 78:934–942, 2006.
116. Zhang SP, Fang WJ, Lu JH, Tan HR, Pan JQ: The experimental study of Radix Puerariae inhibiting glycation in rats induced by D-galactose. *Zhong Yao Cai* 29:266–269, 2006.
117. Kang KA, Chae S, Koh YS, Kim JS, Lee JH, You HJ, Hyun JW: Protective effect of puerariae radix on oxidative stress induced by hydrogen peroxide and streptozotocin. *Biol Pharm Bull* 28:1154–1160, 2005.
118. Xiong FL, Sun XH, Gan L, Yang XL, Xu HB: Puerarin protects rat pancreatic islets from damage by hydrogen peroxide. *Eur J Pharmacol* 529:1–7, 2006.
119. Song CY, Bi HM: Effects of puerarin on plasma membrane GLUT4 content in skeletal muscle from insulin-resistant Sprague-Dawley rats under insulin stimulation. *Zhongguo Zhong Yao Za Zhi* 29:172–175, 2004.
120. Chen WC, Hayakawa S, Yamamoto T, Su HC, Liu IM, Cheng JT: Mediation of beta-endorphin by the isoflavone puerarin to lower plasma glucose in streptozotocin-induced diabetic rats. *Planta Med* 70:113–116, 2004.

121. Hsu FL, Liu IM, Kuo DH, Chen WC, Su HC, Cheng JT: Antihyperglycemic effect of puerarin in streptozotocin-induced diabetic rats. *J Nat Prod* 66:788–792, 2003.
122. Wang JF, Guo YX, Niu JZ, Liu J, Wang LQ, Li PH: Effects of Radix Puerariae flavones on liver lipid metabolism in ovariectomized rats. *World J Gastroenterol* 10:1967–1970, 2004.
123. Yokozawa T, Kim HY, Yamabe N: Amelioration of diabetic nephropathy by dried Rehmanniae Radix (Di Huang) extract. *Am J Chin Med* 32:829–839, 2004.
124. Kuang P, Tao Y, Tian Y: Radix Salviae miltiorrhizae treatment results in decreased lipid peroxidation in reperfusion injury. *J Tradit Chin Med* 16:138–142, 1996.
125. Li S, Wan L: Experimental study on the preventive mechanism of salviae miltiorrhizae against atherosclerosis in rabbits models. *J Huazhong Univ Sci Technolog Med Sci* 24:233–235, 2004.
126. Miura T, Kato A: The difference in hypoglycemic action between polygonati rhizoma and polygonati officinalis rhizoma. *Biol Pharm Bull* 18:1605–1606, 1995.
127. Miura T, Kato A, Usami M, Kadowaki S, Seino Y: Effect of polygonati rhizoma on blood glucose and facilitative glucose transporter isoform 2 (GLUT2) mRNA expression in Wistar fatty rats. *Biol Pharm Bull* 18:624–625, 1995.
128. Kato A, Miura T, Yano H, Masuda K, Ishida H, Seino Y: Suppressive effects of polygonati rhizoma on hepatic glucose output, GLUT2 mRNA expression and its protein content in rat liver. *Endocr J* 41:139–144, 1994.
129. Kato A, Miura T: Hypoglycemic activity of polygonati rhizoma in normal and diabetic mice. *Biol Pharm Bull* 16:1118–1120, 1993.
130. Chen H, Feng R, Guo Y, Sun L, Jiang J: Hypoglycemic effects of aqueous extract of *Rhizoma Polygonati Odorati* in mice and rats. *J Ethnopharmacol* 74:225–229, 2001.
131. Choi SB, Park S: A steroidal glycoside from *Polygonatum odoratum* (Mill.) *Druce.* improves insulin resistance but does not alter insulin secretion in 90% pancreatectomized rats. *Biosci Biotechnol Biochem* 66:2036–2043, 2002.
132. Han LK, Sumiyoshi M, Zhang J, Liu MX, Zhang XF, Zheng YN, Okuda H, Kimura Y: Anti-obesity action of *Salix matsudana* leaves (Part 1). Anti-obesity action by polyphenols of *Salix matsudana* in high fat-diet treated rodent animals. *Phytother Res* 17:1188–1194, 2003.
133. Han LK, Sumiyoshi M, Zheng YN, Okuda H, Kimura Y: Anti-obesity action of *Salix matsudana* leaves (Part 2). Isolation of anti-obesity effectors from polyphenol fractions of *Salix matsudana*. *Phytother Res* 17:1195–1198, 2003.
134. Li HB, Fang KY, Lu CT, Li XE: Study on lipid-regulating function for the extracts and their prescriptions from Semen Cassiae and fructus crataegi. *Zhong Yao Cai* 30:573–575, 2007.
135. Junbao Y, Long J, Jiangbi W, Yonghui D, Tianzhen Z, Songyi Q, Wei L: Inhibitive effect of Semen Cassiae on the weight gain in rats with nutritive obesity. *Zhong Yao Cai* 27:281–284, 2004.
136. Bryans JA, Judd PA, Ellis PR: The effect of consuming instant black tea on postprandial plasma glucose and insulin concentrations in healthy humans. *J Am Coll Nutr* 26:471–477, 2007.
137. Khan SA, Priyamvada S, Arivarasu NA, Khan S, Yusufi AN: Influence of green tea on enzymes of carbohydrate metabolism, antioxidant defense, and plasma membrane in rat tissues. *Nutrition* 23:687–695, 2007.
138. Islam MS, Choi H: Green tea, anti-diabetic or diabetogenic: A dose response study. *Biofactors* 29:45–53, 2007.
139. Zhou X, Wang D, Sun P, Bucheli P, Li L, Hou Y, Wang J: Effects of soluble tea polysaccharides on hyperglycemia in alloxan-diabetic mice. *J Agric Food Chem* 55:5523–5528, 2007.
140. Anandh Babu PV, Sabitha KE, Shyamaladevi CS: Green tea extract impedes dyslipidaemia and development of cardiac dysfunction in streptozotocin-diabetic rats. *Clin Exp Pharmacol Physiol* 33:1184–1189, 2006.
141. Shoji Y, Nakashima H: Glucose-lowering effect of powder formulation of African black tea extract in KK-A(y)/TaJcl diabetic mouse. *Arch Pharm Res* 29:786–794, 2006.
142. Babu PV, Sabitha KE, Shyamaladevi CS: Therapeutic effect of green tea extract on advanced glycation and cross-linking of collagen in the aorta of streptozotocin diabetic rats. *Clin Exp Pharmacol Physiol* 33:351–357, 2006.

143. Li RW, Douglas TD, Maiyoh GK, Adeli K, Theriault AG: Green tea leaf extract improves lipid and glucose homeostasis in a fructose-fed insulin-resistant hamster model. *J Ethnopharmacol* 104:24–31, 2006.
144. Shimada K, Kawarabayashi T, Tanaka A, Fukuda D, Nakamura Y, Yoshiyama M, et al.: Oolong tea increases plasma adiponectin levels and low-density lipoprotein particle size in patients with coronary artery disease. *Diabetes Res Clin Pract* 65:227–234, 2004.

17 Nutritional Antioxidants and Prevention of Cataract

William G. Christen

CONTENTS

17.1 INTRODUCTION

Cataract is a clouding of the lens of the eye that leads to visual impairment and, in some cases, blindness. It is an important public health problem with a number of contributing factors, although the large majority of cataracts are believed to be due to increasing age. Approximately 20.5 million Americans aged 40 years and older show some evidence of age-related cataract [1–3]. Cataracts severe enough to impair vision are estimated to affect 5% of persons aged 65 years and about 50% of persons aged 75 years and older [2,4]. Of added concern, the prevalence of cataract is expected to increase by 50% as the number of elderly persons in the United States increases over the next two decades. Although treatment for cataract is readily available in the form of cataract surgery, this procedure accounts for a large portion of Medicare expenditures [5].

Nutrition is suspected to be one of the factors that play an important role in cataract development and, over the past two decades, a number of epidemiologic studies have examined whether the occurrence of cataract can be related to dietary or plasma levels of a range of nutrients. Because oxidative damage is a prominent feature of age-related cataracts [6–8], a particular focus of these studies has been on nutrients with antioxidant potential, most commonly vitamin C, vitamin E, and beta-carotene. More recent studies have focused on the xanthophyll carotenoids lutein and zeaxanthin, which may also exert antioxidant activity.

This chapter will briefly review the basic science evidence and the evidence from observational studies in humans supporting a possible beneficial effect for antioxidant nutrients in reducing risks of cataract, and will present the findings from completed randomized trials testing antioxidant supplements in cataract prevention.

17.1.1   BASIC SCIENCE AND ANIMAL RESEARCH

Basic science and animal research studies have provided plausible biologic mechanisms by which vitamins with antioxidant properties may exert a protective effect on the human lens. Reactive species of oxygen, generated through photo-oxidation and normal metabolic processes, can damage crystallin proteins and lipids in the lens, disrupt lens fiber membranes, and reduce the functional capabilities of endogenous proteolytic enzymes [9,10]. Supplementation studies in animals further support a possible protective role for antioxidant nutrients in cataract formation. *In vivo* and *in vitro* studies in several animal species have shown that supplementation with antioxidant vitamins, primarily vitamin C [11] or E [12], can prevent or delay cataract development under various conditions of elevated oxidative stress. Antioxidants have also been shown to protect lens proteases, important for the elimination of damaged protein from the lens, from photo-oxidative destruction [13].

17.1.2   OBSERVATIONAL EPIDEMIOLOGIC STUDIES

In observational epidemiologic studies (eg. cross-sectional, case-control, prospective cohort), the investigator merely notes who is exposed to a factor of interest and who is not exposed, and who develops a disease of interest and who remains disease free. Therefore, nutrient status in observational studies reflects the dietary choices made by study participants, and is not influenced in any way by study investigators.

17.1.2.1   Cross-Sectional and Case-Control Studies

Evidence from cross-sectional and case-control studies generally supports a possible beneficial effect for antioxidant nutrients in delaying cataract onset and progression. Most cross-sectional and case-control studies indicate lower risks of at least one cataract type (nuclear, cortical, or posterior subcapsular) for individuals who have high dietary intake or plasma levels of one or more antioxidant nutrients, in particular vitamins C and E [14–42]. However, interpretation of findings from cross-sectional and case-control studies is complicated by inherent limitations of the study design. For example, in cross-sectional studies, information on nutrient status and disease presence or absence is obtained at the same point in time. Therefore, the temporal relationship between nutrient level and cataract occurrence is not possible to address in cross-sectional studies. The temporal relationship between exposure and disease can also be difficult to assess in case-control studies. In addition, case-control studies often must address the possibility of recall bias, which can be difficult to exclude as an alternative explanation for study findings.

17.1.2.2   Prospective Studies

Prospective cohort studies (and case-control studies nested within a prospective cohort) are considered more reliable than cross-sectional and case-control studies because nutrient status, as well as information on other risk factors, is determined before disease occurs. As a result, prospective studies are better able to address the temporal relationship between exposure and disease and thereby provide stronger evidence of a cause–effect relationship. Moreover, because disease has not yet occurred when nutrient status is assessed, recall bias is not a problem in prospective studies. More than a dozen reports from prospective cohorts have examined antioxidant nutrients and cataract [43–56]. Findings of several of the larger studies are shown in Table 17.1 and will be briefly summarized here.

A possible link between higher intake of dietary and supplemental antioxidants and subsequent cataract surgery was examined in three reports from the U.S Nurses Health Study (NHS). In these reports, women provided dietary information by completing a food frequency questionnaire at study entry and at several other times during follow-up. The first report, based on data from more than 50,000 women, included 493 cataract extractions documented during 8 years of follow-up

TABLE 17.1
Prospective Studies of Antioxidants and Cataract

Study	Description	Duration (years)	Endpoint	Findings
Hankinson et al., Nurses' Health Study, 1992 [43]	50,828 female health professionals aged 45–67 yrs	8	493 cataract extractions	Vitamin C supplement use (10 yrs) RR, 0.55; 95% CI, 0.32–0.96 No association with dietary vitamin C or E No association with use of multivitamin supplements
Seddon et al., Physicians' Health Study, 1994 [49]	17,744 male physicians aged 40–82 yrs	5	370 cataracts	Multivitamin supplement use RR, 0.73; 95% CI, 0.54–0.99 No association with use of supplements of vitamin C and/or vitamin E
Leske et al., Longitudinal Study of Cataract, 1998 [50]	744 males and females aged 40 yrs and older	4.6	177 increases in nuclear opacification	Multivitamin supplement use RR, 0.69; 95% CI, 0.48–0.99 Vitamin E supplement use RR, 0.43; 95% CI, 0.19–0.99 Plasma vitamin E high vs. low quintiles: RR, 0.58; 95% CI, 0.36–0.94
Brown et al., Health Professionals Follow-up Study, 1999 [48]	36,644 male health professionals aged 45–75 yrs	8	840 cataract extractions	Dietary lutein and zeaxanthin high vs. low quintiles: RR, 0.81; 95% CI, 0.65–1.01 No association with dietary (α-carotene, (β-carotene, lycopene, or (β-cryptoxanthin
Chasan–Taber et al., Nurses' Health Study, 1999 [47]	50,461 female health professionals aged 45–71 yrs	12	1,471 cataract extractions	Dietary lutein and zeaxanthin high vs. low quintiles: RR, 0.78; 95% CI, 0.63–0.95 No association with dietary (α-carotene, (β-carotene, lycopene, or (β-cryptoxanthin
Chasan–Taber et al., Nurses' Health Study, 1999 [46]	47,152 female health professionals aged 45–71 yrs	12	1,377 cataract extractions	No association with use of multivitamin supplements No association with use of supplements of vitamin C or E
Mares–Perlman et al., Beaver Dam Eye Study, 2000 [53]	2,434 males and females aged 43–86 yrs	5	657 cataracts	Multivitamin supplement use (10 yrs) RR, 0.4; 95% CI, 0.3–0.7 Vitamin C supplement use (10 yrs) RR, 0.4; 95% CI, 0.3–0.6 Vitamin E supplement use (10 yrs) RR, 0.4; 95% CI, 0.3–0.6
Milton et al., Age-related Eye Disease Cohort, 2006 [55]	4,590 males and females aged 55–80 yrs	6.3	1,377* lens events change from baseline or cataract surgery	Multivitamin supplement use Centrum without lutein RR, 0.84; 95% CI, 0.72–0.98
Yoshida et al., Japan Public Health Center–based Prospective Study 2007 [56]	35,186 males and females aged 45–64 yrs	5	767 cataracts 297 cataract extractions	Dietary vitamin C high vs. low quintiles Males: cataract RR, 0.65; 95% CI, 0.42–0.97 cataract extraction RR, 0.70; 95% CI, 0.44–1.20 Females: cataract RR, 0.59; 95% CI, 0.43–0.89 cataract extraction RR, 0.64; 95% CI, 0.41–0.94

* Estimated from report

[43]. Total carotene intake, comparing women in the highest fifth to women in the lowest fifth, was inversely associated with the risk of cataract extraction (relative risk [RR], 0.73; 95% confidence interval [CI], 0.55 to 0.97) after adjustment for other cataract risk factors. There was no association of dietary vitamins C or E with cataract, nor was multivitamin intake associated with cataract. However, use of vitamin C supplements for 10 years or more was associated with a decreased risk of cataract surgery (RR, 0.55; 95% CI, 0.32 to 0.96). Long-term (more than 10 years) use of vitamin E supplements, on the other hand, was shown to be unrelated to the risk of cataract surgery in a second report from that population [46]. A third report examined the association of various carotenoids with cataract surgery. The report was based on 1,471 cataract extractions documented during 12 years of follow-up [47]. Women in the highest quintile of lutein and zeaxanthin intake, compared to women in the lowest quintile, had a 22% lower risk of cataract surgery (RR, 0.78; 95% CI, 0.63 to 0.95) in multivariate analysis. Other carotenoids, including α-carotene, β-carotene, lycopene, and β-cryptoxanthin, were unrelated to risk of cataract surgery.

Similar suggestive findings for lutein and zeaxanthin were reported in a prospective study of 36,644 U.S male health professionals [48]. In that study, a total of 840 cataract extractions were documented during 8 years of follow-up. Compared with men in the lowest quintile of intake, those in the highest quintile of lutein and zeaxanthin intake had a 19% lower risk of cataract surgery (RR, 0.81; 95% CI, 0.65 to 1.01) after adjusting for other cataract risk factors. As in the nurses study, however, intake levels of α-carotene, β-carotene, lycopene, and β-cryptoxanthin were not associated with risk of cataract surgery.

The relation of vitamin supplement use with new diagnoses of cataract was examined in prospective data from Physicians' Health Study I (PHS I). That report included data from 17,744 male physicians who did not report cataract at baseline. A total of 370 cases of visually significant (20/30 or worse) age-related cataract were documented during 5 years of follow-up [49]. Men who reported at baseline that they took only multivitamins, compared with those who used no supplements, had a statistically significant 27% lower risk of cataract (RR, 0.73; 95% CI, 0.54–0.99) after adjustment for other cataract risk factors. Those who reported supplemental use of vitamin C or E alone had a statistically nonsignificant 32% increased risk of cataract (RR, 1.32; 95% CI, 0.85–2.04).

In the Longitudinal Study of Cataract, 177 of 744 men and women showed an increase in the severity of lens nuclear opacities during 5 years of follow-up [50]. The risk of increased opacification was reduced by more than 50% (RR, 0.43; 95% CI, 0.19–0.99) among users of vitamin E supplements, and by 31% (RR, 0.69; 95% CI, 0.48–0.99) among users of multivitamin supplements. Consistent with the findings for vitamin E supplements, the plasma level of vitamin E was inversely associated with risk of nuclear opacification (high vs. low quintile; RR, 0.58; 95% CI, 0.36–0.94). No association was observed for vitamin C intake from diet or supplements in that study.

Prospective data from the Beaver Dam Eye Study also appear to support a possible benefit for antioxidant nutrients in cataract prevention [53]. The study population for that report consisted of 2,434 men and women who were free of cataract at baseline, and who also provided baseline information about diet and vitamin supplement use. Among that subsample, a total of 657 cataracts were documented during 5 years of follow-up. Users of multivitamins for more than 10 years were found to have a statistically significant 60% reduced risk of cataract (RR, 0.4; 95% CI, 0.3–0.7) compared with nonusers. Similar risk reductions were observed for participants who reported using supplements of vitamin C (RR, 0.4; 95% CI, 0.3–0.6) or vitamin E (RR, 0.4; 95% CI, 0.3–0.6) for more than 10 years. In analyses of cataract subtypes, using multivitamins for more than 10 years was associated with a lower risk of nuclear (RR, 0.6; 95% CI, 0.4–0.9) and cortical cataracts (RR, 0.4; 95% CI, 0.2–0.8), but not posterior subcapsular cataracts (RR, 0.9; 95% CI, 0.5–1.9).

A major study objective of the Age-Related Eye Disease Study (AREDS) was to test in a randomized trial the effect of an antioxidant combination (vitamin E, vitamin C, and beta-carotene) on cataract onset and progression in men and women (those results are described below) [57]. In addition to randomized treatment with the antioxidant combination, participants in AREDS were also offered a multivitamin/mineral supplement containing RDA-level dosages (Centrum® without lutein) in order to standardize the usage of nonstudy supplements among the study population. Two-thirds of AREDS participants (3,037 of 4,590) chose to supplement with Centrum. A prospective analysis of these observational data showed that participants who chose to use Centrum had a statistically significant 16% lower risk (RR, 0.84; 95% CI, 0.72–0.98) of any lens opacity progression, which was defined as the occurrence of change from baseline of specified amounts of nuclear, cortical, or posterior subcapsular opacity, or the performance of cataract surgery [55].

Finally, in a recent study of 16,415 men and 18,771 women in Japan, among whom 767 new diagnoses of cataract and 297 cataract extractions were reported during 5 years of follow-up, higher dietary intake of vitamin C from food sources alone (participants reporting any supplement use were excluded from the analysis) was associated with decreased risks of both cataract and cataract extraction [56]. Among men, there was a 35% decreased risk of cataract (RR, 0.65; 95% CI, 0.42–0.97) and a 30% decreased risk of cataract extraction (RR, 0.70; 95% CI, 0.44–1.20). Among women, there was a 41% decreased risk of cataract (RR, 0.59; 95% CI, 0.43–0.89) and a 36% decreased risk of cataract extraction (RR, 0.64; 95% CI, 0.41–0.94).

Taken together, the results of these large prospective cohort studies generally support a possible protective role for antioxidant nutrients in cataract. In fact, including cross-sectional and case-control studies, most observational epidemiologic studies report at least one inverse association between some measure of antioxidant status and one measure of cataract outcome. When the findings are combined across studies and examined more critically, however, it becomes apparent that the data for individual nutrients or individual disease types are very inconsistent. One possible reason for this inconsistency is the presence of chance findings. In studies of nutritional determinants of disease, there is often the opportunity to examine a large number of possible associations in the data. Particularly with cataract, the investigator may explore associations of multiple nutrients with cataract diagnosis or surgery, or with specific subtypes of cataract (eg, nuclear sclerosis, cortical, posterior subcapsular). While it is certainly plausible that nutritional determinants may be different for the various cataract subtypes, the conduct of multiple comparisons within individual studies increases the likelihood of chance findings, and probably contributes to the inconsistent results between studies. Other possible reasons for observed inconsistencies include the use of different methods of nutritional and disease assessment and differences among study populations including differences in nutritional status.

17.1.3   WHY RANDOMIZED TRIALS ARE NEEDED

A particularly important limitation of observational epidemiologic studies is uncontrolled confounding. Because study participants choose their own diets, those who ingest a greater level of antioxidant vitamins, either in the diet or through supplements, are likely to differ from those with less-favorable diets in other important ways, including life-style factors and other dietary practices that may be associated with disease occurrence. In addition, the intercorrelation of nutrients complicates the interpretation of results for individual nutrients in observational studies. Antioxidant vitamins and minerals share common food sources, and high dietary or blood levels of one antioxidant are often associated with high levels of other antioxidants. Thus, an apparent association between a specific antioxidant nutrient and disease may be confounded by other nutrients more directly related to the risk of disease development.

Observational studies can adjust for the effects of known confounders, but not for the effects of unknown or unmeasured confounders. For the small to moderate effects that are hypothesized for antioxidant vitamins, the magnitude of uncontrolled confounding in observational studies can easily be as large as the most plausible benefits or risks that might be expected. Clearly, randomized trials of sufficient size and duration are required to provide reliable data on the specific effect of individual antioxidant vitamins in cataract prevention. If these trials are large enough, randomization will tend to distribute the known and unknown confounding factors evenly among treatment groups.

17.1.4 RANDOMIZED TRIALS OF ANTIOXIDANT SUPPLEMENTS AND CATARACT

Data are available from eight completed randomized trials that examined antioxidant supplements in cataract prevention. The main findings of these trials are presented in Table 17.2 and are briefly discussed here.

The Linxian Cataract Study [58] was an ancillary study of the Chinese Cancer Prevention Study [59], which was conducted in an undernourished population in China. In the Cataract Study, end-of-trial eye examinations conducted among a subset of participants with esophageal dysplasia indicated a reduced prevalence of nuclear cataract in the subgroup of participants aged 65 to 74 years who were randomly assigned to daily treatment with vitamin/mineral supplements (comprising two Centrum tablets plus a 15 mg beta-carotene tablet) compared with those assigned to placebo (OR, 0.57; 95% CI, 0.36–0.90). There was no significant association with nuclear cataract among persons aged 45 to 64 years, nor was there any association with cortical or posterior subcapsular cataract [58].

The Alpha-Tocopherol Beta-Carotene (ATBC) cancer prevention study was the first large-scale randomized trial to test antioxidant vitamins in a well-nourished population [60]. The study population comprised 29,133 Finnish male smokers aged 50 to 69 years who were randomly assigned in a 2 x 2 factorial trial to alpha-tocopherol (50 mg daily) or placebo, and beta-carotene (20 mg daily) or placebo. There have been two reports from the ATBC study that examined the effects of randomized treatment on cataract. In one, which was based on end-of-trial examinations among a random sample of 1,828 participants, supplementation with alpha-tocopherol or beta-carotene was not associated with the end-of-trial prevalence of nuclear (RRs, 0.8 and 0.9, respectively), cortical (RRs, 0.9 and 1.2, respectively), or posterior subcapsular cataract (RRs, 0.9 and 0.7, respectively) [61]. In a second report, based on 425 cataract surgeries documented during more than 6 years of treatment and follow-up of 28,934 men in the cataract surgery population, there was a statistically nonsignificant 9% reduced risk of cataract surgery (RR, 0.91; 95% CI, 0.74-1.11) for those assigned to alpha-tocopherol, and a nonsignificant 3% reduced risk (RR, 0.97; 95% CI, 0.79-1.19) for those assigned beta-carotene [62].

The AREDS tested the effects of a daily antioxidant combination of vitamin E (400 IU), vitamin C (500 mg), and beta-carotene (15 mg) on the development and progression of lens opacities. The findings, based on 2,230 lens events (i.e., increase in opacity grade from baseline or cataract surgery), indicated no apparent benefit of the antioxidant vitamins during the 6.3 years of treatment and follow-up (RR, 0.97; 95% CI, 0.84–1.11) [57].

Physicians' Health Study I was a randomized, double-masked, placebo-controlled, 2 x 2 factorial trial designed to evaluate low-dose aspirin and beta-carotene (50 mg on alternate days) in the primary prevention of cardiovascular disease and cancer among 22,071 U.S. male physicians [63]. The findings in PHS I with respect to cataract indicated that 12 years of beta-carotene treatment, during which 2,015 cataracts were confirmed, had no effect on the overall incidence of cataract (RR, 1.00; 95% CI, 0.91–1.09) [64].

Similar null findings for beta-carotene and cataract were observed in a large trial of female health professionals. The WHS was a randomized, double-blind, placebo-controlled trial using a 2 x 2 x 2 factorial design to test the balance of benefits and risks of beta-carotene (50 mg on alternate days), vitamin E, and aspirin in the primary prevention of cancer and cardiovascular disease [65]. The beta-carotene component of the WHS was terminated early after an average of 2.1 years of treatment and follow-up, primarily because of the null findings on beta-carotene and cancer incidence after 12 years of randomized treatment in PHS I [63]. The findings for cataract in WHS, based on 262 cataracts documented during the 2.1 years of treatment and follow-up, indicated that beta-carotene treatment had no large benefit or harm (RR,0.95; 95% CI, 0.75–1.21) on risk of cataract during the treatment period [66].

The Vitamin E, Cataract, and Age-Related Macular Degeneration (VECAT) study was a small trial of 1,193 men and women who were followed for 4 years during which 142 new cataracts and

TABLE 17.2
Randomized Trials of Antioxidant Supplements and Cataract

Study	Population	Agents tested	Duration (years)	Endpoint	Findings
Chinese Cancer Prevention Trial Linxian, 1993 [58]	2,141Chinese males and females aged 45–74	vitamin/mineral supplements including vitamin E [60 IU/d], vitamin C [180 mg/d], beta-carotene [15 mg/d], or placebo	6.6	160 nuclear, 746 cortical, 45 posterior subcapsular cataracts	nuclear RR, 0.80; 95% CI, 0.57–1.12 45–64 yrs RR, 1.28; 95% CI, 0.57–1.12 65–74 yrs RR, 0.57; 95% CI, 0.36–0.90 cortical RR, 1.05; 95% CI, 0.88–1.26 posterior subcapsular RR, 1.41; 95% CI, 0.75–2.67
Alpha-tocopherol Beta-carotene ATBC Trial, 1997 [61]	1,828 Finnish male smokers aged 50–69	vitamin E 50 mg/d, beta-carotene 20 mg/d, both, or neither	6.6	222 nuclear, 386 cortical, 105 posterior subcapsular cataracts	vitamin E nuclear RR, 0.8; 95% CI, 0.4–1.4 cortical RR, 0.9; 95% CI, 0.6–1.4 posterior subcapsular RR, 0.9; 95% CI, 0.4–1.8 beta-carotene nuclear RR, 0.9; 95% CI, 0.5–1.6 cortical RR, 1.2; 95% CI, 0.8–1.9 posterior subcapsular RR, 0.7; 95% CI, 0.3–1.5
Alpha-tocopherol Beta-carotene ATBC Trial, 1998 [62]	28,934 Finnish male smokers aged 50–69	vitamin E 50 mg/d, beta-carotene 20 mg/d, both, or neither	5.7	425 cataract extractions	vitamin E RR, 0.91; 95% CI, 0.74–1.11 beta-carotene RR, 0.97; 95% CI, 0.79–1.19
Age-related Eye Disease Study AREDS, 2001 [57]	4,596 males and females aged 55–80	antioxidant combination vitamin E [400 IU/d], vitamin C [500 mg/d], beta-carotene [15 mg/d], or placebo	6.3	2,230 lens events ncrease in opacity grade or cataract surgery	RR, 0.97; 95% CI, 0.84–1.11
Physicians' Health Study I PHSI, 2002 [64]	20,968 male U.S physicians aged 40–84	beta-carotene 50 mg on alternate days, or placebo	12	2,015 cataracts	RR, 1.00; 95% CI, 0.91–1.09
Roche European American Cataract Trial REACT, 2002 [68]	297 males and females aged 40 yrs and older	antioxidant combination vitamin E [600 IU/d], vitamin C [750 mg/d], beta-carotene [18 mg/d], or placebo	3	percent increase in opacification	less progression in treated group 1.7% vs 3.3%, p = 0.048 among subset of participants n = 158 with 3 yrs follow–up
Vitamin E, Cataract, and Age-related Macular Degeneration VECAT Study, 2004 [67]	1,193 males and females aged 55–80	vitamin E 500 IU/d or placebo	4	142 cataracts and 168 progressed cataracts	Incidence RR, 1.0; 95% CI, 0.8–1.4 Progression RR, 1.0; 95% CI, 0.7–1.3

TABLE 17.2 (CONTINUED)
Randomized Trials of Antioxidant Supplements and Cataract

Study	Population	Agents tested	Duration (years)	Endpoint	Findings
Women's Health Study WHS, 2004 [66]	36,735 female health professionals aged 45 yrs and older	beta-carotene 50 mg on alternate days, or placebo	2.1	262 cataracts	RR, 0.95; 95% CI, 0.75–1.21
Antioxidants in Prevention of Cataracts APC Study, 2006 [69]	798 males and females aged 35–50 yrs	antioxidant combination vitamin E [400 IU], vitamin C [500 mg], beta-carotene [15mg] 3 times weekly, or placebo	5	cataract progression	no difference in progression rate

168 progressed cataracts were documented. There was no overall benefit of daily vitamin E (500 IU) on cataract incidence (RR, 1.0; 95% CI, 0.8–1.4) or progression (RR, 1.0; 95% CI, 0.7–1.3) in VECAT [67].

The Roche European American Cataract Trial (REACT) tested the effect of an antioxidant combination of daily vitamin E (600 IU), vitamin C (750 mg), and beta-carotene (18mg) on progression of cataract in 297 American and English male and female outpatients with early age-related cataract. Analyses restricted to a subset of participants (n = 158) followed for 3 years indicated that, compared with placebo, those assigned to antioxidant treatment experienced a small benefit (p = 0.048) on progression of cataract as quantified by image analysis [68].

Finally, the Antioxidants in Prevention of Cataracts (APC) Study was a 5-year, triple-masked, placebo-controlled trial conducted in India among 798 males and females, most of whom had significant nuclear cataract at study entry [69]. The APC tested the ability of an antioxidant combination of vitamin C (500 mg), vitamin E (400 IU), and beta-carotene (15 mg) given three times weekly to retard the progression of nuclear opalescence. Analyses indicated no effect of the antioxidant combination on progression of nuclear opalescence during the 5-year treatment period.

In summary, the available evidence from completed trials indicates that treatment with high-dose antioxidant supplements, most particularly beta-carotene [57,58,61,62,64,66,68,69] and vitamin E [57,58,61,62,67–69], but also vitamin C [57, 58, 68, 69], for 3 to 7 years (12 years for beta-carotene in PHS I) has little effect on risk of cataract in older, generally well-nourished populations.

17.1.4 OBSERVATIONAL STUDIES VERSUS RANDOMIZED TRIALS: WHY ARE THE FINDINGS DIFFERENT?

The disappointing findings from randomized trials of antioxidant supplements and cataract contrast with the generally supportive findings from observational studies. Several reasons for the discrepant findings are possible.

If antioxidant nutrients are beneficial in cataract prevention, randomized trials may not have detected the benefit because:

- **Active nutrients not yet identified or tested in trials**: Active nutrients directly responsible for slowing cataract onset and progression may not yet be identified, or if identified, not yet tested in randomized trials. For example, dietary and plasma levels of lutein and zeaxanthin tend to be correlated with levels of antioxidants such as vitamin C, vitamin E, and beta-carotene, and while accumulating observational data support an inverse association with the risk of cataract, lutein and zeaxanthin have not yet been tested in randomized trials.

- **Appropriate doses not yet tested:** Most antioxidant vitamins have been tested at phar-macological doses, well above the minimum daily allowance, which is based on the mini-mal dose required to avoid vitamin deficiency diseases. For most vitamins, however, the optimal dose for maximal health is unknown and remains to be determined. While higher doses may be required to materially affect cataract development, the balance of risks and benefits may also be altered. For example, some reports have suggested significant toxici-ties for pharmacological doses of vitamin E [70], although others have suggested that E and other nutrients are safe across a wide range of doses [71,72].
- **Appropriate durations not yet tested:** Most trials have tested treatment periods of 3 to 7 years, which may be insufficient to alter development of age-related cataract, which is a chronic disease that develops slowly over many years. It is also possible that the inverse association reported in many observational studies is the result of a duration of intake even longer than that recorded by the study, and one that encompasses age ranges representing a 'critical exposure period' (eg. 3rd and 4th decade) for influencing cataract development. If so, then randomized trials, which have tested populations in their 5th decade and older, would be required to test younger populations and follow them for an extended duration, in order to detect a treatment benefit on cataract.

On the other hand, if antioxidant nutrients are not beneficial in cataract prevention, observa-tional studies may have falsely identified a benefit because:

- **Confounding (residual confounding) by other healthy behaviors:** The beneficial effect reported in observational studies may be due instead to other healthy non-dietary behav-iors (eg., avoidance of cigarette smoking) that tend to be associated with a healthful diet.
- **Multiple comparisons and publication bias:** As discussed previously, observational stud-ies often offer the opportunity to examine a large number of possible associations in the data, which increases the likelihood of chance findings. If there is a greater likelihood for studies with positive findings to be reported and published, then the available literature will be biased. This is particularly true in observational studies of nutritional determinants of cataract where multiple comparisons are frequently made, and a significant association(s) between one or more nutrients and one or more cataract endpoint or subtypes may be pref-erentially reported and published to the exclusion of nonsignificant associations.

17.2 CONCLUSION

Randomized trials that have examined the effect of supplementation with individual antioxidant vitamins, or a combination of several vitamins, for 3 to 7 years have provided little evidence of a benefit on cataract development. On-going and recently completed trials will assess the possible benefits of longer term treatment with one or more antioxidant vitamins [73-76], and will provide the first randomized trial data on multivitamin supplementation in generally well-nourished popu-lations [74, 76]. In the meantime, it remains prudent public health policy to encourage increased intake of fruits and vegetables to lower risk for a number of chronic diseases including cataract.

REFERENCES

1. National Eye Institute. Vision Problems in the U.S: Prevalence of Adult Vision. Last accessed February 15, 2006. Available at http://www.nei.nih.gov/eyedata/tables.asp, 2004.

2. Klein, B.E., Klein. R., Linton. K.L. 1992. Prevalence of age-related lens opacities in a population. The Beaver Dam Eye Study. *Ophthalmology* 99, 546–552.

3. Sperduto, R.D., Hiller, R. 1984. The prevalence of nuclear, cortical, and posterior subcapsular lens opacities in a general population sample. *Ophthalmology* 91,815–818.

4. Leibowitz, H.M., Krueger, D.E., Maunder, L.R., Milton, R.C., Kini, M.M., Kahn, H.A., et al. 1980. The Framingham Eye Study monograph: An ophthalmological and epidemiological study of cataract, glaucoma, diabetic retinopathy, macular degeneration, and visual acuity in a general population of 2631 adults, 1973–1975. *Surv. Ophthalmol.* 24 Suppl:335–610.

5. Steinberg, E.P., Javitt, J.C., Sharkey, P.D., Zuckerman, A., Legro, M.W., Anderson, G.F., et al. 1993. The content and cost of cataract surgery. *Arch. Ophthalmol.* 111, 1041–1049.

6. Taylor, A. 1993. Cataract: Relationship between nutrition and oxidation. *J. Am. Coll. Nutr.* 12, 138–146.

7. Spector, A. 1995. Oxidative stress-induced cataract: Mechanism of action. *FASEB J.* 9, 1173–1178.

8. Truscott, R.J. 2005. Age-related nuclear cataract-oxidation is the key. *Exp. Eye. Res.* 80, 709–725.

9. Bunce, G.E., Kinoshita, J., Horwitz, J. 1990. Nutritional factors in cataract. *Ann. Rev. Nutr.* 10, 233–254.

10. Taylor, A. 1999. Nutritional and environmental influences on risk for cataract. In *Nutritional and environmental influences on vision*, A. Taylor, Ed. pp 53–93. CRC Press, Boca Raton, FL.

11. Varma, S.D., Kumar, S., Richards, R.D. 1979. Light-induced damage to ocular lens cation pump: Prevention by vitamin C. *Proc. Natl. Acad. Sci.* 76, 3504–3506.

12. Ross, W.M., Creighton, M.O., Inch, W.R., Trevithick, J.R. 1983. Radiation cataract formation diminished by vitamin E in rat lenses in vitro. *Exp. Eye. Res.* 36, 645–653.

13. Blondin, J., Baragi, V.J., Schwartz, E., Sadowski, J., Taylor, A. 1986. Delay of UV-induced eye lens protein damage in guinea pigs by dietary ascorbate. *Free Radical Biol. Med.* 2, 275–281.

14. Robertson, J. McD., Donner, A.P., Trevithick, J.R. 1989. Vitamin E intake and risk of cataracts in humans. *Ann. N.Y. Acad. Sci.* 570, 372–382.

15. The Italian-American Cataract Study Group. 1991. Risk factors for age-related cortical, nuclear, and posterior subcapsular cataracts. *Am. J. Epidemiol.* 133, 541–553.

16. Leske, M.C., Chylack, L.T., Wu, S.Y. 1991. The Lens Opacities Case-Control Study: Risk factors for cataract. *Arch. Ophthalmol.* 109, 244–251.

17. Jacques, P.F., Chylack, L.T. 1991. Epidemiologic evidence of a role for the antioxidant vitamins and carotenoids in cataract prevention. *Am. J. Clin. Nutr.* 53, 352S–355S.

18. Vitale, S., West, S., Hallfrisch, J., Alston, C., Wang, F., Moorman, C., et al. 1993. Plasma antioxidants and risk of cortical and nuclear cataract. *Epidemiology* 4, 195–203.

19. Wong, L., Ho, S.C., Coggon, D., Cruddas, A.M., Hwang, C.H., Ho, C.P., et al. 1993. Sunlight exposure, antioxidant status, and cataract in Hong Kong fisherman. *J. Epidemiol. Commun. Hlth.* 47, 46–49.

20. Mares-Perlman, J.A., Klein, B.E.K., Klein, R., Ritter, L.L. 1994. Relation between lens opacities and vitamin and mineral supplement use. *Ophthalmology* 101, 315–325.

21. Leske, M.C., Wu, S.Y., Hyman, L., Sperduto, R., Underwood, B., Chylack, L.T., et al. and Lens Opacities Case-Control Study group. 1995. Biochemical factors in the lens opacities. Case–control study. *Arch. Ophthalmol.* 113, 1113–1119.

22. Mares-Perlman, J.A., Brady, W.E., Klein, B.E., Klein, R., Haus, G.J., Palta, M., et al. 1995. Diet and nuclear lens opacities. *Am. J. Epidemiol.* 141, 322–334.

23. Mares-Perlman, J.A., Brady, W.E., Klein, B.E., Klein, R., Palta, M., Bowen, P., Stacewicz-Sapuntzakis, M. 1995. Serum carotenoids and tocopherols and severity of nuclear and cortical opacities. *Invest. Ophthalmol. Vis. Sci.* 36, 276–288.

24. Tavani, A., Negri, E., La Vecchia, C. 1996. Food and nutrient intake and risk of cataract. *Ann. Epidemiol.* 6, 41–46.

25. Jacques, P.F., Taylor, A., Hankinson, S.E., Willett, W.C., Mahnken, B., Lee, Y., et al. 1997. Long-term vitamin C supplement use and prevalence of early age-related lens opacities. *Am. J. Clin. Nutr.* 66, 911–916.

26. Leske, M.C., Wu, S.Y, Connell, A.M., Hyman, L., Schachat, A.P. 1997. Lens opacities, demographic factors and nutritional supplements in the Barbados Eye Study. *Int. J. Epidemiol.* 26, 1314–1322.

27. Delcourt, C., Cristol, J.P., Léger, C.L., Descomps, B., Papoz, L. 1999. Associations of antioxidant enzymes with cataract and age-related macular degeneration. The POLA Study. Pathologies Oculaires Liées à l'Age. *Ophthalmology* 106, 215–222.

28. Simon, J.A., Hudes, E.S. 1999. Serum ascorbic acid and other correlates of self-reported cataract among older Americans. *J. Clin. Epidemiol.* 52, 1207–1211.
29. McCarty, C.A., Mukesh, B.N., Fu, C.L., Taylor, H.R. 1999. The epidemiology of cataract in Australia. *Am. J. Ophthalmol.* 128, 446–465.
30. Nadalin, G., Robman, L.D., McCarty, C.A., Garrett, S.K., McNeil, J.J., Taylor, H.R. 1999. The role of past intake of vitamin E in early cataract changes. *Ophthalmic Epidemiol.* 6, 105–112.
31. Cumming, R.G., Mitchell, P., Smith, W. 2000. Diet and cataract: The Blue Mountains Eye Study. *Ophthalmology* 107, 450–456.
32. Gale, C.R., Hall, N.F., Phillips, D.I., Martyn, C.N. 2001. Plasma antioxidant vitamins and carotenoids and age-related cataract. *Ophthalmology* 108, 1992–1998
33. Jacques, P.F., Chylack, L.T. Jr., Hankinson, S.E., Khu, P.M., Rogers, G., Friend, J., Tung, W., Wolfe, J.K., Padhye, N., Willett, W.C., Taylor, A. 2001. Long-term nutrient intake and early age-related nuclear lens opacities. *Arch. Ophthalmol.* 119, 1009–1019.
34. Kuzniarz, M., Mitchell, P., Cumming, R.G., Flood, V.M. 2001. Use of vitamin supplements and cataract: The Blue Mountains Eye Study. *Am. J. Ophthalmol.* 132, 19–26.
35. Olmedilla, B., Granado, F., Blanco, I., Herrero, C., Vaquero, M., Millan, I. 2002. Serum status of carotenoids and tocopherols in patients with age-related cataracts: A case-control study. *J. Nutr. Health Aging* 6, 66–68.
36. Taylor, A., Jacques, P.F., Chylack, L.T. Jr., Hankinson, S.E., Khu, P.M., Rogers, G., et al. 2002. Long-term intake of vitamins and carotenoids and odds of early age-related cortical and posterior subcapsular lens opacities. *Am. J. Clin. Nutr.* 75, 540–549.
37. Valero, M.P., Fletcher, A.E., De Stavola, B.L., Vioque, J., Alepuz, V.C. 2002. Vitamin C is associated with reduced risk of cataract in a Mediterranean population. *J. Nutr.* 132, 1299–1306.
38. Ferrigno, L., Aldigeri, R., Rosmini, F., Sperduto, R.D., Maraini, G.; The Italian-American Cataract Study Group. 2005. Associations between plasma levels of vitamins and cataract in the Italian-American Clinical Trial of Nutritional Supplements and Age-related Cataract CTNS: CTNS Report #2. *Ophthalmic Epidemiol.* 12, 71–80.
39. Krepler, K., Schmid, R. 2005. Alpha-tocopherol in plasma, red blood cells and lenses with and without cataract. *Am. J. Ophthalmol.* 139, 266–270.
40. Delcourt, C., Carrière, I., Delage, M., Barberger–Gateau, P., Schalch, W.; POLA Study Group. Plasma lutein and zeaxanthin and other carotenoids as modifiable risk factors for age-related maculopathy and cataract: The POLA Study. *Invest. Ophthalmol. Vis. Sci.* 47, 2329–2335.
41. Rodríguez-Rodríguez, E., Ortega, R.M., López-Sobaler, A.M., Aparicio, A., Bermejo, L.M., Marín-Arias, L.I. 2006. The relationship between antioxidant nutrient intake and cataracts in older people. *Int. J. Vitam. Nutr. Res.* 76, 359–366.
42. Vu, H.T., Robman, L., Hodge, A., McCarty, C.A., Taylor, H.R. 2006. Lutein and zeaxanthin and the risk of cataract: The Melbourne visual impairment project. *Invest. Ophthalmol. Vis. Sci.* 47, 3783–3786.
43. Hankinson, S.E., Stampfer, M.J., Seddon, J.M., Colditz, G.A., Rosner, B., Speizer, F.E., Willett, W.C. 1992. Nutrient intake and cataract extraction in women: A prospective study. *Br. Med. J.* 305, 335–339.
44. Knekt, P., Heliovaata, M., Rissanen, A., Aromaa, A., Aaran, R-K. 1992. Serum antioxidant vitamins and risk of cataract. *Br. Med. J.* 305, 1392–1394.
45. Rouhiainen, P., Rouhiainen, H., Salonen, J.T. 1996. Association between low plasma vitamin E concentration and progression of early cortical lens opacities. *Am. J. Epidemiol.* 144, 496–500.
46. Chasan-Taber, L., Willett, W.C., Seddon, J.M., Stampfer, M.J., Rosner, B., Colditz, G.A., Hankinson, S.E. 1999. A prospective study of vitamin supplement intake and cataract extraction among U.S. women. *Epidemiology* 10, 679–684.
47. Chasan-Taber, L., Willett, W.C., Seddon, J.M., Stampfer, M.J., Rosner, B., Colditz, G.A., et al. 1999. A prospective study of carotenoid and vitamin A intakes and risk of cataract extraction in U.S. women. *Am. J. Clin. Nutr.* 70, 509–516.
48. Brown, L., Rimm, E.B., Seddon, J.M., Giovannucci, E.L., Chasan-Taber, L., Spiegelman, D., et al. 1999 A prospective study of carotenoid intake and risk of cataract extraction in U.S. men. *Am. J. Clin. Nutr.* 70, 517–524.
49. Seddon, J.M., Christen, W.G., Manson, J.E., LaMotte, F.S., Glynn, R.J., Buring, J.E., Hennekens, C.H. 1994. The use of vitamin supplements and risk of cataract among U.S. male physicians. *Am. J. Pub. Health* 84, 788–792.

50. Leske, M.C., Chylack, L.T., He, Q., Wu, S.Y., Schoenfeld, E., Friend, J., Wolfe, J., the Longitudinal Study of Cataract Group. 1998. Antioxidant vitamins and nuclear cataract: The longitudinal study of cataract. *Ophthalmology* 105, 831–836.

51. Lyle, B.J., Mares-Perlman, J.A., Klein, B.E.K., Klein, R., Palta, M., Bowen, P.E., Greger, J.L. 1999. Serum carotenoids and tocopherols and incidence of age-related nuclear cataract. *Am. J. Clin. Nutr.* 69, 272–277.

52. Lyle, B.J., Mares-Perlman, J.A., Klein, B.E.K., Klein, R., Greger, J.L. 1999. Antioxidant intake and risk of incident age-related nuclear cataracts in the Beaver Dam Eye Study. *Am. J. Epidemiol.* 149, 801–809.

53. Mares-Perlman, J.A., Lyle, B.J., Klein, R., Fisher, A.I., Brady, W.E., VandenLangenberg, G.M., et al. 2000. Vitamin supplement use and incident cataracts in a population-based study. *Arch. Ophthalmol.* 118, 1556–1563.

54. Jacques, P.F., Taylor, A., Moeller, S., Hankinson, S.E., Rogers, G., Tung, W., et al. 2005. Long-term nutrient intake and 5-year change in nuclear lens opacities. *Arch. Ophthalmol.* 123, 517–526.

55. Milton, R.C., Sperduto, R.D., Clemons, T.E., Ferris, F.L. 3rd; Age-related Eye Disease Study Research Group. 2006. Centrum use and progression of age-related cataract in the Age-related Eye Disease Study: A propensity score approach. AREDS report No. 21. *Ophthalmology* 113, 1264–1270.

56. Yoshida, M., Takashima, Y., Inoue, M., Iwasaki, M., Otani, T., Sasaki, S., Tsugane, S. JPHC Study Group. 2007. Prospective study showing that dietary vitamin C reduced the risk of age-related cataracts in a middle-aged Japanese population. *Eur. J. Nutr.* 46, 118–124.

57. Age-related Eye Disease Study Research Group. 2001. A randomized, placebo-controlled, clinical trial of high-dose supplementation with vitamins C and E and beta-carotene for age-related cataract and vision loss: AREDS report no. 9. *Arch. Ophthalmol..* 119, 1439–1452.

58. Sperduto,R.D., Hu, T.S., Milton, R.C., Zhao, J.L., Everett, D.F., Cheng, Q.F., et al. 1993. The Linxian cataract studies. Two nutrition intervention trials. *Arch. Ophthalmol.* 111, 1246–1253.

59. Blot, W.J., Li, J–Y., Taylor, P.R., Guo, W., Dawsey, S., Wang, G–Q., et al. 1993. Nutrition intervention trials in Linxian, China: Supplementation with specific vitamin/mineral combinations, cancer incidence, and disease-specific mortality in the general population. *J. Natl. Cancer. Inst.* 85, 1483–1492.

60. The Alpha-Tocopherol, Beta-Carotene Cancer Prevention Study Group. 1994 The effect of vitamin E and beta-carotene on the incidence of lung cancer and other cancers in male smokers. *N. Engl. J. Med.* 330, 1029–1035.

61. Teikari, J.M., Virtamo, J., Rautalahti, M., Palmgren, J., Liesto, K., Heinonen, O.P. 1997. Long-term supplementation with alpha-tocopherol and beta-carotene and age-related cataract. *Acta. Ophthalmol. Scand.* 75, 634–640.

62. Teikari, J.M., Rautalahti, M., Haukka, J., Järvinen, P., Hartman, A.M., Virtamo, J., et al. 1998. Incidence of cataract operations in Finnish male smokers unaffected by alpha-tocopherol or beta-carotene supplements. *J. Epidemiol. Commun. Health* 52, 468–472.

63. Hennekens, C.H., Buring, J.E., Manson, J.E., Stampfer, M., Rosner, B., Cook, N.R., et al. 1996. Lack of effect of long-term supplementation with beta-carotene on the incidence of malignant neoplasms and cardiovascular disease. *N. Engl. J. Med.* 334, 1145–1149.

64. Christen, W.G., Manson, J.E., Glynn, R.J., Gaziano, J.M., Sperduto, R.D., Buring, J.E., Hennekens, C.H.. 2003. A randomized trial of beta-carotene and age-related cataract in US physicians. *Arch. Ophthalmol.* 121, 372–378.

65. Lee, I.M., Cook, N.R., Manson, J.E., Buring, J.E., Hennekens, C.H. 1999. Beta-carotene supplementation and incidence of cancer and cardiovascular disease: The Women's Health Study. *J. Natl. Cancer. Inst.* 91, 2102–2106.

66. Christen, W., Glynn, R., Sperduto, R., Chew, E., Buring, J. 2004. Age-related cataract in a randomized trial of beta-carotene in women. *Ophthalmic Epidemiol.* 11, 401–412.

67. McNeil, J.J., Robman, L., Tikellis, G., Sinclair, M.I., McCarty, C.A., Taylor, H.R. 2004. Vitamin E supplementation and cataract: Randomized controlled trial. *Ophthalmology* 111, 75–84.

68. Chylack, L.T. Jr., Brown, N.P., Bron, A., Hurst, M., Kopcke, W., Thien, U., Schalch, W. 2002. The Roche European American Cataract Trial REACT: A randomized clinical trial to investigate the efficacy of an oral antioxidant micronutrient mixture to slow progression of age-related cataract. *Ophthalmic Epidemiol.* 9, 49–80.

69. Gritz, D.C., Srinivasan, M., Smith, S.D., Kim, U., Lietman, T.M., Wilkins, J.H., et al. 2006. The Antioxidants in Prevention of Cataracts Study: Effects of antioxidant supplements on cataract progression in South India. *Br. J. Ophthalmol.* 90, 847–851.

70. Miller, E.R. 3rd, Pastor-Barriuso, R., Dalal, D., Riemersma, R.A., Appel, L.J., Guallar, E. 2005. Meta-analysis: High-dosage vitamin E supplementation may increase all-cause mortality. *Ann. Intern. Med.* 142, 37–46.
71. Hathcock, J.N., Azzi, A., Blumberg, J., Bray, T., Dickinson, A., Frei, B., et al. 2005. Vitamins E and C are safe across a broad range of intakes. *Am. J. Clin. Nutr.* 81, 736–745.
72. Blumberg, J.B., Frei, B. 2007. Why clinical trials of vitamin E and cardiovascular diseases may be fatally flawed. Commentary on The Relationship between Dose of Vitamin E and Suppression of Oxidative Stress in Humans. *Free Radic. Biol. Med.* 43, 1374–1376.
73. Manson, J.E., Gaziano, J.M., Spelsberg, A., Ridker, P.M., Cook, N.R., Buring, J.E., et al., for the WACS Research Group. 1995. A secondary prevention trial of antioxidant vitamins and cardiovascular disease in women: Rationale, design, and methods. *Ann. Epidemiol.* 5, 261–269
74. Christen, W.G., Gaziano, J.M., Hennekens, C.H. 2000. Design of Physicians' Health Study II—A randomized trial of beta-carotene, vitamins E and C, and multivitamins, in prevention of cancer, cardiovascular disease, and eye disease, and review of results of completed trials. *Ann. Epidemiol.* 10, 125–134.
75. Lippman, S.M., Goodman, P.J., Klein, E.A., Parnes, H.L., Thompson, I.M. Jr., Kristal, A.R., et al. 2005 Designing the Selenium and Vitamin E Cancer Prevention Trial SELECT. *J. Natl. Cancer. Inst.* 97, 94–102.
76. CTNS Study Group. 2003. The Italian-American Clinical Trial of Nutritional Supplements and Age-related Cataract CTNS: Design implications. CTNS report no. 1. *Control. Clin. Trials* 24, 815–829.

18 Herbal Treatment of Ischemia

Baowan Lin

CONTENTS

18.1   INTRODUCTION

In this chapter, you will encounter a phytomedicine world that has largely been abandoned by the Western countries during the last 100 years. The significant healing power in the plants, which dates back 4000 years, is still remarkable today. The cultural heritage and wisdom of traditional Chinese medicine (TCM), some of which is presented to readers in this chapter, may offer some helpful information about plant-based herbal compounds that can protect people against ischemia.

For the last 50 years, the Chinese federal government has constantly supported and encouraged studies in TCM. Scientific researchers have isolated and identified the ingredients of many important herbs, testing their effectiveness. A large amount of information on these subjects has been published in the Chinese language.

In this chapter, we will provide information about certain Chinese herbs that have been convincingly analyzed by modern scientific methods. We will briefly review the major Chinese herbs that have been used nutritionally in TCM for combating brain ischemia. However, this chapter is not intended as a treatment manual for this disorder.

Brain ischemia is the third leading cause of death in industrialized countries and is a major cause of permanent disability. With the increase in numbers of the aging population, stroke has become a worldwide major health problem. In the United States, tissue-plasminogen activator (t-PA) is the only thrombolytic drug that has been approved to treat acute brain infarction by blood clot resolution, leading to the restoration of the blood supply. However, t-PA is restricted to administration within 3 hours after the clot formation and has the risk of inducing brain hemorrhage.

Brain injury resulting from the blood flow blockage is difficult to mitigate. Brain infarction is currently irreversible once established. Neurocentric monotherapies of the past 20 years have been failing in clinical applications [1–4], and no effective conventional pharmacotherapy has been established in humans to increase brain repair, nor to reduce infarct volume or neurological deficit in people [4].

Complementary and alternative medicine (CAM) may offer a way to help in combating stroke. Herbal medicine is an important element in the treatment of brain infarction in patients in China, Korea, and Japan. Many people, including doctors, have turned to TCM to help stroke victims. TCM based on herbs is widely involved in stroke treatment [5,6], with about 25% of stroke patients visiting traditional medicine doctors in South Korea [6]. About one third of brain ischemia patients are treated with TCM in China [7]. More than 50% of Chinese people still use traditional herbal prescriptions, particularly when Western medicines (WM) do not produce the desired result. The Chinese government encourages integrating TCM into WM to service patients better, because some diseases that do not respond to WM may be cured by TCM. In the last 50 years, this bedside herbal treatment has been used on patients in WM hospitals in China. These WM hospitals are equipped with apothecaries that dispense Chinese herbs upon request.

The theory and formulas for enhancing the circulation to encourage self-repair in TCM were conceived and tested clinically long before the establishment of laboratory studies of disease models in the United Kingdom and United States. Today, extensive experimental studies have been used to investigate the effectiveness of herbal medication.

This chapter reviews the known disease-fighting compounds of the major herbs and the formulae (or prescriptions) that have been screened for neuroprotection by ischemic model systems. We will discuss how the mechanisms of their neuroprotection on brain ischemia are related to their effectiveness as antioxidants, anti-inflammatory agents, and for anticoagulation and improving blood circulation in the brain.

As an academic neurologist who was trained in WM and practiced in Beijing, and as a neuroscientist working in the United States, I have been constantly attracted by the abundance and richness of the herbal lore available in CM. Thus, for the past 8 years, I have investigated the neuroprotection of a classic formula of TCM applied in a stroke clinic. A formula consisting of nine herbs applied in clinics has been demonstrated to possess significant neuroprotection in animal experimental studies in our lab, Cerebral Vascular Disease Research Center. The nine-herb combination reduced infarct volume, prevented cavitation, accelerated the recovery of paralysis in brain focal ischemia, attenuated neuronal injury, prevented neurodegeneration, and maintained good coordination in global forebrain ischemia (see Section 18.4.3.1). Other effective formulas and herbs are reported by many studies around the world.

18.2   NEUROPATHOLOGY OF CEREBRAL ISCHEMIA

Brain ischemia includes *focal ischemia* i.e. infarction, which is induced by blood flow blockage in cerebral arteries or common carotid arteries with blood clot or embolus, and *global forebrain ischemia*, which usually results from heart attack or cardiac surgery.

In humans, within the infarct the acute neuronal injury is characterized by necrosis. The injury in the penumbra, where the blood flow decline is not as severe as at the core of infarction, includes shrunken neurons and apoptosis [8, 9].

Ischemia precipitates acute inflammation at day 3 with coagulative necrosis and neutrophil infiltration, and then the chronic inflammation begins by infiltration of macrophages and monocytes. Coagulative necrotic tissue is liquefied through lytic enzymes released by leukocytes, so as to remove the dead cells. Finally, the infarct progresses to resorption with neovascularization and cavitation in the brain around 1 month. The infarct ultimately becomes a fluid-filled cavity in 60% of patients at 2 weeks [10].

Endothelial damage in infarcted regions is prominent [11]. Once the endothelium is injured, the blood–brain barrier (BBB) breaks and multiple inflammatory cascades are activated and perivascular neuronal death is initiated. Endothelial injury may result in secondary hypoperfusion via platelet accumulation at the site of the occluded middle cerebral artery and in downstream microvessels associated with loss of microvascular integrity, vasoconstriction, and microthrombus formation [12–15], and peaks at 48 hours. The recirculation impairment exists for 2 weeks [14,15] and leads to scattered microvascular obstruction and microinfarction [16]. This decline in blood supply should promote the death of the injured neurons in the penumbra.

Chronic endothelial damage accompanied by thrombosis continues for weeks after ischemia [17]. The vascular constriction leads to hypoperfusion to induce neuronal degeneration including shrunken neurons (called apoptosis), patches of neuronal loss, and microinfarction in 4 weeks [18]. Therefore, protecting endothelia may attenuate the inflammation and prevent secondary neuronal injury.

Inflammation plays a key role in brain ischemic injury during the healing process. However, acute inflammation may be healed without consequences if inflammation mediators are no longer secreted [19]. Cyclooxygenase-2 (COX2), the key inflammation mediator, converts the released arachidonic acid into prostaglandins (PGs) [20]. PGs are important mediators [19]; toxic PGs instigate tissue damage [20], and are activated by reactive oxygen species (ROS) [21,22]. After ischemia, cyclooxygenase (COX2) is expressed in neurons, glia, infiltrating neutrophils, and endothelia in the human brain [23–26]. Animal experiments show that COX2 is rapidly induced in neurons and later in glia (27) and infiltrating leukocytes (28) for a long time. Neuronal COX2 overexpression is exhibited in the peri-infarct zone [29]. Prohibiting COX2 expression decreases infarct volume [29,30]. Production of ROS markedly increases in the recirculation and in the post-ischemic inflammation; antioxidants decrease infarct volume [22,31].

About 25% of patients develop dementia at 3 months after brain ischemia [32,33]. Delayed encephalopathy has been documented after acute hypoxic-ischemic insult, including brief cardiac arrest and heart surgery [34–36]. A sudden severe dementia, paralysis, and Parkinson syndrome may emerge following a symptom-free period averaging 2 weeks after initial recovery from the primary insult. lesions of the basal ganglia associated with diffuse brain atrophy, infarction, or cortical laminar necrosis are reported in patients experiencing a persistent vegetative state following resuscitation [34–36]. In addition, both β amyloid precursor protein (βAPP) and amyloid β peptide (Aβ), which are the prominent features of Alzheimer's disease (AD), are deposited in cortical and subcortical areas in the brains of nondemented patients following cardiac arrest [37,38]. Animal experimental studies found that inhibiting neuronal COX2 expression may prevent neuronal death at day 3 following global ischemia [39].

Our previous experimental studies establish that, in addition to the expected acute pathological changes, necrosis in hippocampal CA1 sector after transient forebrain ischemia *slowly progressive* alterations also occur in animals. Delayed infarction and neurodegeneration, as well as βAPP and Aβ deposition, occur over a period of many weeks [40–43], which resemble the pathological changes seen in the human brain. The endothelial damage induces secondary damage via thrombosis, infarction, and perivascular neuronal death. The chronic damage is much more severe than the primary injury.

Unfortunately, current studies have been focusing mainly on acute injury in both focal and global ischemia of the brain. Chronic injury has received relatively little attention. No effective conventional pharmacotherapy has yet been successfully established to combat both acute injury and chronic damage following brain ischemia in patients in past decades.

Excess production of ROS, BBB disruption, and postischemic inflammation are considered the key components in the mechanisms of ischemia/reperfusion injury [31,44]. The viewpoint on combating stroke is shifting to combined therapy [8]. Combination of antioxidant and anti-inflammation looks beneficial [4,22,23,45], and prolonging such therapies may augment their effectiveness [46–48]. Scientists are considering that the best approach for combating stroke will be combined therapies to reduce damage and enhance endogenous neurogenesis to replace the dead neurons [8].

18.3 BASIC THEORY ABOUT STROKE IN TCM, CONCEPTION AND TERMS DIFFERENT FROM WESTERN MEDICINE

18.3.1 MECHANISMS OF STROKE IN TCM

Perhaps the most difficult thing for non-Chinese to understand about Chinese herbal medicine is the terminology. TCM emphasizes that blood supply decline or blockage is the major cause of diseases including stroke. Because the symptoms of stroke have the sudden onset of paralysis, numbness, disability in language, and/or loss of consciousness, TCM calls brain ischemia "*wind stroke.*" *Wind* means the stroke emerges as fast as a tornado and is as severely destructive as a tornado. Blood circulation decline induces the *wind*. Improving blood circulation subdues the *wind*. Prompting vascular circulation relieves the symptoms of wind stroke and encourages repair. The causes of the disturbance of blood circulation are hypertension, arteriosclerosis, decreased body function including the disturbed blood circulation due to aging, overwork, dietary problems, or negative emotions such as anger, etc. [49]. To explain the mechanism of diseases, TCM employs the theory about balance between *Yin* and *Yang,* or the opposing forces within the human body.

TCM emphasizes the harmony of body and the balance between Yin and Yang (see Section 18.7.2). As soon as the Yin and Yang are unbalanced, the body's harmony is broken and diseases emerge. The therapeutic principle is to achieve balance between Yin and Yang, thus, to rebuild the body's harmony. Hypertension and arteriosclerosis, the cause of stroke, are termed as exuberant Yang in liver and insufficient Yin in liver, i.e., imbalance of the inner environment of the body.

Excessive Yang in liver induces hypertension and arteriosclerosis, leading to a decrease in the blood supply that causes wind. In addition, TCM realizes the importance of hormones. When people are getting old, the sexual hormone inside the body is decreased. TCM calls it a *deficiency of Yin* in the *kidney**. This induces and enhances the *excessive Yang* in the *liver**. The imbalance of Yin and Yang in the liver and kidney is the fundamental cause of *wind stroke*.

18.3.2 PHILOSOPHY OF DISEASE TREATMENT IN TCM

In contrast to Western medicine's practice of using a single compound to fight stroke, TCM emphasizes team work, i.e., formulae, or combination therapies. The concept of combining one major active herb and several supporting ones to synergize the therapy's pharmacodynamic action and to lessen its adverse effects has been the well established philosophy underlying prescribing practice in CM for more than 2000 years and is supported by knowledge accumulated during those centuries [50]. It was found that combination is more effective than a single herb [50]. Some specific herbs have been among the most popular and widely used drugs in CM over such a long history and have been considered beneficial in improving circulatory disturbances, exerting anti-inflammatory actions, and promoting healing after injury. They have been applied to stroke for generations.

18.4 PHARMACOLOGY OF MAJOR HERBS IN ISCHEMIA TREATMENT

18.4.1 STRATEGY OF STROKE TREATMENT IN TCM

The therapeutic principle of ischemia is to promote blood circulation in the acute stage and to depress the liver's Yang and increase the kidney's Yin to rebuild the Yin–Yang balance in liver and kidney after the acute stage to prevent a new wind stroke attack [49]. In the acute stage, some anti-inflammatory agents are added if the patient has fever.

The combinations for treating stroke focus on improving circulation, removing blood clot, inhibiting inflammation in the acute stage, and maintaining good circulation and adding some herbs to rebuild the Yin–Yang balance in liver and kidney after the acute stage. Thus, the prescriptions contain the herbs to prompt blood circulation, for example, *Astragali, Angelica, Ligusticum wallichii, Carthamus tinctorius, Prunus persica, Gastrodia elata Blume* is to inhibit the liver's Yang, and *Lycium chinense* is to nourish Yin in the liver and kidney. Formulae are more effective than a single herb [50]. There are several formulae for ischemic-stroke treatment.

According to recent studies, herbs contain plenty of nutrition, including vitamins E, A, C, B_{12}, folic acid, and trace elements; some herbs and compounds are neuroprotectant, antioxidant, vasodilator, anticoagulation and anti-inflammatory agents. Following, we will introduce the individual herbs and the formulae.

18.4.2 HERBS

18.4.2.1 *Ligusticum Wallichii (Chuan Xiong, 川芎)*

The root of *ligusticum wallichii* is the part that is used for medicine. Alkaloid tetramethylpyrazine (TMP) is the main active principle [51,52]. Other active components are ferulic acid, ligustilide, folic acid, and vitamin A. *Ligusticum wallichii* is nontoxic [51,53]. It protects endothelial cells against reperfusion injury and improves the microcirculation [54], prevents proliferation of vascular smooth muscle cells [55,56], promotes blood flow, removes blood stasis, and relieves pain. *Ligusticum wallichii* and TMP have been used in treatment of ischemia to treat ischemic stroke and angina pectoris in China since the 1960s.

---

* The liver and kidney in TCM are not the exact organs liver and kidney in WM.

TMP is thought to work in three ways: (1) as an antithrombotic agent, (2) an antagonist of vasoconstriction, and (3) as an anti-inflammatory compound. It decreases vascular resistance to block coronary vasoconstriction, increase blood circulation, and lower blood pressure by reducing the plasma endothelin-1 levels during and after acute ischemia/hypoxia [57,58] and by inhibiting thromboxane-A2 (TAX_2) synthesis after ischemia [51,59,60]. TMP has antithrombotic effects in humans [61] via inhibiting platelet activity [59,62,63]. In addition, TMP is an antioxidant [64], inflammatory inhibitor [65] and calcium antagonist [66]. It reduces the infarct volume through scavenging free radicals and prohibiting neutrophil migration [65]. TMP readily crosses the BBB and is evenly distributed throughout the intact rat brain in 20 minutes after oral administration [67,68]. LD_{50} of TMP is 239 mg/kg i.v. [51]. Ferulic acid inhibits inflammation [69].

18.4.2.2 *Angelica Sinensis (Dang Gui,* 当归)

The root, the medical part of the plant, contains a significant quantity of vitamin B_{12}, E, and folic acid [51]. Other active compounds include ferulic acid, biotin, succinic acid, nicotinic acid, uracil, adenine, and ligustilide. It has seven essential amino acids and 16 essential minerals. *Angelica sinensis* decreases the infarct volume in the brain, and reduces the apoptotic neurons via prohibiting protein BAX [70].

Angelica dilates coronal arteries and increases coronal blood flow [49, 51]. The water extract of *angelica* markedly inhibits platelet action to decrease serotonin (5-HT) release and TAX_2 formation, attenuates myocardial injury from ischemia, lowers blood cholesterol, and reduces atherosclerosis formation [51]. Ferulic acid is the cholesterol-lowing, anti-inflammatory, and antiplatelet aggregation compound. *Angelica* protects humans' vascular endothelia [71] and relaxes arteries [72]. In addition, *angelica* stimulates hematopoiesis in bone marrow because of its high vitamin B_{12} content (0.25–0.4 ug/100 g dried root), folic acid, and biotin [51].

18.4.2.3 *Carthamus Tinctorius (Hong Hua,* 红花)

The flower petal is the usable part of *carthamus tinctorius* (saffron). Its active component is safflower yellow [73,74]. *Carthamus tinctorius* inhibits platelet aggregation and causes vascular dilation [73]. A strong antioxidant, it protects against neuronal degeneration induced by ischemia [49,75–77], and attenuates retinal ischemic damage [76]. It is also a potent channel antagonist that prevents blood coagulation and inhibits platelet aggregation [51,73,74]. The water extract of *carthamus tinctorius* dilates coronary arteries to increase the cells' tolerance to oxygen deprivation and to lower blood pressure. In China, it is used to treat cerebral thrombosis and, in angina pectoris, to increase coronary circulation [51]. *Carthamus tinctorius* lowers plasma cholesterol and triglyceride level [51]. Safflower yellow protects against neuronal degeneration caused by ischemia *in vivo* and *in vitro* (77].

18.4.2.4 *Prunus Persica (Tao Ren,* 桃仁)

The kernel in the seed of *prunus persica* is believed to be the most powerful herb in improving circulation and maintaining the endothelial integrity, although its exact mechanism of action is still unknown. It is thought to inhibit platelet aggregation and coagulation, dilate blood vessels, increase cerebral blood flow (CBF], and decrease capillary permeability [50]. However, *prunus persica* is active only by oral administration. *Prunus persica* contains vitamin B_1 [50] and a lot of oil, which helps to resolve constipation [49]. Overdosage can cause cyanide intoxication [49]. LD_{50} of *prunus persica* is 222.5 ± 7.5g/kg [50].

18.4.2.5 *Astragalus Membranaceus (Huang Qi,* 黄芪)

The root of *astragalus membranaceus* is the medicinal portion and is called *Astragali Radix*. The active components are astragalus saponins, flavonoids, and polysacchararides [51,78]. It contains amino acids. Water extract of *astragali* dilates coronal arteries [49]. *Astragali Radix* promotes DNA synthesis, inhibits platelet aggregation [51] and protects neurons from anoxic damage [79]. *Astragali* has a broad anti-inflammatory effect since it strongly inhibits production of interleukin (IL)-6 and PGE_2, and blocks the effect of IL-1β [80], decreases formation of tumor necrosis factor (TNF)-α and scavenges free radicals [81]. It inhibits fibrosis progression via decrease of transforming growth factor β1 (TGF-β1) [81]. Astragalus saponins scavenge free radicals [78], activate the macrophages, and promote DNA synthesis [51]. Astragaloside IV upregulates t-PA expression in human endothelia after ischemic insult [82]; thus, it is a fibrinolytic potential agent.

When *astragali radix* is working together with *angelica*, estrogenic and antiplatelet aggregation activities are inserted [83] and good angiogenesis of capillaries is encouraged [84]. The five herbs *astragali, angelica, ligusticum wallichii, carthamus tinctorius* and *prunus persica,* constitute the core of therapies for improving circulation in TCM. They are the most important components of the common formula used to treat brain ischemia by inhibiting platelet activity, preventing thrombosis, dilating and protecting blood vessels, and maintaining BBB integrity [49,50]. Their combination prevents neuronal death [88] and works more favorably and effectively than any one of them alone [49,85–87].

18.4.2.6   *Scutellaria Baicalensis (Huang Qin, 黄芩)*

The root of *secutellaria baicalensis* is a very well known antibacterial and anti-inflammatory agent widely used in oriental medicine. *Scutellaria* is multi-functional: an antioxidant, anti-inflammatory and antithrombic agent as well as neuroprotectant, according to recent studies. It has 40 flavonoids [73]. Among them, *baicalin, baicalein, wogonin, oroxylin A,* and *skullcapflavone II* are the active compounds—strong antioxidant, anti-inflammatory and anticoagulation agents [51, 89–92]. Owing to these five compounds, *Scutellaria baicalensis* is defined as the most powerful of all antioxidant preparations [93–99]. It protects neurons in hippocampus CA1 *in vivo* [96, 100] and *in vitro* [96,97,99] from lethal oxidant damage in ischemia/reperfusion.

All of the five flavonoids are powerful antioxidants [73,90,92,96,97,99,101]. Baicalein and baicalin directly scavenge and quench superoxide, hydrogen peroxide, and hydroxyl radicals [96, 101,102]. They enhance Fe^{++} ion oxidation, resulting in inhibition of hydroxyl radical production [103]. They directly scavenge and quench ROS [96,101,102], including nitric oxide (NO) radicals [100,104], and inhibit hydroxyl radical production to protect cellular and mitochondrial membranes [96,98,102,103,105,106].

These five five flavonoids are 5- and 12-lipoxygenase inhibitors [92,97,107] that protect cellular and mitochondrial membranes by effectively inhibiting lipid peroxidation in neurons [96,98, 102,103,105]. Baicalein and baicalin inhibit $(Ca^{2+})_i$ elevations [108]. Thus, neurons are protected after ischemia [96–98,102,103]. Baicalein [96,97,109] and wogonin [110,111] protect neurons from lethal damage in ischemia/reperfusion. Wogonin decreases the volume of brain infarction [112].

Baicalein and baicalin decrease blood cholesterol [73], prevent neurotoxicity induced by glutamate [113] and by amyloid β peptide (Aβ) [114], and protect cortical neurons from Aβ toxicity-induced apoptosis [115]. Part of the Aβ deposition, which converts an acute phase injury response to chronic injury response [118] in the human brain, is released from platelets [116,117]. Additionally, *scutellaria baicalensis* and baicalein protect cardiomyocytes [95,101]and kidney [119] from ischemia.

Scutellaria strongly inhibits inflammation. Baicalin, baicalein, wogonin, and oroxylin A inhibit COX2 expression and the PGE_2 synthesis [89,108,120]. Baicalin binds to inflammatory cytokines IL-1β, -6, and TNF-α to limit their biological functions, and inhibits their production [51,73,100,121,122]. Baicalein and wogonin attenuate induction of free radicals in glia and macrophages in the infarct [123]. Wogonin and oroxylin A inhibit COX2 expression by blocking nuclear factor-kB (NF-kB) activation [89,120,124,125], markedly retards arachidonic acid release, protects the cell membranes against injury [106,126], and reduces microglia and macrophages in the infarct [112].

Baicalein and baicalin inhibit fibrillation and disaggregate the existing fibrils in the brain [127]; baicalein strongly attenuates the inflammation-mediated degeneration of dopaminergic neurons through inhibiting microglial activation [109]. Thus, *scutellaria* has strong anti-inflammatory actions [121,128]. The three strong anti-inflammatory agents are baicalin, baicalein, and wogonin [128].

Scutellaria baicalensis protects the vascular endothelia and prevents thrombotic tendencies by inhibiting TAX_2 release, preventing platelet aggregation [108,129], decreasing the expression of endothelial leukocyte adhesion molecule-1 (ELAM-1) and intercellular adhesion molecule-1 (ICAM-1) [130,131] and $[Ca^{2+}]$ elevation [132], and preventing the decrease of t-PA production [133]. *Scutellaria* and baicalein improve the cellular repair of oxidatively damaged DNA in endothelia [134–136) and inhibit arterial vasoconstriction [137].

Scutellaria is used in the acute stage of ischemia when patients have fever. It is able to work powerfully against bacterial infection. *Scutellaria* is nontoxic when given orally and absorbed quickly by the gastrointestinal tract [51,138,139]. The amount of baicalin in *scutellaria* is 10 times that of baicalein; baicalin is metabolized into baicalein in the human body and by bacteria prior to intestinal absorption, and subsequently metabolized into baicalein [140,141]. Baicalein, baicalin, and wogonin, the aqueous extracts, are absorbed immediately, take action quickly, and provide longer and higher efficacy by oral administration [138,141,142]. Baicalin rapidly appears in plasma and exists for 24 hours [138]. It enters the brain parenchyma—cortex, hippocampus, striatum, thalamus, and brain stem [143]. Baicalein crosses the BBB quickly and evenly distributes throughout the intact rat brain in 20 minutes [51,139].

18.4.2.7   *Paeonia Veitchii* (*Chi Shao,* 赤芍) and *Paeonia Suffruticosa* (*Mu Dan Pi,* 牡丹皮)

The roots of *paeonia veitchii* and the bark of the rhizome of *paeonia suffruticosa* are the portions used for medicine. They are important medicines to attenuate inflammation and reduce capillary permeability to inhibit tissue swelling in TCM. Both have antibacterial properties [51] and include paeonol, paeonoside, paeoniflorin and 1, 2, 3, 4, 6-Penta-O-galloyl-beta-D-glucose (PGG) as the active compounds [51,73,144].

Both *paeonia veitchii* and *paeonia suffruticosa* inhibit COX2 activities [145] and inflammation, prevent fibrosis [51,73], and protect neurons from ROS-mediated death [144]. In addition, *paeonia veitchii* increases endothelium-dependent relaxation, and *paeonia suffruticosa* antagonizes platelet aggregation via inhibiting TAX_2 production [146]. They are absorbed quickly from intestine. The maximal plasma concentration is reached in 20 minutes and 89% of the administered dose is excreted in urine [147,148].

The major components of both *paeonia veitchii* and *paeonia suffruticosa* insert antioxidant and anti-inflammation functions. Paeonol reduces cerebral infarction via scavenging superoxide anion and inhibiting microglia activation and macrophages in infarct [149]. Peaoniflorin and PGG protect neurons by induction of heme oxygenase-1 (HO-1) and scavenging free radicals against ischemic stress [144]. Peaoniflorin blocks sodium current into neurons after ischemic insult [150] and upregulates the expression of heat shock protein (HSP) after the insult to protect neurons [151]. PGG inhibits COX2 activity [145,152], suppresses the expression of ELAM-1 and ICAM-1 to alleviate vascular inflammation [153]. In addition, PGG is a vasorelaxant, which dilates vascular smooth muscle [153]. The median lethal dose (LD_{50}) is: *paeonia suffruticosa,* 3.43 g/kg [51]; paeonol, 4.9 ± 0.47 g/kg [73].

18.4.2.8   *Glycyrrhiza Uralensis* (*Gan Cao,* 甘草)

The root of glycyrrhiza is used to treat diseases. The major active compounds are glycyrrhizin, flavonoid licorice, and ferulic acid [154]. *glycyrrhiza* enhances the absorption of the constituents of *scutellaria baicalensis, paeonia veitchii,* and *paeonia suffruticosa,* and leads to a higher bioavailability of baicalin in the body [142,147,155]. Glycyrrhizin is about 170% sweeter than cane sugar;

therefore glycyrrhiza is the principal adjuvant [51]. It is an antioxidant and inhibits inflammation [51,154] and enhances the heat shock protein (HSP) expression induced by paeoniflorin [151]. Licorice reduces capillary permeability [51].

18.4.2.9   Ginseng (Renshen, 人参)

Ginseng is the root of *Panax ginseng* C.A. Mey. It is the most valued herb widely used in China, Korea, and Japan, and among the Chinese in the United States. For thousands of years, ginseng has been used by the common people as a tonic, and by the rich and nobility as a revitalizing agent. The research on ginseng started in the early 19th century. Some of its chemical structures have been well studied and recognized, but many are not yet fully understood. Ginseng contains multiple active elements. Its component saponins, i.e., ginsenosides, are the principals. It contains maltol, salicylic acid, and vanillic acid; all of these three are antioxidants. Ginseng also contains vitamins. Extract of ginseng lowers serum cholesterol levels and prevents atherosclerosis by the combined action of increasing prostacyclin in the carotid artery and decreasing TAX_2 [51].

Rb$_1$, one of ginsenosides, is the most important for neuroprotective action [49,51]. Rb$_1$ effectively prevents delayed neuronal death and stabilizes the membraneous structure of mitochondria and other organelles in neurons. It reduces the degenerative process of aging, improves behavior and movement activity, and increases learning ability, as well as offers protection against acute myocardial infarction and necrosis [51].

Ginsenosides enhance the biosynthesis of DNA and protein in brain, bone marrow, testis, thymus, and adrenal cortex, and increase sex hormone production. Such increases in biosynthesis of DNA and protein exert some indirect action in prolonging cell life [51]. Ginsenosides increase the synthesis of high-density lipids (HDL) in serum. Ginseng extract increases the biosynthesis of RNA and incorporation of amino acids into the nuclei of hepatic cells, resulting in an increase in serum protein. However, ginseng should not be given to patients who have fever or hypertension.

18.4.2.10   Ginkgo Biloba (*Yin Xing Ye*, 银杏叶)

For decades, the leaf of ginkgo biloba has been used for circulatory disorders to increase peripheral and cerebral blood flow. The leaf has several flavonoid glucosides, including ginkgolide A, ginkgolide B, and bilobalide. It improves the contractile function of the ischemic heart, exerts a protective effect on hypoxic myocardium, increases cerebral blood flow, and exhibits antioxidant activity in animal experimental studies. Ginkgo extract showed neuroprotection on hippocampus in animal studies [51].

18.4.2.11   *Fructus Crataegus Pinnatifida* (*Shan Zha*, 山楂 or Hawthorn Fruit)

The medicinal part is the red fruit of *crataegus pinnatifida*. It is nontoxic and sold on street corners as a popular snack food in northern China. It contains carotene and vitamins C and B$_2$. The active components are chlorogenic, caffeic, citric, crataegolic, maslinic, and ursolic acids, as well as the flavonoids quercetin and vitexin and some saponins.

The herb lowers blood cholesterol by increasing its catabolism to help the surface of the atherosclerotic area in the arterial wall to shrink and become smoother. It increases coronary circulation via increase of blood flow. This reduces oxygen consumption and protects against myocardiac ischemia. It increases myocardial contractility and lowers the blood pressure. In addition, it is very helpful for digesting meat [49,51].

18.4.2.12   *Anemarrhena asphodeloides Bunge* (*Zhi Mu*, 知母)

The rhizome of the plant is the part for medicine. It has six saponins [73]. Recent studies reported that *anemarrhena asphodeloides* decreases the infarct volume through inhibiting neutrophils immigrating into injured brain cortex in the early stage after ischemia insult [156]. Its active component is timosaponins, which lowers blood sugar by increasing the metabolism of glucose and increasing glycogen synthesis in the liver. It also has antibacterial properties and inhibits platelet aggregation [51,73].

18.4.2.13 *Gastrodia Elata* Blume (*Tian Ma,* 天麻)

The rhizome of *Gastrodia elata* Blume is used to subdue the "exuberant Yang" of the liver (see Section 18.3.1), to calm internal wind and relieve convulsions and fainting [51]. Its active elements are gastrodin, vanillyl alcohol, vanillin, vitamin A, and small quantities of the glycoside. This herb has analgesic, anticonvulsive, and sedative effects. It increases coronary and cerebral blood flow, and lowers peripheral blood pressure [50, 51].

Gastrodia elata Blume relieves convulsions and fainting and treats hypertension, dizziness, and headache. Recent studies found it protects neurons in brain ischemia [157, 158]. It should not be used if the patient does not have hypertension.

18.4.2.14 *Lycium Chinense* (*Gou Qi Zi,* 枸杞子)

The red fruit of *Lycium chinense,* or wolfberry, contains vitamins B_1, B_2, C, carotene, nicotinic acid, lycium polysaccharides, Ca, P, and Fe. Its water extract significantly increases nonspecific immunity; lowers blood pressure, plasma cholesterol, and glucose; and improves visual acuity. It increases blood 17-ketosteroids in elderly men [49,51,154]. Lycium polysaccharides reduce the fragmentation of DNA and inhibit apoptosis [51]. According to TCM, *Lycium chinense* strengthens the Yin in the liver and kidney. (As explained earlier, the liver and kidney in TCM have a different meaning from those in Western medicine.)

18.4.2.15 *Epimedium Brevicorum* (*Yin Yang Huo,* 淫羊藿)

The whole plant, excluding the root, is used for medicine and is nontoxic. Its active elements are 28 flavonoids, including icariin and noricariin [51,154], and vitamin E [49]. Water extract of *Epimedium brevicorum* dilates the coronary vessels and increases the coronary flow by reducing vascular resistance. It is commonly used in the treatment of angina pectoris.

Extract of *Epimedium brevicorum* is reputed to have a sexually stimulating effect on men. This herb can stimulate growth of the testis and increase sperm production and excretion of 17-ketosteroids [51]. It lowers blood pressure and decreases blood sugar [49], increases the activity of the immune system [51,154) and enhances the synthesis of DNA and protein [154].

The total flavonoids are antioxidant and slow down the aging process [154]. In addition, icariin is a vasodilatation agent via its Ca^{++} channel blocking action [51], and is reported to be an antioxidant that protects neurons in cerebral ischemia [159]. According to TCM, *Epimedium brevicorum* is a tonic for the Yang in kidney.

18.4.12.16 *Ophiopogon Japonicus* (*Mai Dong,* 麦冬)

The root is the medicinal part. The active components include β-sitosterol, stigmasterol, and ophiopogonin B. *Ophiopogon japonicus* increases coronary blood flow and myocardial contractility, and slowly elevates blood pressure during cardiac shock [51].

18.4.2.17 *Fructus Schisandra Chinensis* (*Wu Wei Zi,* 五味子)

The fruit of *Fructus schisandra chinensis* (*Wu Wei Zi*) is the medicinal part. *Fructus schisandra chinensis* can improve mental function. It contains vitamins A and E. The active compound is γ-schizandrin. Aqueous extract of *Fructus schisandra chinensis* increases myocardial contractility. A combination of *schisandra chinensis, ophiopogon japonicus* and *glycyrrhiza* heals hypotension. The herb is nontoxic. Doses up to 5g/kg do not produce death in mice [51,160].

18.4.2.18   *Cinnamomum Cassia* (*Gui Zhi,* 桂枝)

The twig is the medicinal portion of the plant. The active ingredients are cinnamic aldehyde and cinnamyl acetate. *Cinnamomum cassia* is a condiment with antibacterial and vasodilation functions [49,51]. Working together with *prunus persica* and *paeonia suffruticosa* will yield better effectiveness. If the patient always feels cold, give this herb to make him or her warm and improve blood circulation. Do not give it to patients who have fever.

18.4.2.19   Soybean (*Huang Dou,* 黄豆)

Soybean is one of the major dietary products consumed by both Chinese and Japanese. It is the seed of *Glycine soja*. Its isoflavone ingredients are genistein and daidzein. Both are phytoestrogen and bind to mammary tissue estrogen receptors. Soybean consumption reduces the plasma level of LDL cholesterol and increases HDL cholesterol levels, especially in female monkeys. It lowers total cholesterol level and lessens cardiovascular risk in humans [51]. A recent study reported that dietary isoflavones reduced the infarct volume and improved neurological status in rats [161]. In addition, soybean is very beneficial due to its rich nutrition, including proteins and vitamins.

18.4.3   FORMULAE

Formulae are employed to treat diseases because using a single herb is usually less effective than expected or even has no efficacy. The formulae of Chinese herbal medicine consist of several components having different functions, so the combinations work like teams to fight diseases.

18.4.3.1   Modified Buyang-Huawu Tang (补阳还五汤加减)

Buyang-Huawu Tang, a formula consisting of seven Chinese medicines, is the classic prescription to treat brain infarction in the chronic stage. *Tang* means "decoction" in Chinese language. Withdrawing one medicine from Buyang-Huawu Tang and adding three herbs makes the nine-herb modified Buyang-Huawu Tang, used to treat brain infarction at the acute stage in a clinical setting. The resulting nine herbs are *Ligusticum wallichii*, *Angelica sinensis*, *Carthamus tinctorius*, *Prunus persica*, *astragali*, *Scutellaria baicalensis*, *Paeonia veitchii*, *Paeonia suffruticosa*, and *glycyrrhiza*.

Two animal experimental studies were used to investigate if and how the nine-herb formula works on brain infarction and global ischemia in humans in our lab [162]. Thirty-nine male Sprague-Dawley rats weighing 280–310 g and aged 2.5–2.8 months participated in the focal brain ischemia study. Brain infarction was produced by a 2-hour cerebral middle artery occlusion (MCAo) by intraluminal suture insertion [11]. The rats received the medicine daily up to 28 days by feeding needle that began at 4 hours after the ischemia insult. The results showed promise. The study demonstrated that this nine-herb combination successfully ameliorated the brain injury. The therapy reduced the infarct volume by 53% and 62%, compared with the nontreated groups, at days 3 and 28 respectively, encouraged the recovery of neurological deficit, prevented cavitation, and inhibited inflammation in the infarct, and alleviated scar formation in the peri-infarct zone. The significant recovery of neurological deficit began at 24 hours and recovered at day 28 after treatment. In nontreated rats, neurological function recovery was later and evident deficit persisted at day 28. In addition, the therapy decreased neuronal COX2 expression in the peri-infarct at day 3.

The most interesting sign is that the therapy protected vascular endothelia at day 3 and enhanced the angiogenesis inside the infarcts at day 28. While no normal neurons were seen in the infarcts in nontreated rats at day 28, plenty of normal neurons were observed in the infarcts in all of the treated rats, and these neurons were settled along and around the blood vessels toward the core of infarct from the peri-infarct inner zone. Some of the neurons were differentiated to form axons and dendrites. This implies that the therapy might rescue the newly formed neurons. Additionally, the neuronal proliferation was seen in the top of third ventricle in some treated rats at day 28 while no such activity was observed in nontreated rats. This indicated that the nine-herb formula might have stimulated the neurogenesis after brain infarction.

Our second study was with 70 male Wistar rats weighing 256–405 g and aged 2.8 ± 0.6 months were subjected to 12.5-minute global forebrain ischemia produced by common carotid arteries occlusion plus systemic hypotension [41]. Animals were sacrificed at days 3, 7, 28, and 56. The nine-herb decoction was daily administered by feeding needle initiated at 4 hours after ischemia [162]. The treatment significantly attenuated the neuronal necrosis and inhibited neuronal COX2 expression in hippocampus CA1 sector at day 3. The numbers of normal neurons in hippocampus CA1 were 95 ± 58 (n = 12, treated group) and 28 ± 13 (n = 10, nontreated group) at day 3 (mean ± S.D., $p < 0.05$, ANOVA], while 438 ± 73 in sham rats (n = 4). At days 7–56, in hippocampus CA1, the numbers of normal neurons of treated groups were four times the nontreated groups: 60 ± 41 (n = 7, treated group) vs. 15 ± 8 (n = 8, nontreated group) at day 7, 110 ± 90 (6, treated) vs. 24 ± 8 (6, nontreated) at day 28, 83 ± 27 (6, treated) and 21 ± 5 (7, nontreated) at day 56 ($p < 0.05$). Significantly fewer apoptotic neurons were seen in the treated brains. The numbers of apoptotic neurons of cortex (counted in three standard levels) were 62 ± 44 (n = 6, treated group) and 213 ± 140 (7, nontreated group) at day 56 ($p < 0.05$), 89 ± 44 in sham group (n = 4). These data indicate that the nine-herb therapy attenuated neuronal necrosis and prevented neurodegeneration.

A beam-walking test was employed to detect the rats' coordination after global forebrain ischemia. Time to traverse the 1.5 cm wide and 95 cm long beam at day 56 by the rats were 12 ± 5.9 (non-treated group, n = 7) vs. 4.4 ± 1.6 (treated group, n = 6) seconds ($p < 0.01$), 5.2 ± 0.86 seconds in sham rats (n = 4). The nine-herb therapy encouraged rats' motor movement performance and neurological function recovery.

All 17 28-day and 56-day treated rats in both focal ischemia and global ischemia protocols showed white shining hairs at days 28 and 56 while all 16 survived rats in nontreated groups having brown-yellow hairs on their backs. All four sham rats presented mild color change in the hair [162]. The yellow hair indicates elders, and ischemia accelerated the aging. Treated rats not having brown-yellow hairs meant that stroke-induced aging was delayed or prevented by the medication.

In addition, a five-herb combination consisting of *ligusticum wallichii, angelica sinensis, carthamus tinctorius, prunus persica, astragali* showed similar protective effects at day 56.

These nine herbs are safe and are documented in *Pharmacopoeia of the People's Republic of China*. Their LD_{50} responses were tested and revealed no toxicity [50,51,88,120]. Phytochemical studies found that these herbs are multifunctional, including neuroprotectant [49,75–77,79,96,100], strong antioxidant, anti-inflammatory [51,81,121,128,153], and antiplatelet activities [49,51,73,74,83], as well as anticoagulation and antivasoconstriction properties. Their known disease-fighting compounds are flavonoids; saponins; vitamins E, A, C; folate; ferulic acid; paeonol; paeoniflorin; and PGG (see Table 18.1).

These nine medicines are absorbed quickly by the gastrointestinal tract after ingestion [51,68,138,139,155]. Baicalein, baicalin, and TMP quickly cross the BBB to enter the brain within 20 minutes after oral administration [51,68,139]. *glycyrrhiza* enhances the absorption of other herbs and leads to higher bioavailability of baicalin in the body [147,155].

Six herbs and six compounds in this formula are neuroprotectant. *Scutellaria baicalensis* via baicalein, baicalin, and wogonin [96,97,99,100]; *ligusticum wallichii* via TMP [65]; *paeonia veitchii* and *paeonia suffruticosa* via paeonol [65]; and *angelica sinensis* [70] decrease the infarct volume in the brain. *Carthamus tinctorius* via safflower yellow protects against neuronal degeneration [49,75–77]. *Angelica sinensis* reduces apoptosis [70]. Combination of these herbs prevents neuronal death from ischemia [88].

Five herbs, including *ligusticum wallichii, angelica sinensis, carthamus tinctorius, prunus persica,* and *radix astragalas* are considered the major medicines to improve blood circulation and encourage tissue repair, and are the core of therapy routinely used in TCM to treat ischemia. These five herbs promote circulation by inhibiting blood aggregation, maintaining vascular integrity, and

TABLE 18.1
Latin Names, Chinese Names, Medicinal Part, Nutrition, and Function of Herbs

Latin Name	Chinese Name	Part of Plant	Nutrition	Disease-Fighting Compound	Action
Ligusticum Wallichii	川芎, Chuan Xiong	Rhizome	Vitamin A, folic acid	TMP, ferulic acid ligustilide	Vasodilation, prevents platelet aggregation
Angelica sinensis	当归, Dang Gui	Root	Vitamins A, B_1, B_{12}, E. folic acid, nicotinic acid, biotin, 19 amino acids, 7 essential amino acids, 16 essential minerals	Ferulic acid ligustilide	Vasodilation, prevents neuronal apoptosis
Carthamus tinctorius	红花, Hong Hua	Flower		Safflower yellow	Vasodilation, lowers plasma cholesterol
Astragalus membranaceus	黄芪, Huang Qi	Root	Folic acid, vitamin P, carotene, 25 amino acids trace elements: Co, Se	Astragalus saponins	Antioxidant, dissolves platelet aggregation, promotes cellular DNA repair
Prunus persica	桃仁, Tao Ren	Kernel	Vitamin B_1, oil	Unknown, amygdalin	Increases CBF, anti-inflammation
Scutellaria Baicalensis	黄芩, Huang Qin	Root		Baicalin, baicalin wogonin, oroxylin A	Powerful antioxidant. anti-inflammatory, antibacterial and anti-coagulation agent
Paeonia veitchii	赤芍, Chi Shao	Root		Paeonol, paeoniflorin PGG	Inhibits COX2 activity and inflammation
Paeonia suffruticosa	牡丹皮, Mu Dan Pi	Bark of rhizome		Paeonol, paeoniflorin PGG	Inhibits COX2 activity and inflammation
Glycyrrhiza uralensis	甘草, Gan Cao	Rhizome	Amino acids, biotin, trace minerals: Zn, Co	Glycyrrhizin, licorice	Anti-inflammatory agent
Ginseng	人参, Renshen	Root	Vitamins: C, B_1, B_2, B_{12}, nicotinic acid, trace minerals: Mn, Cu, Co, As	Saponins ginsenosides, salicylic acid	Antioxidant, neuroprotectant
Ginkgo biloba	银杏叶, Yin Xing Ye	Leaf		Flavonoids: ginkgolides	Antioxidant, improves blood circulation
Fructus Crataegus pinnatifida	山楂, Shan Zha	Fruit	Vitamins C, B_2, carotene minerals: Ca, P, Fe.	Chlorogenic acid, caffeic acid, citric acid, flavonoid quercetin	Lowers blood cholesterol, antioxidant
Anemarrhena asphodeloides Bunge	知母, Zhi Mu	Root		Timosaponins	Decreases plasma sugar, inhibits platelet aggregation
Gastrodia elata Blume	天麻, Tian Ma	Rhizome	Vitamin A	Gastrodin	Increases CBF, lowers blood pressure
Epimedium brevicorum	淫羊藿, Yin Yang Huo	Whole plant	Vitamin E	Flavonoids: icariin noricariin	Antioxidant, increases coronary blood flow

TABLE 18.1 (CONTINUED)

Latin Names, Chinese Names, Medicinal Part, Nutrition, and Function of Herbs

Latin Name	Chinese Name	Part of Plant	Nutrition	Disease-Fighting Compound	Action
Fruit of Lycium chinense	枸杞子, Gou Qi Zi	Fruit	Vitamins B$_1$, B$_2$, C, carotene, nicotinic acid, lyceum. minerals: Fe, Zn	Polysaccharides	Inhibits apoptosis, lowers blood pressure, plasma cholesterol and glucose
Ophiopogon japonicus	麦冬, Mai Don	Root	Amino acids	β-sitosterol, ophiopogonin B	Increases coronary blood flow
Fructus Schisandra chinensis	五味子, Wu Wei Zi,	Fruit	Vitamins A, E	γ–schizandrin	Improves mental function
Cinnamomum cassia	桂枝, Gui Zhi	Twig		Cinnamic aldehyde	Vasodilation

vasodilation. It has been demonstrated that the combination of these five herbs works more effectively than any single one of them alone [85].

Sprouting angiogenesis is involved in recovery in the human brain; an increase in neovascularization is correlated with longer survival in patients [163]. When these five herbs work together, they increase angiogenesis [84,164]. A recent study revealed they promote good angiogenesis with the efficacy resembling that of basic fibroblast growth factor (bFGF); the combination is more effective on capillary formation [164].

Four herbs: *scutellaria baicalensis, paeonia veitchii, paeonia suffruticosa,* and *glycyrrhiza* in the formula reduce inflammation to a remarkable degree and improve the healing of wounds [73]. In addition, TMP decreases neutrophils into infarct [65].

ROS markedly increases in the post-ischemia inflammation, and antioxidants decrease infarct volume [22,31]. Seven herbs in the formula are antioxidants, thus they are able to reduce the production of ROS and scavenge the radicals. TMP reduces ROS formation in infarct [65]. *Scutellaria baicalensis, angelica sinensis, astragali, carthamus tinctorius, paeonia veitchii*, and *paeonia suffruticosa* are strong antioxidants via vitamin E, astragalus saponins, safflower yellow, peaoniflorin and PGG [51,77,144]. Astragalus saponins protect neurons and myocardium against injury [51]. Therefore, this therapy targets ROS to ameliorate ischemic injury through protection of mitochondria.

Thus, the nine herbs and their components work as neuroprotectant, antioxidant, anti-inflammatory, and antithrombotic agents, as well as vasoconstriction antagonists. The results of the studies reveal that this formula enhances brain self-repair through inhibiting the detrimental inflammation, protecting endothelia, and encouraging angiogenesis. Finally, some new neurons settle along the blood vessels in the injured regions of the brain.

Note: *Scutellaria baicalensis, paeonia veitchii* and *paeonia suffruticosa* should be removed from the prescription at the beginning of the 2nd month. The five herbs left in the formula are enough for the rehabilitation.

18.4.3.2 Shengmai San (生脉散 or 生脉饮)

Shengmai San consists of ginseng, *Ohiopogon japonicus,* and *Fructus schisandra chinensis*. This formula has been applied to acute myocardial infarction associated with shock in China. This therapy was reported to help elevate blood pressure and improve blood microcirculation and cardiac function in 829 cases in a clinical setting [165]. It was reported that this formula prevented the progression of injury in brain infarction in animal experimental studies [166,167]. The combination of *Fructus schisandra chinensis* and ginseng has been found to be beneficial in memory consolidation in humans [51]. Ginseng extract is effective in reducing inflammation and improves healing of wounds. The mechanism is not clear, but ginseng extract inhibits the increase in capillary permeability (51]. Ginsenosides Rb_1 offers protective action against acute myocardial infarction and necrosis [51], effectively prevents delayed neuronal death, and stabilizes the membraneous structure of mitochondria and other organelles in the hippocampal neurons, reduces the degenerative process of aging, improves behavior and movement activity, and increases learning ability [51].

18.4 NUTRITION AND HEALTH-PROMOTING COMPONENTS OF HERBS' DIETARY INTAKE

The known nutrition and disease-fighting components of these herbs are listed in Table 18.1.

Investigations found that patients with acute ischemic stroke [168] and cerebrovascular diseases [169] have lower plasma concentration of antioxidant vitamins A, C, and E and antioxidant trace minerals Zn and Se, a lack that is associated with poor early outcome. Vitamin E is a major endogenous antioxidant and an inhibitor of intracellular phospholipases A2 (PLA2) [170–172]. Increasing intake of vitamin E [173], vitamin C, and folate [174] reduces the risk of ischemic stroke. Animal experimental study found that pretreatment with vitamin E for 13–16 weeks decreased the brain infarct volume by 56% [175].

Carotenoids, the precursor of vitamin A, decrease in the first 24 hours after the ischemic insult in humans [176]. In acute ischemic stroke patients, the lowered plasma concentrations of carotene [177] and vitamin C [178] are associated with higher levels of inflammation. In addition, inadequate nutrition is common in the aged. Malnutrition, including deficiency of protein-calorie, iron, vitamins, and minerals, impacts on recovery and rehabilitation [179]. Deficiency of vitamins C, A, E, B_1, B_6, B_{12} and folate are encountered very often, and vitamins B_6, B_{12} and folate have important roles in the neuron-cognition function and in the nervous system. In addition, intake of trace mineral Zinc decreases in the elderly [180]. Daily supplementation of antioxidant vitamins and trace elements Zn and Se has a beneficial effect on aging (181]. Therefore, providing elderly patients with nutrition after ischemia is essential. However, herbs listed in this chapter may offer this kind of nutrition.

Phytochemicals are considered as "phytonutrient" by scientists today because they promote health by trapping free radicals and cleaning up toxic wastes before they can damage cells [182]. Phytochemicals, which protect plants against dangers, may save people's lives; antioxidants in plants function as antioxidants in humans as well [182,183]. When people take nutrition from plants, they recruit the health-promoting phytochemicals into their own defense capacity to heal damage. Flavonoids exist widely in plants, help their growth and development, and protect the plants' lives. Saponins have multiple functions [182].

- Vitamin E, the most prevalent antioxidant in cell membrane, prevents the onset of lipidic peroxidation due to ROS, thus preserving the membrane's integrity. *Angelica sinensis,* ginseng, and *Epimedium brevicorum* are rich in vitamin E [51].
- Vitamin C is an antioxidant. Ginseng, *Fructus crataegus pinnatifida*, and fruit of *Lycium chinense* have plenty of vitamin C [51].
- Vitamin A is an antioxidant in cell membranes of lisosomes and microsomes. It prevents the peroxidation induced by ROS in liposomal membranes, maintains the retina's function, and enhances learning ability [182]. Fruit of *Lycium chinense* and *Gastrodia elata Blume* are rich in vitamin A.
- Minerals: *Angelica sinensis* has 16 essential minerals. *Fructus crataegus pinnatifida* contains Ca, P, and Fe. *Glycyrrhiza uralensis* has Zn, Co; fruit of *Lycium chinense* has Fe, Zn; Ginseng has Mn, Cu, Co, and As.

- Flavonoids are potent antioxidants and anti-inflammatory agents. Antioxidants in plants function similarly to antioxidants in people [182,183]. Every herb has flavonoids. *Scutellaria baicalensis*, fruit of *Crataegus pinnatifida* and *Epimedium brevicorum* are rich in flavonoids [51]. Baicalin, baicalein, wogonin, oroxylin A, skullcapflavone II [93–99], and quercetin [182] are the most powerful antioxidants. They are lipoxygenase inhibitors, as well as anti-inflammatory and anticoagulation agents [51,89–92].
- Saponins are multifunctional. They are toxic-waste fighters, antioxidants, and anti-inflammatory agents. Cholesterol aggravates cerebral infarction by hypercholesterolemia in serum and in the brain [185]. Saponins may scoop up cholesterol in the intestinal tract before it is absorbed into the bloodstream. Saponins in *Fructus crataegus pinnatifida* have cholesterol-lowing function. Ginsenosides in *Ginseng* and *Astragalus saponins* in astragali have several functions. Ginsenosides, especially Rb_1, is a strong neuroprotectant [49,51]. Astragaloside IV, one of the astragalus saponins, increases the thrombolytic potential of endothelia by upregulating t-PA expression [82].

Other phytochemicals, for example alkaloid TMP, prevent thrombosis and strongly antagonize platelet aggregation [59,61–63], lower the vascular resistance and increase cerebral blood flow (CBF) [51,57,58,73]. TMP's multifunction includes a free radical scavenger [54,184] and calcium channel blocker [66]. Ferulic acid lowers cholesterol and has an anti-inflammatory effect [69]. Paeoniflorin and PGG alleviate inflammation [51], and protect neurons from oxidative stress [144,150,151]. PGG is a COX2 inhibitor [152], and protects against the inflammation of human endothelia [153]. The prohibition of inflammation attenuates atherosclerosis, thus playing a role in heart disease and stroke [182].

18.5   BENEFITS OF HERBS IN ISCHEMIC DISEASE

- As discussed earlier, the whole herb is more effective than a single component of the herb. We encourage using the whole herb instead of a compound because the benefits could come from as yet unidentified substances in combination with known factors.
- Efficacy of a formula is stronger than a single herb. While the combination of herbs works significantly, each single herb in the formula does not individually show effectiveness [186–189]. For example, shengmai san protects brain ischemia injury, but none of its components independently protect the brain from the insult [189]. Thus, intake of a single herb provides nutrition, not pharmacological efficacy.
- Apply the herbal therapy according to the therapeutic strategy of TCM.
- Some Chinese herbs may supplement nutrition to influence neurogenesis through growth factors [182, 190]. Phytochemicals may encourage self-repair via inhibiting inflammation and improving blood supply in infarct to provide the newborn neurons with an appropriate environment for growth [191].
- After treatment with modified Buyang-Huawu Tang for 4 weeks, stop taking *scutellaria baicalensis, paeonia veitchii,* and *paeonia suffruticosa.* Remove them from the prescription.
- *Ligusticum wallichii, angelica sinensis, carthamus tinctorius, prunus persica, radix astragalas* and ginkgo should be used with caution during pregnancy because they may stimulate uterine constriction and prolong bleeding time during delivery [49–51,192].

18.6   DOSAGES, PREPARATION, AND ADMINISTRATION OF HERBS

The dosages of all of the dry crude herbs for an adult per day are listed in Table 18.2. The dosages are small. However, small amounts of phytochemicals also have a protective effect when they are combined [182]. At these dosages, all of the herbs listed in the chapter are nontoxic. Their LD_{50} was tested and revealed no toxicity [51,73,88,192], except in the case of *Paeonia veitchii* and *Paeonia suffruticosa,* which have very low toxicity. The herbs, except *Scutellaria baicalensis, Paeonia veitchii* and *Paeonia suffruticosa,* are little bit sweet. We may cook them in chicken soup.

TABLE 18.2

Dosage and LD50 of Herbs

Name in Latin	Name in Chinese	Dosage g/day/adult	Toxicity	Possible Side Effect	LD$_{50}$
Ligusticum Wallichii	川芎, Chuan Xiong	3–9	Nontoxic		65.9 ± 31.3g/kg
Angelica sinensis	当归, Dang Gui	6–15	Nontoxic	Bleeding	None
Carthamus tinctorius	红花, Hong Hua	3–9	Nontoxic		None
Astragalus membranaceus	黄芪, Huang Qi	10–15	Nontoxic		None
Prunus persica	桃仁, Tao Ren	6–9	Nontoxic		222.5 ± 7.5 g/kg
Scutellaria Baicalensis	黄芩, Huang Qin	3–9	Nontoxic when given orally	Nausea	None
Paeonia veitchii	赤芍, Chi Shao	6–12	Low toxicity		None
Paeonia suffruticosa	牡丹皮, Mu Dan Pi	6–12	Low toxicity		3.43g/kg
Glycyrrhiza uralensis	甘草, Gan Cao	3–6	Nontoxic		None
Ginseng	人参, Renshen	3–9	Nontoxic		5g/kg
Ginkgo biloba	銀杏叶, Yin Xing Ye		Nontoxic	Nausea, vomiting, appetite loss, headache	7725 mg
Fructus Crataegus pinnatifida	山楂, Shan Zha	10–15	Nontoxic	Nausea, vomiting,	33.8 ml/kg of 10% extract in water
Anemarrhena asphodeloides Bunge	知母, Zhi Mu	3–15	Nontoxic		N/A
Gastrodia elata Blume	天麻, Tian Ma	3–9	Nontoxic		N/A
Epimedium brevicorum	淫羊藿, Yin Yang Huo	10–15	Nontoxic	Nausea, vomiting, dryness of the mouth	N/A
Fruit of Lycium chinense	枸杞子, Gou Qi Zi	9–15	Nontoxic		N/A
Ophiopogon japonicus	麦冬, Mai Don	6–15	Nontoxic	Abdominal distension, gas	N/A
Fructus Schisandra chinensis	五味子, Wu Wei Zi	3–9	Nontoxic		5g/kg in mice do not induce mortality
Cinnamomum cassia	桂枝, Gui Zhi	3–10	Nontoxic		N/A

18.6.1 DECOCTION

Decoction, the medicinal cocktail, is produced by boiling the herbs in water. It is easily prepared in the home. The chosen herbs for 1 day are macerated in 500 ml of cold water and boiled in an inert container. The macerate is brought to a quick boil within 2–3 minutes and then simmered for

45 minutes. Decoction is very popular and widely employed in CM practice [49]. Almost all of the active compounds of herbs can be extracted by this preparation [183]. Decoction leads to a better bioavailability because aqueous extracts are absorbed fast, give a rapid onset of action, and provide longer and higher efficacy than other preparations and administration [140,142,155,193]. The decoction is drunk warm. The microwave oven should be avoided for the preparation of the cocktail.

18.7 GLOSSARY

18.7.1 Definitions Used in Medical Research

Ischemia deficiency of blood in a body part caused functional constriction or actual obstruction of a blood vessel.
Insult in medical field, insult means the injury induced by diseases or trauma. In this chapter, insult indicates the ischemia episode produced by the animal experiments.
Sham rats the rats receive surgery but not ischemia. Thus, their brains have no injury and are normal in an experimental stroke study.
BBB abbreviation for blood–brain barrier. The barrier separates blood from the parenchyma of the central nervous system. It consists of the walls of the blood vessels and the surrounding glial membranes.
ROS reactive oxygen species.
Antioxidant oxidation reactions can produce free radicals that damage cells. Oxidative stress has been implicated in the pathogenesis of stroke, cancer, and neurodegenerative diseases including Alzheimer's disease and Parkinson's disease. Any substance that reduces oxidative damage caused by ROS is antioxidant. Well-known antioxidants include vitamins C, E, and β-carotene, the precursor of vitamin A.
Phytochemicals this word is from the Greek word *phyton*, meaning "plant." Phytochemicals refer to chemicals called flavonoids and saponins, etc., in plants. The do not include proteins, carbohydrates, lipids, vitamins, or minerals.
Anion an ion carrying a negative charge. The anions include all the nonmetals, the acid radicals, and the hydroxyl ion.
Ion an atom having a positive charge.
Hippocampus the region in the brain involved in the control of emotion, attention, and memory. Neurons in hippocampus CA1 are vulnerable to global forebrain ischemia.

18.7.2 TCM Terminology

Yin and Yang a philosophy of ancient China as applied in TCM to explain the mechanisms of diseases and to guide diagnosis and treatment. Yin and Yang are the two fundamental principles in the universe, opposing and supplementing each other. All things have Yin and Yang, the two opposing yet interdependent components. Yin and Yang depend on and control each other. When Yin is excessive, Yang will be too weak, and vice versa. In addition, they create each other, thus, Yin and Yang transform to each other. Ideally, Yin and Yang are always in a state of dynamic balance. Health is the balance between Yin and Yang in the human body. The basic pathogenesis of a disease is the imbalance of Yin and Yang in the body. Diseases are classified as Yin pattern and Yang pattern, which are subdivided into deficient Yin, excess Yin, excess Yang, and deficient Yang patterns. Chinese medicine attempts to achieve a balance between Yin and Yang, thus to restore the body's harmony and to obtain health.
Liver the liver in TCM includes the liver as understood by Western medicine, but also involves part of the central nervous system, the vegetative nervous system, retina, and blood vessels.

Kidney the kidney of TCM includes the kidney, urinary system, reproductive system, part of the endocrine system, and the nervous system.

ACKNOWLEDGMENT

The assistance of Susan B. Peterson, B.A., M.A. in editing the manuscript is gratefully acknowledged.

REFERENCES

1. Pollack A. 2006. AstraZeneca stroke drug fails in a clinical trial. *The New York Times*. October 27:C4.
2. Cheng YD, Al-Khoury L, Zivin JA. 2004. Neuroprotection for ischemic stroke: Two decades of success and failure. *NeuroRx* 1:36–45.
3. Lo EH, Broderick JP, Moskowitz MA. 2004. tPA and proteolysis in the neurovascular unit. *Stroke* 35:354–356.
4. Lo EH, Dalkara T, Moskowitz MA. 2003. Mechanisms, challenges and opportunities in stroke. *Nature Rev Neurosci* 4:399–414.
5. Gong X, Sucher NJ. 2002. Stroke therapy in traditional Chinese medicine (TCM): Prospects for drug discovery and development. *Phytomedicine* 9:478–484.
6. Kim H. 2005. Neuroprotective herbs for stroke therapy in traditional eastern medicine. *Neurological Res* 27: 287–301.
7. Shi FL, Hart RG, Sherman DG, et al. 1989. Stroke in the People's Republic of China. *Stroke* 20:1581–1585.
8. Moskowitz MA, Lo EH. 2003. Neurogenesis and apoptotic cell death. *Stroke* 34:324–326.
9. Ginsberg MD. 2003. Adventures in the pathophysiology of brain ischemia: Penumbra, gene expression, neuroprotection: The 2002 Thomas Willis Lecture. *Stroke* 34: 214–223.
10. Mena H, Cadavid D, Rushing EJ. 2004. Human cerebral infarct: A proposed histopathologic classification based on 137 cases. *Acta Neuropathol* 108:524–530.
11. Lin B, Ginsberg MD. 2000. Quantitative assessment of the normal microvasculature by endothelial barrier antigen (EBA) immunohistochemistry: Application to focal cerebral ischemia. *Brain Res.* 865: 237–244.
12. Garcia JH, Liu KF, Yoshida Y, Chen S, Lian J. 1994. Brain microvessel: Factors altering their patency after the occlusion of a middle cerebral artery (Wistar rat]. *Am J Pathol* 145:728 –740.
13. Garcia JH, Liu KF, Yoshida Y, Lian J, Chen S, del Zoppo GJ. 1994. Influx of leukocytes and platelets in an evolving brain infarct (Wistar rat]. *Am J Pathol* 144:188 –199.
14. Heye N, Paetzold C, Cerbos-Navarro J. 1991. The role of microthrombi and microcirculatory factors in localization and evolution of focal cerebral ischemia. *Neurosurg Rev* 14:7–16.
15. Zhang ZG, Zhang L, Tsang W, Goussev A, Powers C, Ho KL, et al. 2001. Dynamic platelet accumulation at the site of the occluded middle cerebral artery and in downstream microvessel is associated with loss of microvascular integrity after embolic middle cerebral artery occlusion. *Brain Res* 912:181–194
16. Akopov S, Sercombe R, Seylaz J. 1996. Cerebraovascular reactivity: Role of endothelium/platelet/leukocyte interactions. *Cerebrovasc Brain Metab Rev* 8:11–94.
17. Mehta JL, Nicolini FA, Donnelly WH, Nichols WW. 1992. Platelet–leukocyte–endothelial interactions in coronary artery disease. *Am J Cardiol* 69:8B–13B.
18. Kudo T, Takeda M, Tanimukai S, Nishimura T. 1993. Neuropathologic changes in the gerbil brain after chronic hypoperfusion. *Stroke* 24:259–265.
19. Damjanov I. 1996. Inflammation. In *The Pathology for the health-related professions*. Philadelphia: W.B. Saunders Co. pp. 24–43.
20. O'Banion MK. 1999. Cyclooxygenase-2: molecular biology, pharmacology, and neurobiology. *Crit Rev Neurobiol* 13:45–82.
21. Nogawa S, Forster C, Zhang F, Nagayama M, Ross ME, Iadecola C. 1998. Interaction between inducible nitric oxide synthase and cyclooxygenase-2 after cerebral ischemia. *Proc Natl Acad Sci USA.* 95:10966–10971.
22. Iadecola C, Alexander M. 2001. Cerebral ischemia and inflammation. *Curr Opin Neurol* 14:89–94.
23. Iadecola C, Forster C, Nogawa S, Clark HB, Ross ME. 1999. Cyclooxygenase-2 immunoreactivity in the human brain following cerebral ischemia. *Acta Neuropathol* 98:9–14.

24. Michiels C, Arnould T, Knott I, Dieu M, Remacle J. 1993. Stimulation of prostaglandin synthesis by human endothelial cells exposed to hypoxia. *Am J Physiol* 264 (4 Pt 1): C866–874.

25. Sairanen T, Ristimaki A, Karjalainen-Lindsberg ML, Paetau a, Kaste M, Lindsberg PJ. 1998. Cyclooxygenase-2 is induced globally in infarcted human brain. *Ann Neurol* 43:738–747.

26. Tomimoto H, Akiguchi I, Wakita H, Lin JX, Budka H. 2000. Cyclooxygenase-2 is induced in microglia during chronic cerebral ischemia in human. *Acta Neuropathol* 99:26–30.

27. Strauss KI, Barbe MF, Marshall RM, Raghupathi R, Mehta S, Narayan RK. 2000. Prolonged Cyclooxygenase-2 induction in neurons and glia following traumatic brain injury in the rat. *J Neurotrauma.* 17:695–711.

28. Barone FC, Feuerstein GZ. 1999. Inflammatory mediators and stroke: New opportunities for novel therapeutics. *J Cereb Blood Flow Metab* 19:819–834.

29. Hara K, Kong DL, Sharp FR, Weinstein PR. 1998. Effect of selective inhibition of cyclooxygenase-2 on temporary focal cerebral ischemia in rats. *Neurosci Lett* 256:53–56.

30. Dóre S, Otsuka T, Mito T, Sugo N, Hand T, Wu L, et al. 2003. Neuronal overexpression of cyclooxygenase-2 increases cerebral infarction. *Ann Neurol* 54:155–162.

31. Chan PH. 2005. Mitochondrial dysfunction and oxidative stress as determinants of cell death/survival in stroke. *Ann NY Acad Sci* 1042:203–209.

32. Tatemichi TK, Paik M, Bagiella E, Desmond DW, Pirro M, hanzawa LK. 1994. Dementia after stroke is a predictor of long-term survival. *Stroke* 25:1915–1919.

33. Tatemichi TK, Paik M, Bagiella E, Desmond DW, Stern Y, Sano M, et al. 1994. Risk of dementia after stroke in a hospitalized cohort: Results of a longitudinal study. *Neurology* 44:1885–1891.

34. Fujioka M, Okuchi K, Sakaki T, Hiranatsu KI, Miyamoto S, Iwasaki S. 1994. Specific changes in human brain following reperfusion after cardiac arrest. *Stroke* 25:2091–2095.

35. Furlan AJ, Sila CA, Chimowitz MI, Jones SC. 1992. Neurological complications related to cardiac surgery. *Neurol Clin* 10:145–166.

36. Harrison MJ. 1995. Neurologic complications of coronary artery bypass grafting: Diffuse or focal ischemia? *Ann Thorac Surg* 59:1356–1358.

37. Wisniewski HM, Maslinska D. 1996. Beta-protein immunoreactivity in the human brain after cardiac arrest. *Folia Neuropathol* 34:65–71.

38. Jendroska K, Poewe w, Daniel SE, Pluess J, Iwerssen-Schmidt H, Paulsen J, et al. 1995. Ischemic stress induces deposition of amyloid beta immunoreactivity in human brain. *Acta Neuropathol* 90:461–466.

39. Nakayama M, Uchimura K, Zhu RL, Magayama T, Rose M, Stetler RA, et al. 1998. Cyclooxygenase-2 inhibition prevents delayed death of CA1 hippocampal neurons following global ischemia. *Proc Natl Acad Sci USA* 95: 10954–10959.

40. Dietrich WD, Lin B, Globus MY-T, Green EJ, Ginsberg MD, Busto R. 1995. Effect of delayed MK-801 [Dizocilpine] treatment with or without immediate postischemic hypothermia on chronic neuronal survival after global forebrain ischemia in rats. *J Cereb Blood Flow Meteb* 15:960–968.

41. Lin B, Ginsberg MD, Busto R, Dietrich WD. 1998. Sequential analysis of subacute and chronic neuronal, astrocytic and microglial alterations after transient global ischemia in rats. *Acta neuropathol* 95:511–523.

42. Lin B, Schmidt-Kastner R, Busto R, Ginsberg MD. 1999. progressive parenchymal deposition of β-amyloid precursor protein in rat brain following global cerebral ischemia. *Acta neuropathol* 97:359–368.

43. Lin B, Ginsberg MD. 2000. The roles of β-amyloid precursor protein and amyloid β peptide in ischemic brain injury. In *Pharmacology of cerebral ischemia 2000*, J. Krieglstein and S. Klumpp (Eds.) pp. 37–52. Stuttgart: Medpharm Scientific Publishers.

44. Chan PH. 2004. Future targets and cascades for neuroprotective strategies. *Stroke* 35 (suppl I): 2748–2750.

45. Yermakova A, O'Banion MK. 2000. Cyclooxygenases in the central nervous system: Implications for treatment of neurological disorders. *Curr Pharm Des* 6:1755–1776.

46. Block F, Bozdag I, Nolden-Koch M. 2001. Inflammation contributes to the postponed ischemic neuronal damage following treatment with a glutamate antagonist in rats. *Neurosci Lett* 298:103–106.

47. Coimbra C, Drake M, Boris-Moller F, Wieloch T. 1996. Long-lasting neuroprotective effect of post-ischemic hypothermia and treatment with an anti-inflammatory/antipyretic drug. Evidence for chronic encephalopathic processes following ischemia. *Stroke* 27:1578–1585.

48. Davis S, Helfaer MA, Traystman RJ, Hurn PD. 1997. Parallel antioxidant and antiexcitotoxic therapy improves outcome after incomplete global cerebral ischemia in dogs. *Stroke* 28:198–204.

49. Hue ZG. 1994. *Traditional Chinese medicine, the textbook for medical school.* 3rd ed. Beijing: People's Health Publisher (in Chinese).
50. Li R. 1993. Medicines to improve circulation and clean out blood stasis. In *Chinese medicine pharmacology*, 2nd ed. Li YK, and Jiang MY (Eds.), pp.129–146. Beijing: Chinese Medicine of China (in Chinese).
51. Huang KC. 1999. *The pharmacology of Chinese herbs*, 2nd ed. Boca Raton: CRC Press LLC.
52. Watanabe H. 1997. Candidates for cognitive enhancer extracted from medicinal plants: Paeoniflorin and tetramethylpyrazine. *Behav Brain Res* 83:135–141.
53. Ye X. Medicines to improve circulation and clean out blood stasis. 1993, In *Chinese medicine* Ye X (Ed.) pp.377–379. 3rd ed. Shanghai: Shanghai Chinese Medicine School Publisher (in Chinese).
54. Wu W, qiu F. 1994. Experimental study on ischemia and reperfusion injury of rat liver and effects of ligustrazine and salvia compound. *Chin Med Sci J* 9:162–166.
55. Hua J, En-tan G. 1996. Effect of postoperative treatment with a combination of Chuan Xiong and electret on functional recovery of muscle grafts: An experimental study in the dog. *Plast Reconstr Surg* 98:851–855.
56. Li S, Wang JH, Chen SL. 1999. Inhibitory effect of ligustrazine on proliferation of rabbit vascular smooth muscle cells after arterial injury. *Zhonguo Yao Li Xue Bao* 20:917–922.
57. Cao W, Zeng Z, Zhu YJ, Luo W, Demura H, Naruse M, Shi Y. 1998. Effects of tetramethylpyrazine, a Chinese medicine, on plasma endothelin-1 levels during acute pulmonary hypoxia in anesthetized dogs. *J Cardiovasc Pharmacol* 31 Suppl 1:S456–459.
58. Zheng Z, Zhu W, Zhou X, Jin Z, Liu H, Chen X, et al. 1998. Tetramethylpyrazine, a Chinese drug, blocks coronary vasoconstriction by endothelin-1 and decreases plasma endothelin-1 levels in experimental animals. *J Cardiovasc Pharmacol.* 31 suppl1: S313–316.
59. Feng J, Liu R, Wu G, Tang S. 1997. Effects of tetramethylpyrazine on the release of PGI2 and TXA2 in the hypoxic isolated rat heart. *Mol Cell Biochem* 167:153–158.
60. Peng w, Hucks D, Priest RM, Kan YM, Ward JP. 1996. Ligustrazine-induced endothelium-dependent relaxation in pulmonary arteries via a NO-mediated and exogenous L-arginine-dependent mechanism. *Br J Pharmacol* 119:1063–1071.
61. Sheu JR, Hsiao G, Lee YM, Yen MH. 2001. Antithrombotic effects of tetramethylpyrazine in vivo experiments. *Int J Hematol* 73:393–398.
62. Sheu JR, Kan YC, Hung WC, Lin CH, Yen MH. 2000. The antiplatelet activity of tetramethylpyrazine is mediated through activation of NO synthase. *Life Sci* 67:937–947.
63. Sheu JR, Kan YC, Hung WC, Ko WC, Yen MH. 1997. Mechanisms involved in the antiplatelet activity of tetramethlpyrazine in human platelets. *Thromb Res* 88:259–270.
64. Zhang Z, Wei T, Hou J, Li G, Yu S, Xin W. 2003. Iron-induced oxidative damage and apoptosis in cerebellar granule cells: Attenuation by tetramethylpyrazine and ferulic acid. *Eur J Pharmacol* 467:41–47.
65. Hsiao G, Chen YC, Lin JH, Lin KH, Chou DS, Lin CH, Sheu JR. 2006. Inhibitory mechanisms of tetramethylpyrazine in middle cerebral artery occlusion (MCAO)-induced focal cerebral ischemia in rats. *Planta Med* 72:411–417.
66. Pang PK, Shan JJ, Chiu KW. 1996. Tetramethylpyrazine, a calcium antagonist. *Planta Med* 62:431–435.
67. Liang CC, Hong CY, Chen CF, Tsai TH. 1999. Measurement and pharmacokinetic study of tetramethylpyrazine in rat blood and its regional brain tissue by high-performance liquid chromatography. *J Chromotogr B Biomed Sci Appl* 724:303–309.
68. Tsai TH, Liang C. 2001. Pharmacokinetics of tetramethylpyrazine in rat blood and brain using microdialysis. *Int J Pharm* 216:61–66.
69. Ozaki Y. 1992. Anti-inflammatory effect of tetramethylpyrazine and ferulic acid. *Chem Pharm Bull* (Tokyo) 40:954–956.
70. Yang JW, Ouyang JP, Liao WJ, Liu YM, Wang BH, Li K. 2005. The effects of Chinese herb Angelica in focal cerebral ischemia injury in the rat. *Clin Hemorheol Microcirc* 32:209–215.
71. Rhyu MR, Kim JH, Kim EY. 2005. Radix angelica elicits both nitric oxide-dependent and calcium influx-mediated relaxation in rat aorta. *J Cardiovasc Pharmacol.* 46:99–104.
72. Xiaohong Y. Jing–Ping OY, Shuzheng T. Angelica protects the human vascular endothelial cell from the effects of oxidized low-density lipoprotein in vitro. *Clin Hemorheol Microcire* 2000. 22:317–323.
73. Liu C and Hu Y. 1993, Anti-inflammatory herbs. In *Chinese Medicine Pharmacology*, 2nd ed. Li YK, and Jiang MY (Eds.) pp.48–78. Beijing: Chinese Medicine of China (in Chinese).
74. Zhang HL, Nagatsu A, Watanabe T, Sakakibara J, Okuyama H. 1997a. Antioxidative compounds isolated from safflower (*Carthamus tinctorius L.*) oil cake. *Chem Pharm Bull* (Tokyo) 45:1910–1914.

75. Leung AW, Mo ZX, Zheng YS. 1991. Reduction of cellular damage induced by cerebral ischemia in rats. *Neurochem Res* 16:687–692.
76. Romano C, Price M, Bai HY, Olney JW. 1993. Neuroprotectants in Honghua: Glucose attenuates retinal ischemic damage. *Invest Ophthalmol Vis Sci* 34:72–80.
77. Zhu H, Wang Z, Ma C, Tian J, Fu F, Li C, et al. 2003. Neuroprotective effects of hydroxyl safflower yellow a: In vivo and in vitro studies. *Plant Med* 69:429–433.
78. Xue j W, Ichikawa H, Konishi T. 2001. Antioxidant potential of qizhu tang, a chinese herbal medicine, and the effect on cerebral oxidative damage after ischemia reperfusion rats. *Biol Pharm Bull* 24:558–563.
79. He X, Li C, Yu S. 2000. Protective effects of radix astragali against anoxic damages to in vitro cultured neurons. *J Tongii Med Univ* 20:126–127.
80. Shon YH, Nam KS. 2003. Protective effect of astragali radix extract on interleukin 1 beta induced inflammation in human amnion. *Phytother Res* 17:1016–1020.
81. Gui SY, Wei W, Wang H, Wu L, Sun WY, Chen WB, Wu CY. 2006. Effects and mechanisms of crude astragalosides fraction on liver fibrosis in rats. *J Ethnopharmacol* 103(2):154–9.
82. Zhang WJ, Wojta J, Binder BR. 1997b. Regulation of the fibrinolytic potential of cultured human umbilical vein endothelial cells. astragaloside IV downregulates plasminogen activator inhibitor-1 and upregulates tissue-type plasminogen activatior expression. *J Vasc Res* 34:273–280.
83. Song ZH, Ji ZN, Lo CK, Dong TT, Zhao KJ, Li OT, et al. 2004. Chemical and biological assessment of a traditional Chinese herbal decoction prepared from Radix Astragali and Radix *Angelicae Sinensis*: Orthogonal array design to optimize the extraction of chemical constituents. *Planta Med.* 70:1222–1227.
84. Lei Y, Wang JH, Chen KJ. 2003. Comparative study on angiogenesis effect of *Astragalus membranaceus* and *Angelica Sinensis* in chick embryo choriollantoic membrane. *Zhongguo Zhong Yao Za Zhi* 28:876–878 (in Chinese).
85. Cai Q, Li X, Wang H. 2001. Astragali and angelica protect the kidney against ischemia and reperfusion injury and accelerate recovery. *Chin Med J* [Eng] 114:119–123.
86. Xue JX, Yan YQ, Jiang Y. 1994. Effects of the combination of *Astragulus membranaceus* [*Fisch.*] Bge. [AM], *Angelica Sinensis* [Oliv.] diels [TAS], *Cyperus Rotundus L.* [CR], *Ligusticum Chuanxiong* [LC] and *Peaonia Veitchii Lynch* [PV] on the hemorheological changes in "blood stagnation" rats. *Zhongguo Zhong Yao Za Zhi* 19:108–128 (in Chinese).
87. Yim TK, Wu WK, Pak WF, Mak DHF, Liang SM, Ko KM. 2000. Myocardial protection against ischemia-reperfusion injury by a *Polygonum multi-flrum* extract supplemented 'Dang-Gui decoction for enriching blood', a compound formulation, ex vivo. *Phytotherapy Res* 14:195–199.
88. Li X, Bai X, Qin L, Huang H, Xiao Z, Gao T. 2003. Neuroprotective effects of Buyang huanwu decoction on neuronal injury in hippocampus after transient forebrain ischemia in rats. *Neurosci Lett.* 346:29–32.
89. Chen Y, Yang L, Lee TJ. 2000. Oroxylin A inhibition of lipopolysaccharide-induced iNOS and COX-2 gene expression via suppression of nuclear factor-kappaB activation. *Biochem Pharmacol* 59:1445–1457.
90. Lim BO, Yu BP, Kim SC, Park DK. 1999. The antioxidative effect of ganhuangenin against lipid peroxidation. *Phytother Res* 13:479–483.
91. Shieh DE, Liu LT, Lin CC. 2000. Antioxidant and free radical scavenging effects of baicalein, baicalin and wogonin. *Anticancer Res* 20:2861–2865.
92. You KM, Jong HG, Kim HP. 1999. Inhibition of cyclooxygenase/lipoxygenas from human platelets by polyhydroxylated/methoxylated flavonoids isolated from medicinal plants. *Arch Pharm Res* 22:18–24.
93. Hanasaki Y, Ogawa S, Fukui S. 1994. The correlation between active oxygen scavenging and antioxidative effects of flavonoids. *Free Radic Biol Med* 16:845–850.
94. Morimoto S, Tateishi N, Matsuda T, Tanaka H, Taura F, Furuya N, et al. 1998. Novel hydrogen peroxide metabolism in suspension cells of scutellaria baicalensis *Georgi* 273:12601–12611.
95. Shao ZH, Vanden H TL, Qin Y, Becker LB, Schumacker PT, et al. 2002. Baicalein attenuates oxidant stress in cardiomyocytes. *Am J Physiol Heart Circ Physiol* 282:H999–H1006.
96. Hamada H, Hiramatsu M, Edamatsu R, Mori A. 1993. Free radical scavenging action of baicalein. *Arch Biochem Biophys* 306:261–266.
97. Okuda S, Saito H, Katsuki H. 1994. Arachidonic acid: Toxic and trophic effects on cultured hippocampal neurons. *Neuroscience* 63:691–696.

98. Gao D, Tawa R, Masaki H, Okano Y, Sakurai H. 1998. Protective effects of baicalein against cell damage by reactive oxygen species. *Chem Pharm Bull* (Tokyo) 46:1383–1387.

99. Gao Z, Huang K, Yang X, Xu H. 2001. Protective effects of flavonoids in the roots of scutellaria baicalensis georgi against hydrogen peroxide-induced oxidative stress in HS-SY5Y cells. *Pharmacol Res* 43:173–178.

100. Kim YO, Leem K, Park J, Lee P, Ahn DK, et al. 2001. Cytoprotective effect of Scutellaria baicalensis in CA1 hippocampal neurons of rats after global cerebral ischemia. *J Ethnopharmacol* 77:183–188.

101. Shao ZH, Li CQ, Vanden H TL, Becker LB, Schumacker PT, et al. 1999. Extract from *Scutellaria baicalensis Georgi* attenuates oxidant stress in cardiomyocytes. *J Mol Cell Cardiol* 31:1885–1895.

102. Gao Z, Huang K, Yang X, Xu H. 1999. Free radical scavenging and antioxidant activities of flavonoids extracted from the radix of *Scutellaria baicalensis Georgi*. *Biochim Biophys Acta* 1472:643–650.

103. Gao D, Sakkurai K, Katoh M, Chen J, Ogiso T. 1996. Inhibition of microsomal lipid peroxidation by baicalein: a possible formation of an iron-baicalein complex. *Biochem Mol Biol Int* 39:21–25.

104. Tezuka Y, Irikawa S, Kaneko T, Banskota AH, Nagaoka T, et al. 2001. Screening of Chinese herbal drug extracts for inhibitory activity on nitric oxide production and identification of an active compound of *Zanthoxylum bungeanum*. *J Ethnopharmacol* 77:209–217.

105. Gabrielska J, Oszmianski J, Zylka R, Komorowska M. 1997. Antioxidant activity of flavones from *Scutellaria baicalensis* in lecithin liposomes. *Z Naturgorsch* [C] 52:817–823.

106. Yokozawa T, Dong E, Kawai Y, Gemba M, Shimizu M. 1999. Protective effects of some flavonoids on the renal cellular membrane. *Exp Toxicol Pathol* 51:9–14.

107. DeGeorge JJ, Walenga R, Carbonetto S. 1988. Nerve growth factor rapidly stimulates arachidonate metabolism in PC12 cells: potential involvement in nerve fiber growth. *J Neurosci Res* 21:323–332.

108. Kyo R, Nakahata N, Sakakibara I, Kubo M, Ohizumi Y. 1998. Baicalin and baicalein, constituents of an important medicinal plant, inhibit intracellular Ca^{2+} elevation by reducing phospholipase C activity in C6 rat glioma cell. *J Pharm Pharmacol* 50:1179–1182.

109. Li FQ, Wang Z, Liu PB, Hong JS. 2005a. Inhibition of microglial activation by the herbal flavonoid baicalein attenuates inflammation-mediated degeneration of dopaminergic neurons. *J Neural Transm* 112:331–347.

110. Lee H, Kim YO, Kim H, Kim SY, Noh HS, Kang SS, et al. 2003a. Flavonoid wogonin from medicinal herb is neuroprotective by inhibiting inflammatory activation of microglia. *FASEB J* 17: 1943–1944.

111. Son D, Le P, Lee J, Kim H, Kim SY. 2004. Neuroprotective effect of wogonin in hippocampal slice culture exposed to oxygen and glucose deprivation. *Eur J Pharmacol.* 493:99–102.

112. Cho J, Lee HK. 2004. Wogonin inhibits ischemic brain injury in a rat model of permanent middle cerebral artery occlusion. *Biol Pharm Bull* 27:1561–1564.

113. Lee HH, Yang LL, Wang CC, Hu SY, Chang SF, Lee YH. 2003b. Differential effects of natural polyphenols on neuronal survival in primary cultured central neurons against glutamate- and glucose deprivation-induced neuronal death. *Brain Res* 986:103–113.

114. Heo HJ, Kim DO, Choi SJ, Shin DH, Lee CY. 2004. Potent inhibitory effect of flavonoids in *Scutellaria baicalensis* on amyloid beta proteins-induced neurotoxicity. *J Agric Food Chem* 52:4128–4132.

115. Lebeau A, Esclaire F, Rostene W, Pelaprat D. 2001. Baicalein protects cortical neurons from β amyloid (25–35) induced toxicity. *Neuroreport* 12: 2199–2202.

116. Skovronsky DM, Lee V M-Y, Pratico D. 2001. Amyloid precursor protein and amyloid β peptide in human platelets. *J Bio Chem* 276: 17036–17043.

117. Di Luca M, Colciaghi F, Pastorino L, Borroni B, Padovani A, Cattabeni F. 2000. Platelets as a peripheral district where to study pathogenetic mechanisms of Alzheimer disease: The case of amyloid precursor protein. *Eur J Pharmacol* 405:277–283.

118. Cotman CW, Tenner AJ, Cummings BJ. 1996. β-amyloid converts an acute phase injury response to chronic injury responses. *Neurobiol Aging* 17:723–731.

119. Subramanian S, Bowyer MW, Egan JC, Knolmayer TJ. 1999. Attenuation of renal ischemia-reperfusion injury with selectin inhibition in a rabbit model. *Am J Surg* 178:573–576.

120. Chen Y-C, Shen S-C, Chen L-G, Lee TJ, Yang L. 2001. Wogonin, baicalin, and baicalein inhibition of inducible nitric oxide synthase and Cyclooxygenase-2 gene expressions induced by nitric oxide synthase inhibitors and lipopolysaccharide. *Bioch Pharmacol* 61:1417–1427.

121. Li BQ, Fu T, Gong W, Dunlop N, Kung H, yan Y, et al. 2000. The flavonoid baicalin exhibits anti-inflammatory activity by binding to chemokines. *Immunopharmacology* 49:295–306.

122. Krakauer T, Li BQ, Young HA. 2001. The flavonoid baicalin inhibits superantigen-induced inflammatory cytokines and chemokines. *FEBS Lett* 500:52–55.

123. Wakabayashi I. 1999. Inhibitory effects of baicalein and wogonin on lipopolysaccharide-induced nitric oxide production in macrophages. *Pharmacol Toxicol* 84:288–291.

124. Nakamura N, Hayasaka S, Zhang XY, Nagaki Y, Matsumoto M, Hayasaka Y, Terasawa K. 2003. Effects of baicalin, baicalein, and wogonin on interleukin-6 and interleukin-8 expression and nuclear factor-kappa B binding activities induced by interleukin-1 β in human retinal pigment epithelial cell line. *Exp Eye Res* 77:195–202.

125. Piao HZ, Jin SA, Chun HS, Lee JC, Kim WK. 2004. Neuroprotective effect of wogonin: Potential roles of inflammatory cytokines. *Arch Pharm Res* 27:930–936.

126. Shaw S, naegeli P, Etter JD, Weidmann P. 1995. Role of intracellular signaling pathways in hydrogen peroxide-induced injury to rat glomerular mesangial cells. *Clin Exp Pharmacol Physiol* 22:924–33.

127. Zhu M, Rajamani S, Kaylor J, Han S, Zhou, Fink AL. 2004. The flavonoid baicalein inhibits fibrillation of α-synuclein and disaggregates existing fibrils. *J Bio Chem* 279:26846–26857.

128. Lin CC, shieh DE. 1996. The anti-inflammatory activity of *Scutellaria rivularis* extracts and its active components, baicalin, baicalein and wogonin. *Am J Chin Med* 24:31–36.

129. Nakahata N, Kutsuwa M, Kyo R, Kubo M, Hayashi K, Ohizumi Y. 1998. Analysis of inhibitory effects of scutellariae radix and baicalein on prostaglandin E2 production in rat C6 glioma cells. *Am J Chin Med* 26:311–323.

130. Kimura Y, Matsushita N, Yokoi–Hayashi K, Okuda H. 2001. Effects of baicalein isolated from *Scutellaria baicalensis* Radix on adhesion molecule expression induced by thrombi and thrombin receptor agonist peptide in cultured human umbilical vein endothelial cells. *Planta med* 67:331–334.

131. Kimura Y, Matsushita N, Okuda H. 1997a. Effects of baicalein isolated from *Scutellaria baicalensis* on interleukin 1 beta- and tumor necrosis factor alpha-induced adhesion molecule expression in cultured human umbilical vein endothelial cells. *J Ethnopharmacol* 57:63–67.

132. Kimura Y, Okuda H, Ogita Z. 1997b. Effects of flavonoids isolated from scutellariae radix on fibrinolytic system induced by trypsin in human umbilical vein endothelial cells. *J Nat Prod* 60:598–601.

133. Kimura Y, Yokoi K, Matsushita N, Okuda H. 1997c. Effects of flavonoids isolated from scutellariae radix on the production of tissue-type plasminogen activator and plasminogen activator inhibitor-1 induced by thrombin and thrombin receptor agonist peptide in cultured human umbilical vein endothelial cells. *J Pharm Pharmacol* 49:816–822.

134. Higashitani A, Tabata S, Hayashi T, Hotta Y. 1989. Plant saponins can affect DNA recombination in cultured mammalian cells. *Cell Struct Funct* 14:617–624.

135. Ohtsuka M, Fukuda K, Yano H, Kojiro M. 1995. Effects of nine active ingredients in Chinese herbal medicine sho-saiko-to on 2-[2-furyl]-3-[5-nitro-2-furyl] acrylamide mutagenicity. *Jpn J Cancer Res* 86:1131–1135.

136. Chen X, Nishida H, Konishi T. 2003. Baicalin promoted the repair of DNA single strand breakage caused by H_2O_2 in cultured NIH3T3 fibroblasts. *Biol Pharm Bull* 26:282–284.

137. Stanke-Labesque F, Devillier P, Bedouch P, Cracowski JL, Chavanon O, Bessard G. 2000. Angiotensin II-induced contractions in human internal mammary artery: Effects of cyclooxygenase and lipoxygenase inhibition. *Cardiovasc Res* 47:376–383.

138. Akao T, Kawabata K, yanagisawa E, ishihara K, Mizuhar Y, Wakui Y, et al. 2000. Baicalin, the predominant flavone glucuronide of scutellariae radix, is absorbed from the rat gastrointestinal tract as the aglycone and restored to its original form. *J Pharm Pharmacol* 52:1563–1568.

139. Tsai TH, Liu SC, Tsai PL, Ho LK, Shum AYC, Chen CF. 2002. The effects of the cyclosporin A, a P-glycoprotein inhibitor, on the pharmacokinetics of baicalein in the rat: A microdialysis study. *Br J Pharmacol* 137:1314–1320.

140. Lai MY, Chen CC, Hsiu SL, Chao PD. 2001. Analysis and comparison of baicalin, baicalein and wogonin contents in traditional decoctions and commercial extracts of Scutellariae radix. *J Food Drug Analy* 3:145–149.

141. Lai MY, Hsiu SL, Chen CC, Hou YC, Lee Chao PD. 2003. Urinary pharmacokinetics of baicalein, wogonin and their glycosides after oral administration of scutellariae radix in human. *Biol Pharm Bull* 26:79–83.

142. Homma M, Oka K, Taniguchi C, Nitsuma T, Hayashi T. 1997. Systematic analysis of post-administrative Saiboku-To urine by liquid chromatography to determine pharmacokinetics of traditional Chinese Medicine. *Biomed Chromatogr* 11:125–131.

143. Zhang L, Xing D, Wang W, Wang R, Du L. 2006. Kinetic difference of baicalin in rat blood and cerebral nuclei after intravenous administration of scutellariae radix extract. *J Ethnopharmacol* 103:120–125.

144. Choi BM, Kim HJ, Oh GS, Pae HO, Oh H, Jeong S T. et al. 2002. 1,2,3,4,6-Penta-O-galloyl-beta-D-glucose protects rat neuronal cells (Neuro 2A) from hydrogen peroxide-mediated cell death via the induction of heme oxyenase-1. *Neurosci Lett* 328:185–189.

145. Prieto JM, Recio MC, Giner RM, Manez S, Giner-Larza EM, Rios JL. 2003. Influence of traditional Chinese anti-inflammatory medicinal plants on leukocyte and platelet functions. *J Pharm Pharmacol* 55:1375–1282.

146. Goto H, Shimada Y, Tanaka N, Tanigawa K, Itoh T, Terasawa K. 1999. Effect of extract prepared from the roots of *Paeonia lactiflora* on endothelium-dependent relaxation and antioxidant enzyme activity in rats administered high-fat diet. *Phytother Res* 13:526–528.

147. Chen LC, Chou MH, Lin MF, Yang LL. 2002. Pharmacokinetics of paeoniflorin after oral administration of Shao-yao-Gan-chao Tang in mice. *Jpn J Pharmacol* 88:250–255.

148. Yasuda T, Kon R, Nakazawa T, Ohsawa K. 1999. Metabolism of paeonol in rats. *J Nat Prod* 62:1142–1144.

149. Hsieh CL, Cheng CY, Tsai TH, Lin IH, Liu CH, Chiang SY, et al. 2006. Paeonol reduced cerebral infarction involving the superoxide anion and microglia activation in ischemia-reperfusion injured rats. *J Ethnopharmacol* 106:208–205.

150. Zhang GQ, Hao XM, Chen SZ, Zhou PA, Cheng HP, Wu CH. 2003. Blockade of paeoniflorin on sodium current in mouse hippocampal CA1 neurons. *Acta Pharmacol Sinica* 24:1248–1252.

151. Yan D, Saito K, Ohmi Y, Fujie N, Ohtsuka K. 2004. Paeoniflorin, a novel heat shock protein-inducing compound. *Cell Stress Chaperones* 9:378–389.

152. Lee SJ, Lee IS, Mar W. 2003. inhibition of inducible nitric oxide synthase and Cyclooxygenase-2 activity by 1,2,3,4,6-penta-O-galloyl-beta-D-glucose in murine macrophage cells. *Arch Pharm Res* 26:832–839.

153. Kang DG, Moon MK, Choi DH, Lee JK, Kwon TO, Lee HS. 2005. Vasodilatory and anti-inflammatory effects of the 1,2,3,4,6-penta-O-galloyl-beta-D-glucose (PGG) via a nitric oxide-cGMP pathway. *Eur J Pharmacol* 524:111–119.

154. Huang Z, Cui Z. 1993. Tonics. In *Chinese medicine pharmacology*, 2nd ed. Li YK, and Jiang MY (Eds.) pp. 177–205. Beijing: Chinese Medicine of China (in Chinese).

155. Chen LC, Lee MH, Chou MH, Lin MF, Yang LL. 1999. Pharmacokinetic study of paeoniflorin in mice after oral administration of paeoniae radix extract. *J Chromatogr B Biomed Sci Appl* 735:33–40.

156. Oh JK, Hyun SY, Oh HR, Jung JW, Park C, Lee S, et al. 2007. Effects of *Anemarrhena asphodeloides* on focal ischemic brain injury induced by middle cerebral artery occlusion in rats. *Biol Pharm Bull* 30:38–43.

157. Yu SJ, Kim JR, Lee CK, Han JE, Lee JH. 2005. *Gastrodia elata Blume* and an active component, p-Hydroxybenzyl alcohol, reduce focal ischemic brain injury through antioxidant related gene expressions. *Biol Pharm Bull* 28:1016–1020.

158. Kim H, Lee S, Moon K. 2003. Ether fraction of methanol extracts of *Gastrodia elata*, medicinal herb protects against neuronal cell damage after transient global ischemia in gerbils. *Phytothery Res* 17:909–912.

159. Li L, Zhou Q, Shi J. 2005b. Protective effects of icariin on neurons injured by cerebral ischemia/reperfusion. *Chin Med J* 118:1637–1643.

160. Sun S. Wu Wei Zi. 1993. In *Chinese medicine pharmacology*, 2nd ed. Li YK, and Jiang MY (Eds.) pp. 207–208. Beijing: Chinese Medicine of China (in Chinese).

161. Burguete MC, Torregrosa G, Pérez-Asensio FJ, Castelló-Ruiz M, Salom JB, et al. 2006. Dietary phytoestrogens improve stroke outcome after transient focal cerebral ischemia in rats. *Eur J Neurosci* 23:703–710.

162. Lin B. 2008. Integrating comprehensive and alternative medicine into stroke: Herbal treatment of ischemia In: Commentary and alternative therapies and aging population. RR Watson (Ed.) pp. 229–274. New York: Elsevier.

163. Krupinski J, Kaluza J, Kumar P, Kumar S, Wang JM. 1994. Role of angiogenesis in patients with cerebral ischemic stroke. *Stroke* 25:1794–1798.

164. Gao D, Song J, Hu J, Lin J, Zheng L, Cai J, du J, Chen K. 2005. Angiogenesis promoting effects of Chinese herbal medicine for activating blood circulation to remove stasis on chick embryo chorio–allantoic membrane. *Zhong Xi Jie He Za Zhi* 25:912–915.

165. Chen W, Lu YP. Shengmai San. 1993. In *Formulae of Chinese medicine*, 2nd ed. Chen W and Lu YP (Eds.) pp. 200–204. Shanghai: School of Traditional Chinese Medicine of Shanghai.

166. Ichikawa H, Wang L, Konishi T. 2003. Role of component herbs in antioxidant activity of shengmai san—a traditional Chinese medicine formula preventing cerebral oxidative damage in rat. *Am J Chin Med* 31: 509–521.
167. Ichikawa H, Wang L, Konishi T. 2006. Prevention of cerebral oxidative injury by post-ischemic intravenous administration of Shengmai San. *Am J Chin Med* 34: 591–600.
168. Cherubini A, Polidori MC, Bregnocchi M, Pezzuto S, Cecchetti R, Ingegni T, et al. 2000. Antioxidant profile and early outcome in stroke patients. *Stroke* 31:2295–2300.
169. Kwun IS, Park KH, Jang HS, Beattie JH, Kwon CS. 2005. Lower antioxidant vitamins (A, C, and E) and trace minerals (Zn, Cu, Mn, Fe and Se) status in patients with cerebrovascular disease. *Nutr Neurosci* 8:251–257.
170. Clemens JA, Stephenson DT, Smalstig EB, Roberts EF, Johnstone EM, Sharp JD, et al. 1996. Reactive glia express cytosolic phospholipase A2 after transient global forebrain ischemia in the rat. *Stroke* 27:527–535.
171. Farooqui AA, Litsky ML, Farooqui T, Horrocks LA. 1999. Inhibitors of intracellular phospholipase A2 activity: Their neurochemical effects and therapeutical importance for neurological disorders. *Brain Res Bull* 49:139–153.
172. Kramer RM, Stephenson DT, Roberts EF, Clemens JA. 1996. Cytosolic phospholipase A2 [cPLA2] and lipid mediator release in brain. *J Lipid Mediat Cell Signal* 14:3–7.
173. Vokó Z, Hollander M, Hofman A, Koudstaal PJ, Breteler MM. 2003. Dietary antioxidants and the risk of ischemic stroke: the Rotterdam Study. *Neurology* 61:1273–1275.
174. He K, Merchant A, Rimm EB, Rosner BA, Stampfer MJ, Willett WC, Ascherio A. 2004. Folate, vitamin B6, and B12 intakes in relation to risk of stroke among men. *Stroke* 35:169–174.
175. van der Worp HB, Bär PR, Kappelle LJ, de Wildt DJ. 1998. Dietary vitamin E levels affect outcome of permanent focal cerebral ischemia in rats. *Stroke* 29:1002–1005.
176. Chang CY, Lai YC, Cheng TJ, Lau MT, Hu ML. 1998. Plasma levels of antioxidant vitamins, selenium, total sulfhydryl groups and oxidative products in ischemic-stroke patients as compared to matched controls in Taiwan. *Free Radic Res* 28:15–24.
177. Chang CY, Chen JY, Ke D, Hu ML. 2005. Plasma levels of lipophilic antioxidant vitamins in acute ischemic stroke patients: correlation to inflammation markers and neurological deficits. *Nutrition* 21:987–993.
178. Sánchez-Moreno C, Dashe JF, Scott T, Thaler D, Folstein MF, Martin A. 2004. Decreased levels of plasma vitamin C and increased concentrations of inflammatory and oxidative stress markers after stroke. *Stroke* 35:163–168.
179. Moseley MJ. 2001. Nutrition and electrolytes in the elderly. In *Handbook of nutrition in the aged*, 3rd ed. RR Watson (Ed.) pp. 3–13. Boca Raton: CRC Press.
180. Mirie W. 2001. Aging and nutrition needs. In *Handbook of nutrition in the aged*, 3rd ed. RR Watson (Ed.) pp.43–48. Boca Raton: CRC Press.
181. Vicedo TB, Correas FJH. 2001. Antioxidants as therapies of disease of old age. In *Handbook of nutrition in the aged*, 3rd ed. RR Watson (Ed.) pp.343–354. Boca Raton: CRC Press.
182. Joseph JA, Nadeau DA, Underwood A. 2002. Think health–think color. In: *The color code, a revolutionary eating plan for optimum health*, Joseph JA, Nadeau DA, Underwood A (Eds.) New York: Hyperion.
183. Liu X, Wang C. 2005. *Natural products chemistry*. Beijing: Chemical Industry Publisher (in Chinese).
184. Ni JW, Matsumoto K, Watanabe H. 1995. Tetramethylpyrazine improves spatial cognitive impairment induced by permanent occlusion of bilateral common carotid arteries or scopolamine in rats. *Jpn J Pharmacol* 67:137–141.
185. Hayakawa K, Mishima K, Nozako M, Hazekawa M, Aoyama Y, Ogata A, et al. 2007. High-cholesteral feeding aggravates cerebral infarction via decreasing the CB1 receptor. *Neurosci Lett* 414:183–187.
186. Harper JI, Yang SL, Evans AT, Phillipson JD. 1990. Chinese herbs for eczema. *Lancet* 335:795.
187. Atherton D, Sheehan M, Rustin MHA, Budkley C, Brostoff J, Taylor N. 1990. Chinese herbs for eczema. *Lancet* 336:1245.
188. Phillipson JD. 1995. A matter of some sensitivity. *Phytochemistry.* 38:1319–1343.
189. Xuejiang W, Magara T, Konishi T. 1999. Prevention and repair of cerebral ischemia-reperfusion injury by Chinese herbal medicine, Shengmai san, in rats. *Free Radic Res* 31:449–55.
190. Lee J, Duan W, Long JM, Ingram DK, Mattson MP. 2000. Dietary restriction increases the number of newly generated neural cells, and induces BDNF expression, in the dentate gyrus of rats. *J Mol Neurosci* 15:99–108.

191. Lindvall O, Kokaia Z. 2004. Recovery and rehabilitation in stroke. *Stroke* 35 [suppl I]:2691–2694.
192. Dugoua J, Mills E, Perri D, Koren G. 2006. Safety and efficacy of ginkgo (ginkgo biloba) during pregnancy and lactation. *Can J Clin Pharmacol* 13: e277–e284.
193. Zuo F, Zhou ZM, Liu ML. 2001. Determination of 14 chemical constituents in the traditional Chinese medicinal preparation Huangqin-Tang by high performance liquid chromatography. *Biol Pharm Bull* 24:693–697.

Section IV

Fruits and Vegetables to Prevent Illness

19 Can Fruit and Vegetable Consumption Oppose the Negative Health Effects of Tobacco?

Eliane Kellen and Geertruida E. Bekkering

CONTENTS

19.1 INTRODUCTION

Aging is associated with an increased risk of chronic diseases such as cancer and CVD. Smoking increases the risk of such diseases further. The intake of fruit and vegetables is often promoted as part of a healthy lifestyle to prevent chronic diseases. In this chapter we will discuss the health effect of smoking on cancer and CVD, describe the association between fruit and vegetable consumption and these diseases and review whether the negative health effects of smoking can be countered by fruit and vegetable consumption. Our review will focus on studies in the elderly where possible. Studies that reported on nutrients such as antioxidants were not taken into consideration.

Tobacco* contributes to the world's leading killer diseases. If current trends continue, it will kill 100 million people prematurely during this century [1]. According to the Centers for Disease Control and Prevention's Behavioral Risk Factor Surveillance System (BRFSS), an estimated 10% of Americans 65 and older smoked daily in the year 2002 [2].

19.2 HEALTH RISKS OF SMOKING

19.2.1 Cancer

Tobacco is a potent multisite carcinogen, causing cancers of the lung, upper aero-digestive tract, pancreas, stomach, liver, lower urinary tract, kidney and uterine cervix, and causing myeloid leukemia [3]. Smoking is estimated to cause 21% of deaths from cancer worldwide, which indicates that it is a very important preventable cause of cancer mortality. It was calculated that 70% of trachea, bronchus, and lung cancer mortality worldwide is caused by smoking; while smoking accounts for 42% of mouth and oropharynx cancer mortality, 42% of oesophageal cancer mortality, 22% of pancreatic cancer mortality, 28% of bladder cancer mortality and 14% of liver cancer mortality [4]. Evidence of a positive relationship between involuntary passive second-hand smoking, or environmental tobacco smoke and lung cancer in nonsmokers is increasing. This association is biologically plausible, as passive smokers inhale the same carcinogens as active smokers, albeit at a lower dose [5].

Cigarette smoke contains a mixture of more than 60 carcinogens, most of which require metabolic activation to impose their carcinogenic effect; there are competing detoxification pathways. The balance between metabolic activation and detoxification differs among individuals and affects their cancer susceptibility. Persons with higher carcinogen activation and lower detoxification capacity have the highest risk of developing cancer. Metabolic activation of carcinogens leads to the formation of DNA adducts. A DNA adduct is formed when carcinogen metabolites bind to DNA. DNA adducts are absolutely central to the carcinogenic process. If their formation is inhibited or blocked, so is the carcinogenesis. If DNA adducts escape cellular repair mechanisms and persist, they may lead to miscoding, persisting in permanent mutations. Cells with damaged DNA may be removed by apoptosis or programmed cell death. If a permanent mutation occurs in a critical region of an oncogene (genes that stimulate cell division) or tumor suppressor gene (genes that prevent cell division), it can lead to activation of the oncogene or deactivation of the tumor suppressor gene. Multiple events of this type may lead to cells that have lost normal growth control mechanisms and eventually become cancer [6,7]. Furthermore, smoking may impair the immune system, further increasing the risk of cancer [8].

19.2.2 Cardiovascular Disease

Tobacco use is an important cause of acute myocardial infarction worldwide, especially in men [9]. It has been estimated that more than one in every 10 cardiovascular deaths in the world in the year 2000 were attributable to smoking [10]. Quitting smoking will reduce all-cause mortality by 36% among patients with coronary heart disease CHD. [11]. Smoking increases the risk for both ischemic and hemorrhagic stroke and contributes to 12% to 14% of all stroke deaths [12].

Epidemiological evidence indicates a positive association between passive or secondhand smoking and the incidence of CVD [13]. This suggests that even very low levels of cigarette smoke increases the risk. Exposure to environmental tobacco smoke causes a 25% increase in risk of ischemic heart disease. This large effect of such a small exposure is mainly explained by a nonlinear dose–response relation between exposure and risk of heart disease [14]. It has been shown that

---

* In this chapter the terms "tobacco" and "smoking" refer to all forms of tobacco smoking: smoking of cigarettes, pipes, cigars, or bidis which contain tobacco wrapped in the leaf of another plant..

passive smokers have disproportionately increased levels of fibrinogen and homocysteine which are two biomarkers of CVD risk. [15]. Nicotine, and its major metabolites cotinine, carbon monoxide, and thiocyanate are the main biochemical factors responsible for cardiovascular harm [16].

Cigarette smoking impacts all phases of atherosclerosis from endothelial dysfunction to acute clinical events, which are largely thrombotic. Vasomotor dysfunction or impairment of the vasodilatory function, inflammation which is an essential phase, and modification of the lipid profile are components of initiation and progression of artherosclerosis. These three phases precede clinical events. Furthermore, cigarette smoke is associated with dysfunctional thrombohemostatic mechanisms (platelet dysfunction, alteration of antithrombotic and prothrombotic factors, and alteration in fibrinolysis) that promote the initiation and progression of thrombus formation and limit its effective dissolution [17].

Most of the dysfunctions described above can be explained by oxidative stress, which is a consequence of smoking [17]. The anatomical and ultrastructural cardiovascular changes due to smoking are named "smoke cardiomyopathy" [16].

19.3   FRUIT AND VEGETABLE CONSUMPTION IN THE ELDERLY

The intake of fruit and vegetables is often lower than the recommended five or more servings daily. Only $33.3\% \pm 4.9\%$ of the female U.S. population older than 70 met that recommendation in 1999–2000; for the male population older than 70, this was $55.9\% \pm 4.4\%$ [18].

19.4   EFFECTS OF FRUIT AND VEGETABLE CONSUMPTION

A diet of at least 400 grams per day of total fruit and vegetables. has often been promoted as reducing chronic disease risk. However, the epidemiological evidence is not as convincing as was anticipated. In general, cohort studies provide weaker evidence than do case control studies [19]. The differences in result may be partly explained by bias. Retrospective studies are more prone to several types of biases, which may lead to an overestimation of the association, such as (recall bias recall of diet is biased by the diagnosis), selection bias (controls who are willing to participate may be health conscious and thus consuming more fruits and vegetables than those who are not) and bias due to the change of diet and lifestyle following CVD events or being diagnosed with cancer.

19.4.1   EFFECT ON CANCER

The consumption of fruit and vegetables probably decreases the risk of several cancers. This was the conclusion of the largest project ever to investigate the association between diet and cancer, performed by the World Cancer Research Fund (WCRF) and the American Institute for Cancer Research (AICR) [20]. All available evidence was accumulated in one report that concluded that the intake of fruits as well as vegetables decreases the risk of cancers of mouth, pharynx, larynx, esophagus, and stomach. In addition, fruit also reduced the risk of lung cancer. The strength of association was labeled probable, which means there is still uncertainty in the causal relationship. In addition, a suggestive protective association was found between vegetables and cancers of the nasopharynx, lung, colorectum, ovary, and endometrium and between fruit and cancers of the nasopharynx, pancreas, liver, and colorectum.

Based on this report, the WCRF and AICR recommends everybody to consume at least five portions/servings (at least 400 g or 14 oz) of a variety of nonstarchy vegetables and fruits every day [20].

19.4.2 Effect on Cardiovascular Disease

Fruit and vegetable consumption seems to be inversely associated with the occurrence of CHD [19,21] and with a reduced risk of stroke [22]. A high daily consumption (400–500 grams) of fresh fruit and vegetables is recommended to reduce the risk of CHD, stroke, and high blood pressure [23]. Few studies have focused on the elderly. A study among 3588 men and women aged 65 years or older found no association between fruit and vegetable fiber intake and incident CVD [24]. In contrast, a study among 1299 elderly Massachusetts residents found that residents consuming more carotene-containing fruits and vegetables had lower risk of cardiovascular mortality and myocardial infarction [25]. The global mortality attributable to inadequate consumption of fruit and vegetables was estimated to be up to 2.635 million deaths per year [26]. Increasing individual fruit and vegetable consumption to up to 600 g per day could reduce the burden of ischemic heart disease by 31% and ischemic stroke by 19%.

Although no trials have assessed the intake of fruit and vegetables on primary prevention of CHD, there is some evidence on secondary prevention. Ornish et al. 1998. investigated the effect of intensive lifestyle changes in patients with moderate to severe CHD [27]. Lifestyle changes consisted of 10% fat whole foods, a vegetarian diet, aerobic exercise, stress management training, smoking cessation, and psychological support for 5 years. The authors concluded that more regression of coronary atherosclerosis occurred after 5 years than after 1 year in the experimental group. In contrast, in the control group, coronary atherosclerosis continued to progress and more than twice as many cardiac events occurred.

19.5 INTERACTION BETWEEN FRUIT AND VEGETABLE CONSUMPTION AND SMOKING

Chronic diseases are likely to be caused by a combination of environmental factors, genes, and their interaction. For example, only 15% of lifelong smokers in the Western world will develop lung cancer before the age of 75 [28]. This suggests that other factors than smoking alone affect the risk of developing lung cancer.

This section reviews the interaction between fruit and vegetable consumption and smoking. For example, is the protective effect of fruit and vegetables different for smokers than for nonsmokers? Are the antioxidant mechanisms found in fruit and vegetables more important in the presence of high levels of oxidizing DNA-damaging free radicals smoking [29]? And, is the detrimental effect of smoking different for persons who eat more than the recommended five daily servings of vegetables and fruits compared with those who eat less?

19.5.1 Interaction with Cancer

Tobacco-specific nitrosamines and polycyclic aromatic hydrocarbons undergo activation and detoxification processes that are controlled by antioxidants such as quercetin in vegetables and sulforaphane in broccoli [30].

19.5.1.1 Lung Cancer

Several studies assessed the effect of fruit and vegetables in smokers and nonsmokers, but the results on a possible interaction are equivocal. A case-control study found a protective effect of vegetables and apples on lung cancer risk among smokers, but not among nonsmokers [31]. Another case-control study found a fivefold increased risk in lung cancer for smokers reporting a low consumption compared with never smokers reporting high intake of fruit and vegetables, [32]. A large prospective cohort found that lung cancer incidence was lower in smokers with high vegetable intake than in those with a low intake [33]. In contrast, a Swedish case-control study found a protective effect of vegetable consumption on lung cancer risk among both nonsmokers and smokers including former smokers. [34]. Based on a pooled analysis of eight prospective studies, it was suggested that risk of lung cancer in never smokers with high consumption of fruit is decreased by 41% compared with those consuming less fruit. However, this association was not significant. Weaker associations were observed among current and past smokers, while vegetable consumption was negatively associated with lung cancer risk only among current smokers [35].

19.5.1.2 Other Cancers

The risks estimated of tobacco use on the occurrence of gastric cancer seems to be higher among those with low fruit consumption than among frequent fruit-eaters [36]. The protective effects of carotenoids on bladder cancer risk has been found to be confined largely to ever-smokers and were stronger in current than ex-smokers [37]. A case control study suggested that by increasing the daily fruit consumption, the risk of ever-smokers for developing bladder cancer decreased; however it still remained significant [38]. Even in the presence of heavy smoking, a high fruit and vegetable consumption is protective for the risk of head and neck cancer. Forty percent of the cases among ever-smokers appears to be related to the interaction of both risk factors [39].

However, a pooled analysis of two prospective cohort studies found no association between fruit and vegetable consumption and overall cancer risk among never, past, or current smokers except for cruciferous vegetables among male current smokers [40].

A randomized trial investigated the ability of dietary changes in particular diets rich in cruciferous vegetables and flavanoids to increase urinary antimutagenicity and inhibit DNA damage in healthy male smokers at least 15 cigarettes/day for the last 10 years. The data suggested that adherence to a diet rich in cruciferous vegetables and flavanoids was associated with a decrease in adducts after 1 year. However, the authors conclude that smoking is the most important single preventable cause of cancer and that it is unlikely that dietary habits can substantially counteract its effects [41].

19.5.1.3 Cardiovascular Disease

Interaction between fruit and vegetable consumption and smoking for CVD is sparsely examined. To the best of our knowledge, no epidemiological studies assessed whether the effect of smoking on CVD was modified by fruit and vegetable intake. In contrast, several cohort studies assessed whether the effect of fruit and vegetable intake on CVD was modified by smoking. Two cohort studies and a pooled analyses based on two other cohort studies suggested that the protective association was more apparent in current smokers [40,42,43], although the evidence on interaction was weak, if presented. Another cohort observed no clear interaction between smoking and fruit intake [44].

19.6 CONFOUNDING OF THE INTERACTION

As stated above, cohort studies typically provide weaker evidence on the association of fruit and vegetables with chronic disease than do retrospective studies. In addition, results of observational studies may not be confirmed in clinical trials. This has, for example, been shown the relationship between β-carotene and lung cancer. Observational studies showed a protective effect of carotenoids on lung cancer, especially in smokers [46]. However, randomized controlled studies failed to demonstrate reduced lung cancer incidence after prolonged β-carotene supplementation, and even suggested the possibility of harm [47,48]. Bias may partly explain why an effect found in observational studies is not apparent in randomized clinical trials.

19.6.1 Assessment of Fruit and Vegetable Consumption

The consumption of fruit and vegetable is difficult to measure. Estimates of fruit and vegetable intake and disease associations may differ depending on the method used to assess fruit and vegetable intake [49]. For example, food frequency questionnaire-based measures of fruit and vegetable intake have limitations, primarily due to their imprecise assessment of vegetable intake [50]. Also, the majority of observational studies, even cohort studies, note a dietary assessment only at baseline. Any changes to the diet will, therefore, not be taken into account, which may bias the estimate of association.

19.6.2 Clustering of Unhealthy Behaviors

Consumption of fruit and vegetables is typically connected with behavior that is associated with a reduction of cardiovascular and cancer risk. For example, individuals who eat more fruit and vegetables are likely to have lower rates of smoking, a lower intake of salt and saturated fat, higher levels of physical activity, and are less likely to be overweight [44]. Such a clustering of healthy behavior was reported in a European study with subjects aged 60 years or more [51]. Smokers commonly have higher intakes of energy, total fat, saturated fat, cholesterol, and alcohol, and lower intakes of unsaturated fat, fiber, vitamin C, vitamin E, and β-carotene than nonsmokers [52]. Thus, smokers typically have dietary patterns that further exacerbate their smoking-related risk of cancer and CVD, making it difficult to estimate the effect of a single food or nutrient.

19.6.3 Residual Confounding

Inadequate control of confounding may lead to an overestimation of the protective effect of fruit and vegetable consumption in smokers. Especially relevant in this respect is residual confounding, which refers to confounding due to measurement error in a known confounder that is included in a model [53]. This could, for example, arise when results are adjusted for smoking status yes versus no. instead of pack-years, but also when self-reported smoking status is used instead of a biomarker. The risk on residual confounding is especially great when investigating a disease with a very strong risk factor such as lung cancer and smoking. that is inversely associated with the exposure of interest such as fruit and vegetable consumption. or when the exposure of interest is weak compared with the confounder [54]. A simulation study suggested that biases in assessment of smoking exposure between smokers with low versus high β-carotene intake, leading to residual confounding, may plausibly explain much of the observed protective effect of β-carotene levels seen in epidemiological studies [55]. Carefully controlling for residual confounding is indicated in observational studies. After stepwise adjustment for smoking status, duration of smoking, and amount of cigarettes per day, a cohort study found that the negative associations between fruit and vegetable consumption and lung cancer attenuated and remained significant only for people in the highest quartile of vegetable consumption [54].

19.7 BIOCHEMICAL PLAUSIBILITY OF THE INTERACTION BETWEEN FRUIT AND VEGETABLE INTAKE AND SMOKING

Smoking induces oxidative stress. One "puff" exposes the smoker to more than 10^{15} free radicals and additional free radicals and oxidants are found in the tar [56]. Antioxidants are the best protectors of the damage caused by oxidative stress. Two of best-documented categories are the carotenoids and the bioflavonoids. The carotenoids can be found in highly colored fruit and vegetables such as carrots, tomatoes, peppers, and grapefruit. Flavonoids are found in a wide variety of foods—not necessarily colored—such as grapes, cherries, and tea [57]. As mentioned above, clinical trials showed no association between carotene supplements and cancer risk. It has been argued that the complex mixture of micronutrients found in a diet high in fruit and vegetables may be more effective than large supplemental doses of a small number of micronutrients [58]. Future clinical trials should therefore focus on dietary patterns and not on specific vitamins or even food items.

It has been shown that blood concentrations of antioxidants are lower in smokers than in non-smokers. This difference remains after adjustments for dietary differences. It is suggested that this relates to the inflammatory changes due to smoking that are associated with an increased turnover of vitamin C and carotenoid-containing foods [56]. Furthermore, chronic smoking leads to depletion of trace elements such as selenium or zinc, and by interference with the transcription of redox-relevant enzymes. This followed by an up regulation of antioxidative enzymes and factors e.g., gluthathione. After years of smoking, metal catalysts for oxidation reaction accumulate in the vessel wall, and accelerate oxidation reactions, which finally lead to a permanent oxidative deterioration of the cardiovascular system [59]. It is recommended that supplements of trace elements and metal chelating and detoxifying agents should be added to antioxidant supplementation in order to reduce CVD in chronic smokers [59].

Low penetrant genetic conditions may be involved in processes related to diet and smoking. These conditions strongly influence the individual biologic response to environmental carcinogens, which results in a lower or higher susceptibility for certain diseases. In such cases, it can be reasoned that the protective effect of fruit and vegetables, which are important sources of antioxidants, depends on a person's genotype in addition to the amount of oxidative stress. Oxidative stress is a consequence of cigarette smoking. Genetic polymorphisms leading to fast metabolization of smoking carcinogens could lead to less DNA damage from oxidative stress. Hence, the protective effect of the dietary antioxidants may be less in persons of the genotype "fast metabolization." Thus, some subgroups defined by genotype and phenotype may benefit more from dietary strategies. The protective effect of cruciferous vegetable consumption on the risk of myocardial infarction among persons with the *GSTT1*1* allele was greater for current smokers than for non-smokers genetic polymorphism x diet x smoking interaction. It seems that persons with an low functioning *GSTT1* allele may benefit more from the protective effects of cruciferous vegetables than those with higher-activity genotype because the isothiocyanates could remain in the body longer [45]. The field of gene–nutrient interactions is currently under development.

19.8   CONCLUSION

Smoking increases the risk of chronic diseases such as cancer and CVD. The intake of fruits and vegetables seems to have a modest protective effect on the occurrence of these diseases. However, this has been investigated only in observational studies and bias may partly explain the protective association found.

The consumption of fruit and vegetables seems to have a beneficial effect on some cancer risk in smokers. Such an association was weaker, if present, in CVD. To date, no long-term intervention study has determined that increasing fruit and vegetable intake resulted in a decrease in heart disease and cancer incidence and mortality among smokers [60].

The importance of smoking cessation, even at an older age, has been demonstrated. Adhering to a healthy lifestyle in middle age has been shown to lead to a reduction in CVD risk and mortality [61]. Up to 92% of the myocardial infarctions in postmenopausal women may be prevented by consuming a healthy diet high intake of fruit and vegetables, whole grains, fish, and legumes. in combination with moderate alcohol consumption, being physically active, not smoking, and maintaining a healthy weight [62]. Persons who adhere to a Mediterranean type of diet rich in plant foods and cereals and with olive oil as an important fat source, and maintain a healthy lifestyle of nonsmoking, moderate alcohol consumption, and at least 30 minutes of physical activity per day, are less likely to die from all-cause and cause-specific mortality even at ages 70 to 90 years [63].

In conclusion, there is insufficient evidence that increased fruit and vegetable intake can be a substitute for smoking cessation. Therefore, the advice to quit smoking should remain the mainstay of a healthy lifestyle for everybody.

REFERENCES

1. Frieden, T. R. and Bloomberg, M. R. 2007. How to prevent 100 million deaths from tobacco. *Lancet* 369, 1758-1761.
2. National Center for Chronic Disease Prevention and Health Promotion. Behavioral Risk Factor Surveillance System. CDC. 2007.
3. Vineis, P., Alavanja, M., Buffler, P., Fontham, E., Franceschi, S., Gao, Y. T., et al. 2004. Tobacco and cancer: Recent epidemiological evidence. *J. Natl. Cancer Inst.* 96, 99–106.
4. Danaei, G., Vander, H. S., Lopez, A. D., Murray, C. J. and Ezzati, M. 2005. Causes of cancer in the world: Comparative risk assessment of nine behavioural and environmental risk factors. *Lancet* 366, 1784–1793.
5. Hecht, S. S. 2004. Carcinogen derived biomarkers: applications in studies of human exposure to second-hand tobacco smoke. *Tob. Control* 13 Suppl 1, i48–i56.
6. Hecht, S. S. 2003. Tobacco carcinogens, their biomarkers and tobacco-induced cancer. *Nat. Rev. Cancer* 3, 733–744.
7. Wogan, G. N., Hecht, S. S., Felton, J. S., Conney, A. H. and Loeb, L. A. 2004. Environmental and chemical carcinogenesis. *Semin. Cancer Biol.* 14, 473–486.
8. Sopori, M. 2002. Effects of cigarette smoke on the immune system. *Nat. Rev. Immunol.* 2, 372–377.
9. Teo, K. K., Ounpuu, S., Hawken, S., Pandey, M. R., Valentin, V., Hunt, D., Diaz, R., Rashed, W., Freeman, R., Jiang, L., Zhang, X. and Yusuf, S. 2006. Tobacco use and risk of myocardial infarction in 52 countries in the INTERHEART study: A case–control study. *Lancet* 368, 647–658.
10. Ezzati, M., Henley, S. J., Thun, M. J. and Lopez, A. D. 2005. Role of smoking in global and regional cardiovascular mortality. *Circulation* 112, 489–497.
11. Critchley, J. and Capewell, S. 2004. Smoking cessation for the secondary prevention of CHD. Cochrane. *Database. Syst. Rev.*, CD003041.
12. Goldstein, L. B., Adams, R., Alberts, M. J., Appel, L. J., Brass, L. M., Bushnell, C. D., et al. 2006. Primary prevention of ischemic stroke: A guideline from the American Heart Association/American Stroke Association Stroke Council. *Circulation* 113, e873–e923.
13. Raupach, T., Schafer, K., Konstantinides, S., and Andreas, S. 2006. Secondhand smoke as an acute threat for the cardiovascular system: A change in paradigm. *Eur. Heart J.* 27, 386–392.
14. Law, M. R., Morris, J. K., and Wald, N. J. 1997. Environmental tobacco smoke exposure and ischaemic heart disease: An evaluation of the evidence. *BMJ* 315, 973–980.
15. Venn, A. and Britton, J. 2007. Exposure to secondhand smoke and biomarkers of cardiovascular disease risk in never-smoking adults. *Circulation* 115, 990–995.
16. Leone, A. 2005. Biochemical markers of cardiovascular damage from tobacco smoke. *Curr. Pharm. Des.* 11, 2199–2208.
17. Ambrose, J. A. and Barua, R. S. 2004. The pathophysiology of cigarette smoking and cardiovascular disease: An update. *J. Am. Coll. Cardiol.* 43, 1731–1737.
18. Guenther, P. M., Dodd, K. W., Reedy, J., and Krebs-Smith, S. M. 2006. Most Americans eat much less than recommended amounts of fruits and vegetables. *J. Am. Diet. Assoc.* 106, 1371–1379.
19. He, F. J., Nowson, C. A., Lucas, M., and MacGregor, G. A. 2007. Increased consumption of fruit and vegetables is related to a reduced risk of CHD: Meta-analysis of cohort studies. *J. Hum. Hypertens.* 21, 717–728.
20. World Cancer Research Fund/ American Institute for Cancer Research. Food, nutrition, physical activity, and the prevention of cancer: a global perspective. 2007. Washington DC, AICR.
21. Dauchet, L., Amouyel, P., Hercberg, S. and Dallongeville, J. 2006. Fruit and vegetable consumption and risk of CHD: A meta-analysis of cohort studies. *J. Nutr.* 136, 2588–2593.
22. He, F. J., Nowson, C. A. and MacGregor, G. A. 2006. Fruit and vegetable consumption and stroke: Meta-analysis of cohort studies. *Lancet* 367, 320–326.
23. Joint WHO/FAO expert consultation on Diet, Nutrition and the Prevention of Chronic Diseases. Diet, nutrition and the prevention of chronic diseases: report of a joint WHO/FAO expert consultation. WHO technical report series; 916. 2003. Geneva.
24. Mozaffarian, D., Kumanyika, S. K., Lemaitre, R. N., Olson, J. L., Burke, G. L., and Siscovick, D. S. 2003. Cereal, fruit, and vegetable fiber intake and the risk of CVD in elderly individuals. *JAMA* 289, 1659–1666.

25. Gaziano, J. M., Manson, J. E., Branch, L. G., Colditz, G. A., Willett, W. C., and Buring, J. E. 1995. A prospective study of consumption of carotenoids in fruits and vegetables and decreased cardiovascular mortality in the elderly. *Ann. Epidemiol.* 5, 255–260.

26. Lock, K., Pomerleau, J., Causer, L., Altmann, D. R. and McKee, M. 2005. The global burden of disease attributable to low consumption of fruit and vegetables: Implications for the global strategy on diet. *Bull. World Health Organ.* 83, 100–108.

27. Ornish, D., Scherwitz, L. W., Billings, J. H., Brown, S. E., Gould, K. L., Merritt, T. A., et al. 1998. Intensive lifestyle changes for reversal of CHD. *JAMA* 280, 2001–2007.

28. Peto, R., Darby, S., Deo, H., Silcocks, P., Whitley, E. and Doll, R. 2000. Smoking, smoking cessation, and lung cancer in the UK since 1950: Combination of national statistics with two case-control studies. *BMJ* 321, 323–329.

29. Terry, P., Terry, J. B., and Wolk, A. 2001. Fruit and vegetable consumption in the prevention of cancer: An update. *J. Intern. Med.* 250, 280–290.

30. Weisburger, J. H. 1999. Antimutagens, anticarcinogens, and effective worldwide cancer prevention. *J. Environ. Pathol. Toxicol. Oncol.* 18, 85–93.

31. Kubik, A., Zatloukal, P., Tomasek, L., Pauk, N., Havel, L., Dolezal, J. and Plesko, I. 2007. Interactions between smoking and other exposures associated with lung cancer risk in women: diet and physical activity. *Neoplasma* 54, 83–88.

32. Galeone, C., Negri, E., Pelucchi, C., La, V. C., Bosetti, C., and Hu, J. 2007. Dietary intake of fruit and vegetable and lung cancer risk: A case-control study in Harbin, northeast China. *Ann. Oncol.* 18, 388–392.

33. Linseisen, J., Rohrmann, S., Miller, A. B., Bueno-de-Mesquita, H. B., Buchner, F. L., Vineis, P., et al. 2007. Fruit and vegetable consumption and lung cancer risk: Updated information from the European Prospective Investigation into Cancer and Nutrition EPIC. *Int. J. Cancer* 121, 1103–1114.

34. Rylander, R. and Axelsson, G. 2006. Lung cancer risks in relation to vegetable and fruit consumption and smoking. *Int. J. Cancer* 118, 739–743.

35. Smith-Warner, S. A., Spiegelman, D., Yaun, S. S., Albanes, D., Beeson, W. L., van den Brandt, P. A., et al. 2003. Fruits, vegetables and lung cancer: A pooled analysis of cohort studies. *Int. J. Cancer* 107, 1001–1011.

36. Hansson, L. E., Baron, J., Nyren, O., Bergstrom, R., Wolk, A. and Adami, H. O. 1994. Tobacco, alcohol and the risk of gastric cancer. A population-based case-control study in Sweden. *Int. J. Cancer* 57, 26–31.

37. Castelao, J. E., Yuan, J. M., Gago-Dominguez, M., Skipper, P. L., Tannenbaum, S. R., Chan, K. K., et al. 2004. Carotenoids/vitamin C and smoking-related bladder cancer. *Int. J. Cancer* 110, 417–423.

38. Kellen, E., Zeegers, M., Paulussen, A., Van, D. M., and Buntinx, F. 2006. Fruit consumption reduces the effect of smoking on bladder cancer risk. The Belgian case control study on bladder cancer. *Int. J. Cancer* 118, 2572–2578.

39. Boccia, S., Cadoni, G., Sayed-Tabatabaei, F. A., Volante, M., Arzani, D., De Lauretis, A., et al. 2008. CYP1A1, CYP2E1, GSTM1, GSTT1, EPHX1 exons 3 and 4, and NAT2 polymorphisms, smoking, consumption of alcohol and fruit and vegetables and risk of head and neck cancer. *J. Cancer Res. Clin. Oncol.* 134, 93–100.

40. Hung, H. C., Joshipura, K. J., Jiang, R., Hu, F. B., Hunter, D., Smith-Warner, S. A., et al. 2004. Fruit and vegetable intake and risk of major chronic disease. *J. Natl. Cancer Inst.*, 96, 1577–1584.

41. Talaska, G., Al-Zoughool, M., Malaveille, C., Fiorini, L., Schumann, B., Vietas, J., et al. 2006. Randomized controlled trial: Effects of diet on DNA damage in heavy smokers. *Mutagenesis* 21, 179–183.

42. Liu, S., Manson, J. E., Lee, I. M., Cole, S. R., Hennekens, C. H., Willett, W. C., and Buring, J. E. 2000. Fruit and vegetable intake and risk of cardiovascular disease: The Women's Health Study. *Am J. Clin. Nutr.* 72, 922–928.

43. Liu, S., Lee, I. M., Ajani, U., Cole, S. R., Buring, J. E., and Manson, J. E. 2001. Intake of vegetables rich in carotenoids and risk of CHD in men: The Physicians' Health Study. *Int. J. Epidemiol.* 30, 130–135.

44. Bazzano, L. A., He, J., Ogden, L. G., Loria, C. M., Vupputuri, S., Myers, L., and Whelton, P. K. 2002. Fruit and vegetable intake and risk of CVD in US adults: The first National Health and Nutrition Examination Survey Epidemiologic Follow-up Study. *Am J. Clin. Nutr.* 76, 93–99.

45. Cornelis, M. C., El-Sohemy, A., and Campos, H. 2007. GSTT1 genotype modifies the association between cruciferous vegetable intake and the risk of myocardial infarction. *Am. J. Clin. Nutr.* 86, 752–758.

46. Steinmetz, K. A. and Potter, J. D. 1991. Vegetables, fruit, and cancer. I. Epidemiology. *Cancer Causes Control* 2, 325–357.
47. Omenn, G. S., Goodman, G. E., Thornquist, M. D., Balmes, J., Cullen, M. R., Glass, A., et al. 1996. Effects of a combination of beta carotene and vitamin A on lung cancer and CVD. *N. Engl. J. Med.* 334, 1150–1155.
48. Hennekens, C. H., Buring, J. E., Manson, J. E., Stampfer, M., Rosner, B., Cook, N. R., et al. 1996. Lack of effect of long-term supplementation with beta carotene on the incidence of malignant neoplasms and CVD. *N. Engl. J. Med.*, 334, 1145–1149.
49. Smith-Warner, S. A., Elmer, P. J., Fosdick, L., Tharp, T. M., and Randall, B. 1997. Reliability and comparability of three dietary assessment methods for estimating fruit and vegetable intakes. *Epidemiology* 8, 196–201.
50. Kristal, A. R., Vizenor, N. C., Patterson, R. E., Neuhouser, M. L., Shattuck, A. L., and McLerran, D. 2000. Precision and bias of food frequency-based measures of fruit and vegetable intakes. *Cancer Epidemiol. Biomarkers Prev.* 9, 939–944.
51. Bamia, C., Orfanos, P., Ferrari, P., Overvad, K., Hundborg, H. H., Tjonneland, A., et al. 2005. Dietary patterns among older Europeans: The EPIC–Elderly study. *Br. J. Nutr.* 94, 100–113.
52. Dallongeville, J., Marecaux, N., Fruchart, J. C., and Amouyel, P. 1998. Cigarette smoking is associated with unhealthy patterns of nutrient intake: A meta-analysis. *J. Nutr.* 128, 1450–1457.
53. Fewell, Z., Davey, S. G., and Sterne, J. A. 2007. The impact of residual and unmeasured confounding in epidemiologic studies: a simulation study. *Am J. Epidemiol.* 166, 646–655.
54. Skuladottir, H., Tjoenneland, A., Overvad, K., Stripp, C., Christensen, J., Raaschou-Nielsen, O., and Olsen, J. H. 2004. Does insufficient adjustment for smoking explain the preventive effects of fruit and vegetables on lung cancer? *Lung Cancer* 45, 1–10.
55. Stram, D. O., Huberman, M., and Wu, A. H. 2002. Is residual confounding a reasonable explanation for the apparent protective effects of beta-carotene found in epidemiologic studies of lung cancer in smokers? *Am. J. Epidemiol.* 155, 622–628.
56. Northrop-Clewes, C. A. and Thurnham, D. I. 2007. Monitoring micronutrients in cigarette smokers. *Clin. Chim. Acta* 377, 14–38.
57. Furst, A. 2002. Can nutrition affect chemical toxicity? *Int. J. Toxicol.* 21, 419–424.
58. Woodside, J. V., McCall, D., McGartland, C., and Young, I. S. 2005. Micronutrients: dietary intake v. supplement use. *Proc. Nutr. Soc.* 64, 543–553.
59. Bernhard, D. and Wang, X. L. 2007. Smoking, oxidative stress and cardiovascular diseases—do antioxidative therapies fail? *Curr. Med. Chem.* 14, 1703–1712.
60. Kelly, G. S. 2002. The interaction of cigarette smoking and antioxidants. Part I: diet and carotenoids. *Altern. Med. Rev.* 7, 370–388.
61. King, D. E., Mainous, A. G., III ,and Geesey, M. E. 2007. Turning back the clock: Adopting a healthy lifestyle in middle age. *Am. J. Med.* 120, 598–603.
62. Akesson, A., Weismayer, C., Newby, P. K., and Wolk, A. 2007. Combined effect of low-risk dietary and lifestyle behaviors in primary prevention of myocardial infarction in women. *Arch. Intern. Med.* 167, 2122–2127.
63. Knoops, K. T., de Groot, L. C., Kromhout, D., Perrin, A. E., Moreiras-Varela, O., Menotti, A. and van Staveren, W. A. 2004. Mediterranean diet, lifestyle factors, and 10-year mortality in elderly European men and women: The HALE project. *JAMA* 292, 1433–1439.

20 Weight Loss in Elderly People

Aránzazu Aparicio, Laura Mª Bermejo,
Elena Rodríguez-Rodríguez, and Rosa M. Ortega

CONTENTS

20.1 INTRODUCTION

The reduced physical activity undertaken by elderly people, along with the physiological, psychological, social, and often pathological changes they experience, can gradually increase their risk of putting on weight—which could have negative effects on their health and functional capacity. When planning the nutrition of elderly people, care is usually taken to restrict the intake of food with the goal of maintaining body weight. However, such restrictions, which are often inadequately monitored and controlled, can be associated with nutritional and health risks.

20.2 DEFINITIONS OF OVERWEIGHT AND OBESITY

A person who is overweight or obese has an abnormal or excessive accumulation of body fat [1]. The traditional method for deciding whether a person is overweight or obese is to determine his/her body mass index (BMI): the person's body weight (in kg) divided by the square of his/her height in metres (kg/m^2) (Table 20.1). This highly reproducible, easy-to-use index reflects the amount of body fat in most people very well, and has been employed in a great many epidemiological studies. It is also recommended for clinical use by different medical societies and international health organizations. However, the BMI is not a good indication of the amount of body fat carried by athletes or the elderly [2].

TABLE 20.1
BMI Intervals for Degree of Obesity in Adults

Category	BMI intervals (kg/m^2)
Underweight	<18.5
Normal weight	18.5–24.9
Grade I overweight	25–26.9
Grade II overweight (pre-obesity)	27–29.9
Type I obesity	30–34.9
Type II obesity	35–39.9
Type III obesity (morbid)	40–49.9
Type IV obesity (extreme)	≥50

Source: 1,2.

20.3 IDEAL WEIGHT FOR ELDERLY PEOPLE

The official cutoff weights of different organizations establish adults as being overweight when their BMI is between 25 and 29.9 kg/m^2, and as obese when it reaches ≥30 kg/m^2 (Table 20.1). These same cutoffs recognize that being overweight or obese places a person at greater risk of developing health problems, and that within each weight category this risk is further increased when the waist circumference (WC) reaches ≥102 cm in men and ≥88 cm in women [3]. However, controversy surrounds the impact of overweight/obesity on the health of persons aged 65 and over [4].

In 2005, the North American Association for the Study of Obesity and the American Society for Nutrition published a document in which it was recommended that obese persons aged ≥65 years lose weight, but no special recommendation was made for overweight persons [5,6].

Numerous studies report a U- or J-shape relationship between BMI and mortality in adults, but in elderly people this is not so clear [7]. In fact, few recent studies have reported a positive relationship between these variables in the elderly. The 25 kg/m^2 normal limit for BMI may therefore be too restrictive in elderly persons; the appropriate BMI for this age group could be higher [6,7].

Several hypotheses have been put forward to explain the association between BMI and mortality in elderly people. Some suggest this index to be a poor indicator of the quantity and distribution of body fat in people of advanced age since both the fat-free mass and fat mass act as important nutritional reserves during illness. This is of particular importance in elderly people; a higher BMI could help to reduce their risk of dying [8].

Other authors [5,10,11,12] report a negative association between BMI and mortality in persons aged 50–64 years after adjusting for the WC, while WC is positively associated with mortality after adjusting for BMI [9]. They suggest that BMI may reflect the fat free mass of people with the same WC, while WC reflects total and abdominal fat in people with the same BMI. Therefore, a loss of weight (intentional or otherwise) would not necessarily be beneficial in overweight or obese elderly people. Rather, it would be more appropriate to reduce their WC without a loss of weight via exercise. This could be the case irrespective of the BMI interval into which they fall. Nonetheless, more research is needed to confirm these ideas.

20.4 PREVALENCE OF OVERWEIGHT AND OBESITY IN ELDERLY PEOPLE

A high percentage of the world's population is overweight or obese, including members of all age and social groups and both sexes. This situation continues to increase alarmingly and has reached epidemic proportions among some populations. The latest World Health Organization (WHO) data indicate that in 2005 the world was home to 1600 million overweight adults (>15 years of age) and nearly 400 million who were obese. By 2015 these figures are expected to reach some 2030 million and 700 million respectively [1].

With respect to elderly persons, recent studies have shown that 71% of U.S. citizens aged 60 or more to be overweight or obese when classified according to their BMI [13]. Further, more than half of these people have been diagnosed obese according to WC criteria [14]. In Europe, the data are also not quite so alarming. For example, in Spanish citizens aged 65 years or over, the prevalence of overweight is estimated at 44% and obesity at 35% [15].

20.5   FOOD HABITS OF THE ELDERLY

There is an irrefutable relationship between nutrition and health in elderly people. A good nutritional status has a positive effect on mortality, probably via helping to prevent disease and incapacity. The nutritional needs of the elderly are different from those of younger adults; energy needs are lower but the requirements of vitamins and mineral are greater. Any modification of the dietary recommendations for persons of this age group should therefore be moderate; the risk of causing a deficiency could be considerable if the goals sought are very ambitious.

Elderly people may reduce their food intakes for several reasons:

- *Physiological factors*. Modifications in the senses of taste and smell may render acidic or sour foods such as citrus fruits less appetizing. The consumption of fats and sweet foods may, however, increase [16]. The elderly may also experience a lack of appetite or a heightened feeling of satiety. The partial or total loss of teeth could lead to a reduced consumption of fruits and vegetables or meats, and consequently to lower fiber, carotene, and iron intakes, and an increased consumption of fats, oils, and sugars via foods that are easier to chew [17,18]. Xerostomy, or dryness, may also be a problem because the chewing and the swallowing of foods is more difficult.
- *Physical factors* that impede the acquisition or preparation of foods.
- *Psychological factors* such as depression are often associated with a lack of appetite or the rejection of food. Depression in elderly people can also be manifested as a lack of interest in purchasing and preparing food [19,20].
- *Economic factors*: the purchase of certain foods might be limited. The most expensive foods, such as fish and meat, may be purchased less often, while less expensive foods such as milk, chicken, eggs, flour, and cereals may be bought more often [21,22].
- *Social factors*: being a widow or widower and having to eat alone can lead to changes in the diet [23,24].

Most experts also agree that the nutrition of the elderly is generally inadequate [25]. In fact, four out of five elderly have chronic diseases in which diet may play an important role. Further, one out of every five elderly people skips meals, and only about one in 10 consumes the recommended quantities of fruit and vegetables.

Many normal-weight elderly people are aware of the role of good nutrition in health and begin to take more care of what they eat. They may also make changes in their food habits, introducing a stricter control over the intake of heavy meals, especially fatty meals, accompanied by an increase in lighter meals with more white meats, fruits, vegetables, wholemeal cereals, and skimmed milk products. In addition, they may grill, boil, roast, or microwave food rather than fry it (especially in batter). Overweight and obese elderly persons, however, have less healthy food habits. They tend to take more energy from fats and less from carbohydrates, and to consume more meat. They therefore have higher cholesterol intakes. They also consume fewer fruits and vegetables and therefore have poorer vitamin and fiber intakes [26–28]. Finally, elderly people with higher BMIs are reported to consume less-adequate breakfasts and to more frequently skip this meal than their normal-weight counterparts [28].

20.6   THE INFLUENCE OF DIET ON WEIGHT CONTROL

The therapeutic objectives of weight loss in adults are the improvement in or elimination of obesity-associated comorbidity and a reduction in the impact of future complications associated with weight excess. Although a number of weight-loss strategies exist, including lifestyle changes (diet therapy, undertaking physical exercise, behavior modification), pharmacological treatment and bariatric (gastric bypass) surgery [2,29], only the first of these should be used by the elderly. Anti-obesity drugs have not been adequately tested in the elderly and their secondary effects could be serious [30]; bariatric surgery is simply too aggressive in people of advancing age [29].

Among the lifestyle modifications possible, increasing the amount of physical activity undertaken is more advisable than reducing the energy intake since it reduces the WC without weight loss [8,14–16]. In addition, reducing the intake of energy could lead to nutritional deficits [31]. Yet, when elderly people embark on a weight loss program, they are more likely to change their diet than increase the physical activity they undertake [32].

20.6.1   Dietetic Treatment

To design an appropriate weight loss diet for overweight and obese elderly persons it is necessary to bear in mind their gastronomic preferences, timetable, family and previous professional life, economic possibilities, whether meals are taken alone or in company and how (e.g., watching TV or reading while eating), the climate, the degree of physical activity undertaken, his or her clinical history, and other possible complications [33]. Many currently used weight loss diets are based on the restriction of energy intake, yet weight loss appears to be regulated not just by the quantity of energy consumed but also by the composition of the diet [34]; it is therefore necessary to take this into account.

20.6.1.1   Energy Intake

The diets prescribed for the treatment of obesity in the general population should be slightly or moderately hypocaloric and balanced, and should, of course, be personalized. First, energy expenditure needs to be calculated with respect to the sex, age, and physical activity undertaken. This should indicate a diet that provides about 500 kcal less than that required. Such a diet would allow a gradual weight loss that can be maintained over the long term, thus reducing any risks to the patient [29].

In the loss and maintenance of weight it is also important to consider the distribution of energy intake over the day. A number of studies have shown that the greater the number of meals taken daily the smaller the chance of becoming obese [35,36]. Navia & Perea [37] recommend that four to five meals be taken per day.

20.6.1.2   Diet Composition

Studies on overweight and obese people have found them to have food habits different from those of normal-weight people [38], with lower intakes of carbohydrates and fiber (mainly a lower consumption of fruits and vegetables) and a higher intake of fats. Obesity shows a positive correlation with fat intake and a negative correlation with carbohydrate intake [34,39,40]. This suggests that people who are interested in losing weight, rather than simply reducing their energy intake [41] should follow balanced diets with an energy profile close to that recommended, with 55–60% of all energy from carbohydrates and 30–35% from fats and 15% from proteins.

In elderly people of normal weight it is common to see a reduction in the consumption of many foods, and as a consequence their energy intake falls [42]. This could lead to a reduction in the supply of micronutrients—an added problem in older people since their requirements of many of these nutrients (such as calcium, folic acid, vitamin D, and vitamin B_{12}) increase with age. Reducing their intake would only cause nutritional status to deteriorate. Therefore, rather than reducing energy intake in this age group, it would appear better to follow a more balanced diet that includes the recommended number of servings of each food group. This would allow their energy profile to approach that required yet improve the status of many nutrients. Figure 20.1 shows the number of servings and their sizes recommended for each food group. In order to help control body weight, the foods of least energy density within each group would be the best choices.

20.6.1.3 Milk and Milk Products

Weight control diets should include an increase in the consumption of skimmed milk and milk products since they contain less fat, and therefore less energy, than their whole milk counterparts [43,44]. Milk and yogurt would be more advisable than cured or semicured cheeses or milky desserts since the latter contain greater amounts of fat and should be taken in moderation [45]. Elderly people with an inadequate vitamin D intake, or who do not get enough sunshine, should eat milk products enriched with this vitamin [46].

20.6.1.4 Cereals and Pulses

There is evidence that, given their content in complex carbohydrates, fiber, and other minority components, the consumption of cereals [47,48] and pulses [49,50] favors weight loss. Cereals can be eaten either white or wholemeal, although the latter are recommended since they provide more fiber. This provides a sensation of being full and avoids constipation [51,52].

20.6.1.5 Fish, Meat, and Eggs

To favor weight loss, the meat consumed should be lean (chicken, turkey, rabbit, beef) and all fat removed before cooking. Meat derivatives should be avoided [53]. Some studies have shown that substituting fish for meat in hypocaloric diets can lead to greater weight losses; adding fish to the diet is therefore recommendable [54,55]. Either blue or white fish can be eaten because, although blue fish contain more oil, they also have more omega-3 fatty acids. These can help protect against cardiovascular disease [56]. Fish canned in oil should be avoided, however, given its high energy content [29].

20.1.6.6 Fruit and Vegetables

Numerous studies have associated a greater consumption of fruits and vegetables with a lower prevalence of overweight and obesity [57,58]. In an investigation involving 459 healthy men and women enrolled in the Baltimore Longitudinal Study of Aging, Newby et al. [58] reported that those who ate more fruit and vegetables were those who less often saw an increase in their BMI and WC. It would therefore appear essential that these foods be included in weight loss diets [59,60], especially those designed for elderly overweight and obese persons.

Fruits and vegetables have different properties that encourage their inclusion in weight loss diets:

- Their energy density is low. These foods contain large quantities of water; their weight and volume is therefore high but their energy content low. Thus, more of these foods can be eaten for the same energy intake, reducing the hunger experienced when following diets that reduce the number of food servings [60].
- They have high fiber contents. Fiber helps to provide a feeling of satiety; less food is therefore eaten and there is a consequent fall in energy intake [61].
- They are rich in folic acid [62]. This vitamin has been negatively associated with overweight and obesity; the consumption of these foods is therefore advisable in weight loss diets [63–65]. In a study of 182 patients with morbid obesity following a treatment based on lifestyle changes combined with pharmacological treatment, Martínez et al. [65] reported serum folic acid to be the only independent predictor of weight loss. An increase of 1 ng/ mL improved the probability of a successful treatment outcome by 28%.

Food groups	Servings/ day	Foods included in the group	Serving size (g)
Dairy products 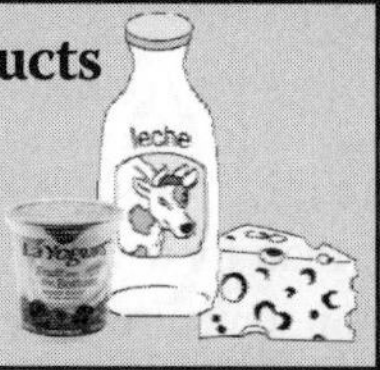	3–4*	Milk Yogurt Fermented milk Low–fat cheese High–fat cheese	200–250 125 125 60–80 40–60
Cereals and pulses 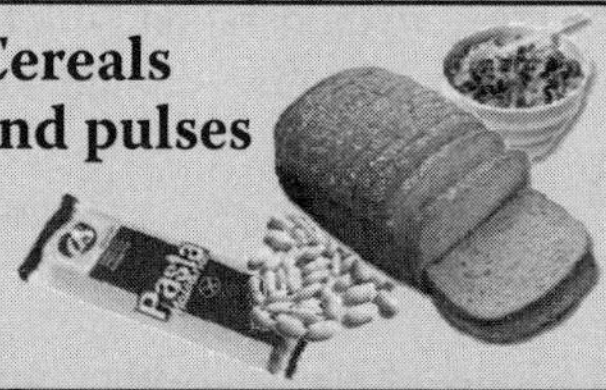	6–8	Bread Breakfast cereals Cookies Rice Pasta Pulses	30–60 30–40 40–50 50–70^r 50–70^r 50–70^r
Meat, fish and eggs 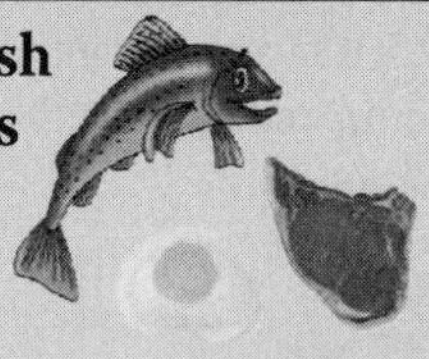	2–3	Meat and meat products Fish and fish products Egg	100–150^r 100–150^r 1 piece
Vegetables 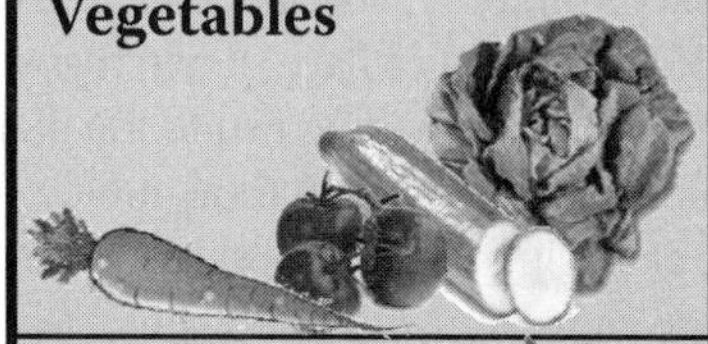	3–5	Vegetables	150–200^r
Fruits 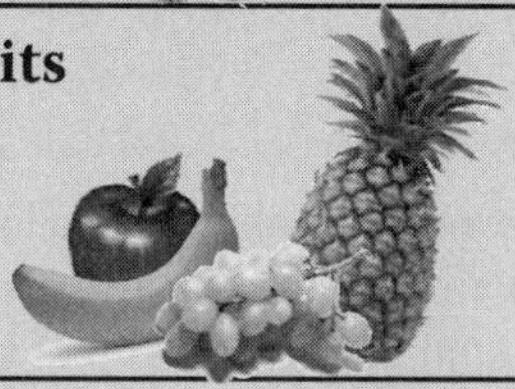	2–4	Juices Fresh fruit	100–150 100–150
Fats and oils 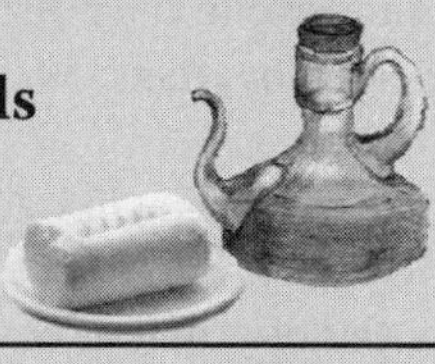	Moderate	Vegetable and seed oils, butter, margarine	<60g/day in total
Sweet things 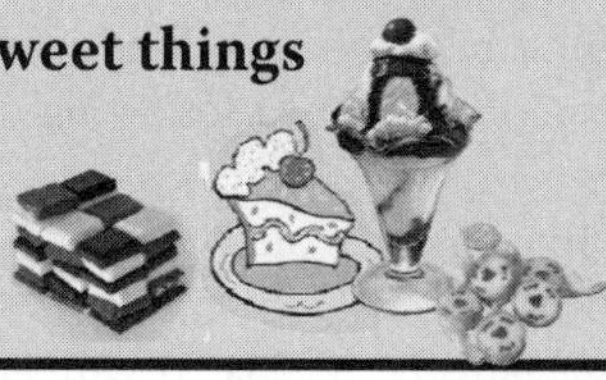	Moderate	Pastries, sugar, sweets	<10% of the total energy intake

FIGURE 20.1 Daily food servings recommended for the elderly (*-preferably skimmed or semi-skimmed; ^{r}-rawfood weight before cooking; the number and weight of servings are an orientation and have been established by one easy application to the dietetic daily practice).

- They have high contents of phytocompounds, including terpenes, steroids, phenolic compounds and glycosinolates etc. [66], all of which have anti-inflammatory properties [67]. Obesity is associated with chronic inflammation, a consequence of the adipose tissue's synthesis of proteins intimately related to the onset of this problem [68].

The consumption of fruit and vegetables by elderly people is also associated with other health benefits. For example, their water content favors hydration; elderly people can experience dehydration since age raises the thirst threshold [69]. The fiber content of fruits and vegetables also helps prevent constipation, which is common in older people due to their use of medications, the presence of certain health problems, and reduced mobility [70]. In addition to reducing the risk of cardiovascular disease, increasing the intake of folic acid via fruits and vegetables also offers protection against cancer and cognitive decline [71]. Finally, the fiber, magnesium, vitamins C and E, carotenoids, flavonoids and phytoestrogens supplied by these foods may help prevent the appearance of diabetes, and again cancer and cardiovascular disease [72]. These compounds certainly reduce blood pressure [73], homocysteine [74], triglyceride, and cholesterol levels [75], and help prevent the oxidation of LDL-cholesterol [76].

20.6.2 OTHER DIETARY RECOMMENDATIONS

The diet should be varied since this is the best way to ensure that all necessary nutrients are obtained in adequate amounts. Many epidemiological studies have shown that a varied diet is associated with a better nutrient intake profile and a reduction in morbidity and mortality [77].

Lipid consumption should be reduced. Foods should be cooked on a hotplate or steamed. Stews and fried foods, especially battered and breaded foods, should be avoided [78].

Food should be well chewed and eaten slowly to give time for satiety signals to develop. This will favor the digestion of food and prevent the appearance of gaseous distension of the stomach or intestine (meteorism) [37].

The use of spices and herbs is recommended since, apart from making food more palatable [79] they may also increase the feeling of satiety and promote thermogenesis. They could therefore be of great use in the treatment of obesity [80]. It has recently been shown that the components of these ingredients reduce the inflammatory response of the adipose tissue in obese persons, perhaps improving the chronic inflammation associated with this disease [81].

Although salt has no calories and thus has little to do with weight loss, it should be used in moderation in order to reduce the high blood pressure so often seen in obese people [82].

20.7 NUTRITIONAL EDUCATION

In general, elderly people have a smaller need of energy but greater vitamin and mineral requirements; the fact that they often eat less means they may face greater nutritional risks. The diets of elderly people are commonly deficient in cereals, pulses, and, above all, fruit and vegetables [31,74]. These supply large quantities of carbohydrate, fiber, vitamins, and minerals; therefore, nutrition experts advocate nutritional education that leads to the diet's containing more adequate amounts of these foods. Although elderly people tend to have strongly rooted food habits and lifestyles, in everyday practice they are also known to be cooperative and capable of changing their food habits and of undertaking other positive activities such as physical exercise, occupational workshops, and cultural activities etc., all of which can improve their quality of life. In nutritional education programs aimed at this age group, caregivers, whether at home or in institutions, play an essential role [83].

Elderly people commonly face problems of calcium, vitamins D and B_{12} deficiency [84], perhaps promoted by loneliness (depression caused by loneliness may lead to less care being taken over the diet), a degree of invalidity, or a lack of knowledge regarding healthy nutrition, etc. Factors such as these should be taken into account when designing nutritional educational programs aimed at this age group. Cooking techniques that adequately prepare food for the elderly should not be overlooked [83].

Food guides are very useful educational tools that allow people to design adequate diets that supply the right quantities of energy and nutrients, meet nutritional objectives, and promote maximum health and functional capacity [46]. Using food guides for adults as a base, nutrition experts have designed guides specifically for the elderly. One of the best known is the USDA Food Guide Pyramid for the Elderly. The base of the pyramid highlights the importance of adequate hydration over the day (eight glasses of liquids). The number of daily servings of the different food groups are then shown, with special emphasis placed on the adequate consumption of cereals, fruits, and vegetables. This guide also includes symbols to highlight the need to consume more foods rich in fiber, such as wholemeal cereals, fruit, vegetables, and pulses. Finally, a flag at the top of the pyramid makes clear that vitamin D and B_{12} supplements in persons over 70 years of age could help promote health [85]. Although an adequate diet should supply all the nutrients necessary for maintaining optimum health, supplements might be advisable for elderly people with low energy intakes or in those suspected of suffering deficiencies [31].

Other countries have also produced nutrition guides specially designed for the elderly. For example, a guide known as *La nutrición correcta en personas mayores* (Correct Nutrition for Elderly People) has been produced in Spain [86]. As well as making clear the recommended number of daily servings from different food groups, it also explains which nutrients are characteristic of each group and suggests serving sizes (Figure 20.1). It also provides a series of criteria to help in correct diet planning [86]. These include:

- Spreading food intake out over four to five meals per day, and not skipping breakfast.
- Monitoring liquid intake; at least two liters per day should be consumed. Water does not make people put on weight, and obese persons should be advised that the goal for them is to lose fat, not water.
- Maintaining a stable weight, avoiding constant gains and losses. In the fight against obesity, excess energy intakes should be avoided and physical activity undertaken.
- Moderating the intake of salt and the consumption of salty foods, as well as alcohol and stimulant drinks such as tea and coffee.
- Avoiding loneliness; it is very important to try to have the company of others and to maintain social contacts as much as possible.
- Taking care with food presentation, avoiding monotony and making meals an agreeable time.

It should be remembered that people are often refractory about using these types of guides since they believe their nutrition is correct and they are often unwilling to analyze any areas that could be improved. To overcome this problem, campaigns have been designed such as that promoting the consumption of five servings of fruits and vegetables per day—a campaign that was generally well accepted [46].

In summary, the diets of elderly people should be designed to ensure they receive the right amounts of energy and nutrients. Given the higher vitamin and mineral requirements of elderly people it is recommended that the overweight and obese elderly not follow restrictive diets since these could lead to nutrient deficiencies. Rather, their diets should be better balanced and they should undertake more physical activity if possible. If a restrictive diet is required, care should be taken that no nutrient deficiencies appear. Finally, appropriate nutritional education material could help elderly people enjoy a healthier old age.

REFERENCES

1. World Health Organization. (2006). Obesity and overweight. Available at: http://www.who.int/media-centre/factsheets/fs311/es/index.html.
2. Salas-Salvadó, J., Rubio, M.A., Barbany, M., Moreno, B., and Grupo Corporativo de la SEEDO. (2007). Consenso SEEDO 2007 para la evaluación del sobrepeso y la obesidad y establecimiento de criterios de intervención terapéutica. *Medicina Clínica* (Barcelona) 128(5), 184–196.
3. National Institutes of Health. Nacional Heart Lung and Blood Institute. (1998). Clinical guidelines on the identification, evaluation, and treatment of overweight and obesity in adults: The evidence report. *Obesity Res.* 6, S51–S210.
4. Janssen, I., Katzmarzyk, P.T., and Ross, R. (2005). Body mass index is inversely related to mortality in older people after adjustment for waist circumference. *J. Am. Geriatr. Soc.* 53, 2112–2118.
5. Villareal, D.T., Apovian, C.M., Kushner, R.F., Klein, S.; American Society for Nutrition; NAASO, and The Obesity Society. (2005). Obesity in older adults: Technical review and position statement of the American Society for Nutrition and NAASO, The Obesity Society. *Obesity Res.* 13(11), 1849–1863.
6. Janssen, I. (2007). Morbidity and mortality risk associated with an overweight BMI in older men and women. *Obesity* 15(7), 1827–1840.
7. Price, G.M., Uauy, R., Breeze, E., Bulpitt, C.J., and Fletcher, A.E. (2006). Weight, shape, and mortality risk in older persons: Elevated waist–hip ratio, not high body mass index, is associated with a greater risk of death. *Am. J. Clin. Nutr.* 84, 449–460.
8. Janssen, I. and Mark, E.A. (2007). Elevated body mass index and mortality risk in the elderly. *Obesity Rev.* 8, 41–59.
9. Bigaard, J., Tjønneland, A., Thomsen, B.L., Overvad, K., Heitmann, B.L., Sørensen, T.I. (2003). Waist circumference, BMI, smoking, and mortality in middle-aged men and women. *Obesity Res.* 11(7), 895–903.
10. Ross, R., Dagnone, D., Jones, P.J., Smith, H., Paddags, A., Hudson, R., and Janssen, I. (2000). Reduction in obesity and related comorbid conditions after diet-induced weight loss or exercise-induced weight loss in men. A randomized, controlled trial. *Ann. Intern. Med.* 133(2), 92–103.
11. Ross, R., Janssen, I., Dawson, J., Kungl, A.M., Kuk, J.L., Wong, S.L., et al. (2004). Exercise-induced reduction in obesity and insulin resistance in women: A randomized controlled trial. *Obesity Res.* 12(5), 789–798.
12. Hardy, R. and Kuh, D. (2006). Commentary: BMI and mortality in the elderly—a life course perspective. *Int. J. Epidemiol.* 35(1), 179–180.
13. Ogden, C.L., Carroll, M.D., Curtin, L.R., McDowell, M.A., Tabak, C.J., and Flegal, K.M. (2006). Prevalence of overweight and obesity in the United States, 1999–2004. *JAMA* 295(13), 1549–1555.
14. Ford, E.S., Mokdad, A.H., and Giles, W.H. (2003). Trends in waist circumference among U.S. adults. *Obesity Res.* 11, 1223–1231.
15. Aranceta, J., Serra, L.l., Foz, M., Moreno, B., and Grupo Colaborativo SEEDO. (2005). Prevalencia de obesidad en España. *Medicina Clínica* (Barcelona) 125, 460–466.
16. Rolls, B.J. (1999) Do chemosensory changes influence food intake in the elderly? *Physiol. Behav.* 66, 193–197.
17. Nowjack–Raymer, R.E. and Sheiham, A. (2007). Numbers of natural teeth, diet, and nutritional status in US adults. *J. Dent. Res.* 86, 1171–5.
18. Sahyoun, N.R, Zhang, X.L., and Serdula, M.K. (2005). Barriers to the consumption of fruits and vegetables among older adults. *J. Nutr. Elder.* 24, 5–21.
19. Thompson, M.P. and Morris, L.K. (1991). Unexplained weight loss in the ambulatory elderly. *J. Am. Geriat. Soc.* 39, 497–500.
20. Sabartés, O. (2002). Factores de riesgo de malnutrición. In: Rubio MA editor. *Manual de alimentación y nutrición en el anciano.* Madrid: SCM, 31–38.
21. US Department of Agriculture. (1990). A decade in review. *Nat Food Review* 13, 1.
22. Moure, L., Puialto, M.J., and Antolín, R. (2003). Cambios nutricionales en el proceso de envejecimiento. *Enfermería Global*, 1–16.
23. Doan, R.M. (1990) The effect of social support on the health and nutrition of rural elderly. Paper presented at the Rural Sociological Association. *J. Rural Comm. Psychol.* 11(2), 3–15.
24. Walker, D. and Beauchene, R.E. (1991) The relationship of loneliness, social isolation, and physical health to dietary adequacy of independently living elderly. *J. Am. Diet. Assoc.* 9, 300–306.

25. Ortega, R.M., Jiménez, A., Andrés, P., Faci, M., Lolo, J.M., Lozano, M.C., et al. (2002). Homocysteine levels in elderly Spanish people: Influence of pyridoxine, vitamin B_{12} and folic acid intakes. *J Nutr. Hlth. Aging* 6, 69–71.

26. Ortega, R.M., Redondo, M.R., Zamora, M.J., López-Sobaler, A.M., and Andrés, P. (1995). Eating behavior and energy and nutrient intake in overweight/obese and normal-weight Spanish elderly. *Ann. Nutr. Metab.* 39, 371–378.

27. Ortega, R.M., Redondo, M.R., Zamora, M.J. López–Sobaler, A.M., Andrés, P., and Encinas–Sotillos, A. (1995). Energy balance and caloric profile in the elderly obese or in those with overweight compared to those of normal weight. *Medicina Clínica* (Barcelona) 104, 526–529.

28. Ortega, R.M. and Andrés, P. (1998). Is Obesity worth treating in the elderly? *Drugs & Aging.* 12, 97–101.

29. Riesco, G., Gómez, C., de Cos, A.I. and Mateo, R. (2002). Obesidad. In: *Manual de alimentación y nutrición en el anciano*, M.A. Rubio, Ed., pp. 121–129. Masson, Barcelona.

30. Cruz, A.J. (1999). Obesidad en los mayores: cuándo actuar y cómo. In: *Alimentación, nutrición y salud en el anciano*, J.M. Ribera and P. Gil, Eds., pp. 157–162. Clínicas Geriátricas, Madrid.

31. Perea, J.M. and Navia, B. (2006). Nutrición del paciente de edad avanzada. In: *Nutriguía: manual de nutrición clínica en atención primaria*, A.M. Requejo and R.M. Ortega, Eds., pp. 72–82. Complutense, Madrid.

32. Horm, J. and Anderson, K. (1993). Who in America is trying to lose weight? *Ann. Int. Med.* 117, 672–676.

33. Díaz, J., Armero, M., Calvo, I., and Rico, M.A. (2000). Obesidad. In: *Nutrición y dietética*, C. Martín, J. Díaz, T. Motilla, and P. Martínez, Eds., pp. 425–452. DAE, Madrid.

34. Ortega, R.M., Requejo, A.M., and Andrés, P. (1999). Influencias dietéticas y control de peso corporal. *Nutrición y Obesidad* 2, 4–13.

35. Toschke, A.M., Küchenhoff, H., Koletzko, B. and von Kries, R. (2005). Meal frequency and childhood obesity. *Obesity Res.* 13, 1932–1938.

36. Zizza, C., Siega-Riz, A.M., and Popkin, B.M. (2001). Significant increase in young adults' snacking between 1977–1978 and 1994–1996 represents a cause for concern! *Prev. Med.* 32, 303–310.

37. Navia, B. and Perea, J.M. (2006). Dieta y control de peso. In: *Nutriguía: manual de nutrición clínica en atención primaria,* A.M. Requejo and R.M. Ortega, Eds., pp. 117–125. Complutense, Madrid.

38. Ortega, R.M., Andrés, P., Requejo, M., López-Sobaler, A.M., Redondo, R.M., and González-Fernández, M. (1996). Hábitos alimentarios e ingesta de energía y nutrientes en adolescentes con sobrepeso en comparación con los de peso normal. *Anales Españoles de Pediatría* 44, 203–208.

39. Astrup A. (2001). The role of dietary fat in the prevention and treatment of obesity. Efficacy and safety of low-fat diets. *Int. J. Obesity. Related Metab. Disorders* 25, S46–S50.

40. Bray, G.A., Paeratakul, S., and Popkin, B.M. (2004). Dietary fat and obesity: A review of animal, clinical and epidemiological studies. *Physiol. Behav.* 83, 549–555

41. Lesi, C., Giaquinto, E., Valeriani, L., and Zoni, L. (2005). Diet prescription in obese patients. *Monaldi Arch. Chest Dis.* 64, 42–44.

42. Zizza, C.A., Tayie, F,A., Lino, M. (2007). Benefits of snacking in older Americans. *J. Am. Diet. Assoc.* 107, 800–806.

43. Ortega, R.M., Requejo, A.M., Carcela, M., Pascual, M.J., and Montero, P. (1999). *Pautas dietético-sanitarias útiles en el control de peso. Madrid: Ayuntamiento de Madrid (Área de Salud y Consumo). Dirección de Servicios de Higiene y Salud Pública, Escuela de Sanidad y Consumo).* Universidad Complutense de Madrid, Madrid.

44. WHO (World Health Organization). (2003). *Development of a WHO global strategy on diet, physical activity and health: European regional consultation.* WHO, Copenhagen.

45. Consejería de Sanidad de la Comunidad de Madrid. (2007). *Control de peso de forma saludable.* Dirección General de Salud Pública y Alimentación, Madrid.

46. Aparicio, A., Bermejo, L. M., López-Sobaler, A. M., and Ortega, R. M. (2007). Guías en alimentación que pueden ser utilizadas como orientación en la planificación de dietas para una semana. In *Nutrición en población femenina: Desde la infancia a la edad avanzada*, R. M. Ortega, Ed., pp. 127–138.

47. Mattes, R.D. (2002). Ready-to-eat cereal used as a meal replacement promotes weight loss in humans. *J. Am. Coll. Nutr.* 21, 570–577.

48. Melanson, K.J., Angelopoulos, T.J., Nguyen, V.T., Martini, M., Zukley, L., Lowndes, J., et al. (2006). Consumption of whole-grain cereals during weight loss: Effects on dietary quality, dietary fiber, magnesium, vitamin B-6, and obesity. *J. Am. Diet. Assoc.* 106, 1380–1388.

49. Anderson, J.W. and Major, A.W. (2002). Pulses and lipaemia, short– and long–term effect: potential in the prevention of cardiovascular disease. *Br. J. Nutr.* 88, S263–S271.

50. Abete, I., Parra, M.D., Martínez, B.E., Pérez, S., Rodríguez, M.C., and Martínez, J.A. (2005). Evaluación del efecto de una dieta hipocalórica, rica en legumbres, sobre la pérdida de peso y sobre marcadores de síndrome metabólico. *Nutrición Hospitalaria* XX(supl.1), 198.

51. Witkowska, A. and Borawska, M.H. (1999). [The role of dietary fiber and its preparations in the protection and treatment of overweight]. *Polski Merkuriusz Lekarski* 6, 224–226.

52. Howarth, N.C., Saltzman, E., and Roberts, S.B. (2001). Dietary fiber and weight regulation. *Nutr. Rev.* 59, 129–139.

53. SENC (Sociedad Española de Nutrición Comunitaria). (2004). Guía de alimentación saludable. Sociedad Española de Nutrición Comunitaria, Madrid.

54. Mori, T.A., Bao, D.Q., Burke, V., Puddey, I.B., Watts, G.F., and Beilin, L.J. (1999). Dietary fish as a major component of a weight-loss diet: Effect on serum lipids, glucose, and insulin metabolism in overweight hypertensive subjects. *Am. J. Clinic. Nutr.* 70, 817–825.

55. Thorsdottir, I., Tomasson, H., Gunnarsdottir, I., Gisladottir, E., Kiely, M., Parra, M.D., et al. (2007). Randomized trial of weight-loss diets for young adults varying in fish and fish oil content. *Int. J. Obesity* 31, 1560–1566.

56. Mozaffarian, D., Bryson, C.L., Lemaitre, R.N., Burke, G.L., and Siscovick, D.S. (2005). Fish intake and risk of incident heart failure. *J. Am. Coll. Cardiol.* 45, 2015–2021.

57. Pérez, C.E. (2002). Fruit and vegetable consumption. *Health Reports* 13, 23–31.

58. Newby, P.K., Muller, D., Hallfrisch, J., Qiao, N., Andres, R., and Tucker, K.L. (2003). Dietary patterns and changes in body mass index and waist circumference in adults. *Am. J. Clinic. Nutr.* 77, 1417–1425.

59. Rolls, B.J., Ello-Martin, J.A., Tohill, B.C. (2004). What can intervention studies tell us about the relationship between fruit and vegetable consumption and weight management? *Nutr. Rev.* 62, 1–17.

60. Ello–Martin, J.A., Roe, L.S., Ledikwe, J.H., Beach, A.M., and Rolls, B.J. (2007). Dietary energy density in the treatment of obesity: a year–long trial comparing 2 weight–loss diets. *Am. J. Clinic. Nutr.* 85, 1465–1477.

61. Gustafsson, K., Asp, N.G., Hagander, B., and Nyman, M (1995). Satiety effects of spinach in mixed meals: Comparison with other vegetables. *Int. J. Food Sci. Nutr.* 46, 327–334.

62. Rampersaud, G.C., Kauwell, G.P., and Bailey, L.B. (2003). Folate: A key to optimizing health and reducing disease risk in the elderly. *Am. J. Clinic. Nutr.* 22(1), 1–8.

63. Tungtrongchitr, R., Pongpaew, P., Phonrat, B., Tungtrongchitr, A., Viroonudomphol, D., Vudhivai, N., and Schelp, F.P. (2003). Serum copper, zinc, ceruloplasmin and superoxide dismutase in Thai overweight and obese. *J. Med. Assoc. Thailand* 86, 543–551.

64. Hirsch, S., Poniachick, J., Avendaño, M., Csendes, A., Burdiles, P., Smok, G., et al. (2005). Serum folate and homocysteine levels in obese females with non-alcoholic fatty liver. *Nutrition* 21, 137–141.

65. Martínez, J.J., Ruiz, F.A., and Candil, S.D. (2006). Baseline serum folate level may be a predictive factor of weight loss in a morbid-obesity-management programme. *Br. J. Nutr.* 96, 956–964.

66. Rao, B.N. (2003). Bioactive phytochemicals in Indian foods and their potential in health promotion and disease prevention. *Asia Pacific J. Clinic. Nutr.* 12, 9–22.

67. Heber, D. (2004). Vegetables, fruits and phytoestrogens in the prevention of diseases. *J. Postgrad. Med.* 50, 145–149.

68. Mehta, S. and Farmer, J.A. (2007). Obesity and inflammation: A new look at an old problem. *Curr. Athero. Rep.* 9, 134–138.

69. Schulz, R.J. (2006). Dehydration in the aged: When thirst is absent. *Pflege Zeitschrift* 59, 758–759.

70. Montero, N.P. and Ribera, J.M. Envejecimiento: cambios fisiológicos y funcionales relacionados con la nutrición. In: *Manual de alimentación y nutrición en el anciano.* M.A. Rubio, Ed., pp. 15–21. Masson, Barcelona.

71. Brzozowska, A., Sicińska, E., Roszkowski, W. (2004). Role of folates in the nutrition of the elderly. *Roczniki Państwowego Zakładu Higieny* 55, 159–164.

72. Liu, S., Manson, J.E., Lee, I.M., Cole, S.R., Hennekens, C.H., Willett, W.C., and Buring, J.E. (2000). Fruit and vegetable intake and risk of cardiovascular disease: The Women's Health Study. *Am. J. Clinic. Nutr.* 72, 922–928.

73. MacGregor, G.A. and He, F.J. (2005). Importance of controlling blood pressure. *Climacteric* 8, S13–S18.

74. Bermejo, L.M., Aparicio, A., Andrés, P., López–Sobaler, A.M., Ortega, R.M. (2007). The influence of fruit and vegetable intake on the nutritional status and plasma homocysteine levels of institutionalized elderly people. *Pub. Hlth. Nutr.* 10, 266–272.

75. Dragsted, L.O., Krath, B., Ravn-Haren, G., Vogel, U.B., Vinggaard, A.M., Bo Jensen, P., et al. (2006). Biological Effects of Fruit and Vegetables. *Proc. Nutr. Soc.* 65, 61–67.

76. Lau, B.H. (2006). Suppression of LDL oxidation by garlic compounds is a possible mechanism of cardiovascular health benefit. *J. Nutr.* 136, 765S–768S.

77. Drewnowski, A., Henderson, S.A., Driscoll, A., Rolls, B.J. (1997). The Dietary Variety Score: Assessing diet quality in healthy young and older adults. *J. Am. Diet. Assoc.* 97, 266–271.

78. Guallar-Castillón, P., Rodríguez-Artalejo, F., Fornés, N.S., Banegas, J.R., Etxezarreta, P.A., Ardanaz, E., et al. (2007). Intake of fried foods is associated with obesity in the cohort of Spanish adults from the European Prospective Investigation into Cancer and Nutrition. *Am. J. Clinic. Nutr.* 86, 198–205.

79. Billing, J. and Sherman, P.W. (1998). Antimicrobial functions of spices: why some like it hot. *Quart. Rev. Biol.* 73, 3–49.

80. Westerterp-Plantenga, M., Diepvens, K., Joosen, A.M., Bérubé–Parent, S., Tremblay, A. (2006). Metabolic effects of spices, teas, and caffeine. *Physiol. Behav.* 89, 85–91.

81. Woo, H.M., Kang, J.H., Kawada, T., Yoo, H., Sung, M.K., Yu, R. (2007). Active spice-derived components can inhibit inflammatory responses of adipose tissue in obesity by suppressing inflammatory actions of macrophages and release of monocyte chemoattractant protein-1 from adipocytes. *Life Sci.* 80, 926–931.

82. Stanton, R.A. (2006). Nutrition problems in an obesogenic environment. *Med. J. Aust.* 184, 76–9.

83. Ortega, R. M., Aparicio, A., and López-Sobaler, A. M. (2005). Educación nutricional. In *Tratado de Nutrición*, A. Gil, Ed., Tomo IV, pp. 523–553. Acción Médica, Madrid.

84. Ortega, R. M. (2002). Necesidades nutricionales del anciano. Bases para establecer unas ingestiones recomendadas adecuadas a este grupo de población. *Formación Continuada Nutrición Obesidad* 5, 163–177.

85. Russell, R. M., Rasmussen, H., and Lichtenstein, A. H. (1999). Modified food guide pyramid for people over seventy years of age. *J. Nutr.* 129, 751–753.

86. Requejo, A. M. and Ortega, R. M. (1995). La Nutrición correcta en personas mayores. *Exmo. Ayto. de Madrid* (Área de Salud y Consumo).

21 Food Intake Regulation and Aging

Roger B. McDonald and Jessica Coppola

CONTENTS

21.1 INTRODUCTION

In the early 1970s clinicians described a set of symptoms associated with an idiopathic decline in health and well-being of individuals who were approaching the end of life. These symptoms included involuntary weight loss, attenuated food intake, increased fragility, depression, and a general lack of social competence. Collectively, these symptoms were referred to as geriatric failure to thrive because the patients did not respond to interventions and they were likely to die within weeks of admission to the hospital [1]. Subsequent clinical and experimental investigations into the mechanism underlying geriatric failure to thrive suggested that involuntary weight loss caused by a decline in appetite (food intake) was the initial manifestation of the disorder. So common and pervasive were the presentation of weight loss/attenuated food intake that the term "anorexia of aging" became a more common descriptor for the collection of signs and symptoms associated with geriatric failure to thrive.

Morley and colleagues were among the first to suggest that a decline in food intake leading to anorexia and significant weight loss might be a normal physiological response to advanced age [2–4]. Their suggestion was based on clinical observations [5] and the results of the first National Health and Nutrition Examination Survey (NHANES), which described a significant decline in energy intake with age and undernutrition in the advanced age groups [6]. The NHANES data were later confirmed by subsequent NHANES Surveys (Table 21.1; [7]), the Continuing Survey of Food Intakes by Individuals (CSFII) (Table 21.1; [8]), The New Mexico Health Study [9], and the

Baltimore Longitudinal Study [10]. The anorexia of aging has become an accepted part of the geriatric vocabulary and is viewed by many as a normal physiological consequence of senescence.

Nonetheless, the mechanism underlying the anorexia of aging remains to be elucidated. Previous research suggests that a disruption in the normal regulation of energy balance (calorie intake – calorie expenditure), psychological and social variables, and pathophysiological conditions all contribute to the development of the anorexia of aging. Several previous reviews have covered extensively the possible mechanism underlying the anorexia of aging and the reader should consult these publications to gain a greater understanding of the condition [11–15]. In this review our discussion will focus only on the regulation of food intake during advanced ages in the absence of pathophysiological conditions. That is, we take the position that the decline in food intake observed in the latter stages of life contributes, in part, to the normal progression of decline observed during aging.

21.2   FOOD INTAKE REGULATION—GENERAL

The importance of regulating food intake in order to meet the energy demands of the human being cannot be overstated. The evolutionary success of the human species reflects, in large part, our ability to extract adequate energy and nutrients from food regardless of choices presented to us within the local environment (that is, humans survive equally well in the tropics as in the polar regions). Humans have also developed an efficient system for storing excess energy that can be called upon in times of inadequate intake. Moreover, the drive to eat comprises a highly redundant neuroendocrine control system that is, arguably, unmatched by any other physiological system. This redundancy ensures that a disruption in only one control mechanism of food intake does not compromise overall energy balance. It is, therefore, no surprise that an age-related breakdown in the regulation of food intake can result in a cascade of effects that lead to frailty and death. A complete description of food intake regulation lies well beyond the scope of this review and the reader should consult previous publications [16–18] for a more thorough description of this process. Nonetheless, a brief overview of the basic features of food intake regulation may be helpful.

One can view the regulation of food intake by dividing it into three general groupings: pre-ingestion, post-ingestion, and storage. While all three groups function independently to regulate food intake, they are interconnected by the message processing centers within the hypothalamus (Figure 21.1). A good way to understand the integration of this system is to follow the process of food intake regulation from hunger to satiation. Let us assume that we are attending a celebration

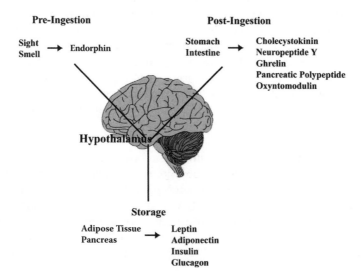

FIGURE 21.1   Signals initiated by affecter organs and the integration of these signals within the hypothalamus.

at which the serving of a large meal may be a tradition. Many people will spend the day leading up to the celebration limiting their food intake in order to enjoy the festive meal completely. As the serving time draws near, blood insulin levels will be low due to the lack of glucose present in the portal vein (see Section 21.5.1). Because insulin inhibits neuropeptide Y (NPY), a food intake stimulatory protein within the hypothalamus, NPY expression increases, resulting in a concomitant enhancement in the drive to eat. Moreover, previous research has found that increased circulation levels of insulin may enhance the secretion (or expression) of the adipose tissue hormone leptin [19], a powerful food intake inhibitory hormone. Low insulin would, therefore, result in a low serum concentration of leptin and the attenuation of the food intake inhibitory function of this hormone—i.e., we will have an increased drive to eat. The lack of food in the stomach or intestine also increases the plasma level of ghrelin, an orexigenic hormone [20].

The increased drive to eat caused by the neuroendocrine response to low insulin and high ghrelin levels are exacerbated by our chemical senses, taste, and smell. The aroma of food cooking and the initial taste of food stimulate the pleasure centers of the brain that secrete opioids and dopaminergic compounds to provide a pleasant sensation associated with the food. In turn, we may begin to salivate and associate the pleasant sensation with a desire to eat. While the mechanisms underlying this so-called cephalic phase of food intake regulation have yet to be elucidated, an increased desire to eat caused by pleasant aromas or flavors most likely involves a complex interaction among structures in the limbic system [21], most notably the amygdala (emotion/reward), the hippocampus (memory), and the hypothalamus (regulation]. Vision can also have an impact on food choices through memory, especially in the area of color and texture [22]. That is, brightly colored food tends to be more appealing and memories tell us whether we should expect the food to be crispy, rough, etc.

Our discussion to this point on the regulation of food intake has focused on the mechanisms that increase our drive to eat. As we swallow our first bite of food our system turns its attention to controlling the amount we eat. To this end, the stomach plays a central role in controlling the amount of food eaten at one setting by detecting changes in internal pressure. As the stomach fills with food, it naturally expands to prevent an increase in internal pressure. When the maximal size of the stomach is reached, additional food will increase the internal pressure, causing mechoreceptors in the wall of this organ to fire. The firing of the mechoreceptors causes neural signals that provide a sensation of satiety—although the mechanism is not well understood—to be sent to the central nervous system (CNS). At the same time, the presence of the stomach chyme in the intestine causes the release of cholecystokinin (CCK), a potent food intake inhibitor. Previous investigations have suggested that the stomach-distension mechanism that inhibits food intake requires the presence of CCK for maximal benefit [23]. Several other food intake inhibitor hormones that are released in response to the presence of food in the gastrointestinal system include peptide YY [24], oxyntomodulin [25], glucogon-like protein 1 [26], and bombasin [18].

21.3 FOOD INTAKE REGULATION—AGING

We have seen that food intake decreases with age (Table 21.1). Interestingly, changes in body weight over the life span to do not correlate with decreasing food intake (Figure 21.2). That is, body weight increases during the third through sixth decades of life, while food intake decreases. An age-related decline in body weight does not begin until approximately the seventh decade of life, although food intake during this period declines at approximately the same rate as that observed in the younger group. The decline in body weight seen during the seventh to ninth and greater decades of life cannot be attributed to increased energy expenditure. Both resting metabolic rate (RMR) [27] and the number of older individuals engaged in regular physical activity [28] decline as compared with the younger ages. Thus, one conclusion that can be drawn for this apparent paradox between food intake and body weight observed throughout the life span is that the "normal" mechanisms associated with energy intake are altered during aging.

TABLE 21.1

Energy Intake by Age and Gender

| | Daily Energy Intake (kcals) | | | |
| | NHANES[a] | | CSFII[b] | |
Age Group	Female	Male	Female	Male
20–29	1957	3025	1841	2821
30–39	1853	2872	1710	2665
40–49	1764	2542	1682	2435
50–59	1629	2341	1600	2270
60–69	1578	2110	1485	2072
70–79[c]	1435	1837	1384	1834
≥80	1329	1776	—	—

[a] Third National Health and Nutrition Examination Survey [7].
[b] Continuing Survey of food Intakes by Individuals [8].
[c] The values in this age group for the CSFII are 70 years and older.

The suggestion that alterations in energy intake regulation constitute a normal aspect of biological aging was tested in a series of studies by Roberts and colleagues [29,30]. In the first study, healthy young (23.7 ± 1.1) and old (70.7 ± 7.1) men were matched for weight, height, body mass index (BMI), and self-reported activity levels. Each age group was fed a diet for 7 days calculated to maintain their body weight and then followed by 21 days of a diet containing 1000 kcals/d greater than the maintenance diet. The overfeeding period was followed by 10 days in which the subjects were instructed to eat as much or as little as they needed to feel satiated. Body weight was followed throughout the experiment. In the second study, reported in the same publication, a similar design was followed except that a group of healthy younger (22.0 ± 3.0) and older (66.0 ± 5.3) men were underfed for 21 days 800 kcals/d less than that fed during maintenance diet. Investigations that incorporate both underfeeding and overfeeding protocols attempt to more closely simulate the day-to-day variation of food intake and the response of the body to maintain stable weight given the variation.

Both young and old men gained weight in response to overfeeding and lost weight during the underfeeding period. There was no significant difference between the age groups in the amount of

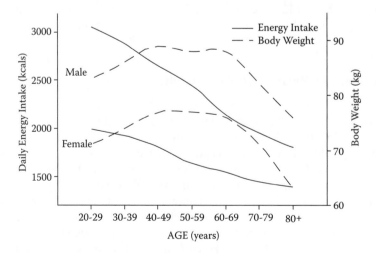

FIGURE 21.2   Daily energy intake [7] and body weight [119] of adults.

weight gained or lost. However, after a 10-day period in which subjects were allowed to eat until they were satiated there were considerable differences in body weight between the young and old groups. Overfed young men returned to their maintenance weight by involuntarily decreasing food intake (all subjects were requested not to diet during this period). In contrast, older men increased their food intake during the voluntary intake phase and gained weight. Underfeeding resulted in significant weight loss in both groups but no difference in the amount lost between the groups. Similar to the pattern observed in the overfeeding study, the young men regained their weight within 10 days following the end of the underfeeding trial. The older men continued to lose or maintain the weight they had lost.

The under- and overfeeding protocol of Roberts and colleagues [30] clearly established that regulation of food intake becomes altered in healthy old men. That is, the old men were unable to involuntarily adjust their food intake to compensate for acute changes in body weight as well as the younger men. The conclusions of Roberts et al. gained support from a short-term, single-meal investigation that used a calorie-preload design [31]. That is, young and old healthy men were provided with a 200 kcal yogurt snack prior to a meal in which they were allowed to eat *ad libitum* to satiation. The caloric intake of young men following the yogurt preload (yogurt + meal) stayed consistently close to caloric intake without the preload (meal only). Conversely, old men ate more calories after the preload (preload + meal) as compared with the no preload conditions.

Given the short-term nature of both the Roberts et al. [30) and Rolls et al. [31] investigations, the effect of a longer period of underfeeding and weight regain remained unclear. These effects were addressed in an investigation in which underfed younger and older men and women were underfed for 6 weeks followed by 6 months of monitoring their body weight and food intake [29]. Old subjects lost considerably more weight than did younger individuals during the 6 weeks of underfeeding. Moreover, old vs. younger subjects were unable to regain the weight to preunderfeeding values, a finding with strong implications for the health of older individuals. That is, voluntary weight loss through a reduction in caloric intake during advanced age may trigger involuntary weight loss leading to the complication of the anorexia of aging.

These investigations [29–31) provide clear evidence that the control mechanisms underlying food intake are altered in aging. The precise nature of these mechanisms remains to be elucidated. Previous investigations have reported that the feeling of satiety occurs sooner during a meal and that the drive to eat is reduced after a fast in older vs. younger subjects [32,33]. For example, Clarkston et al. [32] evaluated the effect of a meal on appetite, hunger, and fullness using subjective measures in young (30 ± 8 years) and old (76 ± 5 years) men and women. While there was no difference between men and women with respect to the measures of satiety, older subjects had reduced hunger and desire to eat throughout the 180 minutes of postprandial evaluation. The attenuated hunger was associated with significantly reduced gastric emptying times, suggesting a physiological correlate to the psychological measures of satiation (see below, Section 21.4.2). Our laboratory has also found alterations in measures of satiation in an rodent model for the anorexia of aging [34]. That is, the size of meals eaten and duration of eating at one meal were significantly less in older rats during their terminal weight loss phase as compared with weight-stable, age-matched rats.

In summary, both human and animal investigations demonstrate that the control of food intake becomes attenuated in the latter stages of life. Older vs. younger individuals lose, in part, the physiological mechanism that regulates the ability to determine the point of satiation (being full) during a single meal. The decline in the ability to determine the satiation point during meals appears to have a major impact on long-term energy balance. That is, short-term alterations in voluntary intake may lead to long-term dsyregulation of food intake and declining body weight in the elderly population. Given the health risk associated with underweight, i.e., frailty and malnutrition, health care workers should monitor closely weight changes in the elderly population.

21.4 PHYSIOLOGICAL AND ANATOMICAL CORRELATES TO DECLINING FOOD INTAKE REGULATION IN AGING

21.4.1 TASTE AND SMELL

It is a common belief that, as humans age, their ability to taste and smell declines, and that this decline may have a negative impact on food intake. Many early reports in humans appeared to confirm this popular perception; however, the majority of these studies were performed on tissue from patients with terminal diseases. More recent studies have attempted to determine if taste and smell decline in normal, healthy elderly people. Because of the subjective nature of these experiments, as well as the challenges of studying humans, the results remain controversial.

In the absence of disease, drugs, or smoking, taste declines only minimally with normal aging [35]. The number of taste buds and papillae do not show a significant age-related decline in function with age in both humans and animals [36,37]. It appears, however, that elderly humans do have significant diminution of function in most low concentration taste/smell detection tasks that have been tested [38,39]. The relevance of these studies has been questioned due to their use of odors at significantly lower concentrations than those commonly found in foods; i.e., no detectable decreases were found in the perception of more concentrated stimuli [40]. In our laboratory, we observed that very old rats fed the same diet for all of their lives will suddenly develop anorexia [34,41]. Enhancing the palatability of their diet by increasing the sugar and fat content or by flavoring the food with vanilla (a preferred flavor in young animals) does not affect the decrease in food intake during age-related anorexia [34].

The relationship between taste/odor perception and increased food intake has not been clearly established, a topic that has been reviewed [42]. If taste and odor perception were responsible for declines in food intake in old age, flavor enhancement of foods would be expected to improve body weight stability. However, the flavor enhancement in foods given to elderly human subjects (average age 85 yrs) with documented deficits in taste and smell did not improve their food intake enough to affect either body weight or body mass index [43]. Longitudinal data will be necessary in order to more accurately characterize sensory alterations in old age and their relationship to food intake. Currently, there is insufficient evidence to support a role for smell or taste deficits as contributing factors to the age-related decline in food intake regulation.

21.4.2 GASTROINTESTINAL

Digestion begins in the mouth through the action of chewing and the initial preparation of food by the salivary glands. Chewing breaks down large pieces of food into smaller ones for ease of swallowing and creates greater surface area for more efficient breakdown by enzymes of the digestive system. The loss of teeth that can occur with age has the potential to affect food intake significantly. In addition, loss of teeth may limit the types of foods eaten and have an impact on proper nutrition. Modern dentistry has eliminated the majority of age-related problems associated with poor dentition, and age-related loss of teeth is not a major disruption to the regulation of food intake. Affordability of dentistry and lack of education as to dental health most likely have a greater impact on poor dentition in the elderly population than does biological aging per se.

The inability to properly and easily swallow food can affect the amount of food eaten. The effect of aging on esophageal function in healthy humans remains controversial, due primary to the limited experimental research in this area. Some research suggests that disorders of the esophagus are more common in elderly subjects than in younger populations and represent a "normal" part of the aging process [44]. Although others agree that the prevalence of swallowing disorders are greater in the aged population, the cause of the dysfunction more likely reflects an association with disease rather than aging per se [45,46]. For example, Kawashima, et al. [46] report that the incidence of dysphasia in a healthy community-dwelling population was highly correlated with a history of stroke. Moreover, disruption of proper swallowing occurs almost universally in age-related neurological disorders such Alzheimer's and Parkinson's Diseases.

Gastrointestinal function may pose yet another potential barrier to normal food intake in elderly humans. Several investigators postulate that elderly humans experience a decrease in stomach elasticity resulting in feelings of fullness that do not correspond to nutritional or energy adequacy [45,47]. Controversy regarding this issue exists due, in large part, to the confounding influence of atrophic gastritis, an acquired disease prevalent in the elderly [48]. Age-related atrophic gastritis generally arises from an infection caused by the bacterium *Helicobacter pylori* (*H. pylori*). This infection causes a reduction or absence in the secretion of hydrochloric acid from the stomach, thereby inhibiting digestion, absorption, and gastric emptying [49]. Several investigations demonstrating impaired gastric function as a consequence of aging have not shown clear evidence that their subjects were free of *H. pylori*. [50–52]. Conversely, investigations using subjects in whom gastric diseases, including atrophic gastritis, were strictly excluded have not demonstrated impairments in gastric acid secretion or transit time [53–56].

Studies of gastrointestinal function in aging rats have produced inconsistent results. Smits [57] compared gastrointestinal transit time in 3, 12, and 24 mo-old male Wistar rats and demonstrated delayed gastric emptying in the oldest group. In contrast, McDougal [58] and Varga [59] observed no significant age differences in rates of gastric emptying. Both of these studies avoided inclusion of rats with evidence of known diseases. It is possible, however, that the contradictory results stem from the heterogeneity that exits within aged animals and the documented physiological transition from presenescence to senescence [60,61]. These studies did not separate the aged animals based on stability of body weight and/or food intake [13].

In summary, it does not appear that taste, smell, or gastrointestinal factors have a major impact on food intake in healthy aged humans. It appears more likely that disease states in the elderly influence reduction in food intake than does biological age per se. For example, atrophic gastritis significantly delays gastric emptying leading to feeling of fullness prior to normal physiological satiation. Age-related neurological disorders can attenuate food take by disrupting normal taste, smell, and swallowing.

21.5 NEURO-HORMONAL CORRELATES TO DECLINING FOOD INTAKE REGULATION IN AGING

21.5.1 Neuropeptide Y

Neuropeptide Y has been widely investigated in its role as an orexic peptide [62]. While secreted peripherally from cells of the small intestine and pancreas, the primary effects of NPY occur within the neural centers of the hypothalamus. The hypothalamic synthesis of NPY takes place in cells of the arcuate nucleus (ARC) and the active peptide is released into the paraventricular nucleus (PVN). Injections of exogenous NPY into the cerebral ventricles or directly into discreet hypothalamic nuclei, such as the PVN, ARC, or ventral medial hypothalamus of rodents will stimulate food intake for up to 24 hours and will result in obesity after repeated injections [60,63,64]. NPY also acts to increase energy storage by decreasing energy expenditure, increasing lipogenic enzymes in adipose tissue and liver, enhancing glucose uptake at adipose, and reducing brown adipose tissue thermogenesis [65]. Additionally, NPY synthesis and release are mediated by leptin, insulin, and glucocorticoids (see below, Section 21.5.2). Evidence of the physiological relevance of NPY includes the fact that changes in hypothalamic NPY production and release are paralleled by natural changes in food intake [66,67].

Although six NPY receptors have been found to date, the ability of NPY to stimulate food intake occurs primarily through two receptors, known as the Y_1 and Y_5 receptors [68]. The receptors are members of the seven-transmembrane-GTP binding protein (G-protein) coupled receptor family that reside on the cell surface while looping in and out of the plasma membrane. The Y_1 receptor is coupled to an inhibitory G-protein and sends its signal by inhibiting adenylate cyclase as well as by opening potassium channels. The Y_5 receptor is coupled to a G-protein that activates the enzyme phospholipase C Stimulation of this pathway by NPY results primarily in the opening of intracellular calcium channels.

Because of its powerful influence on food intake and energy storage, NPY and its Y_1 and Y_5 receptors have been studied extensively as mediators of obesity and anorexia nervosa [18], and have recently been shown to play a role in the anorexia of aging [60,61,69,70]. Injection of NPY into the third ventricle or PVN stimulates food intake of weight-stable, food intake-stable young and old rats. However, in old rats in which spontaneously declining food intake results in a loss of body weight, a rodent model for the anorexia of aging, NPY failed to stimulate food intake to the same degree as that observed in the weight-stable group [69]. The inability of NPY to stimulate food intake in old rats presenting weight loss and declining food intake does not reflect changes in PVN Y1 and Y5 receptor number [61] or specific pathology within the hypothalamus [69]. Some evidence exists to suggest that the attenuated NPY effect on food intake in this model of anorexia of aging reflects a loss in the potentiating effects on NPY by other neural peptides [60].

Measurement of NPY concentrations within rat brain regions and the determination of possible alterations with aging have also been reported [71–73]. Kowalski et al. [72] found that while other neuromodulators showed increased or decreased concentration with age, depending on the brain region, NPY was consistently lower throughout the brain in old (26 mo) compared with young (4 mo) and middle-aged (18 mo) male Wistar rats. From this finding, they proposed that the NPY circuitry might be the most vulnerable of the peptidergic systems to the process of aging. Similarly, Cha et al. [71] documented significant loss of NPY neurons in the cerebral cortex of aged (20 to 29 mo) compared with young (4 to 6 mo) male Sprague Dawley rats.

21.5.2   LEPTIN AND INSULIN

Leptin and insulin are produced in the periphery and inform the brain about adiposity levels of the body. Both are secreted in proportion to the quantity of body fat that the animal possesses, and exogenous administration of either causes declines in food intake in normal animals. This information suggests that leptin and insulin are potential mediators of age-related anorexia. A substantial quantity of research has been conducted on leptin and insulin as well as on their respective receptors in relation to aging.

Leptin, otherwise known as OB protein, is a polypeptide hormone secreted by cells in adipose tissue. It acts on the brain to inhibit food intake and to stimulate thermogenesis [74]. Leptin is transported in the blood on carrier proteins until it reaches the brain, where it influences the neural networks of the hypothalamus that regulate energy balance as well as reproductive capacity. The inhibitory effect of leptin most likely occurs by decreasing gene expression of the orexigenic molecules NPY, agouti related protein (AGRP), and melanin-concentrating hormone (MCH) [74,75] or by increasing the expression and release of the anorexigenic molecules proopiomelanocortin (POMC) and cocaine-amphetamine related transcript (CART) [76,77]. It has been found that serum leptin concentration varies in parallel with body fat stores, rising as adiposity increases in adulthood and falling with the decline in fat stores that occurs with advanced age and senescence [78–81]. Because leptin levels are low in senescence, one would predict NPY levels and food intake to increase as a result of decreased inhibition. However, investigations in aging rodents suggest that leptin has limited impact on the inhibition of NPY [34,69]. In addition, there is evidence that, even in response to exogenous injection of leptin, very old animals do not decrease NPY mRNA levels, as do younger animals [82], suggesting that impaired signal transduction from the leptin receptor in old rats may explain their lack of responsiveness to leptin [83].

Insulin, produced by the pancreas, promotes removal of glucose from the blood, facilitating glucose homeostasis in the circulation. Much evidence suggests that insulin is critical in the maintenance of long-term energy balance [18,27,84]. Similar to leptin, insulin is an anorectic hormone secreted in proportion to adipose stores and communicates with the brain to signal adjustments in energy intake and expenditure [85]. High concentrations of insulin receptors are found within the ARC [86], and intrahypothalamic or ICV administration of insulin affects the gene expression of other food intake modulators in this region [85].

Because of insulin's anorectic effects, its influence on fat storage, as well as its ability to alter gene expression of other neuromodulators in the ARC, it has been a candidate mediator of the anorexia of aging. Research in this area has yielded mixed results, in part due to the use of subjects of varying ages, levels of health, physical activity, and adiposity. Studies of mature, non-obese rats have consistently found that insulin levels do not change with aging [87–90]. Studies in our laboratory have shown that neither insulin levels nor glucose-stimulated insulin secretion are impaired with chronological aging in F344 rats [89]. Research in humans has also demonstrated a lack of alteration in insulin secretion with age in non-obese healthy older humans. After extensive research in this area, Reaven et al. [91–93] concluded that aging in the absence of disease has only minor effects on insulin secretion. These data suggest that currently there is no compelling evidence for a significant role for insulin in aging or the anorexia of aging. Insulin resistance clearly declines with age. However, the effect of age-related insulin resistance on energy balance correlates more precisely with changes in energy expenditure rather than energy intake and will not be covered here. Several recent reviews on this topic are available [94–96].

21.5.3 CHOLECYSTOKININ

Cholecystokinin is a satiating hormone produced in the gastrointestinal tract as well as in the hypothalamus in response to food intake. In the periphery, CCK acts by stimulating pancreatic secretion and gallbladder contraction, promoting intestinal motility, inhibiting gastric emptying, and activating visceral nerves. In the brain, CCK acts as a neurotransmitter that interacts with numerous other chemical mediators to modulate food intake [97,98]. Two distinct types of CCK receptors have been described; CCK_A receptors, which are found in the pancreas, on vagal afferent and enteric neurons, and at a number of brain sites; and CCK_B receptors, which are found in the brain, vagus nerve, and stomach. Both of these receptor subtypes are members of the seven transmembrane G-protein coupled receptor super family, which sends intracellular signals by G-protein mediated signal transduction. CCK has been studied for its potential role in obesity, anorexia nervosa, bulimia, and more recently the anorexia of aging.

Increased release of, or greater sensitivity to CCK has the potential to inhibit food intake in a manner similar to that observed in the anorexia of aging. However, research in this area has provided no consistent evidence for a relationship between CCK levels or potency with age or senescence [99–101]. In fact, under experimental conditions of chronic CCK administration in experimental animals, food intake and body weight are not significantly changed due to caloric compensation via increased frequency of meals [102]. This observation has led to the view that peripheral satiety factors such as CCK are powerful effectors of individual meal size with limited independent influence on long-term energy balance [14].

21.5.4 ENDOGENOUS OPIOIDS

The endogenous opioids, including dynorphin, beta-endorphin, and the enkephalins, are known to function in the body's physiological reward system. They are responsible, in part, for the pleasurable responses experienced after ingestion of high-sugar and high-fat foods [103]. Endogenous opioids act in the brain, primarily in the hypothalamus, amygdala, and the nucleus accumbens [104]. Exogenous injection of opioid receptor agonists increase food intake [105] while injection of opioid receptor antagonists consistently decrease food intake in young animals [106]. In addition, interactions have been demonstrated between opioids and other neuromodulators such as NPY and dopamine, thereby indirectly affecting food intake [107].

Because of their influence on food intake, endogenous opioids have been implicated in the anorexia of aging. Gosnell et al. [103] described an age-related decrease in food intake response to opioid agonists and antagonists injected into the intraperitoneal cavity. Additionally, Martinez et al. [99] demonstrated that, in patients diagnosed with idiopathic senile anorexia, the cerebrospinal fluid contained decreased concentrations of beta-endorphin compared with control subjects of similar age but with normal body weight. However, once a feeding stimulant was given to the anorectic individuals, beta-endorphin levels increased without concomitant improvements in food intake or body weight. This, and the fact that chronic administration of opioid antagonists do not affect food intake or body weight in a long-term manner [108], have led to questions regarding the importance of endogenous opioids in the regulation of food intake.

In contrast to the studies cited above, other investigations have found no significant difference in opioid concentrations from old and young animals within brain areas associated with the control of feeding. In a study by Lau et al. [109], levels of hypothalamic met-enkephalin and beta-endorphin were found to be comparable in Sprague-Dawley rats aged 3, 8, and 23 mos. At least three other investigations have also reported no age-related alterations in the levels of hypothalamic beta-endorphin and met-enkephalin in adult male Sprague Dawley rats [110–112]. Additional data will be necessary to more fully understand the role of endogenous opioids in the development of anorexia associated with advanced age

21.5.5 GLUTAMATE AND GAMMA AMINO BUTYRIC ACID

Glutamate (Glu) and gamma amino butyrate acid (GABA) are the brain's primary excitatory and inhibitory neurotransmitters, respectively. GABA is formed from the decarboxylation of Glu and plays a critical role in preventing overexcitation of neurons under a variety of circumstances. Virtually all neurons in the brain have some combination of the three GABA receptors: GABA A, GABA B, and GABA C. Stimulation of GABA A receptors via benzodiazepines decreases anxiety, stress, and aggression, and increases memory retention along with numerous other known functions.

In the late 1970s, GABA and the GABA A receptor began to be recognized for their role in food intake. The GABA A receptor agonist, muscimol, increases food intake when injected into the PVN or the lateral ventricles [113,114]. Pu et al. [114] demonstrated that although GABA and GABA agonists alone are only mild stimulants of food intake, co-administration of muscimol and NPY elicited a more robust food intake response than either NPY or muscimol alone. Thus, one potential mechanism that may explain attenuated food intake of aged animals infused with NPY may be a decrease in the synergenic effect of GABA. This possibility was explored by our laboratory [60] although the results created more questions than answers. In short, we found that neither NPY, muscimol, nor a combination of NPY and muscimol together produced significant increases in food intake. Although these data support the hypothesis that alterations in GABA or Glu signaling may be a possible mediator of the anorexia of aging, the lack of food intake stimulation from numerous mediators seems to suggest a more wide spread cause.

21.5.6 CYTOKINES

The pro-inflammatory cytokines, such as tumor necrosis factor alpha (TNFα), interleukin 1 beta (IL-1β), and interleukin-6 (IL-6) also alter food intake. Interactions of these cytokines with NPY, leptin, and CCK may play important roles in the inhibition of food intake during injury and illness [115]. It has also been suggested that cytokines might play a role in the anorexia of aging because chronic diseases often accompany old age [116,117]. As discussed above, it is critical to differentiate between aging in the presence of disease and normal aging because the anorexia of aging occurs in humans and experimental animals that appear to be relatively healthy. However, the involvement of cytokines is still a compelling idea in light of the fact that they might act on food intake in senescence, even in the absence of overt disease. In a double blind, placebo-controlled study, Yeh et al. [118] noted that inhibition of cytokine synthesis and release resulted in increased appetite in cachectic geriatric nursing home patients compared to controls. The improvement in appetite did not significantly impact the body weight or body composition of the elderly subjects. This suggests that even in an experiment that studied aging in the presence of disease, decreasing the level of cytokines had minimal benefits. More research will be required to determine the significance of this finding and its impact on the anorexia of aging.

ACKNOWLEDGMENTS

The authors wish to thank Dr. Rodney Ruhe and Jennifer Ruhe for their helpful review.

REFERENCES

1. Hodkinson, H. M. 1973. Non-specific presentation of illness. *Brit Med J* 4: 94–96.
2. Morley, J. E. 1986. Nutritional status of the elderly. *Am J Med* 81: 679–695.
3. Morley, J. E., Mooradian, A. D., Silver, A. J., Heber, D. and Alfin-Slater, R. B. 1988. Nutrition in the elderly. *Arch Intern Med* 109: 890–904.
4. Morley, J. E. and Silver, A. J. 1988. Anorexia in the elderly. *Neurobio Aging* 9: 9–16.
5. Morley, J. E., Silver, A., Fiatarone, M. and Morradian, A. D. 1986. UCLA grand rounds: Nutrition and the elderly. *J Am Geriat Soc* 34: 823–832.
6. Abraham, S., Carroll, M. D. and Dresser, C. M. 1977. Dietary intake of persons 1–74 years of age in the United States. In: Advance data from Vital and Health Statistics of the National Center for Health Statistics Administration, H. R., Ed. Public Health Services, Rockville MD.
7. McDowell, M. A., Briefel, R. R., Alaimo, K., Bischof, A. M., Caughman, C. R., Carroll, M. D., et al. 1994. Energy and macronutrient intakes of persons ages 2 months and over in the United States: Third National Health and Nutrition Examination Survey, Phase I, 1998–1991, Statistics, National Center for Health Statistics., Ed. Advance Data from Vital and Health Statistics, Hyattsville, MD.
8. United States of Department of Agriculture. 1997. Data tables: Results from USDA's 1994–1996 diet and Health Knowledge Survey. CD–ROM, NTIS Accession Number PB98–500457.
9. Koehler, K. M. 1994. The New Mexico Aging Process Study. *Nutr Rev* 52: S34–37.
10. Hallfrisch, J., Muller, D., Drinkwater, D., Tobin, J. and Andres, R. 1990. Continuing diet trends in men: The Baltimore Longitudinal Study of Aging 1961–1987. *J Geronotol* 45: M186–191.
11. Chapman, I. M. 2007. The anorexia of aging. *Clin Geriatr Med* 23: 735–756.
12. Hays, N. P. and Roberts, S. B. 2006. The anorexia of aging in humans. *Physiol Behav* 88: 257–266.
13. Horwitz, B. A., Blanton, C. A. and McDonald, R. B. 2002. Physiologic determinants of the anorexia of aging: Insights from animal studies. *Annu Rev Nutr* 22: 417–438.
14. Morley, J. E. 2002. Pathophysiology of anorexia. *Clin Geriatr Med* 18: 661–673.
15. Wilson, M. M. and Morley, J. E. 2003. Invited review: Aging and energy balance. *J Appl Physiol* 95: 1728–1736.
16. Cummings, D. E. and Overduin, J. 2007. Gastrointestinal regulation of food intake. *J Clin Invest* 117: 13–23.
17. Jequier, E. and Tappy, L. 1999. Regulation of body weight in humans. *Physiol Rev* 79: 451–480.
18. Stanley, S., Wynne, K., McGowan, B. and Bloom, S. 2005. Hormonal regulation of food intake. *Physiol Rev* 85: 1131–1158.
19. Havel, P. J. 2004. Update on adipocyte hormones: Regulation of energy balance and carbohydrate/lipid metabolism. *Diabetes* 53 Suppl 1: S143–151.
20. Cummings, D. E., Purnell, J. Q., Frayo, R. S., Schmidova, K., Wisse, B. E. and Weigle, D. S. 2001. A prandial rise in plasma ghrelin levels suggests a role in meal initiation in humans. *Diabetes* 50: 1714–1719.
21. Petrovich, G. D. and Gallagher, M. 2007. Control of food consumption by learned cues: A forebrain–hypothalamic network. *Physiol Behav* 91: 397–403.
22. Verhagen, J. V. and Engelen, L. 2006. The neurocognitive bases of human multimodal food perception: Sensory integration. *Neurosci Biobehav Rev* 30: 613–650.
23. Kissileff, H. R., Carretta, J. C., Geliebter, A. and Pi-Sunyer, F. X. 2003. Cholecystokinin and stomach distension combine to reduce food intake in humans. *Am J Physiol Regul Integr Comp Physiol* 285: R992–998.

24. Batterham, R. L., Cowley, M. A., Small, C. J., Herzog, H., Cohen, M. A., Dakin, C. L., et al. 2002. Gut hormone PYY3-36 physiologically inhibits food intake. *Nature* 418: 650–654.

25. Cohen, M. A., Ellis, S. M., Le Roux, C. W., Batterham, R. L., Park, A., Patterson, M., et al. 2003. Oxyntomodulin suppresses appetite and reduces food intake in humans. *J Clin Endocrinol Metab* 88: 4696–4701.

26. Verdich, C., Flint, A., Gutzwiller, J. P., Naslund, E., Beglinger, C., Hellstrom, P. M., et al. 2001. A meta-analysis of the effect of glucagon-like peptide-1 7-36 amide on ad libitum energy intake in humans. *J Clin Endocrinol Metab* 86: 4382–4389.

27. Roberts, S. B. and Rosenberg, I. 2006. Nutrition and aging: Changes in the regulation of energy metabolism with aging. *Physiol Rev* 86: 651–667.

28. Barnes, P. M. and Schoenborn, C. M. 2003. Physical activity among adults: United States, 2000 Statistics, National Center for Health Statistics. Advanced Data from Vital and Health Statistics, Hyattsville, MD.

29. Moriguti, J. C., Das, S. K., Saltzman, E., Corrales, A., McCrory, M. A., Greenberg, A. S. and Roberts, S. B. 2000. Effects of a 6-week hypocaloric diet on changes in body composition, hunger, and subsequent weight regain in healthy young and older adults. *J Gerontol A Biol Sci Med Sci* 55: B580–587.

30. Roberts, S., Fuss, P. and Heyman, M. 1994. Control of food intake in older men. *JAMA* 272: 1601–1606.

31. Rolls, B., Dimeo, K. and Shide, D. 1995. Age-related impairments in the regulation of food intake. *Am J Clin Nutr* 62: 923–931.

32. Clarkston, W. K., Pantano, M. M., Morley, J. E., Horowitz, M., Littlefield, J. M. and Burton, F. R. 1997. Evidence for the anorexia of aging: Gastrointestinal transit and hunger in healthy elderly vs. young adults. *Am J Physiol Regul Integr Comp Physiol* 272: R243–R248.

33. Cook, C. G., Andrews, J. M., Jones, K. L., Wittert, G. A., Chapman, I. M., Morley, J. E. and Horowitz, M. 1997. Effects of small intestinal nutrient infusion on appetite and pyloric motility are modified by age. *Am J Physiol Regul Integr Comp Physiol* 273: R755–R761.

34. Blanton, C. A., Horwitz, B. A., Geitzen, D. W., Griffey, S. M., Murtagh-Mark, C. and McDonald, R. B. 1998. Meal patterns associated with the age-related decline in food intake in the Fischer 344 rat. *Am J Physiol Regul Integr Comp Physiol* 275: R1494–R1502.

35. Baker, G. I. and Martin, G. 1997. Molecular and biological factors in aging: the origin, causes, and prevention of senescence. In: *Geriatric medicine*, 3 ed. Cassel, C., Cohen, H., Larson, E., Meier, D., Resnick, N., Rubenstein, L. and Sorenson, L., Eds., pp. 3–28. Springer-Verlag, New York.

36. Miller, I. 1988. Human Taste bud density across adult age groups. *J Geront: Bio Sci* 43: B26–B30.

37. Mistretta, C. 1989. Anatomy and neurophysiology of the taste system in aged animals. *J Neurochem* 40: 20–24.

38. Cain, W. S. and Stevens, J. C. 1989. Uniformity of olfactory loss in aging. *Ann NY Acad Sci* 561: 29–38.

39. Weiffenbach, J. and Bartoshuk, L. 1992. Taste and Smell. *Clinic Geriatr Med* 8: 543–555.

40. Bartoshuk, L. and Duffy, V. 1995. Taste and Smell. In: *Handbook of physiology: Aging* Masoro, E. J., Ed., pp. 363–375. Oxford University Press, New York.

41. McDonald, R. B., Florez-Duquet, M., Murtagh-Mark, C. and Horwitz, B. A. 1996. Relationship between cold-induced thermoregulation and spontaneous rapid body weight loss of aging F344 rats. *Am J Physiol Regul Integr Comp Physiol* 271: R1115–1122.

42. Sorensen, L. B., Moller, P., Flint, A., Martens, M. and Raben, A. 2003. Effect of sensory perception of foods on appetite and food intake: A review of studies on humans. *Int J Obes Relat Metab Disord* 27: 1152–1166.

43. Schiffman, S. S. and Warwick, Z. S. 1993. Effect of flavor enhancement of foods for the elderly on nutritional status: Food intake, biochemical indices, and anthropometric measures. *Physiol Behav* 53: 395–402.

44. Hall, K. E. 2002. Aging and neural control of the GI tract. II. Neural control of the aging gut: Can an old dog learn new tricks? *Am J Physiol Gastrointest Liver Physiol* 283: G827–832.

45. Drozdowski, L. and Thomson, A. B. 2006. Aging and the intestine. *World J Gastroenterol* 12: 7578–7584.

46. Kawashima, K., Motohashi, Y. and Fujishima, I. 2004. Prevalence of dysphagia among community-dwelling elderly individuals as estimated using a questionnaire for dysphagia screening. *Dysphagia* 19: 266–271.

47. Bitar, K. N. and Patil, S. B. 2004. Aging and gastrointestinal smooth muscle. *Mech Aging Dev* 125: 907–910.
48. Green, L. K. and Graham, D. Y. 1990 Gastritis in the elderly. *Gastroenterol Clin N Am* 19: 273–292.
49. Frank, E., Lange, R. and McCallum, R. 1981. Abnormal gastric emptying in patients with atrophic gastritis with or without pernicious anemia. *Gastroenterology* 80: A1151–1157.
50. Brogna, A., Loreno, M., Catalano, F., Bucceri, A. M., Malaguarnera, M., Muratore, L. A. and Travali, S. 2006. Radioisotopic assessment of gastric emptying of solids in elderly subjects. *Aging Clin Exp Res* 18: 493–496.
51. Jones, K. L., O'Donovan, D., Russo, A., Meyer, J. H., Stevens, J. E., Lei, Y., et al. 2005. Effects of drink volume and glucose load on gastric emptying and postprandial blood pressure in healthy older subjects. *Am J Physiol Gastrointest Liver Physiol* 289: G240–248.
52. O'Donovan, D., Hausken, T., Lei, Y., Russo, A., Keogh, J., Horowitz, M. and Jones, K. L. 2005. Effect of aging on transpyloric flow, gastric emptying, and intragastric distribution in healthy humans—impact on glycemia. *Dig Dis Sci* 50: 671–676.
53. Goldschmeidt, M., Barnett, C., Schwarz, B., Karnes, W., Redfern, J. and Feldman, M. 1991. Effect of age on gastric acid secretion and serum gastrin concentrations in healthy men and women. *Gastroenterology* 101: 977–990.
54. Goldschmiedt, M. and Feldman, M. 1993. *Age related changes in gastric acid secretion.* CRC Press, Boca Raton FL.
55. Haruma, K., Kamada, T., Kawaguchi, H., Okamoto, S., Yoshihara, M., Sumii, K., et al. 2000. Effect of age and Helicobacter pylori infection on gastric acid secretion. *J Gastroenterol Hepatol* 15: 277–283.
56. Madsen, J. L. 1992. Effects of gender, age, and body mass index on gastrointestinal transit times. *Dig Dis Sci* 37: 1548–1553.
57. Smits, G. J. and Lefebvre, R. A. 1996. Influence of aging on gastric emptying of liquids, small intestine transit, and fecal output in rats. *Exp Gerontol* 31: 589–596.
58. McDougal, J., Miler, M. and Burks, T. 1980. Intestinal transit and gastric emptying in your and senescent rats. *Dig Dis Sci.* 25: A–15.
59. Varga, F. 1976. Transit time changes with age in the gasterointestinal tract of the rat. *Digestion* 14: 319–324.
60. Coppola, J. D., Horwitz, B. A., Hamilton, J., Blevins, J. E. and McDonald, R. B. 2005. Reduced feeding response to muscimol and neuropeptide Y in senescent F344 rats. *Am J Physiol Regul Integr Comp Physiol* 288: R1492–1498.
61. Coppola, J. D., Horwitz, B. A., Hamilton, J. and McDonald, R. B. 2004. Expression of NPY Y1 and Y5 receptors in the hypothalamic paraventricular nucleus of aged Fischer 344 rats. *Am J Physiol Regul Integr Comp Physiol* 287: R69–75.
62. Beck, B. 2006. Neuropeptide Y in normal eating and in genetic and dietary-induced obesity. *Philos Trans R Soc Lond B Biol Sci* 361: 1159–1185.
63. Stanley, B. G., Leibowitz, S.F. 1985. Neuropeptide Y injected in the paraventricular hypothalamus: A powerful stimulant of feeding behavior. *Proc. Natl. Acad. Sci. USA* 82: 3940–3943.
64. Stanley, B. G., Anderson, K. C., Grayson, M. H. and Leibowitz, S. F. 1989 Repeated hypothalamic stimulation with neuropeptide Y increases daily carbohydrate and fat intake and body weight gain in female rats. *Physiol Behav* 46: 173–177.
65. Kalra, S. P., Dube, M. G., Pu, S., Xu, B., Horvath, T. L. and Kalra, P. S. 1999 Interacting appetite-regulating pathways in the hypothalamic regulation of body weight. *Endocr Rev* 20: 68–100.
66. Kalra, S. P., Dube, M. G., Sahu, A., Phelps, C. P. and Kalra, P. 1991. Neuropeptide Y secretion increases in the paraventricular nucleus in association with increased appetite for food. *Proc Nat Acad Sci USA* 88: 10931–10935.
67. Sahu, A., Kalra, P. S. and Kalra, S. P. 1988. Food deprivation and ingestion induce reciprocal changes in neuropeptide Y concentrations in the paraventricular nucleus. *Peptides* 9: 83–86.
68. Duhault, J., Boulanger, M., Chamorro, S., Boutin, J. A., Della Zuana, O., Douillet, E., et al. 2000. Food intake regulation in rodents: Y5 or Y1 NPY receptors or both? *Can J Physiol Pharmacol* 78: 173–185.
69. Blanton, C. A., Horwitz, B. A., Blevins, J. E., Hamilton, J. S., Hernandez, E. J. and McDonald, R. B. 2001. Reduced feeding response to neuropeptide Y in senescent Fischer 344 rats. *Am J Physiol Regul Integr Comp Physiol* 280: R1052–R1060.
70. Pich, E. M., Messori, B., Zoli, M., Ferraguti, F., Marrama, P., Biagini, G., et al. 1992. Feeding and drinking responses to neuropeptide Y injections in the paraventricular nucleus of aged rats. *Brain Res* 575: 265–271.

71. Cha, C. I., Lee, Y. I., Lee, E. Y., Park, K. H. and Baik, S. H. 1997. Age-related changes of VIP, NPY and somatostatin-immunoreactive neurons in the cerebral cortex of aged rats. *Brain Res* 753: 235–244.

72. Kowalski, C., Micheau, J., Corder, R., Gaillard, R. and Conte-Devolx, B. 1992. Age-related changes in cortico-releasing factor, somatostatin, neuropeptide Y, methionine enkephalin and beta-endorphin in specific rat brain areas. *Brain Res* 582: 38–46.

73. Wang, Z. P., Man, S. Y. and Tang, F. 1993. Age-related changes in the contents of neuropeptides in the rat brain and pituitary. *Neurobio Aging* 14: 529–534.

74. Sahu, A. 1998. Leptin decreases food intake induced by melanin-concentrating hormone MCH, galanin GAL and neuropeptide Y NPY in the rat. *Endocrinology* 139: 4739–4742.

75. Wang, Q., Bing, C., Al-Barazanji, K., Mossakowaska, D. E., Wang, X. M., McBay, D. L., et al. 1997. Interactions between leptin and hypothalamic neuropeptide Y neurons in the control of food intake and energy homeostasis in the rat. *Diabetes* 46: 335–341.

76. Cheng, X., Broberger, C., Tong, Y., Yongtao, X., Ju, G., Zhang, X. and Hokfelt, T. 1998. Regulation of expression of neuropeptide Y Y1 and Y2 receptors in the arcuate nucleus of fasted rats. *Brain Res* 792: 89–96.

77. Kristensen, P., Judge, M. E., Thim, L., Ribel, U., Christjansen, K. N., Wulff, B. S., et al. 1998. Hypothalamic CART is a new anorectic peptide regulated by leptin. *Nature* 393: 72–76.

78. Ahren, B., Larsson, H., Wilhelmsson, C., Nasman, B. and Olsson, T. 1997. Regulation of circulating leptin in humans. *Endocrine* 7: 1–8.

79. Ahren, B., Mansson, S., Gingerich, R. L. and Havel, P. J. 1997. Regulation of plasma leptin in mice: Influence of age, high-fat diet, and fasting. *Am J Physiol Regul Integr Comp Physiol* 273: R113–120.

80. Perry, H. M., Morley, J. E., Horowitz, M., Kaiser, F. E., Miller, D. K. and Wittert, G. 1997. Body composition and age in African-American and Caucasian women: Relationship to plasma leptin levels. *Metabolism* 46: 1399–1405.

81. Ruhl, C. E., Harris, T. B., Ding, J., Goodpaster, B. H., Kanaya, A. M., Kritchevsky, S. B., et al. 2007. Body mass index and serum leptin concentration independently estimate percentage body fat in older adults. *Am J Clin Nutr* 85: 1121–1126.

82. Scarpace, P. J. and Tumer, N. 2001. Peripheral and hypothalamic leptin resistance with age-related obesity. *Physiol Behav* 74: 721–727.

83. Scarpace, P. J., Matheny, M. and Tumer, N. 2001. Hypothalamic leptin resistance is associated with impaired leptin signal transduction in aged obese rats. *Neuroscience* 104: 1111–1117.

84. Woods, S. C., Seeley, R. J., Porte, D., Jr. and Schwartz, M. W. 1998. Signals that regulate food intake and energy homeostasis. *Science* 280: 1378–1383.

85. Schwartz, M. W., Sipols, A. J., Marks, J. L., Sanacora, G., White, J. D., Scheurink, A., et al. 1992. Inhibition of hypothalamic neuropeptide Y gene expression by insulin. *Endocrinology* 130: 3608–3616.

86. Baskin, D. G., Wilcox, B. J., Figlewicz, D. P. and Dorsa, D. M. 1988. Insulin and insulin-like growth factors in the CNS. *Trends Neurosci* 11: 107–111.

87. Hara, S. L., Ruhe, R. C., Curry, D. L. and McDonald, R. B. 1992. Dietary sucrose enhances insulin secretion of aging Fischer 344 rats. *J. Nutr.* 122: 2196–2203.

88. McDonald, R. B. 1990. Effect of age and diet on glucose tolerance in Sprague-Dawley rats. *J. Nutr.* 120: 598–601.

89. Ruhe, R. C., Curry, D. L. and McDonald, R. B. 1997. Altered cellular heterogeneity as a possible mechanism for the maintenance of organ function in senescent animals. *J Gerontol A Biol Sci Med Sci* 52: B53–58.

90. Starnes, J. W., Cheong, E. and Matschinsky, F. M. 1991. Hormone secretion by isolated perfused pancreas of aging Fischer 344 rats. *Am J Physiol Endocrinol Metab* 260: E59–66.

91. Reaven, E., Wright, D., Mondon, C. E., Solomon, R., Ho, H. and Reaven, G. M. 1983. Effect of age and diet on insulin secretion and insulin action in the rat. *Diabetes* 32: 175–180.

92. Reaven, G. M. and Reaven, E. P. 1980. Effects of age on various aspects of glucose and insulin metabolism. *Mol Cell Biochem* 31: 37–47.

93. Reaven, G. M. and Reaven, E. P. 1985. Age, glucose intolerance, and non-insulin-dependent diabetes mellitus. *J Am Geriat Soc* 33: 286–290.

94. Buijs, R. M. and Kreier, F. 2006. The metabolic syndrome: a brain disease? *J Neuroendocrinol* 18: 715–716.

95. Frisard, M. and Ravussin, E. 2006. Energy metabolism and oxidative stress: impact on the metabolic syndrome and the aging process. *Endocrine* 29: 27–32.

96. Kreier, F., Kalsbeek, A., Sauerwein, H. P., Fliers, E., Romijn, J. A. and Buijs, R. M. 2007. Diabetes of the elderly and type 2 diabetes in younger patients: Possible role of the biological clock. *Exp Geront* 42: 22–27.

97. Reidelberger, R., Varga, G. and Liehr, R.-M. 1994. Cholecystokinin suppresses food intake by a nonendocrine mechanism in rats. *Am J Physiol Regul Integr Comp Physiol* 267: R901–R908.

98. Reidelberger, R. D. 1994. Cholecystokinin and control of food intake. *J. Nutr.* 124: 1327S–1333S.

99. Martinez, M., Arnalich, F. and Hernanz, A. 1993. Alterations of anorectic cytokine levels from plasma and cerebrospinal fluid in idiopathic senile anorexia. *Mech Aging Develop* 72: 145–153.

100. Miyasaka, K., Kanai, S. and Masuda, M. 1995. Gene expression of cholecystokinin CCK and CCK receptors, and its satiety effect in young and old male rats. *Arch Gerontol Geriatr* 21: 147–155.

101. Miyasaka, K., Kanai, S., Ohta, M. and Funakoshi, A. 1997. Aging impairs release of central and peripheral cholecystokinin CCK in male but not in female rats. *J Gerontol A Biol Sci Med Sci* 52: M14–18.

102. Crawley, J. and Beinfeld, M. 1983. Rapid development of tolerance to the behavioral actions of cholecystokinin. *Nature London* 302: 703–706.

103. Gosnell, B. A., Levine, A. S. and Morley, J. E. 1983. The effects of aging on opioid modulation of feeding in rats. *Life Sci* 32: 2793–2799.

104. Vaccarino, A. L. and Kastin, A. J. 2001. Endogenous opiates: 2000. *Peptides* 22: 2257–2328.

105. Morley, J. E. and Levine, A. S. 1983. Involvement of dynorphin and the kappa opioid receptor in feeding. *Peptides* 4: 797–800.

106. Echo, J. A., Lamonte, N., Ackerman, T. F. and Bodnar, R. J. 2002. Alterations in food intake elicited by GABA and opioid agonists and antagonists administered into the ventral tegmental area region of rats. *Physiol Behav* 76: 107–116.

107. Rudski, J. M., Grace, M., Kuskowski, M. A., Billington, C. J. and Levine, A. S. 1996. Behavioral effects of naloxone on neuropeptide Y-induced feeding. *Pharmacol Biochem Behav* 54: 771–777.

108. Brands, B., Thornhill, J. A., Hirst, M. and Gowdey, C. W. 1979. Suppression of food intake and body weight gain by naloxone in rats. *Life Sci* 24: 1773–1778.

109. Lau, S. M. and Tang, F. 1995. The effect of haloperidol on met-enkephalin, beta-endorphin, cholecystokinin and substance P in the pituitary, the hypothalamus and the striatum of rats during aging. *Prog Neuropsychopharmacol Biol Psychiatr* 19: 1163–1175.

110. Gambert, S. R., Garthwaite, T. L., Pontzer, C. H. and Hagen, T. C. 1980. Age-related changes in central nervous system beta-endorphin and ACTH. *Neuroendocrinology* 31: 252–255.

111. Missale, C., Govoni, S., Croce, L., Bosio, A., Spano, P. F. and Trabucchi, M. 1983. Changes of beta-endorphin and Met-enkephalin content in the hypothalamus-pituitary axis induced by aging. *J Neurochem* 40: 20–24.

112. Tang, F., Tang, J., Chou, J. and Costa, E. 1984. Age-related and diurnal changes in Met5-Enk-Arg6-Phe7 and Met5-enkephalin contents of pituitary and rat brain structures. *Life Sci* 35: 1005–1014.

113. Horvath, T. L., Pu, S., Dube, M. G., Diano, S. and Kalra, S. P. 2001. A GABA-neuropeptide Y NPY interplay in LH release. *Peptides* 22: 473–481.

114. Pu, S., Jain, M. R., Horvath, T. L., Diano, S., Kalra, P. S. and Kalra, S. P. 1999. Interactions between neuropeptide Y and gamma-aminobutyric acid in stimulation of feeding: A morphological and pharmacological analysis. *Endocrinology* 140: 933–940.

115. Langhans, W. and Hrupka, B. 1999. Interleukins and tumor necrosis factor as inhibitors of food intake. *Neuropeptides* 33: 415–424.

116. Morley, J. E. 2001. Decreased food intake with aging. *J Gerontol A Biol Sci Med Sci* 56: 81–88.

117. Morley, J. E 2001 Anorexia, body composition, and ageing. *Curr Opin Clin Nutr Metab Care* 4: 9–13.

118. Yeh, S., and Schuster, M. 1999. Geriatric cachexia: The role of cytokines. *Am J Clin Nutr* 70: 183–197.

119. McDowell, M. A., Fryar, C. D., Hirsch, R., and Ogden, C. L. 2005. Anthropometric reference data for children and adults: U.S. Population, 1999–2002 Statistics, National Center for Health Statistics, Hyattsville, MD.

Index

A